EAI/Springer Innovations in Communication and Computing

Series Editor

Imrich Chlamtac, European Alliance for Innovation, Ghent, Belgium

The impact of information technologies is creating a new world yet not fully understood. The extent and speed of economic, life style and social changes already perceived in everyday life is hard to estimate without understanding the technological driving forces behind it. This series presents contributed volumes featuring the latest research and development in the various information engineering technologies that play a key role in this process. The range of topics, focusing primarily on communications and computing engineering include, but are not limited to, wireless networks; mobile communication; design and learning; gaming; interaction; e-health and pervasive healthcare; energy management; smart grids; internet of things; cognitive radio networks; computation; cloud computing; ubiquitous connectivity, and in mode general smart living, smart cities, Internet of Things and more. The series publishes a combination of expanded papers selected from hosted and sponsored European Alliance for Innovation (EAI) conferences that present cutting edge, global research as well as provide new perspectives on traditional related engineering fields. This content, complemented with open calls for contribution of book titles and individual chapters, together maintain Springer's and EAI's high standards of academic excellence. The audience for the books consists of researchers, industry professionals, advanced level students as well as practitioners in related fields of activity include information and communication specialists, security experts, economists, urban planners, doctors, and in general representatives in all those walks of life affected ad contributing to the information revolution.

Indexing: This series is indexed in Scopus, Ei Compendex, and zbMATH.

About EAI - EAI is a grassroots member organization initiated through cooperation between businesses, public, private and government organizations to address the global challenges of Europe's future competitiveness and link the European Research community with its counterparts around the globe. EAI reaches out to hundreds of thousands of individual subscribers on all continents and collaborates with an institutional member base including Fortune 500 companies, government organizations, and educational institutions, provide a free research and innovation platform. Through its open free membership model EAI promotes a new research and innovation culture based on collaboration, connectivity and recognition of excellence by community.

Parul Agarwal • Kavita Khanna
Ahmed A. Elngar • Ahmed J. Obaid
Zdzislaw Polkowski
Editors

Artificial Intelligence for Smart Healthcare

Springer

EAI
RESEARCH MEETS INNOVATION

Editors
Parul Agarwal
Computer Science and Engineering
Jamia Hamdard
New Delhi, India

Kavita Khanna
Delhi Skill and Entrepreneurship University
Dwarka, Delhi, India

Ahmed A. Elngar
Faculty of Computers and Artificial Intelligence
Beni-Suef University
Beni-Suef City, Egypt

Ahmed J. Obaid
Faculty of Computer Science and Mathematics
University of Kufa
Najaf, Iraq

Zdzislaw Polkowski
Jan Wyzykowski University
Polkowice, Poland

ISSN 2522-8595 ISSN 2522-8609 (electronic)
EAI/Springer Innovations in Communication and Computing
ISBN 978-3-031-23601-3 ISBN 978-3-031-23602-0 (eBook)
https://doi.org/10.1007/978-3-031-23602-0

This Springer imprint is published by the registered company Springer Nature Switzerland AG
The registered company address is: Gewerbestrasse 11, 6330 Cham, Switzerland

Preface

The healthcare sector has a huge amount of data to be processed and needs attention. Artificial intelligence and related technologies like machine learning, deep learning, IoT, big data analysis, neural networks, expert systems, physical robots, automated robotic processes, and several other technologies have the potential to revolutionize the current and future of smart healthcare by dynamically accessing information, connecting stakeholders like people, clinics/hospitals related to healthcare, and then actively managing and generating responses to the needs of the medical ecosystem in an intelligent manner. Each of these technologies has its own domain of application. The range of applications they possess is imaging analysis, patient-centric care, cloud-based network, connected staff and infrastructure, disease diagnosis and treatment, patient engagement, and others. Though the process has already begun, still a lot more needs to be done. Efficient algorithms and models that can find solutions to the above applications can break the barriers in their adoption in the healthcare sector. COVID-19 has led the medical practitioners, pharma companies, and scientists in identifying vaccines and drugs and providing optimal care to the patients. To save the world from such unprecedented times, forecasting models and prediction algorithms are the need of the hour.

This book shall to the best cover these aspects related to healthcare and also identify the challenges and find solutions for the same. Intended as a power-packed book, it shall explore not only the current state but also find effective solutions using these technologies for the future. An insightful read shall yield the audience a platform to exchange ideas and innovations by diving into the current and the future scenarios. One-to-one healing between the patient and the doctor shall change the way healthcare works.

This book is divided into three major parts. Part I: Fundamentals and Applications of AI and Enabling Technologies in Various Sectors, Part II: AI-Enabled Innovations in the Health Sector, and Part III: Security and Privacy Concerns. Part I focuses on applications of AI, deep learning, neural networks, etc. in various domains and helps the reader to gain an insight into how these technologies find their applications. Part II primarily discusses the applications of AI in the healthcare sector. Its applications for brain-related problems, disease diagnosis, smart health education, etc. are discussed in this part. Part III has contributions that discuss the security and privacy-related issues associated with it. There are 30 chapters in all. A summary of each of the parts and the chapters is provided below.

Part I: Fundamentals and Applications of AI and Enabling Technologies in Various Sectors

Chapter "A Secured Data Sharing Protocol for Minimization of Risk in Cloud Computing and Big Data in AI Application"

The study proposes a mystery allocation gathering key administration convention (SSGK) for the purpose of preventing unauthorized access to the communication measure and shared information. There's a gathering key and a secret allocation map that distributes it. This reduces the risk of allocation information in dispersed storing and recoveries by 12%. SSGK technique with 98.25% accuracy, 97.92% sensitivity, and 93.89% recall has been established.

Chapter "Predictive Modelling for Healthcare Decision-Making Using IoT with Machine Learning Models"

An overview of machine learning techniques and their applications in the health industry is discussed. Deep learning (DL) using neural networks has lately shown promise in healthcare. A small group of people is used to anticipate how many days off employees will have. Factors such as check-in time, days away from home, and augmentation strategies in boosting the F1-score.

Chapter "Artificial Intelligence for Smart in Match Winning Prediction in Twenty20 Cricket League Using Machine Learning Model"

This study predicts the outcome of T20 matches. Cricket matches have lot of impact on the mind of the audience. A good prediction can help people accept the match's results and avoid them putting in stress, as well as, emotional trauma. This chapter uses Machine learning techniques for a better prediction of the outcomes of the match. Several factors can be analysed including the behavioural patterns of the players. Cricketers who are self-assured typically have a high sense of mastery over their abilities, expect things to go their way and hold themselves to a higher performance standard. Mental skills such as multitasking and flexible thinking are needed to keep a cricketer's mind from becoming overwhelmed by any complexity.

Guided athlete reflection after the performance was promoted as a valuable tool in developing and applying idiographic coping behaviors that could improve perceptions of control and self-confidence while influencing stress and emotion processes.

Chapter "Comparative Analysis of Handwritten Digit Recognition Investigation Using Deep Learning Model"

This chapter uses the CNN framework for handwritten digit recognition. It analyses and compares the performance of various conventional machine learning classifiers to the Deep learning-based Convolutional neural networks. This work can be applied in the healthcare sector, where, usually doctors are prescribing medicines through paper slips and the handwriting recognition poses a problem to the patient as well as the pharmacist. MNIST data was used to improve machine learning training and categorization.

Chapter "An Investigation of Machine Learning-Based IDS for Green Smart Transportation in MANET"

This research uses ML to distribute characteristics to IDS for MANET Green Smart Transportation. The performance of ML-IDSs may be used to detect incursions while learning about the MANET. ML optimized KDD IDS. Each controlled packet earned an anomaly score. With MANETs, datasets are scarce. The IDS for Green Smart Transportation was built using a working prototype and ML approaches. Using IDS and ML to detect and prevent MANET abuse is the approach used. This work adds to the body of information about IDSs.

Chapter "A Critical Cloud Security Risks Detection Using Artificial Neural Networks at Banking Sector"

This study focused on cloud banking developers and IT managers. The best ANN integration approach anticipates and minimizes significant security and cloud challenges. This chapter explores the use of Artificial neural networks for predicting critical cloud computing security issues in the banking sector. Optimistic predictions of significant cloud security issues can lead to better performance of the cloud-based baking sector. It holds relevance as on today in the healthcare sector, as most of the transactions made by patients are performed online. Thus, the technology proposed in the current research provides better confidence and security. Consequently, a Critical Cloud Security Risks Detection Using Artificial Neural Networks at Banking Sector would make healthcare system efficient. Optimistic projections of major cloud security issues would boost cloud-based banking performance. Performance measurements including accuracy 98.76%, sensitivity 97.34%, recall 94.53%, and F measure 97.82% were achieved. The result is better than the present methods.

Chapter "A Solution to Pose Change Challenge: Real-Time, Robust, and Adaptive Human Tracking Systems Using SURF"

The present requirement in the healthcare system is the development of smart hospitals. Reports suggest that one in twenty-five patients suffer from hospital acquire infections. It's a major task to track down the healthcare staff, patients, visitors etc. Presently, RFID is used to track people in hospitals, and for that manual tagging of humans to be tracked is done. This is done by wearing special wristbands, gloves, or external badges to register their position at specific events of interest. This chapter presents a revolutionary GRABCUT implementation on the interest point-based method. This approach removes background descriptors from the object model, which is then utilized by a SURF-based tracker. An auto-tuned classifier is then used to distinguish between posture change and occlusion. This chapter's algorithm is adaptable, resilient, and real time. The tests are done both inside and outdoors.

Chapter "Analysis on Identification and Detection of Forgery in Handwritten Signature Using CNN"

The Forgery of Handwritten Signature is a critical task but hackers sometimes copied the information easily. Many standard approaches like evolutionary algorithm, Random-forest optimization, Xboosting machine learning, and SVM cannot solve signature forging. The Forgery of Handwritten Signature is a critical task but hackers sometimes copied the information easily. This chapter concentrate on Identification and Detection of Forgery in Handwritten using CNN deep learning technology. The available medical with digital information has been used train the CNN architecture. The testing process has been initiated through testing block in CNN deep intelligence. The privacy, ethical and legal issues of Forgery has been identified and suggested which data is original. The document writer checks the falsified signature. Existing approaches struggle to identify fake documents and signatures. The average accuracy is 83.3%, sensitivity 99.2%, recall 98.24%, F score 97.23%, and throughput 98.91%. These enhanced findings outperformed prior models.

Chapter "Experimental Analysis of Internet of Technology-Enabled Smart Irrigation System"

The new Cloud-enabled Smart Agri-Handling Strategy (CSAHS) is presented. The CSAHS technology will allow farmers to remotely monitor their crops and get weather alerts. For this study, the IoT connects farm smart land equipment to a distant cloud server. The ARM IoT-Web Module has Wi-Fi. It uses data (like PH, soil moisture, rain, temperature, and humidity) from smart sensors to operate agricultural smart equipment. This IoT-enabled agricultural gadget saves water. The outcome is optimum crop irrigation at the right time. The CSAHS reduces labor, reduces agricultural losses, and provides timely weather information.

Chapter "Analysis on Exposition of Speech Type Video Using SSD and CNN Techniques for Face Detection"

The use of multimedia has led to more and more videos being generated. Thus, their storage, management, and mapping becomes a serious problem. This paper employs a two step process for emotions detection. Face Detection is done using SSD (Single Shot Multibox Detector) and emotion classification is done using CNN. Face-SSD employs fully CNN to identify video uploads. This study used CNN-based speech type video extraction and face identification to estimate storage and simplify content indexing. Finally, performance metrics like 98.45% accuracy, 97.34% sensitivity, 94.23% recall, and throughput have been calculated

Part II: AI-Enabled Innovations in the Health Sector

Chapter "Depressive Disorder Prediction Using Machine Learning-Based Electroencephalographic Signal"

Early detection of depression is crucial. This chapter uses EEG signals from a publicly available database to evaluate sleep disorders and alcoholism. Its classifier tools may assist classify topics with disorders. Frequency bands (Apha, Delta, Theta, and Beta) provide the parameters.

Chapter "Generation of Masks Using nnU-Net Framework for Brain Tumor Classification"

By dealing with the dataset assortment seen in the medical domain datasets, this paper proposes a technique called nnU-Net with adjustments in the encoder-decoder design. The MRI dataset is used to mine the shape from the radiometric properties. Pre-processing, network architecture, training, and post-processing for every new job and pragmatic choices are automatically configured.

Chapter "A Brain Seizure Diagnosing Remotely Based on EEG Signal Compression and Encryption: A Step for Telehealth"

The need for e-health and remote health is increasing andrequires information to be transmitted between the patients and the healthcare stakeholders. as such,data compression and encryption becomes crucial. This work presents both EEG data reduction and encryption techniques. The Huffman adaptive coding and encryption technique using 256-bit AES (CBC) is performed. It improves compression and encryption performance on the CHB-MIT Scalp EEG database.

Chapter "A Deep Convolal Neural Network-Based Heart Diagnosis for Smart Healthcare Applications"

Coronary artery diseases were classified using hybrid filtering (HCAD). A probabilistic Adaptive Random Forest classifier was utilized to predict HCAD data. This study classified CTA/heart images using level set formulation and GHSB (Gaussian Hue, Saturation, and Brightness). For cardiac disorders, GHSB employs fusion. This method is slow and inaccurate. Adaptive filters and threshold segmentation can identify HCAD faster. It increases True positives using adaptive machine learning. Heart disease is predicted by RFO segmentation and classification. Application of DCNN-based feature selection and image net classification in healthcare is necessary for healthcare applications. This research employs GHSB and RFO models on MRI cardiac scans. This model finds and extracts the CAB from the image. Thus, the blockade's breadth and length are determined. Last but not least, 99.74% accuracy, 98.81% precision, 98.14% recall, 94.87% F1 score, 59.26% PSNR, 0.0989% CC, and 99.45% sensitivity were attained.

Chapter "A Dynamic Perceptual Detectors Module-Related Telemonitoring for the Intertubes of Health Services"

An evaluation of intellectual data approaches for computer systems with restricted resources is investigated by dynamically configuring the vehicle's hardware and software to the required operating mode. To test this method, a low-power microcontroller and a neural network model are used. Using the MIT-BIH Arrhythmia testbed, adapting the node design to the strain during execution reduces power use by 50%. A quantized neural network could detect arrhythmias with 98% accuracy.

Chapter "ConvNet-Based Deep Brain Stimulation for Attack Patterns"

An algorithm for identifying Parkinson's disease using limited cross-sectional brain structural MRI data was developed and validated in this work. To encode prediction and classification, a type of RNN called LSTM may learn order dependence. Computational linguistics and voice recognition are two examples. Deep learning LSTMs are challenging. An LSTM predicts the highest trembling speed of fake and real stimuli. Assault patterns were recognized by the architecture, alerting the doctor.

Chapter "Web-Based Augmented Reality of Smart Healthcare Education for Machine Learning-Based Object Detection in the Night Sky"

The authors suggested Space360, a virtual planetarium for people who cannot go to the planetarium due to COVID. Space360 allows users to observe every celestial body in the night sky at any time. Space360 is about stargazing and seasonal constellations and provides knowledge on the celestial body. This feature will display details such as visibility, declination, etc. This applies to all 88 visible constellations and eight planets in our solar system.

Chapter "The Role of Augmented Reality and Virtual Reality in Smart Health Education: State of the Art and Perspectives"

AR and VR can improve teaching by providing immersive multimodal environments with different sensory characteristics. The chapter finishes with several novel approaches to challenges and research topics for future educators interested in these new technologies.

Chapter "Estimation of Thyroid by Means of Machine Learning and Feature Selection Methods"

This study uses KNN, naive Bayes, and SVM to categorize thyroid datasets. Comparing several machine learning algorithms helps forecast illness. The E.S.T. D.D. Model is better for future thyroid ailment detection. Existing applications were not suitable for pre-stage thyroid diagnosis. So, a complex model is necessary. Accuracy of 98.53%, recall of 97.23%, the throughput of 98.34%, and sensitivity of 99.23% were attained.

Chapter "A Multiuser-Based Data Replication and Partitioning Strategy for Medical Applications"

This research provides a real-time cloud computing hybrid multi-user data replication and partitioning solution for medical applications. Two stages are used in this study: data replication and multi-user partitioning. To retrieve data, numerous servers' machine decision patterns are replicated. This stage partitions cloud data. Data replication and partitioning outperform previous solutions on large medical decision patterns. A wide range of replicant protocols exist. A review of distributed storage and content management system replication approaches is presented. The test has 98.23% accuracy, 94.53% sensitivity, and 92.29% recall.

Chapter "A Deep Study on Thermography Methods and Applications in Assessment of Various Disorders"

This research examines numerous thermography methods and their usefulness. The temperature of an object influences its infrared emission. Thermal imaging is utilized in medical diagnostics, mechanical and electrical maintenance, as well as building heat loss measurement. This chapter concentrates on temperature measurement and non-destructive testing. An overview of infrared thermography, temperature measurement, and non-destructive testing is provided. Recent advances in these fields are also addressed. This study's accuracy was 98.67%, sensitivity was 94.45%, and recall was 92.34%.

Chapter "A Smart Healthcare Cognitive Radio System for Future Wireless Commutation Applications with Test Methodology"

Determining the whole system rather than simply individual components is challenging due to the lack of a device-independent design. To overcome this problem, this study proposes the CORATM Cognitive Radio Research Technique using MICR. MICR advises PU and SU to use behavior-based node assessment to assess cognition. Assessing both main and secondary user success may be highly beneficial. This study's results include accuracy 98.34%, sensitivity 98.56%, recall 98.51%, F scores 98.65%, and throughput 99.32%. It competes with 4G and 5G.

Chapter "Indication of COVID-19 and Inference Employing RFO Classifier"

Pandemic origins have left many jobless in developing countries and beyond. Managing the GDP is challenging. Obvious limitations must be addressed in order to determine COVID-19 impact. So, we employ the RFO machine learning model. The model categorizes variables affecting unemployment. This performance measure attained metrics like accuracy 98.45%, recall 97.235%, sensitivity 95.345%, F measure 93.785%, and sensitivity 99.325%. These measures outperform techniques in data sensitivity estimations. The RFO-based COVID-19 unemployment estimates social and ethical characteristics. This application tests machine learning techniques in today's economy.

Chapter "Magnetic Resonance Images for Spinal Cord Location Detection Using Deep Learning Model"

Deep learning is used to predict MRI images of spinal cord damage. The suggested deep learning model is CONN; the layers are max-pooling, hidden, dense, normalized, and ReLu. This model has 13 layers and performed better than previous models. 97.23% recall, 95.12% precision, and 98.71% accuracy were achieved.

Chapter "COVID-19 Recognition in X-Ray and CTA Images Using Collaborative Learning"

COVID-19 is a serious illness that may be fatal. This research proposes Otsu thresholding under random forest optimization machine learning to diagnose COVID-19 X-ray images. Finally, estimation accuracy 99.46%, sensitivity 99.48%, recall 99.36%, and F1 score of 99.42% were achieved.

Chapter "Artificial Intelligence for Enhancement of Brain Image Using Semantic Segmentation CNN with IoT Classification Techniques"

The major goal is to use a medical database to show how various brain imaging variables affect malignancies. Methods enhance data segmentation, feature extraction, and classification. To assess the proposed semantic segmentation, deep convolution neural network classification algorithms are used. This approach and medical data model may be scalable according to experimental results.

Part III: Security and Privacy Concerns

Chapter "A Novel Framework for Privacy Enabled Healthcare Recommender Systems"

The authors suggested a two-tier structure to explore it in this study. The patient's identity is first anonymized, then data is randomly generated using homomorphic encryption. The presented framework serves two purposes. It is free of third-party participation and promotes privacy by integrating two-layer design for patient data protection. Also, the proposed solution may aid as a standard for protecting patients' privacy and integrity.

Chapter "An Evaluation of RSA and a Modified SHA-3 for a New Design of Blockchain Technology"

This research added a new criterion for evaluating the RSA algorithm used in blockchain technology. To improve hashing speed, a redesigned hash algorithm (SHA3) was developed by replacing AND and NOT by ADD. The major result was less memory use and faster RSA method complexity and hashing. Finally, compression between proposed algorithms (amendment RSA and modified SHA-3) improved memory, security, and speed.

Chapter "Quality of Smart Health Service for Enhancing the Performance of Machine Learning-Based Secured Routing on MANET"

The goal is to enhance routing performance for ad hoc networks utilizing multipath and a hop count-based routing parameter. Better routing services for congested applications, particularly multimedia apps can be achieved through this model. On the CSMA/CA approach, EED and PLR are evaluated in MAC layer associations. These variables are used with application QoS needs to build additional routing parameters. Typical multipath protocols avoid application-layer route preferences under varying congestion circumstances by using constant routing parameters. The suggested approach outperforms the AOMDV standard in terms of PDR, congested overheads, and EED for application congestion types.

Chapter "Spoof Attacks Detection Based on Authentication of Multimodal Biometrics Face-ECG Signals"

Face and ECG biometric authentication is the purpose of this project. Face and ECG multimodality system has the best statistical performance. ECG has been shown to improve the anti-spoofing capabilities of conservative biometric-based systems. It describes an ECG-based authentication mechanism. Awica Wavelet Transformation techniques are required alongwith an improved method of authentication. The results were 94% accuracy, 98% FAR, 7.93% FRR, and 14.99-minute process time.

This book intends to provide the reader with extensive coverage of AI, its enabling technologies in the healthcare sector. We wish to thank whole-heartedly the entire team of Springer, particularly Eliška Vlčková, Managing editor, EAI, for her constant support and guidance. We also extend our thanks to all the contributors and reviewers. They are the major stakeholders in the editing of a book. Our gratitude to our family and friends. Last but not the least, we bow before the Almighty for his blessings throughout the journey.

New Delhi, India — Parul Agarwal
Dwarka, Delhi, India — Kavita Khanna
Beni-Suef, Egypt — Ahmed A. Elngar
Najaf, Iraq — Ahmed J. Obaid
Polkowice, Poland — Zdzislaw Polkowski

Contents

Part I
Fundamentals and Applications of AI and Enabling Technologies in Various Sectors

A Secured Data Sharing Protocol for Minimisation of Risk in Cloud Computing and Big Data in AI Application

Vijay Prakash Sharma, Kailas S. Patil, G. Pavithra, Sangeetha Krishnan, and Anju Asokan

1 Introduction

This section designs a brief cloud computing-based data-sharing protocol with the goal of minimising risk. Administration-based cloud security is performed through a minimum risk estimation model. When compared to other techniques, the combination of the secret sharing group key management (SSGK) proposed model provides a 12% additional benefit. Rising advances in large data, such as cloud processing [1], business intellect [2], data removal [3], mechanical evidence combination engineering (industrial information integration engineering (IIIE)) [4], and the Web of Things [5], have opened the door for upcoming initiative structures (enterprise systems (ES)) [6]. Distributed computation is an additional processing prototype by the entire asset on the Internet's construction of a cloud benefit pool for allocating to numerous submissions and, additionally, benefiting significantly. A large assumption was secured in comparison to and expected to disseminate the plan.

V. P. Sharma (✉)
Department of IT, Manipal University, Jaipur, Rajasthan, India

K. S. Patil
Department of ECE, Sharnbasva University, Kalaburagi, Karnataka, India

G. Pavithra
Department of ECE, Dayananda Sagar College of Engineering (DSCE), Bangalore, Karnataka, India

S. Krishnan
Department of CSE, Panimalar Engineering College, Chennai, Tamil Nadu, India

A. Asokan
Sri Krishna College of Technology, Coimbatore, Tamil Nadu, India
e-mail: anjuasokan@skct.edu.in

P. Agarwal et al. (eds.), *Artificial Intelligence for Smart Healthcare*,
EAI/Springer Innovations in Communication and Computing,
https://doi.org/10.1007/978-3-031-23602-0_1

Furthermore, it carries extraordinary flexibility, flexibility, and effectiveness aimed at task implementation. By utilising cloud computing administrations, the numerous labour advantages in building and custodial zing a super computation or lattice registering condition for keen submissions are significantly reduced. Regardless of this preference, safety fundamentals significantly improve when knocking goes adjacent to a cloud-recognisable household [7, 8] yield the benefit authorised by massive data progress, protection, and defence problems [9, 10], as they were originally inclined to. These promotion-directorial consistency issues move sensitive data to a suitable space by unifying planetary.

A construction safety structure for dispersed storage is not a humble assignment. Securing collective information from unapproved cancellation, medication, and creation is troublesome. As a result, collective information on the cloud is outside the controller's scope of genuine associates, making mutual statistics practical based on the concentration of genuine customers. Similarly, the growing quantity of assemblies, devices, and submissions linked by the cloud reminds us of the dangerous progress of passages, making it extra difficult to yield legitimate admission controllers. Finally, collective information on the haze cannot be lost or incorrectly changed by cloud providers or organisation aggressors. Customarily, there are two separate strategies to advance the safety of the distribution framework. To benefit from the common information, a single admittance controller [11, 12] is used, with only approved clients being recorded in the entrance control counter. The added strategy is bunch key administration [13, 14], in which a gathering key is utilised to ensure mutual information. Even though access control lets the information get to real members, it can't shield them from the assault of cloud suppliers [15, 16].

In the current gathering key sharing frameworks, the gathering key is, by and large, overseen by a free outsider. Such strategies assume that the outsider is consistently genuine [17, 18]. Nevertheless, the supposition isn't always genuine, particularly in distributed storage. The paper will include a puzzle imparting key organisational gathering to address the safety issue of the distribution of information on dispersed storage. Using systems would allow us to gather with assistance while also preventing fakes. To make common data useful when soliciting legitimate clients, symmetric encryption calculations [19] must be used to encode the majority of the data. When you stop implying that one data proprietor needs to impart data to various people, the coding fact directs the genuine sharers toward the data proprietor. Furthermore, the entry that unravels the most data controls the doorway's acceptance of imparted data. The data encryption calculations [20] would use to encode the encrypted message.

Furthermore, making true parts might unravel the entrance. Third, if there is a chance that the conveyed majority of the data is referred to by unapproved clients, these gathering uses puzzle offering arrangements to consign the true parts [21, 22]. We procure a careful security cloud, including security parts with standardly arranged mists. Also, certification provides security by claiming the majority of the data imparted by disseminated stockpiling. Building a security framework before disseminating capacity may accelerate the path of a cloud clinched alongside critical business circumstances.

Data influence in the cloud is a technique that enables operators to quickly and accurately admit data into the cloud. Because of the cost savings and extensive features of cloud services, the data owner outsources their information to the cloud. Because the cloud examination contributor is a third-party contributor, the information holder has no control over their data [23, 24]. The primary problem with storing data in the cloud is the lack of privacy and security, and various solutions are available. This study focuses on several contracting systems involving threatened data sharing, such as data involvement through forwarding safety, protected statistics sharing for energetic groups, quality-based data sharing, encrypted data sharing, and common effects [25–31], founded on a set of privacy-preserving verification directions for the right to use and handle subcontracted data [32].

Emerging big data technologies, including cloud computing, business intelligence, data mining, industrial information integration engineering (IIIE), and the Internet of Things (IoT), have ushered in an innovative era for upcoming enterprise systems (ES) [33–37]. Cloud computing is a novel computing model in which all Internet resources are pooled into a cloud reserve pool and dynamically assigned to various requests and facilities. Compared to traditional distribution systems, it saves significant money and provides superior job execution elasticity, scalability, and efficiency. The multiple company investments in establishing and maintaining a supercomputer in an otherwise grid computing atmosphere for smart requests can be efficiently condensed by leveraging cloud computing services [38–41]. Despite these benefits, security requirements skyrocket when storing personally identifiable information in the cloud. Regulatory compliance difficulties arise because sensitive data is moved from the federated domain to the disseminated domain [42], and before reaping the benefits of big data technologies, first and foremost, security and privacy concerns must be addressed. It's not straightforward to create a security mechanism for cloud storage [43–45]. Since shared information on the cloud is beyond the regulatory reach of authorised contributors, a solution should be found to make collective information usable on request through genuine operators.

Furthermore, as the number of parties, strategies, and apps using the cloud grows, so does the number of access opinions, making it increasingly problematic to maintain adequate access regulators [46]. Finally, cloud-based data can be lost or erroneously updated by the cloud provider or network intruders. It's tough to keep shared data safe from unwanted deletion, modification, or falsification [47].

Cloud computing is quickly gaining traction because of the provisioning of elastic, flexible, and on-demand storage and processing resources for clients [48–50]. Cloud computing is a great way to save on capital and operating expenses. This monetary gain is a crucial factor in cloud acceptance [51]. On the other hand, security and privacy are major considerations in adopting cloud technology for data storage. Cryptography, in which documents are typically encrypted before being stored in the cloud, is one way to address these concerns [52]. While cryptography ensures data safety in the cloud, when data is common amongst a group, cryptographic services must be flexible enough to deal with individual clients, exercise access to manage keys, and control keys powerfully to ensure data confidentiality. Group data management offers more beneficial properties than two-party communication or data handling by a single person. Current, departed, and newly hired organisation members may pose an insider threat, jeopardizing data confidentiality and privacy. The lack of control over statistics and computation while using the cloud for garages presents various security concerns for businesses. The absence of control over data and the storage platform also encourages cloud clients to keep access to data to influence it (personal information and the facts shared amongst a collection of customers via the general public cloud). Before storing data in the cloud, the customer encrypts it, ensuring that the cloud does not learn any information about its records. Access rights are granted to one-of-a-kind users via a dispensing key for encryption. However, this may place an undue burden on clients. By putting a third birthday celebration between the client and the cloud and transferring all operational responsibilities to a third party, the consumer's burden will be reduced. However, there is a chance that 1/3 of the birthday party will engage in harmful behaviour while doing so.

In this research, we suggest protected data sharing in clouds, which provides safety, as mentioned earlier, by limiting agreements with the third-party server. It helps limit the number of things to consider at the third birthday celebration. This strategy ensures statistical confidentiality by assigning a few operational tasks to a third party. In this case, layer encryption is utilised, with the lower-layer encryption completed by the record owner and the top layer encryption completed by a third party. The owner grants the user access to the record by demonstrating the key used for lower-layer encryption during the report's encryption or decryption. As a result, returning control of activities to the statistics owner aids in maintaining confidentiality. Because the departing member cannot obtain a key used for lower-layer encryption from the owner of the records, he or she will be unable to decrypt the statistics independently. For new customer inclusion or person exit, no frequent decryption and encryption are required.

1.1 Cloud Storage for Big Data

Aside from allowing users to store all their data in the cloud, cloud storage also provides a wide range of record-keeping services. Clients do not have to buy and maintain their own IT centres because scale-parallel computing runs on low-cost goods hardware in a pre-configured configuration; cloud-based, completely big data enterprises have inherent accessibility, scalability, and cost efficiency. Data is continually produced due to the rapid progress of science and technology. The big data era has arrived in modern society [36]. Business industries have developed different applications to extract meaningful information from big data. However, these data sources operate in distinct environments and use different formats. It's difficult to get relevant information from these. Cloud services are now used by small, medium, and large businesses to store and analyse data. When needed, these cloud services offer a pay-as-you-go (PAYG) strategy for businesses. Cloud services offer important advantages for big data, including low computational costs, storage, automated tools, and reprogrammable virtualised resources. It is extremely beneficial to huge corporations in terms of expanding their operations. Simultaneously, most data-mining methods necessitate a significant number of computer properties in order to examine this vast data. As a result, businesses must pay cloud service providers excessively large sums of money. In addition, businesses and organisations will have to wait longer to analyse massive data and extract insights from it. As a result, small- and medium-sized businesses are particularly vulnerable. The suggested research aims to develop a more lightweight data analysis paradigm. We'll need to create a data deduplication technique for this. The deduplication procedure saves storage space and time while processing data.

1.2 Techniques

Writing text messages is one of the stages in steganography, and one of the options is to encrypt the textual content message. The text is then hidden in the chosen medium and sent to the recipient. The reverse system retrieves the original text message when the receiver is turned off. Creating various bits of textual content in a picture or other media is one of the several tactics employed in steganography. Considering the preceding, documents are required, including the image record and the information's textual content file. The LSB (least significant bit) mechanism is the most common way to hide the facts in the message's least significant bit (LSB). Because LSB affects the eight bits' slightest modifications, it reduces the snapshot to its bare essentials. However, one of its main drawbacks is the limited amount of information that can be contained in such images using LSB alone. LSB is quite vulnerable to attacks.

In contrast to 8-bit formats, LSB approaches applied to 24-bit formats are difficult to find. Masking and filtering are two other options. It is commonly associated with JPEG. This technology extends the life of image records by overlaying secret facts on top of them. It also relies on the files that will be integrated. As a result, experts no longer consider this a form of steganography. All algorithms used for any type of layout have advantages and disadvantages and depend on the environment in which they are utilised. Various evolving techniques were compared.

1.3 Extraction

The extraction process occurs on the getting side when the additional party accepts the Stego image and uses it with the withdrawal programme to extract the game message's name without any errors or modifications.

The embedding approach is currently used to move from the cover image to the mystery message to the Stego photograph. In contrast, the removal method goes from cover copy to secret communication toward Stego photographs. The Stego

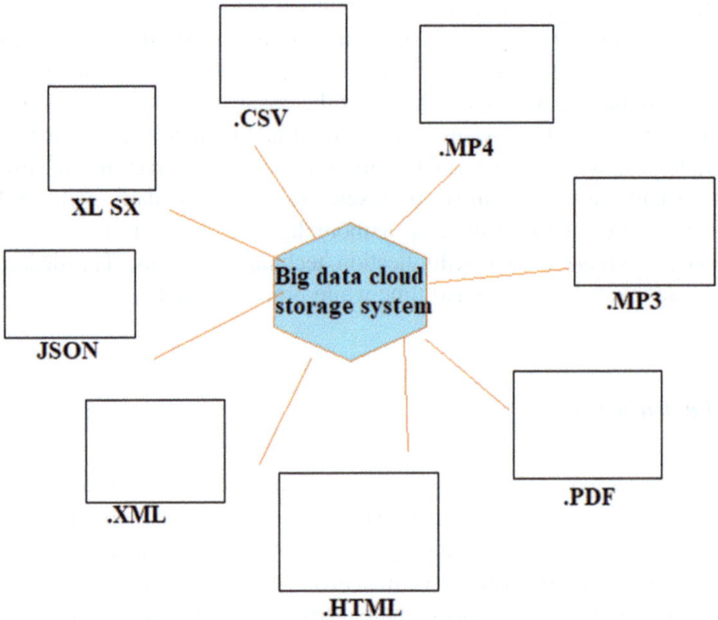

Fig. 1 Big data stored in public cloud storage system

photograph is entered first; earlier, the secret messages were removed, as shown in Fig. 1. The cloud-based big data application provides valuable material; here, all modifications are performed through format type. The available formats are .pdf, XML, DOC, and so on, with this cloud ID providing security.

2 Existing Methods

Ghosh, S [19] proposed a safe allocation strategy for individual well-being accounts in distributed computation based on ciphertext policy-based ascribed basis encryption (CP-ABE) [20]. Its focus is on limiting unapproved customers' access to private information. Limbadri, K. et al. [21] proposed an entry controller plan for the human being accounted in dispersed computation based on CP-ABE. Only one entirely assumed main specialist in the framework is responsible for key administration and key age in [22]. This work provided a novel public significant encoding by accepted equity permits on the entire ciphertext or a predetermined ciphertext.

To reinforce the creation's confidence regarding the prerequisite, Wu et al. [23] projected a productive and protected character-dependent encryption conspire by the balance test in the dispersed calculation. This framework [24] proposed a CP-ABE that employs bilinear blending to provide customers with ciphertext and fine-grained admittance organisation. In this framework, [25] projected a plan termed ACPC that pointed toward a generous, safe, proficient, and powdered information admission controller in a P2P stockpiling cloud. This framework proposed another structure, Reverse Address Adaptive Controlling (RAAC), to alleviate the single-point execution bottleneck of the remaining CP-ABE-built admittance control plans for public distributed storing. However, these plans utilise personality security by utilising quality-based strategies, which neglect to ensure client property protection. AWS (Amazon Web Services) is currently working on addressing security issues in the cloud. This framework proposed System Application Protocol for Data Sampling (SAPDS), a security-focused information-sharing plan. It combines the characteristic of relying on encryption with intermediary re-encryption and mystery key refreshing abilities without requiring any trust in an outsider. However, quality encryption conspires to choose the capacity and correspondence above SAPDS. In the current work, there is no gathering-based admission control framework. The framework's security is extremely low because of the absence of solid cryptography strategies.

3 Proposed System

In SSGK, an effective agreement is projected to address the safe difficulties of information allocation in dispersed storage without dependence on slightly trusted strangers. To prevent the key from being used to translate the frequent information by unapproved customers, previous uses of symmetrical encryption calculations [11] to scramble the mutual information, topsy-turvy calculations [12], and mystery allocating plans are used to allocate strategy is attainable together. This framework [31] was created concurrently in 1979 as a response to the need to protect steganography answers. A mystery is isolated by n dividends from a seller and collective amongst n sponsors in a mystery distribution plan. They expanded the idea of the first mystery allocation and introduced the idea of the obvious mystery allocation variable single source (VSS). The assets of obviousness imply that investors can check whether their offers are predictable. The information proprietor is completely trusted and will never be tainted by enemies. The framework is stronger because the mystery-sharing plan successfully disseminates the gathering key. The gathering individuals can assemble their sub-mystery offers to reproduce the gathering key.

Format wise file separation, file chunking, hash value finding, and grouping hash values are the four key mechanisms of the planned scheme. Figure 2 depicts the proposed system's design. The architecture of the projected organisation is first described in this section. We then went over the proposed method's process flow and algorithm.

Figure 3 explains the registration details of the proposed GUI design: user id, user name, email id, password, confirmed password, and DOB. Using these details, authors can be registered easily.

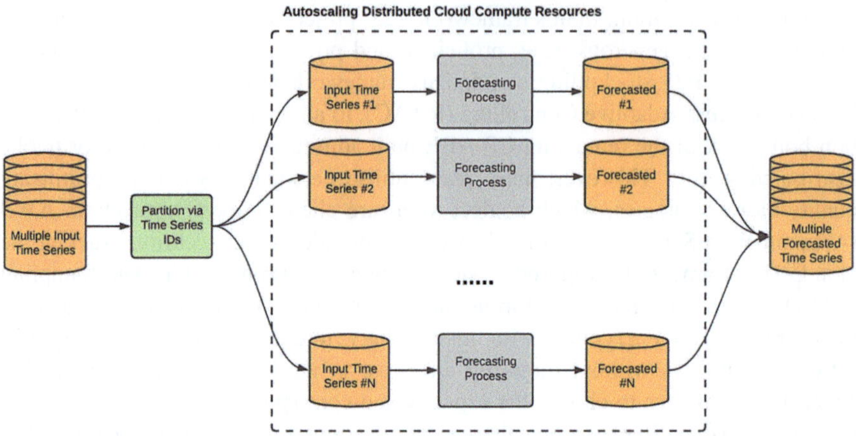

Fig. 2 Projected system

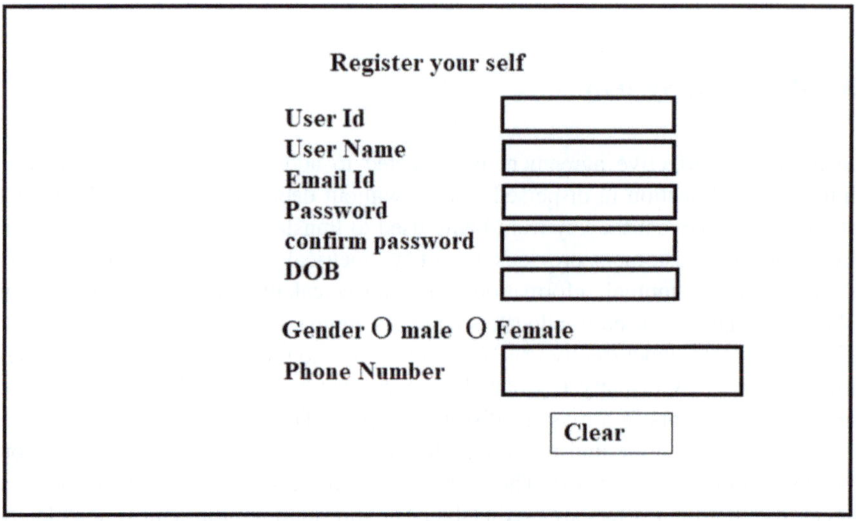

Fig. 3 Registration details

3.1 Module Implementation

3.1.1 Cloud Provider

Cloud provider gives a public stage for information proprietors to store and offer their encoded information. The cloud supplier does not direct information access regulators to proprietors. Any client can download the scrambled data without restriction.

3.1.2 Data Owner

Describes the entry strategy and encodes its data using symmetric encryption calculations and a gathering key. The individuals who fulfilled the entrance strategy established a sharing gathering. The proprietor then employs a mystery-sharing strategy to appropriate the encryption input to the distribution gathering. Gathering people: each gathering part, including the information proprietor, is assigned by extraordinary and a couple of keys.

3.1.3 The Assembly Members

The gathering individuals have openly become intrigued by encoded information in the public cloud. If the client obtains the information decoding key from the proprietor, the information is unscrambled.

4 Results and Analysis

This explains a brief discussion of the Secured Data Sharing Protocol for Minimisation of Risk in Cloud Computing and Big Data. Cloud provider login system gives confidential security to a database like a server or cloud. The dashboard section's main menu and all transactions have been identified using the proposed SSGK model.

The registration page for the user and owner enters their details like email, name, password, mobile number, user ID, etc., as shown in Fig. 4.

Figures 5 and 6 explain the welcome and main menu GUIs. All step-by-step processes are validated here by the owner and a group member. The transaction id, type, time, and type of transaction are verified with proper constraints.

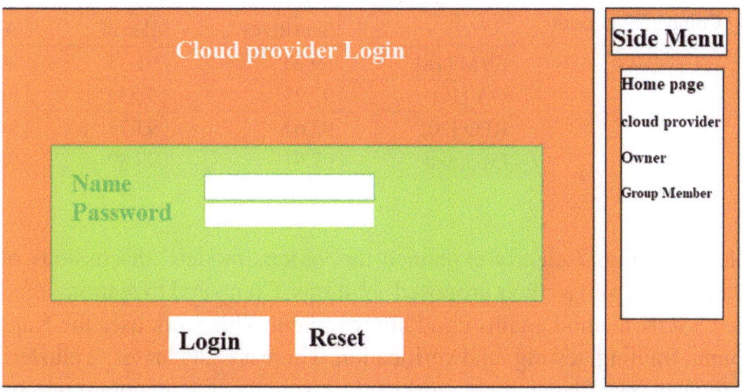

Fig. 4 The login page for the admin user and owner

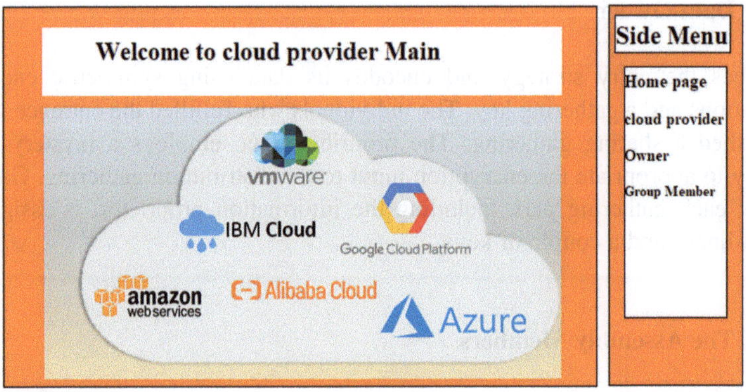

Fig. 5 After logging into the cloud provider, check all the users' and owner's information, uploaded information, etc.

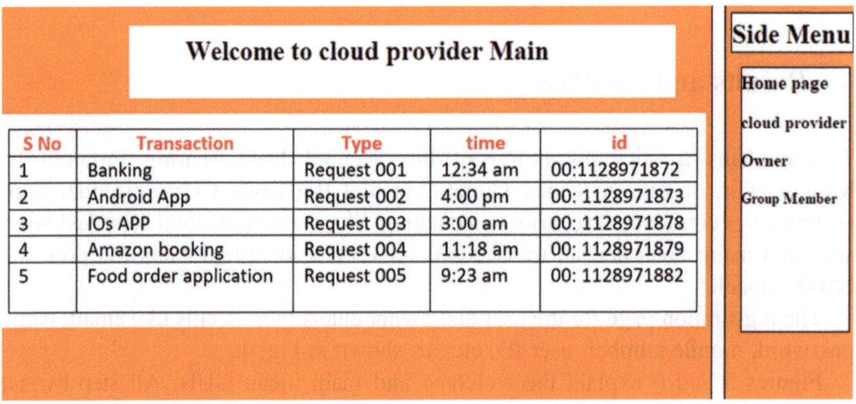

Fig. 6 Here, we can get all the transactions made by the owner and user in the application, which the cloud worker monitors

Table 1 Comparative result

	Sensitivity	Recall	Accuracy
SVM [18]	89.23	91.35	89.93
GA [19]	91.23	95.32	91.45
RFO [20]	93.67	93.78	94.98
Proposed	97.91	93.89	98.25

Table 1 and Fig. 7 clearly explained the various models' discussions of SVM, GA, and RFO, as well as their proposed solutions. Compared to reaming models, the proposed SSGK method attains good improvement. This work uses the Kaggle data set for input training, testing, and verification. There are 24 classes, 2 clustering, and 10,000 rows of .csv files in these workloads. Using this file, maintain preprocessing and feature extraction as well as classification.

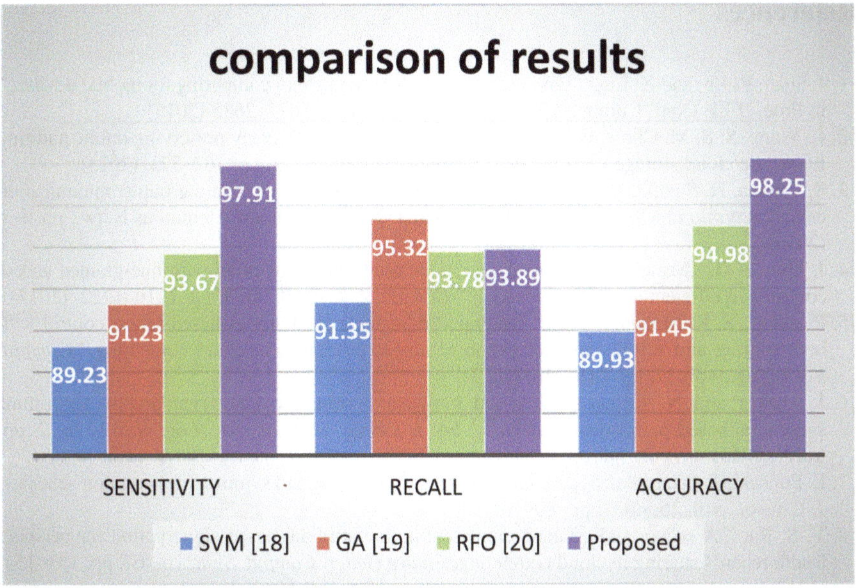

Fig. 7 Comparison of results

5 Conclusion

In this study, we propose a new key administration meeting aimed at information participants in dispersed storage. In SSGK, in addition to checked mystery allocation, we use RSA to source the information manager in order to achieve fine-grained control over the reappropriated information without relying on any stranger. Likewise, we provide an itemised examination of possible attacks and related protections that demonstrates the GKMP is safe beneath extra-fragile assumptions. We also show that our convention has less capacity and more unpredictability. The safety instrument in our plan guarantees network information safety in distributed storage. Encryption ensures the dissemination of information on the public network; a patterned safety plot variety of the information in the framework has only recently grown to be accepted at gatherings. The improved presentation concerning capacity and calculation makes our plan more grounded. The forwarding and reverse security issues in group key administration may necessitate a few changes to our convention. An effective and unique instrument for gathering individuals remains an upcoming effort. The SSGK method secured cloud and big data security, providing accuracy 98.25%, sensitivity 97.92%, and recall 93.89%. The proposed model attains more improvement compared to earlier models.

References

1. J. Shao, R. Lu, and X. Lin.: "Fine-grained data sharing in cloud computing for mobile devices," in Proc. IEEE Conf. Comput. Commun. (INFOCOM), pp.2677–2685 (2015)
2. C. Wang, S. S. M. Chow, Q. Wang, K. Ren, and W. Lou.: "Privacy preserving public auditing for secure cloud storage," IEEE Trans. Comput., vol. 62, no. 2, pp. 362–375, (2013).
3. S. Tanada, H. Suzuki, K. Naito, and A. Watanable, Proposal for secure group communication using encryption technology, Proc. 9th Int. Conf. Mobile Comput. Ubiquitous Netw., pp. 1–6 (2016).
4. J. Zhou et al.: "Securing outsourced data in the multi-authority cloud with fine-grained access control and efficient attribute revocation," *Comput. J.*, vol. 60, no. 8, pp. 1210–1222, (2017).
5. R. Ahuja, S. K. Mohanty, and K. Sakurai.: "A scalable attribute-set-based access control with both sharing and full-fledged delegation of access privileges in cloud computing," *Comput. Elect. Eng.*, vol. 57, pp. 241–256, (2017).
6. J. Thakur and N. Kumar.: 'AES and blowfish: Symmetric key cryptography algorithms simulation-based performance analysis,' *Int. J. Emerg. Technol. Adv. Eng.,* vol. 1, no. 2, pp. 6–12, (2011).
7. E. Fujisaki, T. Okamoto.: Secure integration of asymmetric and symmetric encryption schemes, *J. Cryptol.,* vol. 26, no. 1, pp. 80–101, (2013).
8. Y. S. Rao.: A secure and efficient ciphertext-policy attribute-based signcryption for personal health records sharing in cloud computing, *Future Gener. Comput. Syst.,* vol. 67, pp. 133–151, (2017).
9. S. Jin-Shu, C. Dan, W. Xiao-Feng, and S. Yi-Pin.: Attributed-based encryption schemes, *J. Softw.*, vol. 22, no. 6, pp. 1299–1315, (2011).
10. H. Liu, Y. Huang, and J. K. Liu.: Secure sharing of Personal Health Records in cloud computing: Ciphertext-Policy Attribute-Based Signcryption, *Future Gener. Comput. Syst.,* vol. 52, pp. 67–76, (2015).
11. K. Huang et al.: PKE-AET: Public key encryption with authorized equality test, *Comput. J.,* vol. 58, no. 10, pp. 2686–2697, (2015).
12. Saikumar, K. Rajesh V.: Coronary blockage of artery for Heart diagnosis with DT Artificial Intelligence Algorithm. *Int J Res Pharma Sci,* 11(1), 471–479 (2020).
13. Saikumar, K., Rajesh, V.: A novel implementation heart diagnosis system based on random forest machine learning technique *International Journal of Pharmaceutical* 12(1), 85–88 (2020).
14. Alekhya, N., & Kishore, N. P.: performance comparison of gfrp composite i section with an aluminum I section. *International Journal of Civil Engineering and Technology*, 8(4), 278–286 (2017).
15. Shankar, K. S., Ganesh, M., & Kumar, K. S.: Combustion Chamber Analysis Using CFD for Operation Condition. In IOP Conference Series: Materials Science and Engineering, Vol. 455, No. 1, p. 012032, IOP Publishing (2018).
16. Kalavagunta, V., & Hussain, S.: Wing Rib Stress Analysis of DLR-F6 aircraft. In IOP Conference Series: Materials Science and Engineering, Vol. 455, No. 1, p. 012033. IOP Publishing (2018).
17. Ebenezer, N. G. R., Ramabalan, S., & Navaneethasanthakumar, S.: Advanced design optimization on straight bevel gears pair based on nature inspired algorithms. *SN Applied Sciences*, 1(10), 1–9 (2019).
18. Vagdevi, K., Jyothirmai, B., Devi, V. R., & Rao, K. V.: Study of band gap engineering in graphene based electrode materials by density functional calculations: A search for high performance graphene based devices. In AIP Conference Proceedings, Vol. 2200, No. 1, p. 020010. AIP Publishing LLC (2019).
19. Ghosh, S. K., Mehedi, J., & Samal, U. C.: Sensing performance of energy detector in cognitive radio networks. *International Journal of Information Technology*, 11(4), 773–778, (2019).

20. Bhanuprakash, L., Parasuram, S., & Varghese, S.: Experimental investigation on graphene oxides coated carbon fibre/epoxy hybrid composites: Mechanical and electrical properties. *Composites Science and Technology*, 179, 134–144, (2019).
21. Limbadri, K., Singh, S. K., Satyanarayana, K., Singh, A. K., Ram, A. M., Ravindran, M., ... & Suresh, K.: Effect of processing routes on orientation-dependent tensile flow behavior of Zircaloy-4 at elevated temperatures. Metallography, *Microstructure, and Analysis*, 8(3), 393–405 (2019).
22. Kishore, N. P., Shaik, T., Himagireesh, C., Prasad, K. D., & Alekhya, N.: Cryogenic heat treatment process for D2 steel & M2 steel. In AIP Conference Proceedings, Vol. 2269, No. 1, p. 030082. AIP Publishing LLC.1 Research 12, pp. 3904–3916 (2020).
23. Raju K., Chinna Rao B., Saikumar K., Lakshman Pratap N.: An Optimal Hybrid Solution to Local and Global Facial Recognition Through Machine Learning. In: Kumar P., Obaid AJ, Cengiz K., Khanna A., Balas V.E. (eds) A Fusion of Artificial Intelligence and Internet of Things for Emerging Cyber Systems. Intelligent Systems Reference Library, vol 210. Springer, Cham. https://doi.org/10.1007/978-3-030-76653-5_11 (2022).
24. Sankara Babu B., Nalajala S., Sarada K., Muniraju Naidu V., Yamsani N., Saikumar K.: Machine Learning Based Online Handwritten Telugu Letters Recognition for Different Domains. In: Kumar P., Obaid AJ, Cengiz K., Khanna A., Balas V.E. (eds) A Fusion of Artificial Intelligence and Internet of Things for Emerging Cyber Systems. Intelligent Systems Reference Library, vol 210. Springer, Cham. https://doi.org/10.1007/978-3-030-76653-5_12 (2022).
25. Kiran Kumar M., Kranthi Kumar S., Kalpana E., Srikanth D., Saikumar K.: A Novel Implementation of Linux Based Android Platform for Client and Server. In: Kumar P., Obaid AJ, Cengiz K., Khanna A., Balas V.E. (eds) A Fusion of Artificial Intelligence and Internet of Things for Emerging Cyber Systems. Intelligent Systems Reference Library, vol 210. Springer, Cham. https://doi.org/10.1007/978-3-030-76653-5_8 (2022).
26. Nora Omran Alkaam, Ahmed J. Obaid, Mohammed Q. Mohammed.: A Hybrid Technique for Object Detection and Recognition Using Local Features Algorithms, Journal of Advanced Research in Dynamical and Control Systems, Vol. 10, No. 2: 2330–2344 (2018).
27. K. Balachander, S. Ramesh, Ahmed J. Obaid.: Simulation Of 1KW Multi-Level Switch Mode Power Amplifier, *International Journal of Innovations in Scientific and Engineering Research*, Vol. 5, No. 9: 85–92 (2018).
28. Saba Alyasiri, Ahmed J. Obaid.: A New Approach for Object Detection, Recognition and Retrieving in Painting Images, *Journal of Advanced Research in Dynamical and Control Systems,* Vol. 10, No. 2: 2345–2359 (2018).
29. Dilip Kumar Sharma.: "Some Generalized Information Measures: Their characterization and Applications", Lambert Academic Publishing, Germany, 2010. ISBN: 978-3838386041 (2010).
30. D. K. Sharma, B. Singh, R. Regin, R. Steffi and M. K. Chakravarthi.: Efficient Classification for Neural Machines Interpretations based on Mathematical models, 2021 7th International Conference on Advanced Computing and Communication Systems, 2021, pp. 2015–2020, (2021).
31. F. Arslan, B. Singh, D. K. Sharma, R. Regin, R. Steffi and S. S Rajest.: "Optimization Technique Approach to Resolve Food Sustainability Problems," 2021 International Conference on Computational Intelligence and Knowledge Economy, 2021, pp. 25–30 (2021).
32. G. A. Ogunmola, B. Singh, D. K. Sharma, R. Regin, S. S. Rajest and N. Singh.: "Involvement of Distance Measure in Assessing and Resolving Efficiency Environmental Obstacles," 2021 International Conference on Computational Intelligence and Knowledge Economy, pp. 13–18 (2021).
33. D. K. Sharma, B. Singh, M. Raja, R. Regin and S. S. Rajest. An Efficient Python Approach for Simulation of Poisson Distribution, 2021 7th International Conference on Advanced Computing and Communication Systems, pp. 2011–2014 (2021).
34. D. K. Sharma, B. Singh, E. Herman, R. Regine, S. S. Rajest and V. P. Mishra, "Maximum Information Measure Policies in Reinforcement Learning with Deep Energy-Based Model," 2021 International Conference on Computational Intelligence and Knowledge Economy, pp. 19–24 (2021).

35. D. K. Sharma, N. A. Jalil, R. Regin, S. S. Rajest, R. K. Tummala and T. N.: "Predicting Network Congestion with Machine Learning," 2021 2nd International Conference on Smart Electronics and Communication, pp. 1574–1579 (2021).
36. Pandya, S., Wandra, K., Shah, J., A Hybrid Based Recommendation System to overcome the problem of sparcity, International Conference on emerging trends in scientific research, December, (2015).
37. Mehta, P., Pandya, S.: A review on sentiment analysis methodologies, practices and applications, *International Journal of Scientific and Technology Research*, 9(2), pp. 601–609 (2020).
38. Yousaf, A., Umer, M., Sadiq, S., Ullah, S., Mirjalili, S., Rupapara, V., & Nappi, M.: Emotion Recognition by Textual Tweets Classification Using Voting Classifier (LR-SGD). *IEEE Access,* 9, 6286–6295. https://doi.org/10.1109/access.2020.3047831 (2021).
39. A.K. Gupta, Y.K Chauhan, and T Maity.: A new gamma scaling maximum power point tracking method for solar photovoltaic panel Feeding energy storage system, IETE Journal of Research, vol.67, no.1, pp.1–21, (2018).
40. Sadiq, S., Umer, M., Ullah, S., Mirjalili, S., Rupapara, V., & Nappi, M. Discrepancy detection between actual user reviews and numeric ratings of Google App store using deep learning. Expert Systems with Applications, 115111. https://doi.org/10.1016/j.eswa.2021.115111 (2021).
41. Rupapara, V., Narra, M., Gonda, N. K., Thipparthy, K., & Gandhi, S.: Auto-Encoders for Content-based Image Retrieval with its Implementation Using Handwritten Dataset. 2020 5th International Conference on Communication and Electronics Systems, 289–294, (2020).
42. A. Jain, R. Dwivedi, A. Kumar, and S. Sharma.: Network on chip router for 2D mesh design, *Int. J. Comput. Sci. Inf. Secur.,* vol. 14, no. 9, p. 1092, (2016).
43. A. Jain, A. K. AlokGahlot, and S. K. S. RakeshDwivedi.: "Design and FPGA Performance Analysis of 2D and 3D Router in Mesh NoC," *Int. J. Control Theory Appl.*, pp. 0974–5572, (2017).
44. A. Bhardwaj, S. Kaur, A. P. Shukla, and M. K. Shukla.: Performance Comparison of De-speckling filters on the Basis of Incremental Iteration in Ultrasound Imaging, in 2019 International Conference on Power Electronics, Control and Automation, pp. 1–5 (2019).
45. G. S. Sajja, K. P. Rane, K. Phasinam, T. Kassanuk, E. Okoronkwo, and P. Prabhu.: "Towards applicability of blockchain in agriculture sector," Materials Today: Proceedings, (2021).
46. H. Pallathadka, M. Mustafa, D. T. Sanchez, G. Sekhar Sajja, S. Gour, and M. Naved, "Impact of machine learning on management, healthcare and agriculture," Materials Today: Proceedings, (2021).
47. Guna Sekhar Sajja, Malik Mustafa, R. Ponnusamy, Shokhjakhon Abdufattokhov, Murugesan G., P. Prabhu.: "Machine Learning Algorithms in Intrusion Detection and Classification", Annals of RSCB, vol. 25, no. 6, pp. 12211–12219, (2021).
48. S. K. Sharma, A. Jain, K. Gupta, D. Prasad, and V. Singh.: An internal schematic view and simulation of major diagonal mesh network-on-chip, *J. Comput. Theor. Nanosci.,* vol. 16, no. 10, pp. 4412–4417, (2019).
49. D. Ghai, H. K. Gianey, A. Jain, and R. S. Uppal.: Quantum and dual-tree complex wavelet transform-based image watermarking, *Int. J. Mod. Phys.* B, vol. 34, no. 04, p. 2050009, (2020).
50. D. S. Gupta and G. P. Biswas, "A novel and efficient lattice-based authenticated key exchange protocol in C-K model," *Int. J. Commun. Syst.,* vol. 31, no. 3, art. no. e3473 (2018).
51. Rajendran, S., Mathivanan, S. K., Jayagopal, P., Janaki, K. P., Bernard, B. A. M. M., Pandy, S., & Somanathan, M. S.: Emphasizing privacy and security of edge intelligence with machine learning for healthcare. International Journal of Intelligent Computing and Cybernetics (2021).
52. Surinder Singh and Hardeep Singh Saini.: "Security approaches for data aggregation in Wireless Sensor Networks against Sybil Attack," 2018 Second International Conference on Inventive Communication and Computational Technologies, pp. 190–193, Coimbatore, India. https://doi.org/10.1109/ICICCT.2018.8473091 (2018).

Predictive Modelling for Healthcare Decision-Making Using IoT with Machine Learning Models

Rajasekar Rangasamy, Thayyaba Khatoon Mohammed, Mageshkumar Chinnaswamy, and Ramachandran Veerachamy

1 Introduction

The common problem in a health prediction system is the rapid changes in hospital patient flow. To create a communication between the virtual computer and physical things, the Internet of Things (IoT) is created [1]. Microprocessor chips are enabled to collect the information as soon as possible. Without individual patient flow data, healthcare facilities frequently find it challenging to meet demand, while neighbouring facilities have private patients. It is worth noting that the healthcare or medical industry is improved, and health is preserved by diagnosing and preventing disorders. The machine-learning software to overcome chronic conditions is referred to as innovative healthcare decisions. ML, machine reasoning, and robotics are the exclusive approaches and techniques involved in Artificial Intelligence (AI) (Fig. 1) [2]. Through the fast-developing applied sciences like Cloud computing environment, mobile communication, and big data tools, ML models benefit from those applications to serve healthcare sectors. With the help of the technologies mentioned earlier, ML is efficient in making precise predictive results, and it also helps produce human-centred intelligent solutions [3].

Ultimately, these technologies play an irreplaceable role in strengthening the healthcare industry and benefits like offering centralised healthcare services for the countryside and impoverished zones. This chapter emphasises ML algorithms and

R. Rangasamy (✉) · M. Chinnaswamy · R. Veerachamy
Department of Computer Science and Engineering, GITAM School of Technology, GITAM (Deemed to be University), Bengaluru Campus, Bengaluru, India

T. K. Mohammed
Department of Computer Science and Engineering-AIML, Malla Reddy University, Hyderabad, India
e-mail: hodaiml@mallareddyuniversity.ac.in

P. Agarwal et al. (eds.), *Artificial Intelligence for Smart Healthcare*, EAI/Springer Innovations in Communication and Computing,
https://doi.org/10.1007/978-3-031-23602-0_2

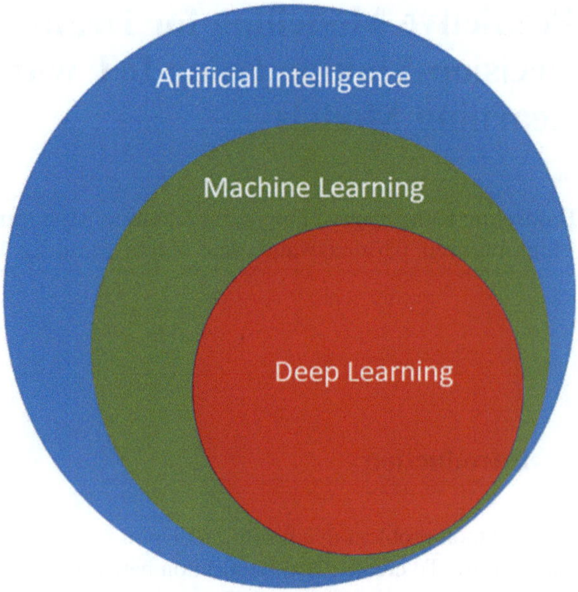

Fig. 1 State-of-the-art of machine learning approach

their classification and prediction of IoT data in the healthcare sector. It mainly focuses on the application of ML in different healthcare activities. We have examined the workings by comparing them on various parameters. The next step in the investigation will be to compare available studies, distinguish features and drawbacks, and identify possible shortfalls in each methodology for choosing appropriate ML to develop an efficient statistical method. Through this research, we know that k-Nearest Neighbour (KNN) may be the most popular algorithm for classification and prediction tasks. It takes longer to produce the output [4]. In order to improve both systems' performance, recurrent neural networks (RNN) and long short-term memory (LSTM) are combined. The challenges are researched in this investigation: To what extent can predictive health models be improved by combining IoT data with ML-based computational methods? [5]. In short, this chapter presents the following contributions:

(a) This chapter presents an outline of ML models and their typical applications and the development of ML pipelines for accuracy in healthcare and to detect causes of risk factors at each phase.
(b) This chapter emphasises many standard security and privacy-related issues related to taking up ML models and offers capable results for the powerful tool of ML techniques, especially for healthcare service applications.
(c) This chapter highlights multiple open research/open scholarship challenges and problems that need additional examination.

The chapter's organisation, Segment 2, deals with ML models and their classification in healthcare. Section 3 discusses the application of ML algorithms in prediction applications and various causes of vulnerability and issues related to the use of ML.

Section 4 focuses on multiple potential solutions to ensure privacy and security to IoT and ML users in the healthcare sector. Section 5 throws light on the discussion and results of the Healthcare Prediction Performance analysis. Finally, Sect. 6 concludes the chapter with multiple directions for further research.

2 Related Works

Traditional big data techniques, which are used to discover patterns in massive databases, are no longer up to the task of extracting knowledge from such distributed, extensive, and wide-ranging data sets. Data mining techniques help support the data processing and the transformation of that data into actionable insights [6]. In the healthcare industry, many forecasting and recommender systems have been researched. An experiment was conducted to investigate the best method for predicting heart attack or stroke and measure the findings. The genetically optimised CNN is being used to identify breast cancer. Other knowledge extraction and data mining in which systems have been suggested [7]. ML is one of the most cutting-edge ideas when it comes to AI. ML is a strategic platform to establish automated, highly complex, and objective predictive techniques for multi-view and dimensional biomedical/computational data analysis. The ML algorithms can access and reconfigure their structure based on measured data by enhancing a set of parameters or an objective. Numerous symptoms can be diagnosed, detected, contained, and treated with the help of ML [8, 9]. The reviews thus far indicate that ML and other AI techniques have been critical in predicting, diagnosing, and containing the COVID-19 pandemic, which can help mitigate the incredible responsibility on already-scarce medical systems [10]. To our experience and understanding, no research has been published in Mexico that uses prevalence and incidence labelled datasets for adaptive and maladaptive COVID-19 cases to advance the supervised Classification model for COVID-19 infectious disease prediction. As a result, the current study attempts to add in these gaps.

ML was innovated to control the machine to act intelligently by gaining knowledge from their environment. As mentioned in the previous section, ML allows computers to perform from previous experiences fully autonomous using different datasets, completeness of information algorithms to estimate future behaviours and actions and make intelligent decisions. ML is typically divided into three categories: supervised / unsupervised / reinforcement learning [11]. ML works with labelled extracted features. On the other hand, RL is trained in a real-world environment with real-world data. Its goal is to learn about a given scenario and determine the appropriate methodologies to use in that environment. It's mainly used in robotics, navigation, and video games. Furthermore, ML algorithms have training program data requirements. ML can create regression models to find relationships between the variables, classify mislabelled datasets, and cluster data into categories [12].

3 Machine Learning Models and Classification in Healthcare Applications

Machine learning is the study of understanding how computers learn from data and continuously upgrade themselves. ML is mighty compared to other statistical methodologies, especially in decision-making [13]. Features refer to the information collected from a dataset given to the algorithm. Features with premium quality supplied to the algorithm are essential because the prediction accuracy created by a model depends on it. In the beginning, it is necessary to have an idea about ML and its various approaches (Fig. 2) and know about algorithms used in ML for clustering and classification [14].

3.1 Supervised Machine Learning

In this approach, a training set is given with suitable objectives. Supervised Learning is divided into two groups called Classification and Regression. These methods build the connection between the inputs and outputs using labelled training data. In a task, the discrete output is known as classification, and if it is a continuous output variable, the task would be regression. Supervised machine learning ultimately aims for predicting a known output based on a common dataset. Binary and multiclass are the two forms of classification. Former deals with two sets of classes [15]. The input data are arranged in two groups of classes. For instance, they classified Spam and no Spam in emails and made "YES/NO" predictions. These classes are described as 0 and 1. To its contrast, multiclass classification deals with three or more predictable classes. Identification of cancer stages would be the perfect example of the classes as it is defined as 0, 1, 2, etc.

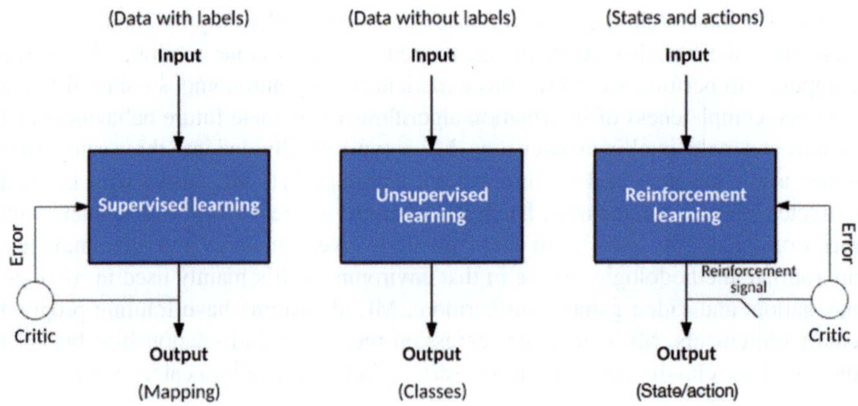

Fig. 2 Models of machine learning

3.2 *Unsupervised Learning*

One of the functions of unsupervised ML is labelling hidden structures within unlabeled data. The most prevalent examples of unsupervised ML methods are forming a group of data points using a similarity metric and dimensionality depletion of high dimensional data to lower-dimensional subspaces. In addition to that, it can also be used to detect abnormalities—Ex.: Clustering [16–18].

3.3 *Semi-supervised Learning*

This method is used when labelled and unlabelled test data sets are feasible for training, commonly a small and large volume of unlabelled data. To get significant learning accuracy, minor marked data should be used with large amounts of unmarked data in real-life circumstances. Human involvement is essential for attaching datasets. Tagging requires much time, and hence, it may obstruct the creation of fully labelled training and bring out heavy expenditure. Therefore, semi-supervised ML is considered a better solution [19, 20].

3.4 *Reinforcement Learning*

Based on specific observations, the performance of actions and rewards over a certain period is known as Reinforcement Learning (RL). Nowadays, RL is widely implemented in healthcare applications where the disease is diagnosed earlier and the symptoms are identified. Go Game is the best example to illustrate the efficiency of RL in healthcare applications. In Go Game, PCs use RL incorporated with supervised and unsupervised ML methods to beat a human champion competitor [21].

The difference between the supervised, unsupervised, and semi-supervised ML models is shown in Table 1.

ML technique is applied to predict or detect disease at its early stages. Hence, this technique increases the possibility of patients being cured, and the treatments would

Table 1 Comparative analysis of different ML Models [11]

Learning class	Class type	Model of class	Performance of accuracy
Supervised	Labelled	Classification regression	High
Unsupervised	Unlabelled	Clustering transformations	Low
Semi-supervised	Labelled & unlabelled	Classification clustering	Medium
Reinforcement learning	Labelled & unlabelled	Classification and clustering	Hybrid High & low

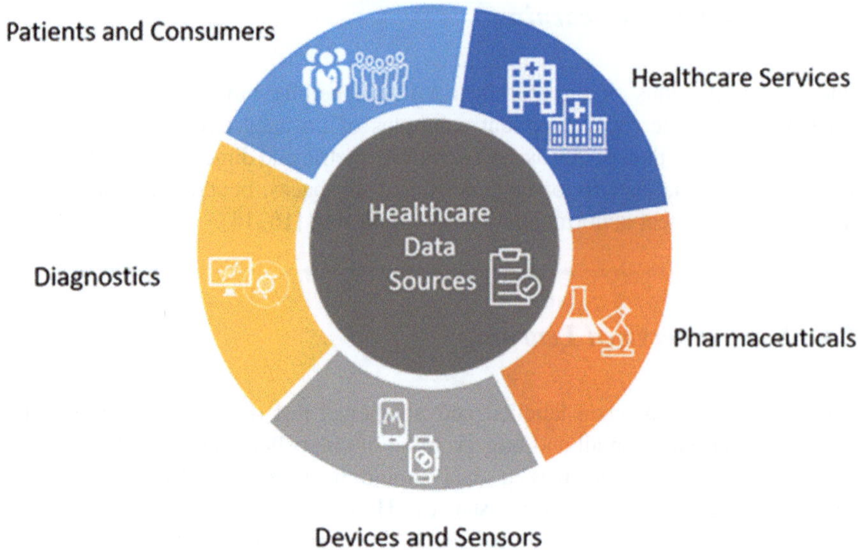

Fig. 3 Representation of miscellaneous sources help in healthcare data

be uncomplicated because the disease is diagnosed earlier. Data accuracy is driven by numerous factors including the algorithm, feature set, training dataset, and diseases being analysed. In this segment, a selected disease will be discussed as example with its significance of spotting at an early stage. ML methods are applied to detect the disease and the various properties involved in predictions [22].

In a clinical setting, forecasting the advancement of disease is called prognosis. It involves spotting symptoms and the different stages of diseases, whether it becomes worse, better, or remains at the same stage for a specific time and monitoring the patients' health problems, irrespective of their incapability of doing day-to-day activities and their survival [23]. A few of the various multi-modal data related to patients are phenotypic, genomic, proteomic, pathology tests logs, medical image sets, etc., are collected in a clinical test setting. These multi-modal data help us to perform prognosis, diagnosis, and the treatment of disease (Fig. 3).

4 Healthcare Applications of ML in Diagnosis

In a complete medical history, hospitals and other healthcare sectors bring out various data consisting of Electronic Health Records (EHRs) and composed of structured and unstructured data of patients daily. ML-based methods promoted in the extraction of clinical properties help in the diagnosis process [24]. Various imaging methods produce the economic and successful extraction of data from medical images. The different types of imaging techniques include Magnetic

Resonance Imaging (MRI), Computed Tomography (CT), ultrasound, and Positron Emission Tomography (PET), etc. These imaging techniques bring us preliminary information based on the different parts of the body that are functional and anatomical information. It plays a dynamic role in the analysis and detection of irregularities of the body [25].

5 Secure and Privacy-Preserving Use of Healthcare Measures on IoT and ML

5.1 Sources of Vulnerabilities in ML

The ML technique that demands a considerable amount of data is applied (HER). Since the data collected are so large, it leads to time absorption and more human support. Indeed, in regular practice, we can manage accurate clinical data to diagnose effectively. But the working condition of the ML is affected by various threats [26–29].

5.2 Vulnerabilities Due to Data Annotation

Data Annotation allocates labels to every data or information sample (e.g., Medical Image). Expert clinicians always carry out data Annotation to make the enhanced domain datasets. In the medical field, improving the ML models has become more critical. It is disclosed that ML without grip would be a failure [30].

5.3 Vulnerabilities in Model Training

In modal training, there are many threats, and some of them are unsuitable or partial training, non-observance, model corruption and stealing [31–34]. In some circumstances, inappropriate variables like learning rate, epochs, and batch size are skilled in ML models, producing improper or incomplete training. In the case of privacy flaws, including cyberattacks, data and model corruption attacks, and others like these, there is a significant risk with machine learning (ML) models [35–41]. These vulnerabilities disturb the ML models to a greater extent. Protecting the ML systems in critical applications is necessary to provide a safe and virtuous ML system [42].

6 Results and Discussion

The function of ML models is presented and compared by predicting the number of patients injured and the persons leaving work [43–47]. There are two types of results. On the type part, we forecast the number of persons injured. The parameters such as Logistic Regression (LR), Decision Tree (DT), Random Forest (RF), and Artificial Neural Network (ANN) (with fixed field and injury narratives as input) are observed [48].

6.1 Healthcare Diagnoses Outcome

Tools like DT, LR, RF, and ANN are applied to bring out the injury results [49]. Fixed field entries and injury narratives are the two inputs used for finding results [50–53]. As shown in Table 2, some field entries are treated as having 100% accuracy and the F1-score is used as the input value for work-related injury discourses, which is not fair. For instance, ANN on the complete accuracy is 68.11%, and LR and RF level accuracy is 68.19% and 68.11%. Further, to find out the F1-score, the most compactable model is ANN. The F1-score of ANN is 0.681, and the F1-scores of LR and RF are 0.65 and 0.66. Comparing both models, the best performance could be derived from ANN for its improved performance level. F1 score of DT is 0.58, and hence, it has less precision level. Table 2 implies the F1-score and precision level of RF and ANN skilled in imbalanced injury narratives. Random forest is inbuilt with uppermost F1-score and accuracy [54, 55]. Figure 4 shows the prevailing uncertain conditions of RF trained on the injury narrative. In the balanced and unbalanced datasets, the F1-score of ANN, after the augmentation of the F1-score in the subset Classes 1, 5, 8, and 9, is enhanced. In comparison, there is no data augmentation in Classes 2, 3, 4, and 7. For Classes 2, 3, and 7, the F1-score has decreased, and in Class 4, there are no traces of the F1-score. On the whole, the F1-score of ANN on the unbalanced test dataset is 0.62; after augmentation, the F1-score has reduced to 0.60 (Fig. 5a, b).

Table 2 Each ML model's accuracy and F1-score are summarised

	Fixed field entries		Imbalanced narratives	
Model	F1-score	Accuracy (%)	F1-score	Accuracy (%)
LR	0.68	68.19	0.88	92.25
DT	0.59	59.28	0.93	93.45
RF	0.69	59.18	0.94	94.91
ANN	0.68	59.92	0.62	93.19

Positive	Prediction Label									
Label	I	II	III	IV	V	VI	VI	VIII	IX	X
I	290	21					8	11		
II		161717					536			
III			7273							81
IV		101		4353			414			
V					289				45	
VI			245			189				
VII							12819			
VIII								672		
IX		21			726				412	
X							8338			516

Fig. 4 Matrix of confusion for ML experts on injury histories

6.2 Feature Predictions

Since the text narratives are unstructured, it cannot find the valuable features to forecast the target class. We are implementing the ANN skill on fixed fields to examine the feature significance. ANN is practised each time by discarding the one predictor variable from the data. ANN calculates the F1 score of ANN practised on all values of the entire dataset, and the ANN is practised on one missing variable. This variation shows the feature significance. Table 3 presents the importance of each feature in a sorted array.

7 Conclusions and Future Work

Compared with all other sectors, the most responsible and complex sectors are nothing but healthcare. ML models are used in clinical applications to change traditional healthcare service delivery. This chapter outlines risk factors and issues in developing ML pipelines in healthcare sectors. It also offers solutions for security and privacy conserving ML for safety applications in healthcare. This chapter compiles the ML algorithms and their applications in the medical field to predict future IoT and ML codes trends. This research drives towards investigating novel data collection techniques to improve the standard and enhance the features of work incidents and happenings in mining. In addition, this research provides models based on traits of the incident in mining for predicting the worker's number of days absent

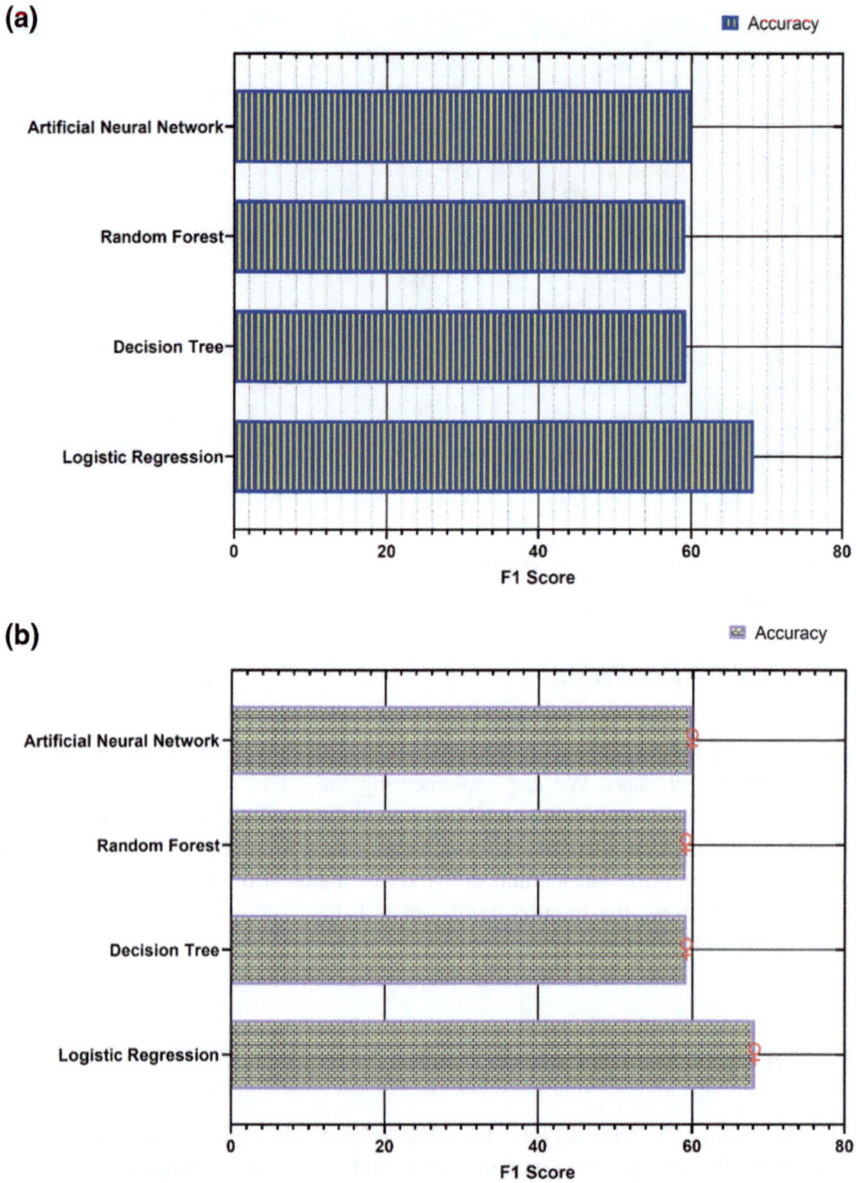

Fig. 5 Shows the (**a**) Fixed Field values and (**b**) Imbalance Narratives based on F1-score of Artificial Intelligence

Table 3 In determining the relative importance, predictor variable, and their characterisations

Feature	Injury characterisation
Type of the injury	Describes the severe injuries based on their main physical attributes
Classification	Identifies the variables that were most responsible for the accident that resulted in those factors
Patient's body part injured	Defines the part of the human body which has been seriously wounded
Source of injury	Identifies the entity, toxins, awareness, or genital motion that caused the serious injuries

from work. CNN's and Recurrent Neural Networks (RNN) are the promising techniques in DL that have shown the best output in text allocation. Based on such DL models, there is a place for extensive research. In recent times, the adversarial network has been implemented in text generation. Finally, an in-depth study could be done in the field of safety management in workplaces where GANs help overcome data imbalance issues.

References

1. B. Nithya and V. Ilango, "Predictive analytics in health care using machine learning tools and techniques," *2017 International Conference on Intelligent Computing and Control Systems (ICICCS)*, 2017, pp. 492–499.
2. S. M. Sasubilli, A. Kumar and V. Dutt, "Machine Learning Implementation on Medical Domain to Identify Disease Insights using TMS," *2020 International Conference on Advances in Computing and Communication Engineering (ICACCE)*, 2020, pp. 1–4.
3. Das, Z. Nayeem, A. S. Faysal, F. H. Himu and T. R. Siam, "Health Monitoring IoT Device with Risk Prediction using Cloud Computing and Machine Learning," *2021 National Computing Colleges Conference (NCCC)*, 2021, pp. 1–6.
4. Kaparthi, S.; Bumblauskas, D. Designing predictive maintenance systems using decision tree-based machine learning techniques. Int. J. Qual. Reliab. Manag. 2020, 37, 659–686.
5. Kaparthi, S.; Bumblauskas, D. Designing predictive maintenance systems using decision tree-based machine learning techniques. Int. J. Qual. Reliab. Manag. 2020, 37, 659–686.
6. Zhang, W.; Yang, D.; Wang, H. Data-Driven Methods for Predictive Maintenance of Industrial Equipment: A Survey. IEEE Syst. J. 2019, 13, 2213–2227.
7. Yoo, Y.; Park, S.H.; Baek, J.G. A Clustering-Based Equipment Condition Model of Chemical Vapor Deposition Process. *Int. J. Precis. Eng. Manuf.* 2019, 20, 1677–1689.
8. C. Liao, R. Chen, and S. Tai, Emotion stress detection using EEG signal and deep learning technologies - *IEEE Conference Publication, 2018 IEEE Int. Conf. Appl. Syst. Invent.,* no. 2, pp. 9093, 2018.
9. F.P. An, "Medical image classification algorithm based on weight initialisation-sliding window fusion convolutional neural network," *Complexity,* vol. 2019, Article ID 9151670, 2019.
10. K. Muthumayil, R. Karuppathal, T. Jayasankar, B. Aruna Devi, N. Prakash, S. Sudhakar, A Big Data Analytical Approach for Prediction of Cancer Using Modified K-Nearest Neighbour Algorithm, *Journal of Medical Imaging and Health Informatics,* Vol. 11, No. 8, August 2021, pp. 2120–2125.

11. L. Arokia Jesu Prabhu, Sudhakar Sengan, G.K. Kamalam, J. Vellingiri, Jagadeesh Gopal, Priya Velayutham, V. Subramaniyaswamy, Medical Information Retrieval Systems for e-Health Care Records using Fuzzy Based Machine Learning Model. *Microprocessors and Microsystems*, https://doi.org/10.1016/j.micpro.2020.103344.
12. Sengan Sudhakar, V. Priya, A. Syed Musthafa, Ravi Logesh, Palani Saravanan, V. Subramaniyaswamy, A fuzzy-based high-resolution multi-view deep CNN for breast cancer diagnosis through SVM classifier on visual analysis, *IOS Press-Journal of Intelligent & Fuzzy Systems*, pp. 1–14, 2020.
13. S. Sudhakar and S. Chenthur Pandian "Secure packet encryption and key exchange system in mobile ad hoc network", *Journal of Computer Science*, vol. 8, no. 6, pp. 908–912, 2012.
14. S. Sudhakar and S. Chenthur Pandian, "Hybrid cluster-based geographical routing protocol to mitigate malicious nodes in mobile ad hoc network", *International Journal of Ad Hoc and Ubiquitous Computing*, vol. 21 no. 4, pp. 224–236, 2016.
15. A. U. Priyadarshni and S. Sudhakar, "Cluster-based certificate revocation by cluster head in mobile ad-hoc network", *International Journal of Applied Engineering Research*, vol. 10, no. 20, pp. 16014–16018, 2015.
16. S. Sudhakar and S. Chenthur Pandian, "An efficient agent-based intrusion detection system for detecting malicious nodes in MANET routing", *International Review on Computers and Software*, vol. 7, no. 6, pp. 3037–304, 2012.
17. S. Sudhakar and S. Chenthur Pandian, "Authorised node detection and accuracy in position-based information for MANET", *European Journal of Scientific Research*, vol. 70, no. 2, pp. 253–265, 2012.
18. Sengan Sudhakar, L. Arokia Jesu Prabhu, V. Ramachandran, V. Priya, Ravi, Logesh, V. Subramaniyaswamy, Images super-resolution by optimal deep AlexNet architecture for medical application: A novel DOCALN, *IOS Press-Journal of Intelligent & Fuzzy Systems*, pp. 1–14, 2020.
19. Avuthu Sai Meghana, Sudhakar S, Arumugam G, Srinivasan P, Kolla Bhanu Prakash, Age and Gender prediction using Convolution, ResNet50, and Inception ResNetV2, *International Journal of Advanced Trends in Computer Science and Engineering*, Vol. 9, No. 2, 2020, pp: 1328–1334.
20. C. Cao, F. Liu, H. Tan et al., "Deep learning and its applications in biomedicine," *Genomics, Proteomics & Bioinformatics*, vol. 16, no. 1, pp. 17–32, 2018.
21. S. Latif, A. Qayyum, M. Usama, J. Qadir, A. Zwitter, and M. Shahzad, "Caveat emptor: The risks of using big data for human development," *IEEE Technology and Society Magazine*, vol. 38, no. 3, pp. 82–90, 2019.
22. Solares, J.R.A.; Raimondi, F.E.D.; Zhu, Y.; Rahimian, F.; Canoy, D.; Tran, J.; Gomes, A.C.P.; Payberah, A.H.; Zottoli, M.; Nazarzadeh, M.; et al. Deep learning for electronic health records: A comparative review of multiple deep neural architectures. *J. Biomed. Inform.* 2020, 101, 103337.
23. Zame, W.R.; Bica, I.; Shen, C.; Curth, A.; Lee, H.-S.; Bailey, S.; Weatherall, J.; Wright, D.; Bretz, F.; Van Der Schaar, M. Machine learning for clinical trials in the era of COVID-19. *Stat. Biopharm. Res.* 2020, 12, 506–517.
24. P. Manta, S. Chandra Singh, A. Deep, and D. N. Kapoor, "Temperature-regulated gold nanoparticle sensors for immune chromatographic rapid test kits with reproducible sensitivity: a study," *IET Nanobiotechnol.*, no. nbt2.12024, 2021.
25. O. M. Abo-Seida, N. T. M. El-dabe, A. Refaie Ali and G. A. Shalaby, "Cherenkov FEL Reaction With Plasma-Filled Cylindrical Waveguide in Fractional D-Dimensional Space," in *IEEE Transactions on Plasma Science*, vol. 49, no. 7, pp. 2070–2079, 2021.
26. P. Manta et al., "Analytical approach for the optimization of desiccant weight in rapid test kit packaging: Accelerated predictive stability (APS)," *Systematic Reviews in Pharmacy,* vol. 11, no. 8, pp. 102–113, 2020.
27. Osama M. Abo-Seida, N.T.M. Eldabe, Ahmed Refaie Ali, & Gamil.Ali Shalaby. (2020). Far-Field, Radiation Resistance and temperature of Hertzian Dipole Antenna in Lossless

Medium with Momentum and Energy Flow in the Far- Zone. *Journal of Advances in Physics*, 18, 20–28.
28. P. Manta, R. Chauhan, H. Gandhi, S. Mahant, and D. N. Kapoor, "Formulation rationale for the development of SARS-COV-2 immunochromatography rapid test kits in India," *J. Appl. Pharm. Sci.* DOI: https://doi.org/10.7324/JAPS.2021.1101017
29. N.T.M. El-Dabe, A. Refaie Ali, A.A. El-shekhipy, Influence of Thermophoresis on Unsteady MHD Flow of Radiation Absorbing Kuvshinski Fluid with Non-Linear Heat and Mass Transfer, *American Journal of Heat and Mass Transfer* 2017, DOI: https://doi.org/10.7726/ajhmt.2017.1010
30. P. Manta, D. N. Kapoor, G. Kour, M. Kour, and A. K. Sharma, "critical quality attributes of rapid test kits - a practical overview," *Journal of Critical Reviews*, vol. 7, no. 19, pp. 377–384, 2020.
31. Osama M. Abo-Seida, N.T.M. Eldabe, M. Abu-Shady, A. Refaie Ali, "Electromagnetic non-Darcy Forchheimer flow and heat transfer over a nonlinearly stretching sheet of non-Newtonian fluid in the presence of a non-uniform heat source', *Solid State Technology*, Vol. 63 No. 6 (2020).
32. P. Manta, N. Wahi, A. Bharadwaj, G. Kour, and D. N. Kapoor, "A statistical quality control (SQC) methodology for gold nanoparticles based immune-chromatographic rapid test kits validation," *Nanosci. Nanotechnol.*-Asia, vol. 11, no. 6, pp. 1–5, 2021.
33. N.T. El-dabel; A. Refaie Ali; A. El-shekhipy, A.; and A. Shalaby, G. (2017) "Non-Linear Heat and Mass Transfer of Second Grade Fluid Flow with Hall Currents and Thermophoresis Effects," *Applied Mathematics & Information Sciences*: Vol. 11: Iss. 1, Article 73.
34. G. S and S. R. Raja. T, "A Comprehensive Survey on Alternating Fluids Used For The Enhancement of Power Transformers," 2021 IEEE International Conference on the *Properties and Applications of Dielectric Materials*, 2021, pp. 57–60.
35. Dr. C. Saravana Murthi, Dr. C. R. Rathish, J. Indirapriyadharshini, Deepak V, Dr. A. Sagai Francis Britto, A Novel and Effective Method for Automatic Paper Trimming and Cutting process in Paper Industries, *International Journal of Advanced Science and Technology*, 2020, Volume 29, Issue No 6, pages 4136–4143.
36. A. Sagai Francis Britto C. R. Rathish, C. Saravana Murthi, J. Indirapriyadharshini, Deepak V, A Novel and Effective Method for Automatic Paper Trimming and Cutting process in Paper Industries, *International Journal of Advanced Science and Technology*, 2020, Volume 29, Issue 6, Pages 4136–4143.
37. Rathish Radhakrishnan & Karpagavadivu Karuppusamy, Cost Effective Energy Efficient Scheme for Mobile Adhoc Network, *International Journal of Computing*, 2020, Volume 19, Issue 1, Pages 137–146.
38. C.R. Rathish, Hybrid Mobile Ad-Hoc Delay Tolerant Network for Optimum Routing in Wireless Sensor Networks, *International Journal of Innovative Technology and Exploring Engineering,* 2019, Volume 8, Issue 11, Pages 1303–1308.
39. K. Karthikayan Dr. Siva Agora Sakthivel Murugan, Rathish. C. R, Natraj. N. A, An Enhanced Localization Scheme for Mobile Sensor Networks, *International Journal of Computational Engineering Research*, 2013, Volume 3, Issue 7, Pages 36–43.
40. Dr. Siva Agora Sakthivel Murugan, Rathish. C. R, Natraj. N. A, K. Karthikayan, A Compact T-Fed Slotted Microstrip Antenna for Wide Band Application, *International Journal of Scientific & Technology Research*, 2013, Volume 2, Issue 8, Pages 291–294.
41. C. R Rathish, P Devasundar, A High Throughput Pattern Matching Using Byte Filtered Bit_Split Algorithm, *Networking and Communication Engineering*, 2012, Volume 4, Issue 6, Pages 316–319.
42. C. R. Rathish, Dr. A. Rajaram, Hierarchical Load Balanced Multipath Routing Protocol for Wireless Sensor Networks, *International Journal of Inventions in Computer Science and Engineering,* April 2016, Volume 3, Issue 4, pp: 2348–3539.

43. Siva Agora Sakthivel Murugan, K. Karthikayan, Natraj. N. A, Rathish. C. R, An Enhanced Localization Scheme for Mobile Sensor Networks, *International Journal of Computational Engineering Research*, 2013, Volume 03, Issue 7, pages 36–43.
44. M. Govindaraj, R. Rathinam, C. Sukumar, M. Uthayasankar and S. Pattabhi, "Electrochemical oxidation of bisphenol-A from aqueous solution using graphite electrodes," "*Environmental Technology*", 2013: 34:4, 503–511.
45. R. Rathinam, M. Govindaraj, K. Vijayakumar and S. Pattabhi, "Decolourization of Rhodamine B from aqueous by electrochemical oxidation using graphite electrodes", *"Desalination and Water Treatment*", 2016, 57:36, 16995–17001.
46. R. Rathinam, M. Govindaraj, K. Vijayakumar and S. Pattabhi "Removal of Colour from Aqueous Rhodamine B Dye Solution by Photo electrocoagulation Treatment Techniques", "*Journal of Engineering, Scientific Research and Application*", 2015, 1: 2, 80–89.
47. K. Jayanthi, R. Rathinam and S. Pattabhi, "Electrocoagulation treatment for removal of Reactive Blue 19 from aqueous solution using Iron electrode", "Research Journal of Life Sciences, Bioinformatics, *Pharmaceutical and Chemical Sciences*", 2018, 4:2, 101–113.
48. R. Rathinam and S. Pattabhi, "Removal of Rhodamine B Dye from Aqueous Solution by Advanced Oxidation Process using ZnO Nanoparticles", *Indian Journal of Ecology,* 2019, 46:1: 167–174.
49. Żywiołek, J.; Rosak-Szyrocka, J.; Jereb, B. Barriers to Knowledge Sharing in the Field of Information Security. *Management Systems in Production Engineering* 2021, 29, 114–119.
50. T. A. Al-asadi and A. J. Obaid, "Object Based Image Retrieval Using Enhanced SURF," *Asian Journal of Information Technology*, vol. 15, no. 16, pp. 2756–2762, 2016.
51. M. Umadevi, R. Rathinam, S. Poornima, T. Santhi and S. Pattabhi," Electrochemical Degradation of Reactive Red 195 from its Aqueous Solution using RuO2/IrO2/TaO2 Coated Titanium Electrodes", "Asian Journal of Chemistry", 2021, 33:8, 1919–1922.
52. C. Meshram, R. W. Ibrahim, A. J. Obaid, S. G. Meshram, A. Meshram and A. M. Abd El-Latif, "Fractional chaotic maps based short signature scheme under human-centered IoT environments," *Journal of Advanced Research*, 2020.
53. A. J. Obaid, K. A. Alghurabi, S. A. K. Albermany and S. Sharma, "Improving Extreme Learning Machine Accuracy Utilizing Genetic Algorithm for Intrusion Detection Purposes," in *Advances in Intelligent Systems and Computing*, Springer, Singapore, 2021, pp. 171–177.
54. ThirumalaiRaj Brindha, Ramasamy Rathinam, Sivakumar Dheenadhayalan, "Antibacterial, Antifungal and Anticorrosion Properties of Green Tea Polyphenols Extracted Using Different Solvents" "*Asian Journal of Biological and Life Sciences*", 2021, 10:1, 62–66.
55. R. Rathinam and M. Govindaraj, "Photo electro catalytic Oxidation of Textile Industry Wastewater by RuO2/IrO2/TaO2 Coated Titanium Electrodes", *"Nature Environment and Pollution Technology",* 2021, 20:3, 1069–1076.

Artificial Intelligence for Smart in Match Winning Prediction in Twenty20 Cricket League Using Machine Learning Model

Maheswari Subburaj, Ganga Rama Koteswara Rao, Binayak Parashar, Indirapriyadharshini Jeyabalan, Hemalatha Semban, and Sudhakar Sengan

1 Introduction

Since football and cricket are probably respected and recognised by many worldwide, cricket is perhaps the most cherished game in India. Vast volumes of technical studies have been distributed in the past few years, and different researchers have predicted the cricket world cup winner using factors influencing final scores. They use the Support Vector Machine (SVM) model to detect final scores, such as linear regression, support vector machines, decision trees, logistic regression, and random

M. Subburaj (✉)
Department of Computer Science and Engineering, Vellore Institute of Technology, Chennai, Tamil Nadu, India
e-mail: maheswari.s@vit.ac.in

G. R. K. Rao
Department of Computer Science and Engineering, Koneru Lakshmaiah Education Foundation, Vaddeswaram, Andhra Pradesh, India

B. Parashar
Department of Computer Science and Engineering, Ajay Kumar Garg Engineering College, Ghaziabad, Uttar Pradesh, India

I. Jeyabalan
Department of Mechatronics Engineering, Sri Krishna College of Engineering and Technology, Coimbatore, Tamil Nadu, India

H. Semban
Department of Computer Science and Engineering, Sri Shakthi Institute of Engineering and Technology, Coimbatore, Tamil Nadu, India

S. Sengan
Department of Computer Science and Engineering, PSN College of Engineering and Technology, Tirunelveli, Tamil Nadu, India

P. Agarwal et al. (eds.), *Artificial Intelligence for Smart Healthcare*,
EAI/Springer Innovations in Communication and Computing,
https://doi.org/10.1007/978-3-031-23602-0_3

forest, to allow access. Cricket is one of the world's most prominent games. The T20 format is ubiquitous, as it is an unrelenting game that pulls the audience to the ground and viewers to their residences. The Indian Premier League (IPL) [1] is an expert T20-IPL directed by the Board of Control for Cricket. The IPL is scheduled to be held in a city in India. Frequent contact is an independent variable that influences the outcome, and sponsorship has provided advertising and a massive market, similar to many mobile prediction apps. The team's recommendations, ability, system, and other regular factors are essential in assuming the cricket coordinates' follow-up precision. As innovation develops and applications like Dream 11 and wagering locales become well-known, individuals will utilise the Artificial Intelligence (AI) model's forecasts [2]. The use of AI makes life simpler in numerous aspects. This helps the user predict the winner when betting on the teams [3]. The Indian Premier League (IPL) is a well-known T20 cricket league worldwide, including India. After ICC tournaments, the Indian Premier League (IPL) is India's most prominent domestic league. As a result, creating a model that can predict the impact of the match is a real-world machine learning challenge. Many factors influence the outcome of a T20 match in cricket, including the stadium, toss winner, and runs scored in the Powerplay. As a result, we predict game outcomes based on these features. A tested training dataset consists mainly of all matches between 2008 and 2020 (Fig. 1).

This article is organised so that Sect. 1 helps the user; as a result, we predict game outcomes based on each feature. A dataset consists mainly of all the matches between 2008 and 2020. Section 2 is a review of related literature on IPL match win-win situations. Section 3 recommends the proposed data preprocessing, cleaning, preparation, and encoding model. Section 4 mentions the result and discusses the analysis of the top two teams based on the number of matches they have won against each other and how the venue affects them.

2 Related Works

Based on games won between 1995 and 1997, an experiment was done to determine the outcome (win, lose, or draw) of football games played by a highly qualified English Premier League (EPL) team, Tottenham Hotspurs. The Bayesian net model had a prediction accuracy of 59.21% [4]. Bayesian networks underperformed other ML algorithms such as MC4-a Decision Tree, Naïve Bayesian Learner, Data-Driven Bayesian, and K-Nearest Neighbour (KNN). Major League Baseball's (MLB) technological development has encountered significant segments over the last few decades. Usually, human analysis does not recognise these. Occasionally, ball-by-ball information and specific knowledge and insight are critical [5, 6].

Consequently, skilled MLB leagues now use ML methods to get and use statistics [7]. The research begins in Nairobi, Kenya, and lasts for 7 months. The review is an attempt, and its actions were comprehensively observed in all classes of persons, from youths to senior citizens. Respective models were constructed to monitor the person's brief stance and behavioural intention for the Android phones, such as smartphone cash stimulation and the technological innovation model. The findings

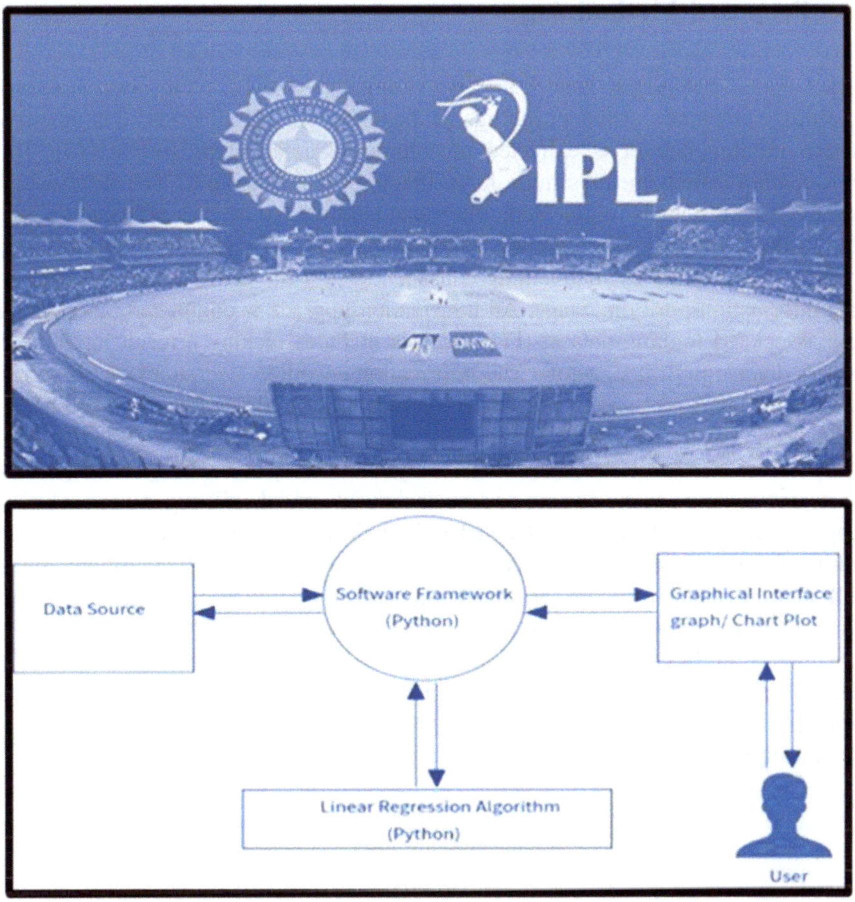

Fig. 1 Block diagram of predicted IPL score using ML

[8] for sports betting and the steps required to make progress assessments of population security issues [9] were predicted.

With the advancement of cricket, sports commentators have become a hot topic. Much research has been conducted on cricket, but they have yet to make a breakthrough in predicting match winners due to inconsistent and complicated tested training datasets. Most approaches have been used to determine match winners, such as KNN, logistic regression, SVM, and Naïve Bayes, but nothing has been accurate [10, 11]. Many statistical techniques have been introduced to data source production, and many classified algorithms have been tried to model the 1-day cricket match (50 over). With 80% accuracy, the author predicted the winning team. The expected 1-day international tournament contributes by ensuring ICC player rating data, ICC pace bowlers' and batsmen's total points, the home key component, ICC evaluation disparities, and ground impacts on the tournament [12].

3 Proposed Methodology

The model comprises American Sign Language (ASL): data preprocessing, cleaning, preparation, and encoding. At first, the ten IPL periods' continuously tested training dataset is extracted in comma-separated value format [13]. The information arrangement is huge for achieving ideal outcomes. The information preprocessing stage is fragmented, noisy, and conflicting [14, 15]. Information is to be loaded with missing qualities and corrected for irregularities. Information approval is finished by maintaining consistency over the tested training dataset in the information purifying stage. An information upgrade is completed by counting the associated training dataset (Fig. 2). This includes picking a result measure to assess diverse indicator factors. The information encoding stage marks each period with short tags and encodes players as mathematical qualities for future display as actualised beneath [16–18].

The Scikit-Learn Label Encoder is a Python library that changes straight-out factors over to numeric factors and an insightful model utilising a nonexclusive capacity called a class model that takes boundary model indicators' information results from unsurprising elements [19]. The tested training dataset contributes to the ML algorithms and assesses various situations like throw victory, throw choice, and group victory. In this way, new information is acquired with the last forecast. Distinctive multi-arrangement calculations, for example, linear regression (LR), Decision Tree (DT), and random forest (RF), are executed to predict the precision and cross-validation score. Out of these grouping calculations, the RF algorithm is the most precise.

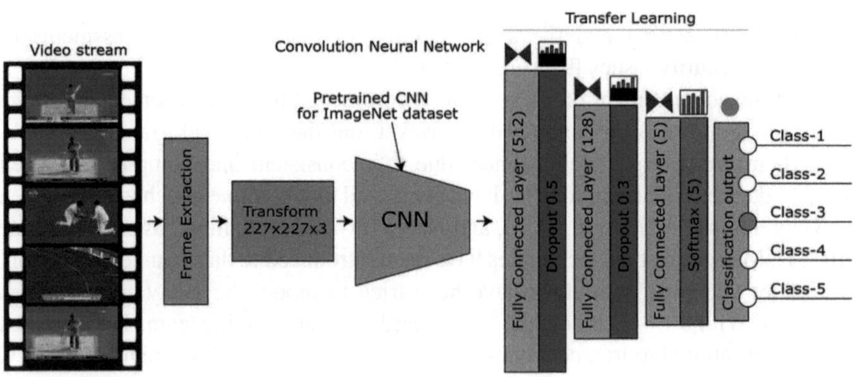

Fig. 2 The proposed model architecture

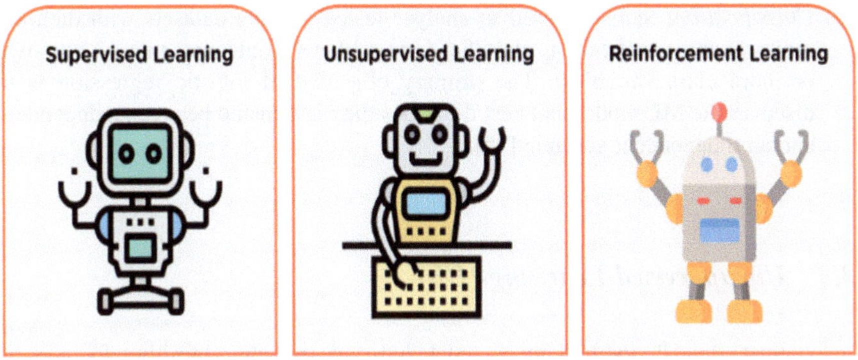

Fig. 3 Machine learning classification

Table 1 Test analysis

Team A	Team B	Location	Toss winner	Toss decision	Date	Winning state
CSK	MI	Mumbai	CSK	1	4 April 2020	CSK
KXIP	RR	Chennai	RR	0	8 April 2020	RR
KKR	CSK	Delhi	KKR	1	14 April 2020	KKR
MI	DC	Kolkata	DC	0	24 April 2020	DC
DC	CSK	Ahmadabad	CSK	1	27 April 2020	CSK

3.1 *Machine Learning Classification*

There are three types of learning: supervised, unsupervised, and reinforcement (Fig. 3).

3.2 *Supervised Learning (SL)*

The algorithm in an SL model comes to understand specific data to generate a reliable prediction for the result of new data (Table 1). (a) Regression and (b) Classification [19–29]:

(a) *Regression*: A regression model, such as a mathematical formula, predicts a linear function. We believe you're forecasting match scores based on the game's characteristics, such as run, match, etc. Another typical example is estimating a player's score based on the matches they have played. Regression is defined as $Y = a + bX$, where Y stands for a score, X for player name and age, and a and b for equation coefficients [30–34].

(b) *Classification*: Statistics used to analyse tested training datasets with dichotomous outcomes are called “classification problems” (outcomes may be only two or more class variables). The primary objective of logistic regression is to discover the ML model that best describes the relationship between a dependent and an independent variable [35].

3.3 Unsupervised Learning (UL)

In contrast, the UL method gives unlabeled data that the algorithm focuses on understanding by automatically extracting co-occurrence and statistical properties. For I Clustering, II Anomaly Detection, III Association, and IV Autoencoders, we use the ML technique.

3.4 Reinforcement Learning (RL)

RL simulates a game-like situation in which the computer performs the trial-and-error technique [36–39]. For the decisions it requires, the AI is determined. Less-supervised RL relies on the learning advisor to assess performance solutions by attempting numerous solutions in order to find the best one [40].

First, the winner is tossed, and the winners add up. The second is the possibility of playing a tournament by winning a toss (Figs. 4, 5, 6, 7, 8, 9, and 10).

4 Result and Discussions

Top 2 team analysis based on the number of matches won against each other and how the venue affects them [41–46]. Previously, we noticed that CSK won 79 matches and RCB won 70 matches. Now let us compare the venue with a match between CSK and RCB. In MA Chidambaram Stadium, Chepauk, Chennai, researchers found that CSK won many games against RCB. RCB has not defeated CSK at St George’s Park or Wankhede Stadium but has defeated them at Kingsmead and New Wanderers Stadium. It demonstrates that when attempting to play against RCB at Chepauk Stadium, CSK has an excellent chance to win. It shows that venue is an important factor in predictability [47–51].

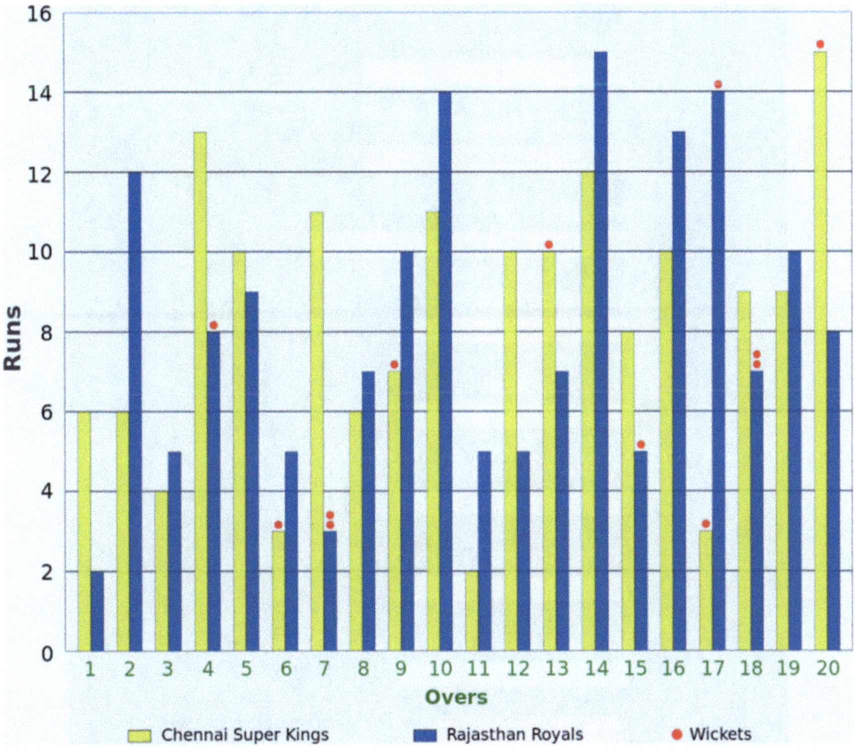

Fig. 4 IPL T20 analysis

4.1 Linear Regression (LR)

Linear regression is a statistical method that determines the average relationship between two or more continuous factors in response and features different factors (Figs. 11 and 12) [52–54]. In other words, the goal of LR analysis is to understand the relationship between the two multiple regressions so that it can be used to forecast the future by identifying the most likely value of the predictor variable given a specific value of independent factors (Table 2).

4.2 Step-by-Step Process of Machine Learning Classifications

Step 1—Collection of training dataset

We used the training sets from "www.kaggle.com/nowke9/ipldata" when collecting and analysing. The tested training dataset is divided into two files: matches.csv, which encompasses tournament information from 2008 to 2020, and deliveries.csv, which includes ball-by-ball relevant data for each game.

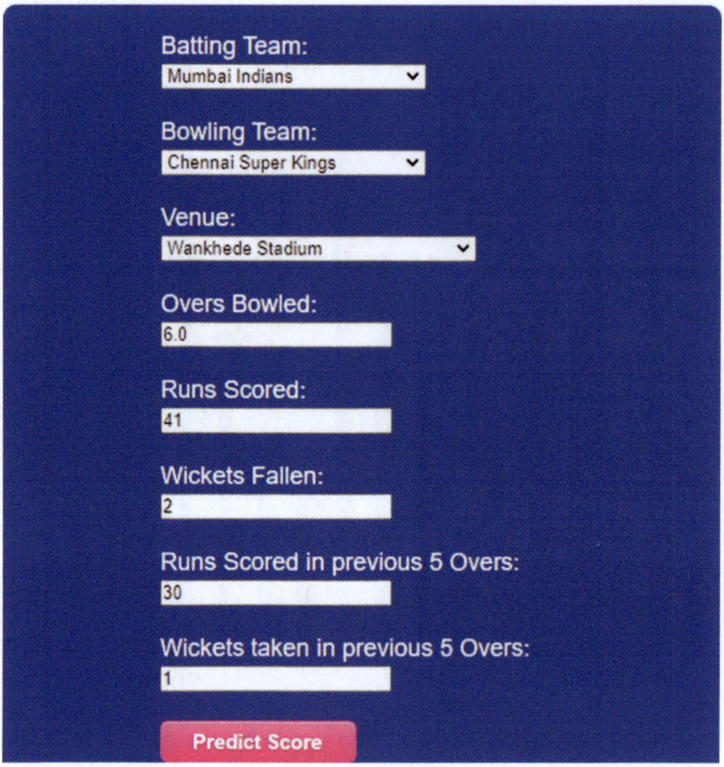

Fig. 5 Mobile app screen

```
[46] predicted_winner=[]
     for i in out:
         #print(list(dicval.keys())[list(dicval.values()).index(i)])
         predicted_winner.append(list(dicval.keys())[list(dicval.values()).index(i)])

[47] ipl=pd.read_csv('test.csv')
     ctr=0
     k=0
     total=len(ipl['winner'])
     for i in ipl['winner']:
         if i==predicted_winner[k]:
             ctr=ctr+1
         k=k+1
     print(ctr)
     print("Accuracy of our prediction of recent IPL is ", (ctr/total)*100)

     4
     Accuracy of our prediction of recent IPL is 80.0

[48] predicted_winner

     ['MI', 'RR', 'MI', 'CSK', 'CSK']
```

Fig. 6 Prediction result

```
import matplotlib.pyplot as plt
fig = plt.figure(figsize=(8,4))
ax1 = fig.add_subplot(121)
ax1.set_xlabel('toss_winner')
ax1.set_ylabel('Count of toss winners')
ax1.set_title("toss winners")
temp1.plot(kind='bar')

ax2 = fig.add_subplot(122)
temp2.plot(kind = 'bar')
ax2.set_xlabel('winner')
ax2.set_ylabel('Count of match winners')
ax2.set_title("Match winners")
```

```
Text(0.5, 1.0, 'Match winners')
```

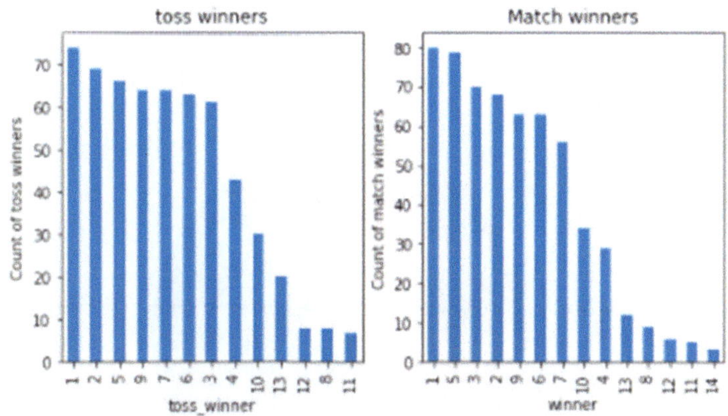

Fig. 7 This image is a graph

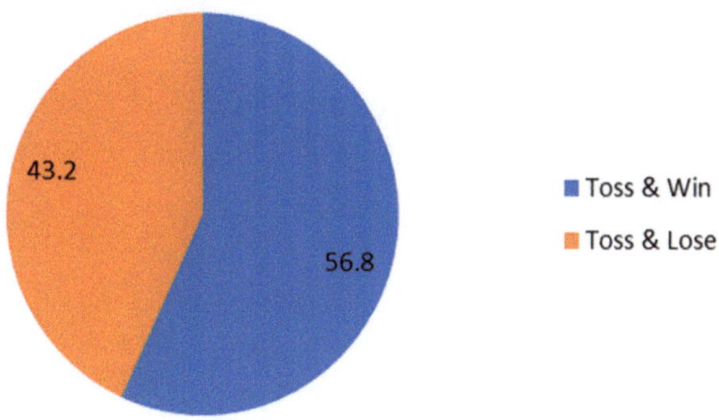

Fig. 8 Winning the CSK toss by the chance of a tournament

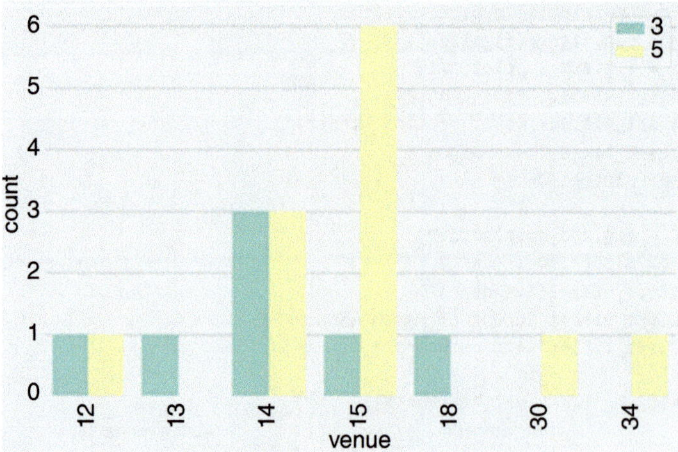

Fig. 9 Winning opportunity of a game by making the playoffs the ML toss

Fig. 10 Evidence of location is an essential component in forecasting

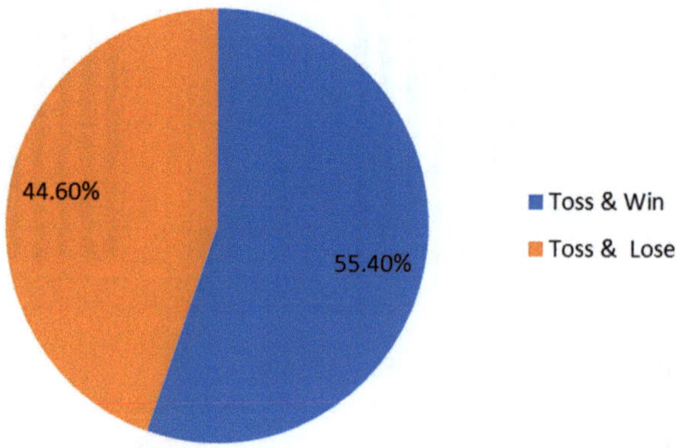

Fig. 11 Linear regression

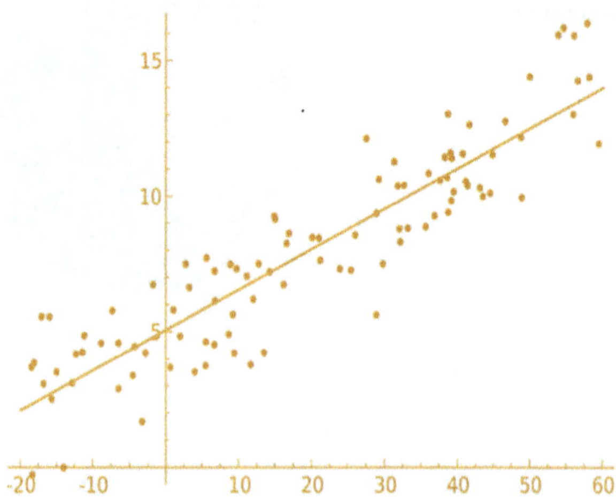

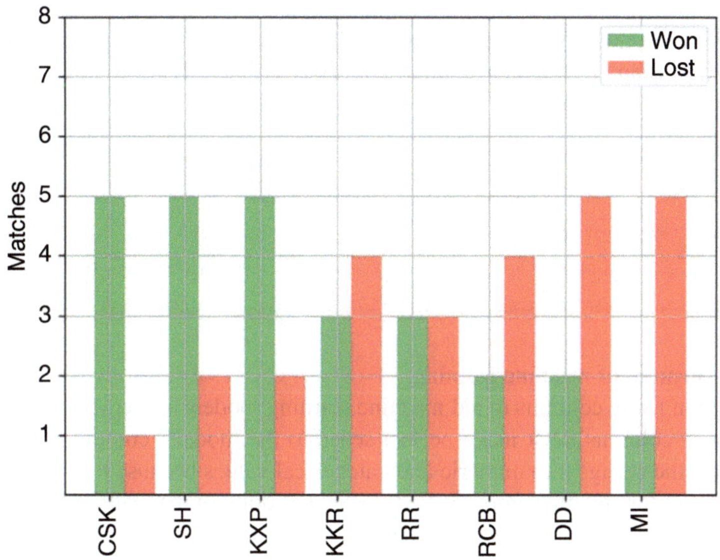

Fig. 12 Matches each team has won in total

Table 2 Demonstrate the win and loss count of team

Teams	Match	Win	Loss	Tied	Points	NRR
A	2	1	1	0	3	0.878
B	3	2	0	1	4	0.242
C	3	2	1	0	2	0.1329
D	4	1	2	1	4	−1.192
E	5	2	1	2	1	0.202
F	6	3	2	1	2	0.3728
H	1	1	0	0	2	−0.231
I	2	1	1	0	3	−1.29

Step 2—Obtaining and summarising data in the play area

This study reads the CSV file using ".read csv()." The ".read csv()" function takes an absolute or a relative path. As a result, the file was saved in Google Collaboratory, where it was used as an ML tool.

```
#Importing Libraries
import pandas as pd

#Reading data from CSV file
matches=pd.read_csv("/content/drive/My Drive/Colab Notebooks/matches.csv")
```

Step 3—Further preprocessing the training datasets

With the tested training dataset, we discovered an intriguing redundancy. In columns Team 1, Team 2, Winner, and Toss Winner, Team Rising Pune Super Giants was duplicated.

```
#Replacing the Rising Pune Supergiant with Rising Pune Supergiants
matches["team2"]=matches["team2"].replace("Rising Pune Supergiant","Rising Pune Supergiants")
matches["team1"]=matches["team1"].replace("Rising Pune Supergiant","Rising Pune Supergiants")
matches["winner"]=matches["winner"].replace("Rising Pune Supergiant","Rising Pune Supergiants")
matches["toss_winner"]=matches["toss_winner"].replace("Rising Pune Supergiant","Rising Pune Super
```

Step 4—Feature of machine learning

When using columns to aid machine learning models in prediction, the values in those columns must make perfect sense to the models' computers. We must encode the strings into numeric and categorical values because they can't understand or infer anything from the text. Instead of doing it manually, we can use the Scikit-Learn library's Label Encoder.

```
#encoding the numeric values
encoder= LabelEncoder()
matches["team1"]=encoder.fit_transform(matches["team1"])
matches["team2"]=encoder.fit_transform(matches["team2"])
matches["winner"]=encoder.fit_transform(matches["winner"].astype(str))
matches["toss_winner"]=encoder.fit_transform(matches["toss_winner"])
matches["venue"]=encoder.fit_transform(matches["venue"])
```

What relationship is there between the Toss Winner and Winner variables containing the winning teams' names? The only thing they would have in common is that they would have the same value, which is insufficient to make them logical. Additionally, Toss Decision could refer to either bat or field, but which team are they referring to? To address this issue, we will create three new columns, Team1 Win, Team1 Toss Win, and Team1 Batting, to correspond to the columns Winner, Toss Winner, and Toss Decision, respectively. These tables will show the correlation with column 1, "Team".

```
#outcome variable team1_win as a probability of team1 winning the match
matches.loc[matches["winner"]==matches["team1"],"team1_win"]=1
matches.loc[matches["winner"]!=matches["team1"],"team1_win"]=0

#outcome variable team1_toss_win as a value of team1 winning the toss
matches.loc[matches["toss_winner"]==matches["team1"],"team1_toss_win"]=1
matches.loc[matches["toss_winner"]!=matches["team1"],"team1_toss_win"]=0

#outcome variable team1_bat to depict if team1 bats first
matches["team1_bat"]=0
matches.loc[(matches["team1_toss_win"]==1) & (matches["toss_decision"]=="bat"),"team1_bat"]=1
```

Step 5—Feature selection

Based on the machine learning knowledge we had, we hand-picked many options. However, we lack statistical evidence to claim that the chosen features are significant in our tested training dataset. Feature Selection, a Scikit-Learn module, gives us a few choices for classification algorithms. We'll begin by seeing if any of the columns have duplicated values in other columns. We must first create a correlation matrix to find the connections between the columns. Correlation can tell us whether two columns share characteristics if the correlation is high enough in absolute terms.

Step 6—Testing of ML models

Multiple ML models can train the classifier according to the statistical information we have and, using the configuration, analyse the outcome of certain input variables for a classification problem that exists. DT, RF, LR, and SVM classifiers will be measured, and the most effective ML algorithm will be selected. After being built, validating the model with values not associated with exposure to the ML model is crucial. As an outcome, we have been using Scikit's "Train Test Split" to learn a class that partitions data into two parts with an 80–20 variation. 80% of the available information is used to validate the algorithm, and the remaining 20% is used.

5 Conclusion

The best performance in cricket necessitates that the winning team be an integrated component. The manuscript's primary goal is to research the training dataset for Indian Premier League cricket and assess the players' behavior. Here, three feature computations are used, and the most accurate analyses are compared. Anaconda and Jupiter's Notebooks are the systems to be used. Random Forest has a maximum performance of 89.15% and will provide the most incredible performance. This metadata will be used in the future to prevent future glorious victory teams from violating the preceding Indian Premier League tournament provisions. Consequently, it can be predicted to use this prediction too.

References

1. Abhishek, S., Ketaki, V., Patil, P., Yuktha., Meghana, S.: Predictive Analysis of IPL Match Winner using Machine Learning Techniques. International Journal of Innovative Technology and Exploring Engineering, 9 (1), 430–435, (2019).
2. Aneem-Al-Ahsan Rupai, Md. Saddam Hossain Mukta, and Najmul Islam A. K. M.: Predicting Bowling Performance in Cricket from Publicly Available Data. In Proceedings of the International Conference on Computing Advancements. Association for Computing Machinery, New York, NY, USA, Article 58, 1–6, (2020)

3. Barot H, Kothari A, Bide P, Ahir B and Kankaria R.: Analysis and Prediction for the Indian Premier League, International Conference for Emerging Technology, Belgaum, India, 1–7, (2020).
4. Ch Sai, Abhishek., Ketaki V.Patil., Yuktha, P., Meghana, K.S., Sudhamani, M.V.: Predictive Analysis of IPL Match Winner using Machine Learning Techniques. International Journal of Innovative Technology and Exploring Engineering, 9(2S), (2019).
5. Daniel Mago, Vistro., Faizan, Rasheed., Leo Gertrude, David.: The Cricket Winner Prediction with Application of Machine Learning and Data Analytics. International Journal of Scientific & Technology Research, 8 (9), (2019).
6. Deep, Prakash., Dayalbagh, C., Patvardhan, C., Vasantha Lakshmi, C.: Data Analytics based Deep Mayo Predictor for IPL-9. International Journal of Computer Applications, 152 (6), 6–11. (2016).
7. Pabitra Kumar, Dey., Gangotri, Chakraborty., Purnendu, Ruj., Suvobrata, Sarkar.: A Data Mining Approach on Cluster Analysis of IPL. International Journal of Machine Learning and Computing, 2 (4), 351–354, (2012).
8. Parag, Shah.: Predicting Outcome of Live Cricket Match using Duckworth-Lewis Par Score. International Journal of Latest Technology in Engineering, Management and Applied Science, 6 (7),72–75, (2017).
9. Rameshwari, Lokhande, Chawan, P.M.: Live Cricket Score and Winning Prediction. International Journal of Trend in Research and Development, 5 (1), 30–32, (2018).
10. Raza Ul Mustafa., Saqib Nawaz, M., Ikram Ullah Lali, M., Tehseen, Zia., Waqar, Mehmood.: Predicting the Cricket Match outcome using Crowd Opinions on Social Networks: A Comparative Study of Machine Learning Methods. Malaysian Journal of Computer Science, 30 (1), 63–76, (2017).
11. Sonu, Kumar., Sneha, Roy.: Score Prediction and Player Classification Model in the Game of Cricket using Machine Learning. International Journal of Scientific and Engineering Research, 9 (2), 237–242, (2018).
12. Sudhamathy, G., Raja Meenakshi, G.: Prediction on IPL Data Using Machine Learning Techniques in R Package. ICTACT Journal on Soft Computing, 11 (1), (2020).
13. Tyagi S, Kumari R, Makkena S.C, Mishra C and Pendyala, V.S.: "Enhanced Predictive Modeling of Cricket Game Duration Using Multiple Machine Learning Algorithms," *International Conference on Data* (2020).
14. S. Sudhakar and S. Chenthur Pandian, "Hybrid cluster-based geographical routing protocol to mitigate malicious nodes in mobile ad hoc network," *International Journal of Ad Hoc and Ubiquitous Computing*, vol. 21 no. 4, pp. 224–236, (2016).
15. A. U. Priyadarshni and S. Sudhakar, "Cluster-based certificate revocation by cluster head in a mobile ad-hoc network," *International Journal of Applied Engineering Research*, vol. 10, no. 20, pp. 16014–16018, (2015).
16. S. Sudhakar and S. Chenthur Pandian, "Investigation of attribute aided data aggregation over dynamic routing in wireless sensor," *Journal of Engineering Science and Technology*, vol. 10, no. 11, pp. 1465–1476, (2015).
17. S. Sudhakar and S. Chenthur Pandian, "Trustworthy position-based routing to mitigate against the malicious attacks to signifies secured data packet using geographic routing protocol in MANET", WSEAS *Transactions on Communications*, vol. 12, no. 11, pp. 584–603, (2013).
18. S. Sudhakar and S. Chenthur Pandian, "A Trust and co-operative nodes with affects of malicious attacks and measure the performance degradation on geographic aided routing in mobile ad hoc network", Life *Science Journal*, vol. 10, no. 4s, pp. 158–163, (2013).
19. Thowfeek MH, Samsudeen, SN, Sanjeetha, MBF. Drivers of Artificial Intelligence in Banking Service Sectors, Solid State Technology; 63(5): 6400 – 6411 (2020).
20. Samsudeen SN, Thowfeek MH, Rashida, MF. School Teachers' Intention to Use E-Learning Systems in Sri Lanka: A Modified TAM Approach, International Journal of Information and Knowledge Management, 5(4), 55–59 (2015).

21. Samsudeen, SN, Thowfeek, MH. Small Medium Entrepreneurs' Intension to Use Cloud Computing: Reference to Eastern Province of Sri Lanka, Journal of Management, 11(1), 1–10 (2014).
22. Thowfeek, MH. Salam, MNA. Students' Assessment on the Usability of E-learning Websites. Procedia-Social and Behavioral Sciences, 141; 916–922 (2014).
23. Samsudeen, S. N. Acceptance of cloud of things by small and medium enterprises in Sri Lanka, Journal of Advanced Research in Dynamical and Control Systems, 12(2), 2276–2285 (2020).
24. Thowfeek, MH, Samsudeen SN. Readiness of Resources for Flipped Classroom. In Proceedings of the 2019 8th International Conference on Educational and Information Technology, pp. 92–96 (2019).
25. Jalil, N.A., P Prapinit, M Melan, AB Mustaffa. Adoption of Business Intelligence-Technological, Individual and Supply Chain Efficiency. Proceedings of the 2019 International Conference on Machine Learning, Big Data and Business Intelligence. Year: 2019, Volume: 1, Pages: 67–73 (2019).
26. Nasir Abdul Jalil, Ha Jin Hwang, and Norazryana Mat Dawi. Machines Learning Trends, Perspectives and Prospects in Education Sector. In Proceedings of the 2019 3rd International Conference on Education and Multimedia Technology. Association for Computing Machinery, New York, NY, USA, 201–205 (2019).
27. Jalil, N.A., Hwang, H.J. Technological-centric business intelligence: Critical success factors. International Journal of Innovation, Creativity and Change, Volume 5, Issue 2, Pages 1499 to 1516 (2019).
28. O. M. Abo-Seida, N. T. M. El-dabe, A. Refaie Ali and G. A. Shalaby, "Cherenkov FEL Reaction with Plasma-Filled Cylindrical Waveguide in Fractional D-Dimensional Space," in IEEE Transactions on Plasma Science, vol. 49, no. 7, pp. 2070–2079, (2021).
29. Nasir Abdul Jalil and Koay Kian Yeik. Systems, Design and Technologies Anxieties Towards Use of Self-service Checkout. In Proceedings of the 2019 3rd International Conference on Education and E-Learning. Association for Computing Machinery, New York, NY, USA, 122–127 (2019).
30. B. Singh, N. A. Jalil, D. K. Sharma, S. R. K. Kumar and D. Jebakumar immanuel, "Computational systems overview and Random Process with Theoretical analysis," 2021 7th International Conference on Advanced Computing and Communication Systems, pp. 1999–2005 (2021).
31. Osama M. Abo-Seida, N.T.M. Eldabe, Ahmed Refaie Ali, & Gamil.Ali Shalaby. Far-Field, Radiation Resistance and temperature of Hertzian Dipole Antenna in Lossless Medium with Momentum and Energy Flow in the Far-Zone. Journal of Advances in Physics, 18, 20–28 (2020).
32. Roy Setiawan, Luigi Pio Leonardo Cavaliere, KartikeyKoti, Gabriel Ayodeji Ogunmola, N. A. Jalil, M. Kalyan Chakravarthi, S. S Rajest, R. Regin, Sonia Singh, "The Artificial Intelligence and Inventory Effect on Banking Industrial Performance" Turkish Online Journal of Qualitative Inquiry. Volume 12, Issue 6, 8100–8125 (2021).
33. Roespinoedji, D., Juniati, S., Hasan, H., Jalil, N.A., Shamsudin, M.F. Experimenting the long-haul association between components of consuming renewable energy: ARDL method with special reference to Malaysia. Int. J. Energy Econ. Policy 9, 453–460 (2019).
34. N.T.M. El-Dabe, A. Refaie Ali, A.A. El-shekhipy, Influence of Thermophoresis on Unsteady MHD Flow of Radiation Absorbing Kuvshinski Fluid with Non-Linear Heat and Mass Transfer, American Journal of Heat and Mass Transfer (2017).
35. D. K. Sharma, N. A. Jalil, V. K. Nassa, S. R. Vadyala, L. S. Senthamil and T. N, "Deep learning Applications to classify Cross-Topic Natural Language Texts Based on Their Argumentative Form," 2021 2nd International Conference on Smart Electronics and Communication, pp. 1580–1586, (2021).
36. D. K. Sharma, N. A. Jalil, R. Regin, S. S. Rajest, R. K. Tummala and T. N, "Predicting Network Congestion with Machine Learning," 2021 2nd International Conference on Smart Electronics and Communication, pp. 1574–1579 (2021).

37. Osama M. Abo-Seida, N.T.M. Eldabe, M. Abu-Shady, A. Refaie Ali, "Electromagnetic non-Darcy Forchheimer flow and heat transfer over a nonlinearly stretching sheet of non-Newtonian fluid in the presence of a non-uniform heat source", Solid State Technology, Vol. 63 No. 6 (2020).
38. NT. El-dabel; A. Refaie Ali; A. El-shekhipy, A.; and A. Shalaby, G. "Non-Linear Heat and Mass Transfer of Second Grade Fluid Flow with Hall Currents and Thermophoresis Effects," Applied Mathematics & Information Sciences: Vol. 11: Iss. 1, Article 73 (2017).
39. K. Karthikayan Dr. Siva Agora Sakthivel Murugan, Rathish. C. R, Natraj. N. A, An Enhanced Localization Scheme for Mobile Sensor Networks, International Journal of Computational Engineering Research, Volume 3, Issue 7, Pages 36–43 (2013).
40. Dr. Siva Agora Sakthivel Murugan, Rathish. C. R, Natraj. N. A, K. Karthikayan, A Compact T-Fed Slotted Microstrip Antenna for Wide Band Application, International Journal of Scientific & Technology Research, Vol. 2, no. 8, Pp. 291–294 (2013).
41. C. R Rathish, P Devasundar, A High Throughput Pattern Matching Using Byte Filtered Bit_Split Algorithm, Networking and Communication Engineering, Vol. 4, no. 6, Pp.316–319 (2012).
42. Renuka J Bathi, Sameena Parveen, Neeraj Taneja, Oral Tuberculous Ulcer – A Report of Two Cases, Journal of Indian Academy of Oral Medicine and Radiology, Volume 15, Issue 2, Pages 62–65 (2003).
43. N. Keerthana, Viji Vinod and S. Sudhakar, "A Novel Method for Multi-Dimensional Cluster to Identify the Malicious Users on Online Social Networks", Journal of Engineering Science and Technology Vol. 15, No. 6, pp: 4107–4122, (2020).
44. A. U. Priyadarshni and S. Sudhakar, "Cluster Based Certificate Revocation by Cluster Head in Mobile Ad-Hoc Network", International Journal of Applied Engineering Research, Vol. 10, No. 20, pp. 16014–16018, (2015).
45. S. Sudhakar and S. Chenthur Pandian, "Investigation of Attribute Aided Data Aggregation Over Dynamic Routing in Wireless Sensor," Journal of Engineering Science and Technology Vol.10, No.11, pp:1465–1476, (2015).
46. S. Sudhakar and S. Chenthur Pandian, "Authorized Node Detection and Accuracy in Position-Based Information for MANET", European Journal of Scientific Research, Vol.70, No.2, pp.253–265,(2012).
47. T. Radhika K Mohideen, C Krithika, N Jeddy, S Parveen, A Meta-Analysis in Assessing Oxidative Stress Using Malondialdehyde in Oral Submucous Fibrosis, European Journal of Dentistry, (2021).
48. Parveen S Taneja N, R Bathi, Serum Glycoproteins as Prognosticator in Head and Neck Cancer Patients – A Follow Up Study, Oral Oncology Head and Neck Oncology, Vol. 47 (2011).
49. K. Ganesh Kumar and S. Sudhakar, Improved Network Traffic by Attacking Denial of Service to Protect Resource Using Z-Test Based 4-Tier Geomark Traceback, Wireless Personal Communications, Vol.114, No. 4, pp:3541–3575, (2020).
50. J. Kubiczek and B. Hadasik, "Challenges in Reporting the COVID-19 Spread and its Presentation to the Society," J. Data and Information Quality, vol. 13, no. 4, pp. 1–7, (2021).
51. Sameena Parveen, Impact of Calorie Restriction and Intermittent Fasting on Periodontal Health, Periodontology 2000, Vol. 87, no. 1, Pp. 315–324 (2021).
52. D. S. Q. Al-Yasiri and A. J. Obaid, "A New Approach for Object Detection, Recognition and Retrieving in Painting Images," Journal of Advance Research in Dynamic and Control System, vol. 10, no. 2, pp. 2345–2359, (2018).
53. T. A. Al-asadi and A. J. Obaid, "Object detection and recognition by using enhanced speeded up robust feature," International Journal of Computer Science and Network Security, vol. 16, no. 4, pp. 66–71, (2016).
54. Parveen S. Bathi R, Taneja N, Dermoid Cyst in The Floor of The Mouth-A Case Report, Karnataka State Dental Journal, Vol. 25, Issue 2, pp. 52–54, (2006).

Comparative Analysis of Handwritten Digit Recognition Investigation Using Deep Learning Model

Joel Sunny Deol Gosu, Balu Subramaniam, Sasipriyaa Nachimuthu, Kamalanathan Shivasankaran, Arjun Subburaj, and Sudhakar Sengan

1 Introduction

A Convolutional Neural Network provides the convenience of extracting and using feature vectors over other ANN to evaluate the awareness of 2D form with a significantly lower degree of accuracy and no translation, balancing/manipulations. Initially, this research was addressed in their object. Convolutional Neural Networks was a control layer by the author to determine the digit and character [1]. CNN technology is simple, making it easy to install. We might well take the MNIST set of data for training and identification. This set of data aims primarily at characterising

J. S. Deol Gosu
Present Address: Department of Computer Science and Engineering, Kallam Haranatha Reddy Institute of Technology, Guntur, Andhra Pradesh, India

B. Subramaniam
Department of Computer Science and Engineering, Vivekanandha College of Engineering for Women, Namakkal, Tamil Nadu, India

S. Nachimuthu
Department of Computer Science and Engineering, Kongu Engineering College, Perundurai, Tamil Nadu, India
e-mail: sasipriya@kongu.ac.in

K. Shivasankaran
Department of Multimedia, School of Design, Vellore Institute of Technology, Vellore, India
e-mail: kamalanathan.s@vit.ac.in

A. Subburaj
Tranxit Technology Solutions Private Limited, Chennai, Tamil Nadu, India
e-mail: aj@sentientlabs.io

S. Sengan (✉)
Department of Computer Science and Engineering, PSN College of Engineering and Technology, Tirunelveli, Tamil Nadu, India

P. Agarwal et al. (eds.), *Artificial Intelligence for Smart Healthcare*,
EAI/Springer Innovations in Communication and Computing,
https://doi.org/10.1007/978-3-031-23602-0_4

articles 1–10. Therefore, we have a total of 85,000 images for training and validation. Each digit is described by 32 grey image pixels [2]. The quantities are transferred to the Convolutional Neural Networks input layers, and afterwards, the hidden layers usually contain two sets of the convolutional layer. After this, it is visualised to the fully connected layers, and a SoftMax classification scheme is presented to dial the numbers. Researchers will use Python, OpenCV, Django, or TensorFlow to incorporate this classification [3]. To achieve accuracy with decreased operating uncertainty and costs, the Convolutional Neural Networks framework is proposed. To express the best learning parameters to set up a CNN, the complete innovative database identifies the investigator applying the review process for HDR and the mathematical collection of neural networks. The cohesive hybrid set of mathematical and geometric features aims to accomplish local and global sample numbers' characteristics [4]. The process utilises genetic modification algorithms to select the best attributes and a neighbour to evaluate the handwritten digit dataset's endurance. Regarding the purpose of isolated handwritten words [5], suggested a deep CNN. The proposed method is an excellent way of extracting practical visual attributes from an image frame. The approach assumes two handwritten datasets (IAM and RIMES) under several experiments to determine the model's optimal parameters [6].

1.1 Abbreviations and Acronyms

- CNN – Convolution Neural Network
- NN – Neural Network

1.1.1 Units

- *Fully Connected Multi-layer Neural Network:* The multi-layer CNN can label data points in the MNIST training dataset at a failure of less than 4.42% on the validation dataset with one or more neural networks [7]. This channel extracts the features that encompass the practical spatial domain of the image data, and therefore extraordinarily high dimensions are required. Such CNN is questionable because such networks' criteria are more than 200,000, which is unacceptable if complex and complicated faults have collaborated with large data sets [8].
- *Data Sets:* The classification of specific character recognition is investigated in this problem. The MNIST database provided an example of training. This research created a database of 50,000 training sets and 20,000 test results, including census responses extracted. The original images are 64 × 64 standardised in size; however, they contain grey images because of the Graphical User Interface [9].

The image pixel resolution results are computed as −0.1 in shadow (white) and 1.275 in the middle of the photo (black)—the actual outcomes in a measured input of 0 and a difference of roughly 1. The decision variables are 15 grey images of 15 × 8 digits developed by hand. But only data variables were used in this case [10]: the background and foreground (−1) result in binary images. Such images were configured to provide adequate imbalance features for discriminatory practices in each '0'.

2 Related Works

HSD of minimal security has indeed formed significant improvements. Several papers were published with research and development of new handwritten numerals, characters, and English word categorisation [11]. The 3-layer Deep Belief Network (DBN) with a greedy algorithm for the MNIST dataset was evaluated, and a precision of 98.75% was described. In the aim of improving the efficiency of recurrent neural networks (RNN), the procedures and principles for deactivating were adapted in recognition of unpredictable handwriting. The reviewer significantly improved RNN efficiency, reducing the Character Error Rate (CER) and Word Error Rate (WER) [12]. The experiment explained that he might have been sufficient to attain an extremely high degree of precision using DL. The accuracy of the CNN with Keras and Theano was 98.72% [13]. Consequently, CNN operations that have used Tensorflow performance in an exceedingly better outcome of 99.70%. Even though the method and guidelines seem more complex and challenging than standard ML algorithms, precision becomes apparent. The investigator focuses on the various pre-processing methods used to recognise characters by respective classes of images, from easy, handwritten verification and information with a vibrantly coloured, cluttered background and wide-ranging complexity. This describes specific pre-processing methodologies, including skew detection and identification, stretching of the image, character recognition, deletion of noise, widespread acceptance and differentiation, and morphological diagnostic methods [14]. It was concluded that together we could process the image completely using a single pre-processing approach. However, a pre-processing module could not achieve complete precision even after implementing all these methodologies. CNN can be used for the acknowledgement of English character recognition. The features are considered from threshold mapping and its Fourier descriptors. The character is described by researching its template and attributing its attributes. To have access, a test was conducted to determine the number of hidden layer nodes to attain the network's maximum performance. For handwritten English alphabets with a minor test set, 94.13% accuracy was mentioned [15].

3 Proposed CNN Image Classification

Classified images are not a simple problem that can be managed to achieve by various methods. Nevertheless, many ML systems have been effectively implemented in recent times. Researchers consequently recommended dramatic CNNs to direct and evaluate our handwritten figures throughout that work. Building Convolutional Neural Networks plays an essential role in effectiveness and cost factors. So, after thoroughly reading its boundary conditions, we have established a chic CNN in our execution. Usually, critical elements described below have included Convolutional Neural Networks for HDR: Prepare patterns before feeding CNN. Before actually accessing the network, all images are pre-processed [16–18]. CNN is constructed for the size of 64 × 64 pixels in our experimental tests. Subsequently, all images were cut to the same size to feed the model. They are provided to the deep model to prepare images to retrieve characteristics. As relatively recently shown, a clear CNN is used throughout the experiment to extract powerful features used in the ultimate decision to support their classification [54–56]. The last layer, SoftMax, minimises the variance at the highest possible CNN level [19, 20].

3.1 PReLU

A Parametric Rectified Linear Unit (PReLU) is an intuitionistic fuzzy rectified unit with a curve for zero value. Lawfully: $f(B_i) = B_i$ if $B_i \geq 0 f(B_i) = A_i B_i$ if $B_i \leq 0$.

- Feature Extraction: LR Image
- *CNN Layer 1:* 56 Filters of 1 × 5 × 5 Image Size Extraction
- *Activation Function:* ReLU
- *Result:* 56 Map Feature Set
- *Limits:* 1 × 5 × 5 × 56

3.2 Shrinking

Reduces the function vectors' size (by limiting parameters) using reduced filters (compared to the number of filters used for image feature extraction).

- *Conv. Layer 2:* Shrinking 12 filters of size 56 × 2 × 2
- *Activation Function:* PReLU
- *Result:* 12 Feature Maps
- *Limits:* 56 × 2 × 2 × 12

3.3 Non-linear Mapping

Maps the LR to HR patches image features. This procedure is performed with many map-based layers relatively small than SCRNN (Fig. 1).

- *Conv. Layers 3–6:*
- Mapping
- 4 × 12 Filters of Size 12 × 4 × 4
- *Activation Function:* PReLU
- *Result:* HR Feature Maps
- *Limits:* 4 × 12 × 4 × 4 × 12

3.4 Expanding

Determines the complexity of the feature vector. The whole procedure performs the complete reverse function as the decreasing layers produce the HR image more reliably.

- *Conv. Layer 7:*
  - Increasing
  - 56 Filters of Size 12 × 2 × 2

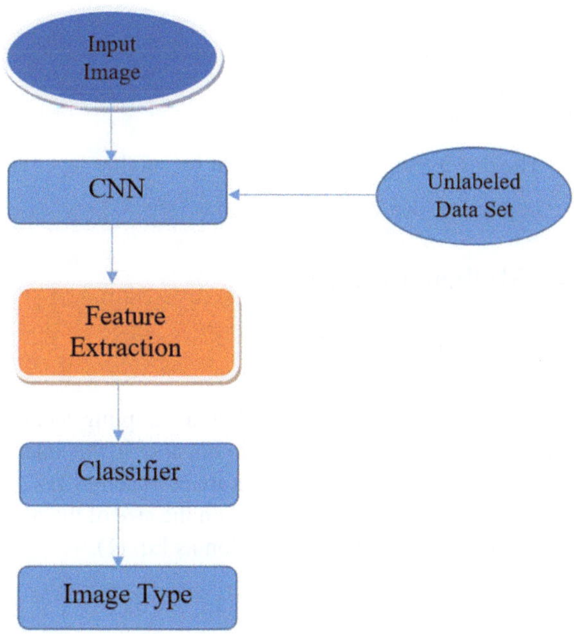

Fig. 1 Process of image function extraction

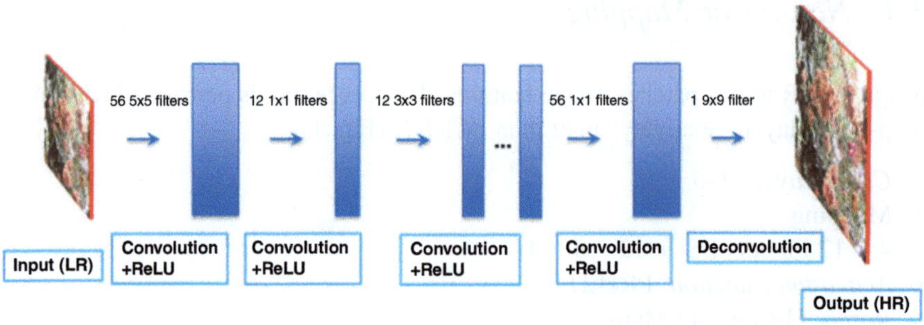

Fig. 2 Image processing

- *Activation Function:* PReLU
- *Result:* 12 Feature Maps
- *Limits:* 12 × 2 × 2 × 56

3.5 Deconvolution

Produces the HR image from HR features

- *DeConv Layer 8:*
  - Deconvolution
  - One filter of size 56 × 8 × 9
- *Activation Function:* PReLU
- *Output:* 13 Feature Maps
- *Parameters:* 56 × 8 × 9 × 1

  The down-sampling layer might be another layer and is often hidden (Fig. 2).

4 Mathematical Model

4.1 Subsampling Layer

The sub-sampling function applies a sampling technique on the input maps. The input and output visualisations do not alter in this interface. For instance, if there are N input maps, there are N output maps exactly [21–29]. The test operation reduces the size of the feature maps based on the size of the mask [30–34]. The two different shows are used in this investigation as Eq. (1).

$$\text{Image}_j^i = \text{MapFunction}\left[\beta_j^i \text{DownSampling}\left(\text{Image}_j^{i-1}\right) + B_j^i\right] \tag{1}$$

where (·) is a sub-sampling feature. This predominant source encapsulates the estimated value or n to block the actual accuracy of the input image maps [35–41]. Therefore, the map output dimension significantly decreases to n periods for both feature vector components. The output maps are ultimately triggered as linear/non-linear [42–47].

5 Result and Discussion

In this case, the digital image of the handwritten digit is the pattern x, and0–9 is the category y. We use 1500 of 64 × 64 gray scaled images as a dataset, and we separate this dataset into 1200 for training data and 300 for testing data. For pattern x, we reshape 64 × 64 gray scaled images to 4096-dimension vectors [48–53]. Therefore, we apply LDA on a Gaussian model with 4096-dimension Gaussian distribution (Figs. 3, 4, 5, 6, 7, 8 and 9).

6 Conclusion

The proposed Handwritten Digital Recognition has shown us that traditional neural networks training can distribute comparatively more minor fault rates that aren't too far from several other trailing results that focus on deep Convolutional Neural Networks. Convolutional Neural Networks has the advantage of being able to extract and use feature data. This research's significance would address all the Convolutional Neural Networks model features that deliver the best precise

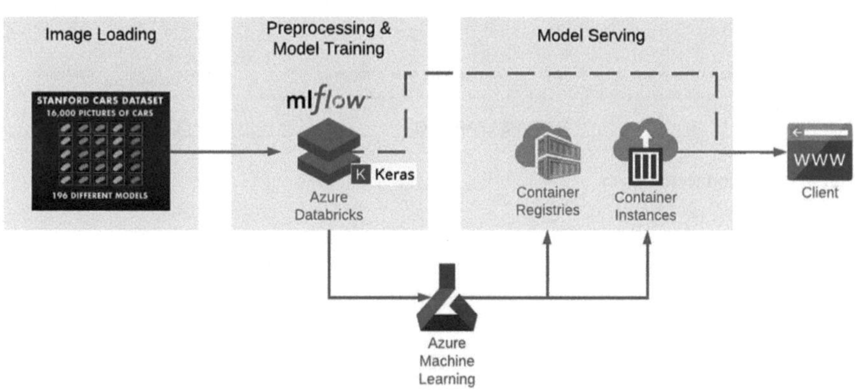

Fig. 3 Convolution Neural Framework

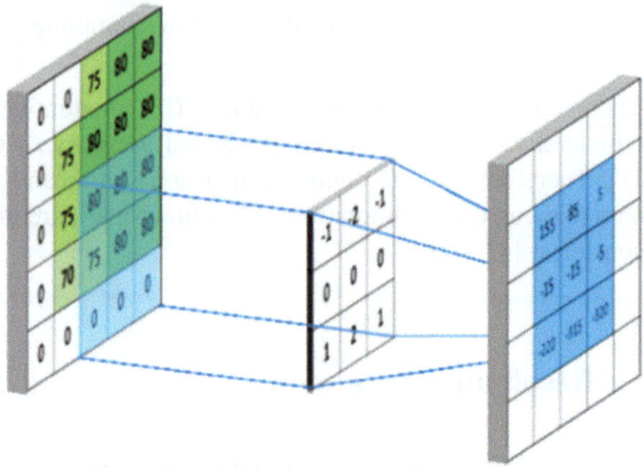

Fig. 4 Input Image and the function

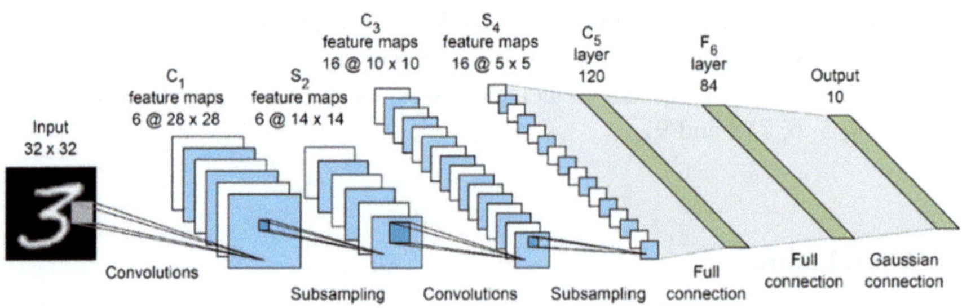

Fig. 5 The use of six images increases the final image size

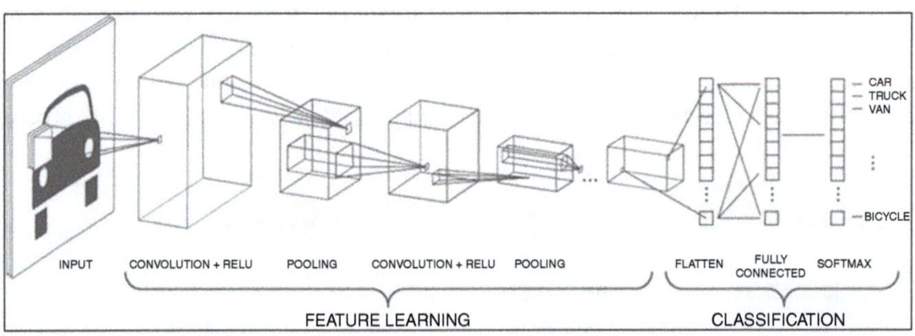

Fig. 6 Fully connected layer

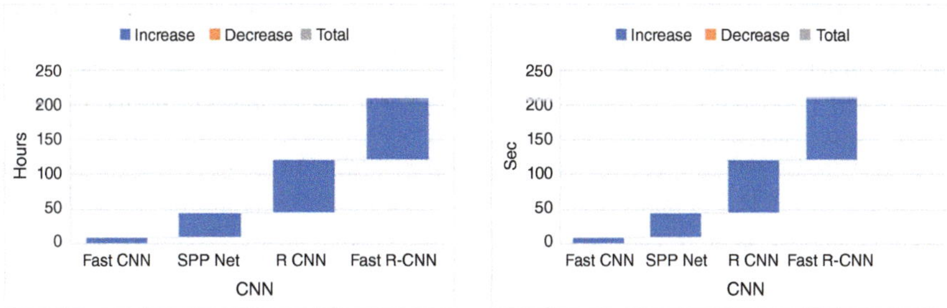

Fig. 7 Accuracy Rate at each level

Fig. 8 Tensorflow using CNN

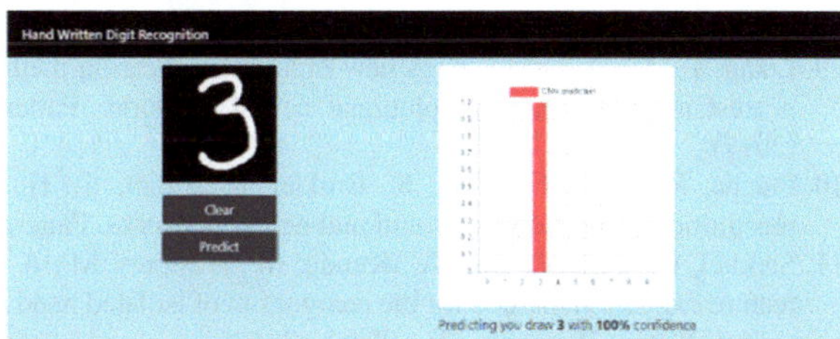

Fig. 9 Open CV using Django

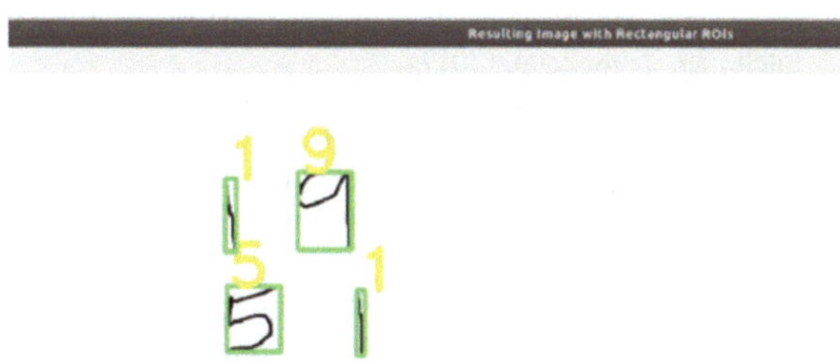

assessment for an MNIST dataset. The model's metadata of dissimilar methodologies and error frequency is ordered as follows: (a) Random Forest Classifier is 1.32%, (b) K-Nearest Neighbours is 4.34%, (c) Support Vector Machine is 4.134%, (d) Convolutional Neural Networks is 5.28%, (e) TensorFlow is appropriate and provides a maximum 100% presentation similar to OpenCV.

References

1. Ahlawat, S., Rishi, R.: A genetic algorithm-based feature selection for handwritten digit recognition. Recent Pat. Comput. Sci., 12, 304–316, (2019)
2. Aparna, KH, Vidhya, Subramanian., Kasirajan, M., Vijay Prakash, G., Chakravarthy, V.S., Sriganesh Madhvanath.: Online Handwriting Recognition for Tamil. Proceedings. 9th International Workshop on Frontiers in Handwriting Recognition, Proceedings. 438–443, (2004).

3. Avita, Ahlawat., Amit, Choudhary., Anand, Nayyar., Saurabh, Singh., Byungun, Yoon.: Improved Handwritten Digit Recognition Using Convolutional Neural Networks (CNN). Sensors, 20, 3344, (2020).
4. Boufenar, C., Kerboua, A., Batouche, M.: Investigation on deep learning for off-line handwritten Arabic character recognition. Cogn. Syst. Res., 50, 180–195, (2018).
5. Chen, L.C., Papandreou, G., Kokkinos, I., Murphy, K., Yuille, A.L.: Deep Lab: Semantic image segmentation with deep convolutional nets, atrous convolution, and fully connected CRFs. IEEE Trans. Pattern Anal. Mach. Intell., 40, 834–848, (2018).
6. Devi R. K and Elizabeth Rani G.: "A Comparative Study on Handwritten Digit Recognizer using Machine Learning Technique," IEEE International Conference on Clean Energy and Energy Efficient Electronics Circuit for Sustainable Development, 1–5, (2019).
7. Elanwar, R., Qin, W., Betke, M.: Making scanned Arabic documents machine-accessible using an ensemble of SVM classifiers. Int. J. Document Anal. Recognit., 21 (1–2), 59–75, (2020).
8. Garg, N.K., Kaur, D.L., Kumar, D.M.: Segmentation of handwritten Hindi text, Int. J. Comput. Appl., 1 (4), 22–26, (2010).
9. Liang, T., Xu, X., Xiao, P.: A new image classification method based on modified condensed nearest neighbor and convolutional neural networks. Pattern Recognit. Lett., 94, 105–111, (2017).
10. Ptucha, R., Such, F., Pillai, S., Brokler, F., Singh, V., Hutkowski, P.: Intelligent character recognition using fully convolutional neural networks. Pattern Recognit., 88, 604–613, (2019).
11. Sarkhel, R., Das, N., Das, A., Kundu, M., Nasipuri, M.: A multi-scale deep quad tree-based feature extraction method for the recognition of isolated handwritten characters of popular indic scripts. Pattern Recognit., 71, 78–93, (2017).
12. Shi, B., Bai, X., Yao, C.: An End-to-end trainable neural network for image-based sequence recognition and its application to scene text recognition. IEEE Trans. Pattern Anal. Mach. Intell., 39, 2298–2304, (2017).
13. Sueiras, J., Ruiz, V., Sanchez, A., Velez, J.F.: Offline continuous handwriting recognition using sequence to sequence neural networks. Neurocomputing, 289, 119–128, (2018).
14. Vashist P.C, Pandey A and Tripathi A.: A Comparative Study of Handwriting Recognition Techniques, International Conference on Computation, Automation and Knowledge Management, 456–461, (2020).
15. Wu, Y.C., Yin, F., Liu, C.L., Improving handwritten Chinese text recognition using neural network language models and convolutional neural network shape models. Pattern Recognit., 65, 251–264, (2017).
16. S. Sudhakar and S. Chenthur Pandian "Secure packet encryption and key exchange system in mobile ad hoc network", Journal of Computer Science, vol. 8, no. 6, pp. 908–912, (2012).
17. S. Sudhakar and S. Chenthur Pandian, "Hybrid cluster-based geographical routing protocol to mitigate malicious nodes in mobile ad hoc network", International Journal of Ad Hoc and Ubiquitous Computing, vol. 21 no. 4, pp. 224–236, (2016).
18. A. U. Priyadarshni and S. Sudhakar, "Cluster-based certificate revocation by cluster head in mobile ad-hoc network", International Journal of Applied Engineering Research, vol. 10, no. 20, pp. 16014–16018, (2015).
19. S. Sudhakar and S. Chenthur Pandian, "Investigation of attribute aided data aggregation over dynamic routing in wireless sensor," Journal of Engineering Science and Technology, vol. 10, no. 11, pp. 1465–1476, (2015).
20. T. A. Al-asadi and A. J. Obaid, "Object Based Image Retrieval Using Enhanced SURF," Asian Journal of Information Technology, vol. 15, no. 16, pp. 2756–2762, (2016).
21. C. Meshram, R. W. Ibrahim, A. J. Obaid, S. G. Meshram, A. Meshram and A. M. Abd El-Latif, "Fractional chaotic maps based short signature scheme under human-centered IoT environments," Journal of Advanced Research, (2020).
22. A. J. Obaid, K. A. Alghurabi, S. A. K. Albermany and S. Sharma, "Improving Extreme Learning Machine Accuracy Utilizing Genetic Algorithm for Intrusion Detection Purposes," in Advances in Intelligent Systems and Computing, Springer, Singapore, pp. 171–177 (2021).

23. Ishaq, A., Sadiq, S., Umer, M., Ullah, S., Mirjalili, S., Rupapara, V., & Nappi, M. Improving the Prediction of Heart Failure Patients' Survival Using SMOTE and Effective Data Mining Techniques. IEEE Access, 9, 39707–39716 (2021).
24. Surinder Singh and Hardeep Singh Saini "Security approaches for data aggregation in Wireless Sensor Networks against Sybil Attack," 2018 Second International Conference on Inventive Communication and Computational Technologies, pp. 190–193, Coimbatore, India (2018).
25. Rustam, F., Khalid, M., Aslam, W., Rupapara, V., Mehmood, A., & Choi, G. S. A performance comparison of supervised machine learning models for Covid-19 tweets sentiment analysis. PLOS ONE, 16(2), e0245909 (2021).
26. Surinder Singh and Hardeep Singh Saini "Security Techniques for Wormhole Attack in Wireless Sensor Network", International Journal of Engineering & Technology, Vol. 7, No. 2.23, 59–62 (2018).
27. Yousaf, A., Umer, M., Sadiq, S., Ullah, S., Mirjalili, S., Rupapara, V., & Nappi, M. Emotion Recognition by Textual Tweets Classification Using Voting Classifier. IEEE Access, 9, 6286–6295 (2021).
28. Surinder Singh and Hardeep Singh Saini, "Learning-Based Security Technique for Selective Forwarding Attack in Clustered WSN", Wireless Pers Commun 118, 789–814 (2021).
29. Sadiq, S., Umer, M., Ullah, S., Mirjalili, S., Rupapara, V., & NAPPI, M. Discrepancy detection between actual user reviews and numeric ratings of Google App store using deep learning. Expert Systems with Applications, 115111 (2021).
30. A.K. Gupta, Y. K. Chauhan, and T Maity, "Experimental investigations and comparison of various MPPT techniques for photovoltaic system," Sādhanā, Vol. 43, no. 8, pp. 1–15, (2018).
31. A. Jain, A. K. Gahlot, R. Dwivedi, A. Kumar, and S. K. Sharma, "Fat Tree NoC Design and Synthesis," in Intelligent Communication, Control and Devices, Springer, 2018, pp. 1749–1756 (2018).
32. A.K. Gupta, "Sun Irradiance Trappers for Solar PV Module to Operate on Maximum Power: An Experimental Study," Turkish Journal of Computer and Mathematics Education, Vol. 12, no. 5, pp. 1112–1121, (2021).
33. N. R. Misra, S. Kumar, and A. Jain, "A Review on E-waste: Fostering the Need for Green Electronics," in 2021 International Conference on Computing, Communication, and Intelligent Systems, 2021, pp. 1032–1036 (2021).
34. A.K. Gupta, Y.K Chauhan, and T Maity and R Nanda, "Study of Solar PV Panel Under Partial Vacuum Conditions: A Step Towards Performance Improvement," IETE Journal of Research, pp. 1–8, (2020).
35. A. Jain, A. K. AlokGahlot, and S. K. S. RakeshDwivedi, "Design and FPGA Performance Analysis of 2D and 3D Router in Mesh NoC," Int. J. Control Theory Appl., pp. 0974–5572, (2017).
36. A.K. Gupta, Y.K Chauhan, and T Maity, "A new gamma scaling maximum power point tracking method for solar photovoltaic panel Feeding energy storage system," IETE Journal of Research, vol. 67, no. 1, pp. 1–21, (2018).
37. Joshi M., Agarwal A.K., Gupta B. Fractal Image Compression and Its Techniques: A Review. In: Ray K., Sharma T., Rawat S., Saini R., Bandyopadhyay A. (eds) Soft Computing: Theories and Applications. Advances in Intelligent Systems and Computing, vol 742. Springer, Singapore (2019).
38. Agarwal, A. Implementation of Cylomatrix complexity matrix. Journal of Nature Inspired Computing, 1 (2013).
39. A. K. Gupta et al., "Effect of Various Incremental Conductance MPPT Methods on the Charging of Battery Load Feed by Solar Panel," in IEEE Access, vol. 9, pp. 90977–90988, (2021).
40. Saleem A., Agarwal A.K. Analysis and Design of Secure Web Services. In: Pant M., Deep K., Bansal J., Nagar A., Das K. (eds) Proceedings of Fifth International Conference on Soft Computing for Problem Solving. Advances in Intelligent Systems and Computing, vol 437. Springer, Singapore (2016).

41. N. Gupta and A. K. Agarwal, "Object Identification using Super Sonic Sensor: Arduino Object Radar," 2018 International Conference on System Modeling & Advancement in Research Trends, pp. 92–96 (2018),
42. S. Shukla, A. Lakhmani and A. K. Agarwal, "A review on integrating ICT based education system in rural areas in India," 2016 International Conference System Modeling & Advancement in Research Trends, 2016, pp. 256–259 (2016).
43. Agarwal A.K., Rani L., Tiwari R.G., Sharma T., Sarangi P.K. Honey Encryption: Fortification Beyond the Brute-Force Impediment. In: Manik G., Kalia S., Sahoo S.K., Sharma T.K., Verma O.P. (eds) Advances in Mechanical Engineering. Lecture Notes in Mechanical Engineering. Springer, Singapore (2021).
44. Khullar V, Singh HP, Agarwal AK. Spoken buddy for individuals with autism spectrum disorder. Asian J Psychiatr; 62 102712 (2021).
45. Hassan, M.I., Fouda, M.A., Hammad, K.M. and Hasaballah, A.I. Effects of midgut bacteria and two protease inhibitors on the transmission of Wuchereria bancrofti by the mosquito vector, Culex pipiens. Journal of the Egyptian Society of Parasitology. 43(2): 547–553 (2013).
46. Surinder Singh and Hardeep Singh Saini, "Detection Techniques for Selective Forwarding Attack in Wireless Sensor Networks", International Journal of Recent Technology and Engineering, Vol. 7, Issue-6S, 380–383 (2019).
47. Fouda, M.A., Hassan, M.I., Hammad, K.M. and Hasaballah, A.I. Effects of midgut bacteria and two protease inhibitors on the reproductive potential and midgut enzymes of Culex pipiens infected with Wuchereria bancrofti. Journal of the Egyptian Society of Parasitology. 43(2): 537–546 (2013).
48. Surinder Singh and Hardeep Singh Saini "Security for Internet of Thing (IoT) based Wireless Sensor Networks", Journal of Advanced Research in Dynamical and Control Systems, 06-Special Issue, 1591–1596 (2018).
49. Hasaballah, A.I. Toxicity of some plant extracts against vector of lymphatic filariasis, Culex pipiens. Journal of the Egyptian Society of Parasitology. 45(1): 183–192 (2015).
50. J. Kubiczek and B. Hadasik, "Challenges in Reporting the COVID-19 Spread and its Presentation to the Society," J. Data and Information Quality, vol. 13, no. 4, pp. 1–7, Dec. (2021).
51. Hasaballah, A.I. Impact of gamma irradiation on the development and reproduction of Culex pipiens. International journal of radiation biology. 94(9): 844–849 (2018).
52. Sajja, G. S., Rane, K. P., Phasinam, K., Kassanuk, T., Okoronkwo, E., & Prabhu, P. Towards applicability of blockchain in agriculture sector. Materials Today: Proceedings (2021).
53. Pallathadka, H., Mustafa, M., Sanchez, D. T., Sekhar Sajja, G., Gour, S., & Naved, M. Impact of machine learning on management, healthcare and agriculture. Materials Today: Proceedings (2021).
54. Guna Sekhar Sajja, Malik Mustafa, R. Ponnusamy, Shokhjakhon Abdufattokhov, Murugesan G., P. Prabhu. Machine Learning Algorithms in Intrusion Detection and Classification. Annals of the Romanian Society for Cell Biology, 25(6), 12211–12219 (2021).
55. Arcinas, Myla & Sajja, Guna & Asif, Shazia & Gour, Sanjeev & Okoronkwo, Ethelbert & Naved, Mohd. Role of Data Mining in Education For Improving Students Performance For Social Change. Turkish Journal of Physiotherapy and Rehabilitation. 32. 6519 (2021).
56. Hasaballah, A.I. Impact of paternal transmission of gamma radiation on reproduction, oogenesis, and spermatogenesis of the housefly, Musca domestica L. International Journal of Radiation Biology. 97(3): 376–385 (2021).

An Investigation of Machine Learning-Based IDS for Green Smart Transportation in MANET

C. Edwin Singh and J. Amar Pratap Singh

1 Introduction

For many research findings, wireless communication for Green Smart Transportation has become the optimal method. Green Smart Transportation helps promote Connectedness, collaboration, adaptability, and profitability will all benefit from green manoeuvrability and intelligent transportation technologies. Furthermore, new trend methods enable advanced technology to be retained with every application, making them more accessible. Mobile Ad hoc Networks (MANET) are wireless technologies with a high node mobility level because of the limited-range wireless communication and increased network node mobility. MANET is a self-configuring network of mobile routers connected by wireless links with no access point. In MANET, breaking communication links is very frequent, as nodes are free to move anywhere. Unlike other cellular networks, MANETs don't really necessitate a permanent framework. Nodes should work together to provide essential communication, with the high connection constantly evolving to meet MANET needs. Since the protocols that allow MANET operations are complex, they are well adapted to severe or unpredictable Green Smart Transportation environments. MANETs are now a common research domain, with applications in various fields, including Green Smart Transportation, emergencies, tactical operations, environmental management, and military services.

Methods of machine learning have been applied for maliciousness and anomaly-based. ML methods focus on algorithms that can learn from data without being specifically developed. Given the wide variety of network traffic, machine learning is extremely useful. Despite ML characteristics, IDS approaches are rarely used in

C. E. Singh (✉) · J. A. P. Singh
Department of CSE, NICHE, Nagercoil, Tamil Nadu, India
e-mail: japs@niuniv.com

P. Agarwal et al. (eds.), *Artificial Intelligence for Smart Healthcare*,
EAI/Springer Innovations in Communication and Computing,
https://doi.org/10.1007/978-3-031-23602-0_5

the actual world, and harmful detection still reigns supreme. The substantial Fake Positive Rate (FPR) issue is frequently regarded as the primary driver of IDS adoption. Indeed, on a high-traffic network, even an FPR of 1.08% might generate so many false alarm rate that MANET becomes impossible to process. This research proposes to improve the IDS by deploying real MANETs for Green Smart Mobility using machine learning approaches. Improving IDS accuracy on existing training datasets isn't adequate to complete this study because the results aren't applicable to real-world MANETs. Indeed, rather than traffic monitoring, machine learning techniques learn the traffic in a dataset. The traffic in a dataset is what machine learning models learn, not how much traffic there is. Retraining them on the monitored network is necessary, but it is not achievable because it calls for tagged training datasets that contain assaults on the MANET environment. We proposed an efficient architecture for IDS on KDD using ML models. The following optimisation methods are used in this framework: (a) data augmentation, (b) parameter estimation, and (c) supervised learning. This method obtained a maximum prediction performance of 94.48% on the KDD test data collection with a low Probability of 1.98%. Consider simple metrics like Precision, Recall, and F-Score when assessing particular ML effectiveness for IDS types.

2 Related Works

Massive IDS methods have been anticipated to minimise security issues in MANET to improve effective IDS performance. However, these approaches have challenges increasing prediction performance, and presently MANET remains challenging due to the security challenges such as energy usage and Packet Delivery Ratio. An penetration testing system is a computing device that detects the system's software behaviour in the MANET to identify intruders. Since information technology can be vulnerable to security flaws, it is cost-effective challenging to network setup that is not resistant to threats. IDSs accurately find and defend against attacks by monitoring nodes and user misbehaviour. IDS have been considered an integral part of solutions for preventing recent trends. Yongguang et al. [1] developed a systematic IDS and solution framework for MANETs in innovative research in wireless IDS study. MANET concentrated on policies for creating IDS that can identify attacks instantly. The mobile node has an administrator connected to it, and every node in the system interacts in the IDS. To promote collaboration of neighbouring nodes, shared IDS is recommended. To develop the standardised profile, [2] introduces an innovative aspect of data processing approach that uses "hybrid-feature" analytics to obtain the intelligent system standard forms of MANET traffic.

Standard of Care is a network and switched function that optimizes traffic so that the most relevant traffic gets through first. The performance of critical systems has improved. The switch's QoS changes depending on its level; the greater the platform's level, the better the internet access layer it supports. The network connection's QoS manages packet loss and decreases latency and jitters. Service quality is a collection of capabilities that function on a network to ensure that the high programs and traffic run reliably even when network bandwidth is constrained. Based on the QoS, anomaly-based IDS can be divided into sub-categories. These are mathematical and ML-based types. Nonparametric, multi-variable, and time sequence statistics are used in statistical data. Case and N-based, expert classifications, and ML are examples of knowledge-based devices that use finite-state models and laws. Buczak and Guven [3] recommend DL algorithm selection based on problem-solving. ANNs, grouping, Genetic Algorithms, and other algorithms are examples of algorithms. Specification-based is a hybrid model that combines the strengths of both trademark and anomaly-based models. Yin et al. [4] used a Recurrent Neural Network (RNN) to evaluate the NSL-KDD datasets, and the RNN's output correlated to that of other ML classification models such as J48, SVM, and RF. It is used to classify single- and multi-data and has a higher amount of IDS performance. Since RNN processing takes longer, researchers have investigated, so in the coming years, Long Short-Term Memory (LSTM)/Gated Recurrent Unit (GRU) is being used to solve the problem [5].

ML is a sub-domain of AI that exploits data's inherent information to identify ML methods and help with decision-making automatically [6]. Various algorithms and techniques synthesise a powerful tool for designing intelligent predictive systems for a broad spectrum of business tasks. In cyber security, specifically IDS, we use classification algorithms to discover anomalies and offensive incidents in a secured network [7]. The strength of machine learning (ML) depends on its capacity to identify patterns based on a variety of variables within enormous amounts of network traffic data, which would normally need manual mining with the help of an experienced user [8]. The extracted patterns are used to build generalised models, predicting the legitimacy of future network traffic instances automatically/determining their proximity to anomalous/legitimate behaviours. Hence, ML-based IDSs go beyond standard-setting thresholds, monitor specific metrics, and adapt to demanding MANET environments [9].

Ad-hoc network service security is a difficult problem to solve. The first step in building robust cybersecurity solutions is always to understand probable attackers. The secured transfer of information in MANET relies heavily on security. MANETs are more sensitive to virtual than wired networks due to the lack of a central planning tool and a wireless transmission medium. Several attacks affect MANET. In MANET, security Assault on the Protocol Stack, Malicious Code, and Repudiation are all possible. Threats on the Packet Filtering Session include theft and SYN Overflow. Drowning, Black Hole, and Grey Hole are all terms used to describe the in-network layer. Attacks such as Worm Hole and Link Spoofing occur. Deep packet inspection and surveillance take place at the Data Link Layer. In Physical Layer, Traffic Jamming, Eavesdropping occurs. IDS detects the system's software behaviour in the MANET to identify intruders.

3 Proposed ML-Based Green Smart Transportation IDS

ML methods create an explicit or implicit framework that categorises the patterns analysed. The requirement for class labels to exercise the behavioural model [10], a technique that applied reflective training on resources, is a unique feature of these strategies. While the former is centred on creating ML models that enhance efficiency based on existing research investigations [11] [12], ML ideas' efficacy also correlates with statistical approaches. As an outcome, ML-IDS can adapt its methodology as new knowledge is acquired [13]. While this feature can make it more attractive to use such strategies in all Green Smart Transportation network environments, MANET resource-intensive scheduling is a key drawback. IDS have been subjected to many ML-based approaches. This research article presents the most significant advantages and disadvantages of Machine Learning on MANET (Fig. 1).

The primary investigation of ML-IDS is to recognise and classify the nodes' observable misbehaviour patterns using IDS and the necessary ML features as inputs. As a result, effective IDS system design and implementation following the application's problems is another significant issue [14, 15]. MANET architecture necessitates maximum energy efficiency. As a result, IDS processes can use less energy consumption while achieving the desired outcomes [16, 17]. Comparing all the most commonly utilised ML models concerning the critical key factors when determining the IDS for MANETs is summarised in Table 1 [18].

In addition to the regular mentioned above, specific IDS could help deal with the volume of trained datasets. Analysing the Primary Components is a strategy for reducing a dataset's difficulty [19]. PCA is an intermediate detecting system rather

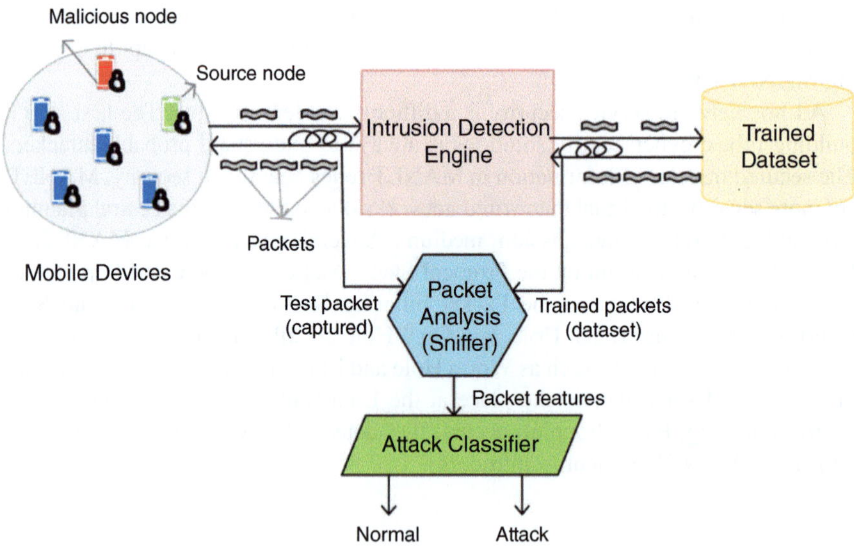

Fig. 1 Architecture of ML-based IDS

Table 1 Taxonomy of machine learning

ML types	Suitability in MANETs		
	Accuracy	Training time	Resource constraint
ANN	Strong	Strong	Good
Bayesian network	Good	Weak	Strong
Markov model	Strong	Good	Good
SVM	Strong	Weak	Weak

than a detection scheme itself. PCA is a translation method that uses 'n' correlated variables to describe PCA. PCA fetches the total factors down to DS > n. And the next step is to find associations between different extracting features from the trained dataset using association-rule mining. For example, internal links among data consistent with a specific relationship can be opened using ML association rules. Knowledge Discovery in Databases (KDD) hit the scene in the 1990s, promising to "define fresh, true, particularly effective, and clear and understandable patterns for data." [20, 21]. Data exploration methods emerged as a subset of KDD, consisting of "applying DL to massive databases to explore valuable knowledge immediately". KDD and ML are widely utilised to compare network traffic instances in network-related repositories as a particular application. The phrase "data mining" is commonly used to categorise and relate various IDS decision bases as a standard wildcard assessment method [22].

3.1 Pre-processing and Data Augmentation

The research has consistently criticised the KDD for its shortcomings and rectified inconsistency and redundancy. Links and threats in these databases are indeed not a clear reflection of a network's fraudulent activities and attacks. The proposed architecture is applied to the entire MANET. The chapter implies that the practicality of our solution is demonstrated by evaluating its outcomes to state-of-the-art examples. The researchers conclude that these datasets' detection rates cannot be generalised to real MANET [23].

3.2 Parameters Optimization

Parameters are the neural net factors set before practice. Simulation parameters include the number of nodes, packet size, optimisation method, learning rate, and features. Hyperparameters are also individually adjusted, or all possible variations of a value set are tested. This method, glorious as facility hunting [24, 25], has the vantage of object planetary optimal values. H. The combination of parameters that offer the best classification results. Nevertheless, is stubborn to use in implementation because there are umpteen parameters identified by a giant explore squad. We choose two faster and statesman late algorithms: Random Look and Tree-structured Parzen Estimator. Exploring imbalanced collection is a creation machine acquisition problem. In our test case, the number of links in the normal and DoS groups is decreased. Two primary ways to restructure classes available are R2L and U2R classes: under and oversampling [26, 27].

3.3 Ensemble Learning

Ensemble learning is a technique of improving overall predictive efficiency by integrating multiple frameworks. The core concept is that a group of base learners is more successful than a single dominant learner, improving the prediction's ability. Many ML techniques, like KDD, observed outcomes with the Ensembling learning approach.

3.4 Algorithm 1 for ML Classification for Malicious Node Detection

Step 1. **Initialize** Vector v, b = 0
Step 2. **Set** Data Set = $(D_1, D_2), \ldots, (D_n, D_n)$
    Train SVM to learn decision function
Step 3. **For** each Data Set is D **Do**
    Classify D_i using decision function $f_x(D_i)$
Step 4. **If** (Function Margin < 1) **Then**
Step 5. Compute
Step 6. **For** Sample Data for reducing errors to predict **Do**
    $f_x = (HyperPlane^T D^i + LengthofIntercept)$
    $FunctionM\ arg\ in(FM) = (HyperPlane^T D^i + LengthofIntercept)$
Step 7. **If** (Prediction is Accurate) **Then**
    Do Next
Step 8. **Else**
    Train SVM
Step 9. **End If**
Step 10. **End If**
    Classify D_i as Malicious Nodes
Step 11. **End**

3.5 Algorithm 2 for Optimal Solution for Acceptable Error Rate

Step 1. **Begin**
Step 2. **Set** Network Nodes
Step 3. Assess appropriateness for discrete nodes
Step 4. **While** (! Check State) **Do**
Step 5. Proceed the Cross over Process
Step 6. Proceed the Mutation Process
Step 7. Evaluate the new node
Step 8. Select individual to substitute nodes
Step 9. Update Node State
Step 10. **End**
Step 11. Return Optimal Solution for Path Selection
Step 12. **End**

3.6 Algorithm 3 for Packet Anomaly Prediction

Step 1. The Input of the Network Packet
Step 2. Output for Packet Anomaly
Step 3. Extract Protocol Headers from Data Packet
Step 4. **For** Network Protocol Header **Do**
  Choice the Parameters
  Translate Unconditional into Mathematical Features
  Normalize Features is {0 , 1}
Step 5. **End For**
Step 6. **If** CNN Protocol Header is Trained **Then**
  Set Anomaly Scores
Step 7. **Else**
  Training Data Set on Neural Network
  Set Anomaly Scores
Step 8. **End If**
Step 9. **End**

The SVM algorithm is used to train the dataset to detect the malicious node in machine learning classification. SVM trains on a set of label data. SVM is used for both classification and regression problems. SVM draws a decision boundary that is a hyperplane between any two classes to separate them or classify them. It imports the dataset and then splits it into training and test samples. It classifies the target and then initialises the Support Vector Machine to fit the training data. The classes for the test set have been predicted, and then the prediction is attached to the test set for comparing; thus, the prediction result is determined, and the malicious node is detected.

The main idea for packet anomaly prediction is to train the historical data and identify and recognise outlier data according to previous streams patterns and trends. Anomaly Detection is the technique of identifying rare events or observations which can raise suspicions by being statistically different from the rest of the observations. The SVM algorithm clusters the normal data behavior using a learning area in anomaly detection. Then, the testing example identifies the abnormalities that go out of the learned area. Fitting a neural network involves using a training dataset to update the model weights to create a good mapping of inputs to outputs. Training a neural network involves using an optimisation algorithm to find a set of weights to best map inputs to outputs. The iterative training process of neural networks solves an optimisation problem that finds parameters that result in a minimum error or loss when evaluating the training dataset.

4 Mathematical Model of ML Process

For the proposed ML method, we formulate a statistical approach. Each intelligent metre contributes to the prevalence of unique characteristics viewed for this time-space in a 3D matrix, $M_i = (M_{i1}, M_{i2}, M_{i3})$. Here, the certain effective rutting period and a "HELLO" data packet connection to the 1-hop neighbourhood are encompassed in each channel. We measure the centre matrix of M with N time frames by using Eq. (1).

$$\overline{M} = \frac{1}{N}\sum_{i=0}^{N}[M_{i1}, \ldots, M_{i3}] \tag{1}$$

Then researchers measured the error to the mean vector from input sample data M, Eq. (2).

$$D(M) = \left[M - \overline{M}\right]^2 \tag{2}$$

If the routing time is significantly higher than the $[D(M) > T]$, this implies that it is not inside the acceptable range traffic and are therefore considered as a threat. Here, the optimum projection path from the ML data set is processed, Eq. (3)

$$\begin{aligned} &T = D(M_i) \\ &\text{where, } i = \text{ArgMax}[D(M_i], M_i \in D \end{aligned} \tag{3}$$

ML is assessing the 'T' threshold and constructing training data for our ML models using this mathematical formula in MANET Routing Protocol for Green Smart Transportation. This 'T' extends only to N slots, and the 'T' will then be updated according to network security settings on MANET. Each intelligent metre

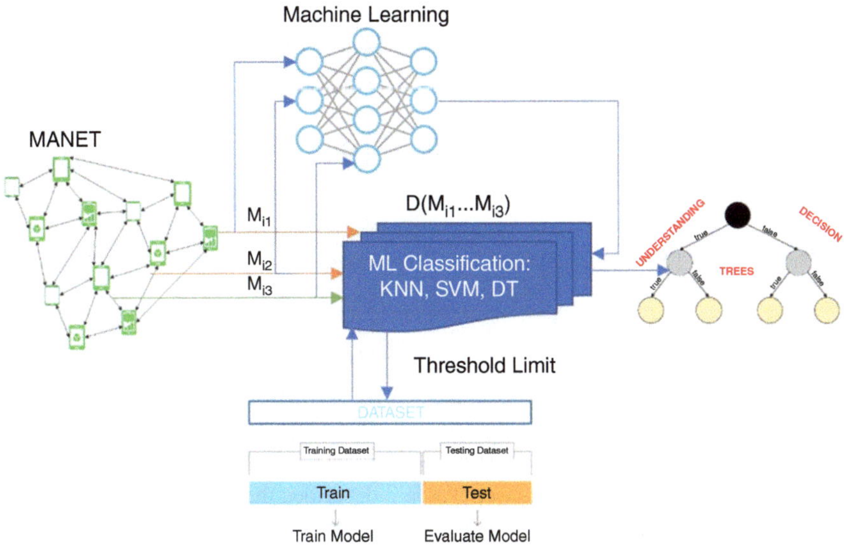

Fig. 2 ML-IDS decision flow

can therefore perform within an adaptive 'T' range. Hello, packet, RREQ, and RREP route optimisation data are now evaluated for every successive congestion control in an ML framework to estimate $D(M)$. For our ML model, classifiers, including the ML algorithm, are considered test data $D(M)$ and its comparative three distinct features. Our proposed model's complete flow charts are exposed in Fig. 2.

5 Result and Discussion

5.1 Simulations

The simulation is conducted on the open-source Waikato Environment for Knowledge Analysis (WEKA), which is a data analysis platform that offers a simple GUI for training and testing ML with different parametric settings. It contains features for information pre-processing, correlation, grouping, association rules, and other ML implementation tools. It's ideal for creating advanced ML models.

5.1.1 Findings of KDD

For evaluating Dendron using the KDD, this research adopted a set of pre-processing steps broadly used in the literature study. We randomised the datasets to make them smaller while maintaining their characteristic state. Furthermore, all redundancy is

Table 2 Training and test dataset using KDD

Class	Training data set	Test data set
Normal	9192	81,292
DoS	5819	51,345
PRB	250	2241
R2L	123	928
U2R	39	49

Table 3 Values for each dataset's test parameters

Symbol	Parameters	KDD data set
Class	List of class	8
F	List of features	27
σ	SD	4
I	No. of iterations	1500
β	Beta value	45

avoided from the incomplete dataset. Table 2 describes the occurrences used in our findings' research training data sets. Except for the U2R class, whereby 51.45% of the test cases are considered, the training data set includes 11.34% of each type's instances. Dendron is evaluated using the KDD dataset to construct a training dataset comprising 10.12% of the preliminary cases, with the remaining 90.86% used in the testing process. Table 2 shows instances used in the training and test set included in the simulation results.

Since the optimisation process is not probabilistic, these two variables challenge the testing. As a result, the ML method would not produce the same result for each variable, regardless of the discrepancies in the outcomes between the different data distributions. The appropriate optimisation process was designed to obtain the end's ID rules. The parameters and values used to evaluate the design for each dataset are given in Table 3. We suggested our model's appropriateness using the Mean-F-Measure (σ-FM) method. The aim is to optimise this standard metric such that Dendron considers all of the dataset's classes evenly. FM was designed to calculate the correlation among Recall and Precision measures amongst all dataset groups in the sense of multi-classification issues. The False Negative Rate and Positive Rate of a class are taken into account by the Recall and Precision measures. As a result, FM is a good measure for balancing detection and false reports. Also, under the measures, equate Dendron's efficiency to that of "Rule of Thumb" algorithms. We may confidently assert that our methodology can provide adequate and consistent intrusion prevention rules to help a violation detection method using case-based analysis. Dendron achieved high efficiency to test data, demonstrating that FM is a proper investigation metric. The increased values of the mean metrics of FM, Maximum Precision, and Threat Accuracy show that Dendron achieved a high detection rate for all dataset categories.

6 Performance Analysis

The performance measures are considered when assessing and comparing the QoS model.

- **Precision (P)** = TP/(TP + FP), which is the percentage of classification intrusions that indeed occur
- **Recall (R)** = TP/(TP + FN), which would be the proportion of correctly predicted intrusions to the total intrusions
- **F-Score(F)** = (2/(1/P) + (1/R)), to determine the prediction performance, a trade-off regarding classification accuracy was achieved.

We used different ML algorithms with many evaluation strategies to analyse the KDD dataset and the appropriate subgroups related to performance measures. A reliability subset assessor with the most acceptable search is used to paradigm the datasets. ML frameworks are used to develop and analyse ML methods. The regression metrics are Precision, Recall, and F-Score for unknown testing datasets, shown in Table 4 and Fig. 3.

The technique mentioned in the preceding section combines the features of ML to generate semantically understandable and reliable IDS rules that can predict known attacks of Green Smart Transportation. Furthermore, Dendron can address the

Table 4 Simulation test results

ML classification	Precision	Recall	Accuracy	Test time in seconds
Naive Bayes	0.718	0.682	0.929	37.18
Multilayer Perception	0.827	0.729	0.937	50.18
NBTree	0.891	0.791	0.948	102.34
Random Forest	0.918	0.9387	0.993	367.238

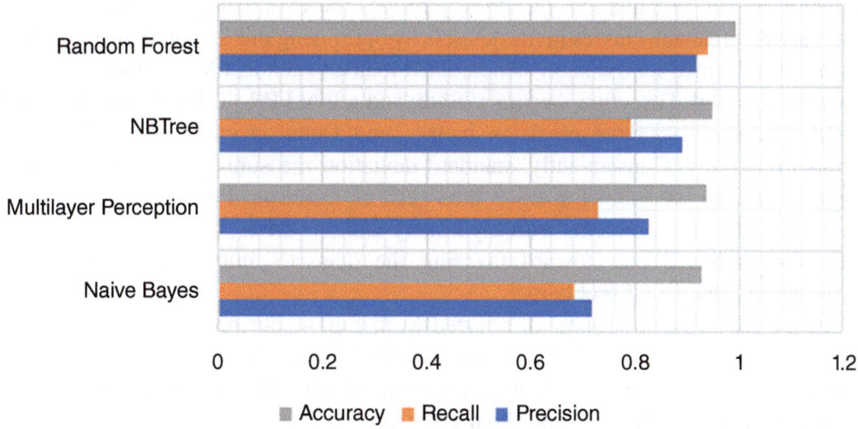

Fig. 3 Analysis of simulation

Table 5 Dendron metrics of training data set in %

Training data set	Accuracy	μ-FM	Average Accuracy	Attacks Accuracy	Attack Detection Rate	False Attack Rate
KDD	98.12	87.19	91.21	89.36	98.91	0.89
NB15	91.16	67.18	71.28	67.19	89.10	0.68

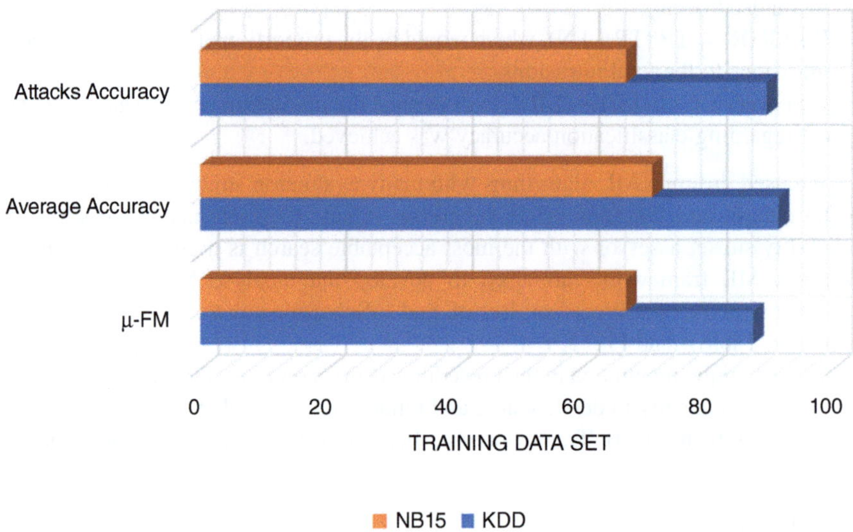

Fig. 4 σ-FM of IDS accuracy

problems network traffic faces according to ML methodologies in MANET. When mixed with the α, β, and γ weights, the distribution possibility function is balanced ML algorithms' propensity to be partial toward the dataset's significant elements of threats—the overall detection measure of σ-FM, which was used as an optimal function in this ML method. Dendron improves the DTs to improve the detection ratio across all attack classes in the datasets by optimising this standard measure. Our plan outperformed its rivals on standardised metrics such as FM, Average, Attacks Accuracy, a high Detection Accuracy Rate, and a low FPR (Table 5). On the other hand, Dendron lacks the precision metric, and Dendron emphasises all dataset groups relatively. Consequently, standard deviation measures become much more significant than precision for algorithms such as Dendron. Prediction accuracy in multi-classification problems with asymmetry datasets arises, for example, when an ML system has a bias toward favoring the dataset's important groups while disregarding the trivial problems.

In the MANET environment, referred to in Fig. 4, our proposed methodology outperforms the standard ML approach. In 98.12% of the regions, the proposed method exceeded the passive approach in terms of reliability. The static method has an accuracy rate of 91.21%, and the **σ** error rate is 87.19%.

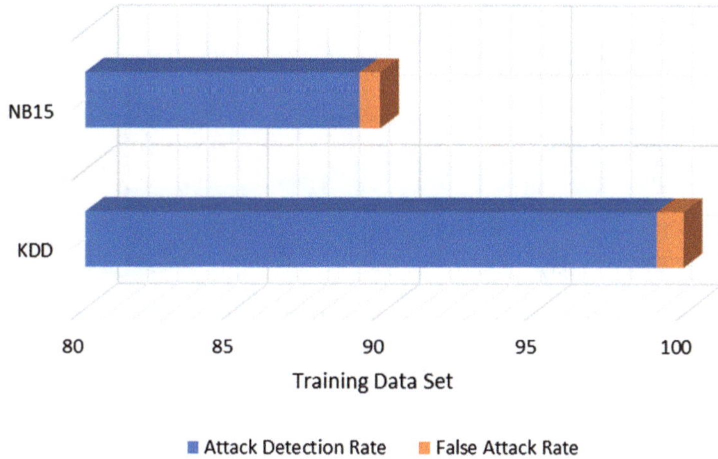

Fig. 5 Attack Detection vs. False Attack Rate

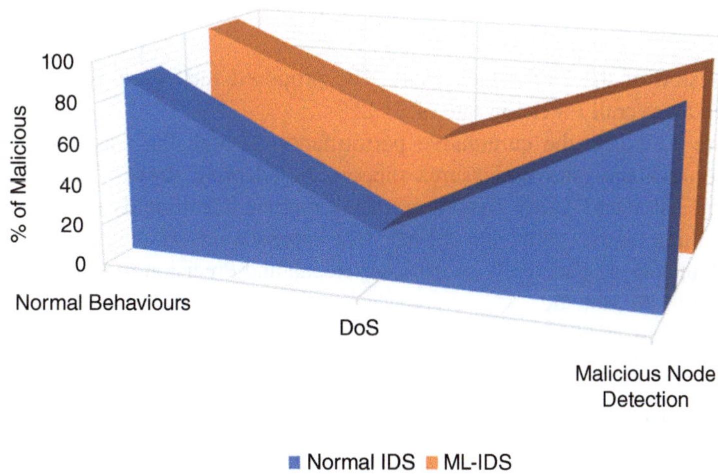

Fig. 6 Performance analysis of Recall

Figure 5 shows the efficiency of the Attack Detection Rate in every 100 nodes. Remember that the Attack Detection Rate demonstrates harmful incidence detectability by explicitly measuring the precision of identifying threats cases. Overall, the adaptive solution achieves a 98.91% of Attack Detection Efficiency.

Besides, Fig. 6 illustrates the total Recall for each class used in the trained datasets. We provide an adjacent comparison of the results of fixed and adaptive approaches to every type. And for the Normal level, the precision of the ML techniques is virtually equal. There are indeed 0.45% variance outcomes in dynamic analysis, and this variation is defined small as if this precision is the mean of the Recall throughout 100 nodes. On the other hand, there is a considerable contrast in

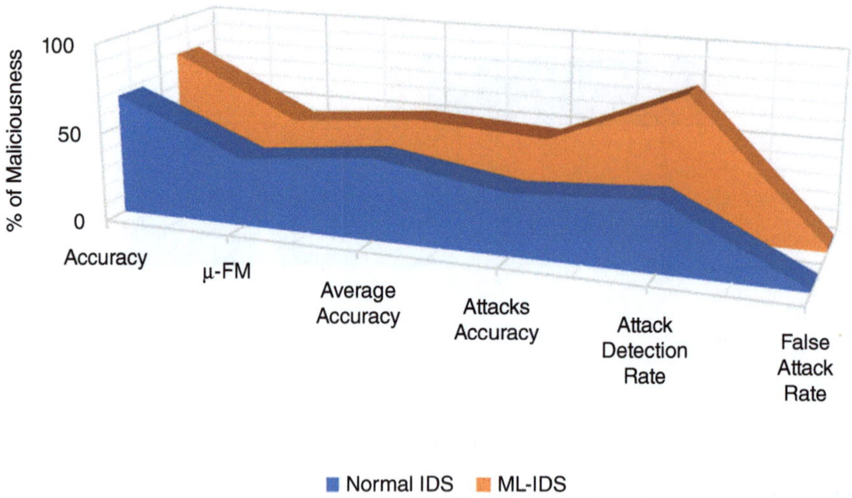

Fig. 7 Performance analysis % of maliciousness

the precision of the DoS attack class. The proposed methodology, in particular, achieved an overall Precision rate of 91.21%.

Figure 7 depicts the cumulative performance of both the adaptive and static processes. All prevention measures support the adaptive strategy's reign. Except for the precision and Attack Detection Ratio parameters thoroughly discussed above, the remaining metrics show that our ML-IDS approach is outstanding. The proposed ML-IDS technique effectively coordinates Recall and Precision in all dataset classes according to the statistic.

7 Conclusion

We required the ML-IDS detection method to use behavioural features to classify faulty events in a Green Smart Transportation MANET environment. Albeit briefly, in this study, the primary IDS, along with its key architecture, enables identification for each targeted 'Maliciousness' system. The evolutionary computing organisation has successfully provided ML-IDS on different test cases. MANET investigates the current state of the art in ML classifiers of KDD. A structured cascade design used to lower the FPR and boost TPR accuracy is 88.39% and 1.94% FPR on KDD by building a series of meta-specialists. Also, ML techniques incorporate modified techniques and are merged to generate meta-specialists. Our research findings ensure our concept's ability to adapt to the new Green Smart Transportation network MANET environment, obtaining ratings that exceed fixed IDS by increasing 73.37%. We claim that our MANET analysis provides new ADR guidelines, as an automatic retraining mechanism can substantially reduce human interference.

References

1. Y. Zhang and W. Lee, "Intrusion Detection in Wireless Ad Hoc Networks," Proceedings of the 6th Annual International Conference on Mobile Computing and Networking (ACM MobiCom'00), Boston, MA, pp. 275–283, Aug. 2000.
2. Y. Huang, W. Fan, W. Lee, and P. S. Yu, "Cross-Feature Analysis for Detecting Ad-hoc Routing Anomalies," Proceedings of the 23rd International Conference on Distributed Computing Systems, Providence, RI, pp. 478–487, May 2003.
3. L. Buczak and E. Guven, "A survey of data mining and machine learning methods for cybersecurity intrusion detection." IEEE Communications Surveys Tutorials, vol. 18, no. 2, pp. 1153–1176, 2016.
4. Yin, C., Zhu, Y., Fei, J., & He, X. (2017). A deep learning approach for intrusion detection using recurrent neural networks. IEEE Access,5, 21954–21961.
5. Tao Ma, Fen Wang, Jianjun Cheng, Yang Yu, and Xiaoyun Chen. A hybrid spectral clustering and deep neural network ensemble algorithm for intrusion detection in sensor networks. Sensors, 16(10), 2016.
6. Sudhakar Sengan, S. Chenthur Pandian, Trustworthy Position-Based Routing to Mitigate against the Malicious Attacks to Signifies Secured Data Packet using Geographic Routing Protocol in MANET, WSEAS Transactions on Communications, vol. 12, no. 11, pp: 584–603, (2013).
7. M. H. Bhuyan, D. K. Bhattacharyya, and J. K. Kalita. Network anomaly detection: Methods, systems, and tools. IEEE Communications Surveys Tutorials, 16(1):303–336, First 2014.
8. Mahbod Tavallaee, Ebrahim Bagheri, Wei Lu, and Ali A. Ghorbani. A detailed analysis of the kdd cup 99 data set. In Proceedings of the Second IEEE International Conference on Computational Intelligence for Security and Defense Applications, CISDA'09, pages 53–58, Piscataway, NJ, USA, 2009. IEEE Press.
9. R. Panigrahi and S. Borah, "A detailed analysis of cicids2017 dataset for designing intrusion detection systems," vol. 7, pp. 479–482, 01 2018.
10. S. Sudhakar, S. Chenthur Pandian, "A Trust and Co-Operative Nodes with Affects of Malicious Attacks and Measure the Performance Degradation on Geographic Aided Routing in Mobile Ad Hoc Network. Life Science Journal, vol. 10, no. 4s, pp: 158–163, (2013).
11. F. Palenzuela, M. Shaffer, M. Ennis, J. Gorski, D. McGrew, D. Yowler, D. White, L. Holbrook, C. Yakopcic, and T. M. Taha, "Multilayer perceptron algorithms for cyberattack detection," pp. 248–252, 2016 IEEE National Aerospace and Electronics Conference and Ohio Innovation Summit, 7 2016.
12. S. Thombre, R. Ul Islam, K. Andersson, and M. S. Hossain, "IP based Wireless Sensor Networks: Performance Analysis using Simulations and Experiments," Journal of Wireless Mobile Networks, Ubiquitous Computing, and Dependable Applications, 7(3):53–76, September 2016.
13. A. L. Buczak and E. Guven, "A Survey of Data Mining and Machine Learning Methods for Cyber Security Intrusion Detection,". IEEE Communications Surveys & Tutorials, 18(2): 1153–1176, October 2015.
14. S. Sudhakar, S. Chenthur Pandian, Secure Packet Encryption and Key Exchange System in Mobile Ad hoc Network, Journal of Computer Science, vol. 8, no. 6, pp: 908–912, (2012)
15. S.Sudhakar, S. Chenthur Pandian, Hybrid Cluster-based Geographical Routing Protocol to Mitigate Malicious Nodes in Mobile Ad Hoc Network, International Journal of Ad Hoc and Ubiquitous Computing, vol. 21, no. 4, pp: 224–236, (2016).
16. Mahbod Tavallaee et al. "A detailed analysis of the KDD CUP 99 data set". In: IEEE Symposium. Computational Intelligence for Security and Defense Applications, CISDA 2 (July 2009).
17. R. Sommer and V. Paxson. "Outside the Closed World: On Using Machine Learning for Network Intrusion Detection". In: 2010 IEEE Symposium on Security and Privacy. May 2010, pp. 305–316.

18. S. Sudhakar, S. Chenthur Pandian.: An Efficient Agent-Based Intrusion Detection System for Detecting Malicious Nodes in MANET Routing, International Review on Computers and Software, vol. 7, no. 6, pp: 3037–304, (2012).
19. S. Sudhakar, S. Chenthur Pandian.: Authorized Node Detection and Accuracy in Position-Based Information for MANET, European Journal of Scientific Research, vol. 70, no. 2, pp: 253–265, (2012).
20. Monowar Bhuyan, Dhruba K Bhattacharyya, and Jugal Kalita. Network Traffic Anomaly Detection and Prevention: Concepts, Techniques, and Tools. Jan. 2017.
21. Tracy Camp, Jeff Boleng, and Vanessa Davies. Wireless Communication and Mobile Computing: Special issue on Mobile Ad Hoc Networking: Research, Trends and Applications. IEEE International Conference on Distributed Computing Systems, 2(5):483–502, September 2002.
22. Dong Seong Kim, Khaja Mohammad Shazzad, and Jong Sou Park. A framework of survivability model for wireless sensor network. IEEE Proceedings of the First International Conference on Availability, Reliability and Security, February 2006.
23. Rahul C. Shah and Jan M. Rabaey. Energy-Aware Routing for Low Energy Ad Hoc Sensor Networks. IEEE Wireless Communications and Networking Conference, 1:350–355, March 2002. Berkeley Wireless Research Center, University of California, Berkeley.
24. Manel Guerrero Zapata and N. Asokan. Secure Routing for Mobile Ad hoc Networks. Proceedings of the 1st ACM workshop on Wireless security, pages 1–10, 2002.
25. Keerthana, N., Viji, Vinod., Sudhakar, Sengan.: A Novel Method for Multi-Dimensional Cluster to Identify the Malicious Users on Online Social Networks, Journal of Engineering Science and Technology, vol. 15, no. 6, pp: 4107–4122, (2020).
26. Priyadarshni, A.U., Sudhakar, S.: "Cluster-Based Certificate Revocation by Cluster Head in Mobile Ad-Hoc Network", International Journal of Applied Engineering Research, vol. 10, no. 20, pp. 16014–16018, (2015).
27. K. Jayanthi, R. Rathinam and S. Pattabhi, "Electrocoagulation treatment for removal of Reactive Blue 19 from aqueous solution using Iron electrode", "Research Journal of Life Sciences, Bioinformatics, Pharmaceutical and Chemical Sciences", 4:2, 101–113 (2018).

A Critical Cloud Security Risks Detection Using Artificial Neural Networks at Banking Sector

R. Velmurugan, R. Kumar, D. Saravanan, Sumagna Patnaik, and Siva Kishore Ikkurthi

1 Introduction

Even though there has been a lot of study and development in cloud computing ventures, many fail miserably, particularly in banking. However, before cloud infrastructure can be broadly adopted, many serious cloud security concerns such as data confidentiality and privacy, quality of services (QoS), portability and interoperability, and mobility must remain managed and mitigated [1]. Furthermore, although cloud infrastructure has several benefits, cloud computing in banking organizations is plagued by numerous cloud protection concerns. Cloud risk assessment aims to detect and assess cloud risks protection problems early on to forecast the extent of cloud computing security [2]. Cloud infrastructure risk assessment has become a common standard for successful banking organizations. New studies have contributed to the cloud computing vulnerability field in enhancing development processes and security. The software project manager and staff will use risk assessment to better cloud infrastructure risks. Both consumer and business customers are

R. Velmurugan (✉) · R. Kumar
Department of Computer Science (PG), Kristu Jayanti College, Bengaluru, India
e-mail: velmurugan@kristujayanti.com; rkumar@kristujayanti.com

D. Saravanan
Department of CSE, IFET College of Engineering, Villupuram, India

S. Patnaik
Department of Information Technology, JB Institute of Engineering and Technology, Hyderabad, India

S. K. Ikkurthi
Department of Civil Engineering, Koneru Lakshmaiah Educational Foundation, Guntur, Andra Pradesh, India
e-mail: i.sivakishore@kluniversity.in

P. Agarwal et al. (eds.), *Artificial Intelligence for Smart Healthcare*,
EAI/Springer Innovations in Communication and Computing,
https://doi.org/10.1007/978-3-031-23602-0_6

rapidly implementing cloud storage. It allows for quick and fast user access, efficiently addresses users' complex and scalable needs, and offers convenient metered use for its services. It may be the ideal solution for healthcare infrastructure. Until Cloud storage can be broadly embraced, many serious concerns surrounding stability, data confidentiality and ownership, service efficiency, and mobility must be addressed. To overcome these challenges, this chapter suggests a new approach that incorporates a technology network specifically tailored to address the problems that arise in an assistive healthcare system. The cloud framework provides a high degree of abstraction within this assistive health architecture, and its resources can be accessed efficiently by consumers through a simple web interface. The current approach involves methods for managing energy demand while ensuring care quality to solve the power constraint problem. An auto-switch network or algorithm may efficiently manage the monitoring duration. Data contexts and context-sensitive implementations would be the newest strategy for dealing with abnormalities in physiological state variations.

To address data ownership, security, and privacy issues, MoCAsH adopts a federated Cloud architecture. MoCAsH presents a federated P2P cloud paradigm to solve data security, ownership, and anonymity. An Assistive Healthcare Infrastructure Mobile Cloud is suggested here. This new design addresses our prior Active Grid infrastructure's flaws. User-friendly connection, elastic resources, infrastructure scaling, and resource metered usage and accounting are all included in the Cloud storage capabilities. Data protection and ownership and concerns about security and privacy are often addressed in the most recent Cloud design. Encryption and data security are addressed using the P2P approach for federating cloud resources belonging to diverse service providers. Parts of the Active Grid infrastructure have been constructed and moved to be used. While there is a lot of study and improvement in cloud computing, many cloud computing initiatives, especially in the banking sector, have a high mistake rate. Furthermore, while cloud computing has many advantages, security concerns are currently plagued. These days, the client's most pressing concern is security. If a customer wishes to benefit from cloud computing fully, the client's information, facilities, and applications must all be secure. However, cloud technology has become the major focus of commercial businesses, which depend on cloud-based applications, storage capacity, and other cloud-based services such as data centers to operate. Cloud technology has a large and beneficial impact on banks since it allows them to be more flexible and analyze and handle services more efficiently.

Cloud risk management has become a common practice among today's most successful banking institutions (Fig. 1). Recent surveys have identified a cloud computing hazard region in the growing effort to improve design methods and safety. Cloud computing hazards may be mitigated more effectively with the help of risk management. Massive processing and storage capacity is provided by integrating numerous shared assets in cloud computing, which has lately advanced quickly. For example, "cloud computing" refers to the ability to satisfy real-time user storing, processor, and program needs over a computer network. The finance department rents a cloud computing system that includes hardware, software, and

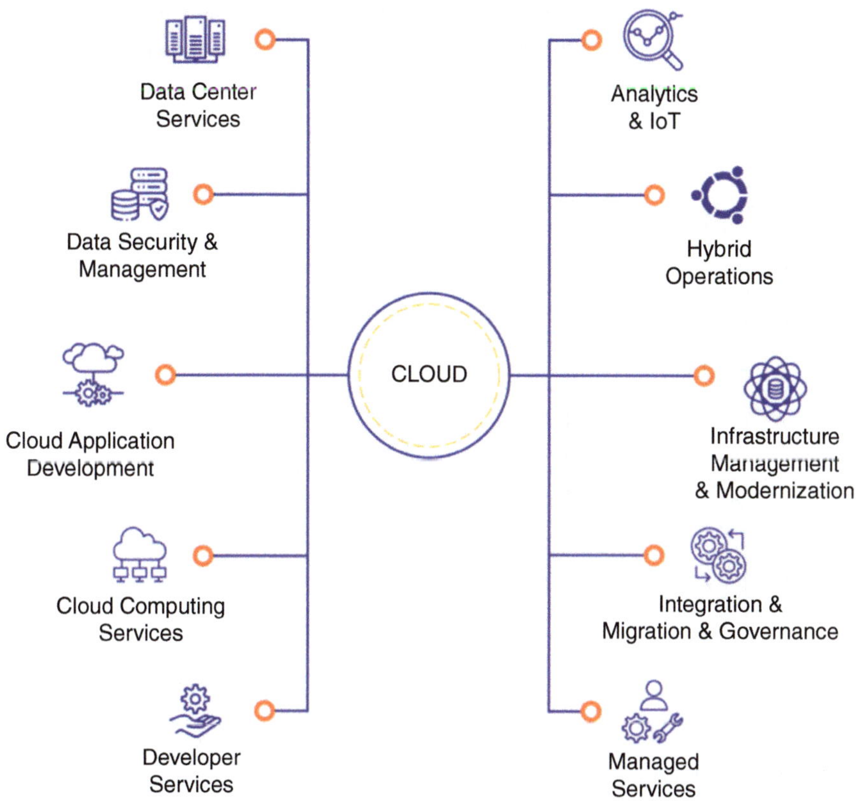

Fig. 1 Critical cloud risk

processes for real-time usage in this scenario. The system is accessible to anybody in the department and from any location using several devices (i.e., PCs, laptops, mobile devices, etc.). Finally, based on secondary research, our chapter aims to identify the major concerns and challenges that banking organizations face in cloud computing. Artificial neural networks (ANNs) remain equivalent to our neural organizations and give a somewhat decent strategy for tackling arrangement and forecast issues. ANN is an assortment of numerical models that may copy organic neural framework properties like versatile human learning. ANNs are comprised of handling components considered neurons associated by joints that incorporate weight coefficients that go about as neurotransmitters in our sensory system. The neurons are typically comprised of three layers: an information layer, at least one hidden layer, and a hidden layer (Fig. 2). The ANN process has been used to learn the process like training, recall, and eliminating the risk related to the cloud application. As a result, neural networks may solve complicated problems like classification and prediction.

ANNs have been effectively employed to tackle various hard and real-world issues in various applications. ANN was proven to be more effective and accurate

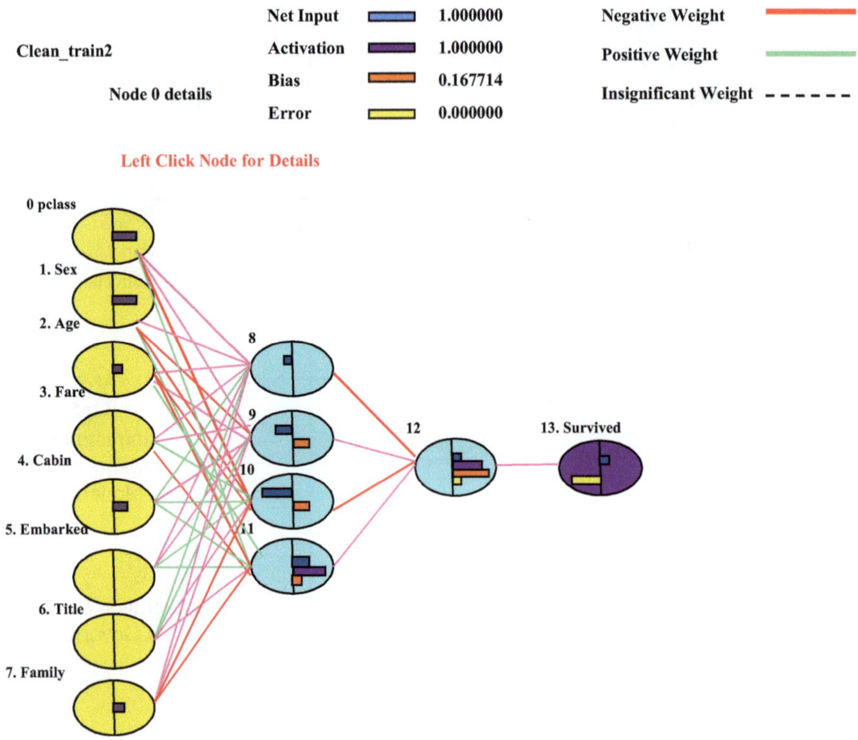

Fig. 2 ANN architecture

than other classification approaches. The categorization of a neural network is separated into two steps. The network must be trained on a dataset initially. The organization is then assessed towards distinguishing the characterizations of a new dataset by changing the associations between neurons. The current work utilized around 70% of the information for network preparation and 30% for network approval. While a wide range of ANNs has been created, feedforward neural networks (FNNs) are the most pervasive and generally utilized. The objective of preparing an FNN numerically is to limit a blunder work E or to recognize a minimizer $w = (w_1, w_2, \ldots, w_n)$ to such an extent that $w = \min E(w)$. When preparing the dataset into a CSV file, some mistakes can be found, which were detected through the classification process.

2 Artificial Neural Networks

Artificial Neural Networks (ANNs) are a subfield of AI (ANN). It's a mathematical model that's aided thru biological brain networks' organization and functioning features. A neural network comprises a connected group of artificial neurons that

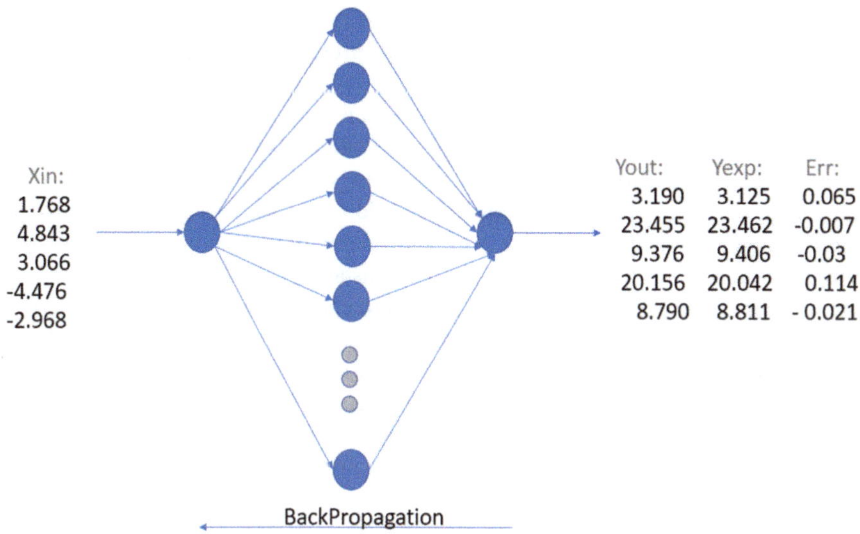

Fig. 3 Neural networks: understanding the non-linearity

process data in a connectionist fashion. In general, an ANN is a self-organizing framework that calibrates its construction dependent on outer or inward information that goes through the organization throughout the learning interaction.

The latest Neural Network model is non-linear; those are finding problems in cloud risk effectively (shown in Fig. 3). They're typically employed to represent complex interactions between inputs and outputs or towards finding data patterns. ANN has been used in a variety of applications with great success. For example, ANN has proven to be effective in prediction, handwritten character recognition, and housing price evaluation. Layers of neurons are common in the brain. Layers are gatherings of neurons that execute comparable capacities. Layers may be divided into three categories. Customer programmers continue to contribute to the data layer, which is still a layer of neurons. Customers' applications get data from neurons in the yield layer. In addition, there are layers of protection between them. The secret layer neurons are linked to different neurons, and they never work straightforwardly with the customer program. Every neuron in a neurological organization can influence handling at any layer. In neuronal organizations, the secret layers are optional. Although the info and yield layers are required, a single layer that serves as both an information and yield layer is viable.

There are two types of ANN learning: directed and undirected. Giving the neural organization an assortment of test information and the normal yields from each of these examples are alluded to as coordinated preparing. The most predominant sort of neural organization preparing is coordinated preparing. The neural organization goes through various cycles, or ages, as coordinated preparing proceeds until the genuine yield approaches the expected yield with a sensible blunder rate. One pass through the preparation tests comprises one emphasis. Undirected preparing is identical to coordinated preparing, yet there are no projected yields. When the neural organization orders the contributions to various groups, this is known as undirected training. As with directed training, the training develops through numerous epochs. As preparation advances, the neural organization finds characterization classifications [3]. The way toward allotting these association loads is known as preparing. The weight framework is generally loaded up with arbitrary numbers in most preparing strategies. The neural network's validity is then checked. The loads are then changed depending on how well the neural organization performed. This progression is rehashed until the approval mistake is under a certain threshold [4]. A neural network should remain assessed to check whether it remains prepared for genuine use when it has been prepared. This last stage is essential in deciding if additional preparation is required. Approval information records should be segregated from preparing information to approve a neural organization [5] effectively. In this chapter, practically 80% of all-out example information was utilized for network preparation. About 20% of the complete example information was utilized for system validation.

3 Literature Survey

The concept "cloud computing risk management" applies to the computing technologies, protocols, and methods that may be utilized to mitigate the risk of cloud computing failure. Risk control is becoming increasingly relevant in several IT-related areas, such as networks, banking data management, and cloud storage [6]. Furthermore, the cloud banking platform is based on economic philosophies and is a resource management model. Its position in the loan and deposit industry is similar to that of commercial banks [7]. Cloud protection is a broad term that refers to any set of rules, controls, and technology used to protect data, resources, and networks from various threats. Furthermore, recent analysis has concentrated on security solutions rather than market characteristics such as service reliability, affordability, and consistency [8]. This research will forecast critical cloud problems in Malaysian banking institutions. They suggested a conceptual architecture for cloud security banking, encompassing banking security, legal, privacy, enforcement, and regulatory concerns [9]. To begin with, versatility refers to the ability to move and take part in various places and at different times using some portable computers, such as mobile phones, PDAs, and wireless notebooks. Finally, CDM can be divided into four distinct types: A third party providing cloud services makes public cloud services available to the public or a large business community [9]. A single entity or corporation operates and owns a private cloud, which focuses on managing virtualizing infrastructure and automating facilities that remain utilized and customized for several lines of business and important classes. In terms of the target audience, community clouds dip somewhere between public and private clouds [10]. This model uses a select community of individuals inside an organization who have the same concerns, priorities, or protection standards [11]. Hybrid cloud

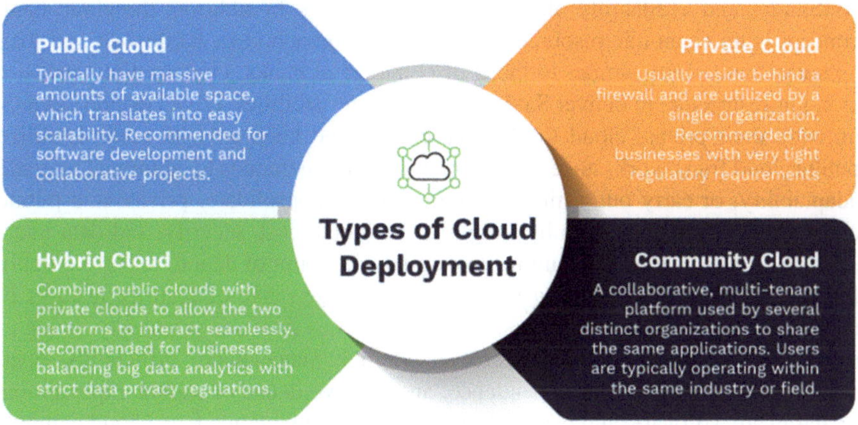

Fig. 4 Types of cloud deployment

combines public and private cloud approaches, blending the technical notions of public cloud systems with the private cloud's foundation. Fourth, Cloud Risk Management (CRM): risk must be considered in all stages of interactions and examined at any operation level about the belongings that must be covered in Cloud computing [12]. Aside from that, there are a variety of risks that bank management should be aware of. The biggest risk for many banks is credit risk, but there are many other threats with which supervisory authorities must inform banks and compel them to comply [13]. One of the determining variables is the Cloud Portal since the success of the whole framework is largely reliant on the simplicity with which customers will access provided resources. Registered users can check the status and data of remote sensors. The cloud platform may be used to monitor distant mobile devices, update context-aware rules, alter emergencies, and perform other vital tasks. Only registered clients access the portal, which resembles a website's back-end operations center and connects to a back-end servers network. Furthermore, medical data in healthcare settings is sensitive, and its security must be ensured. Policy-driven policies must be implemented depending on the program, climate, and user situations to address this issue. When a nurse or doctor needs rapid access to "hidden" data to offer proper emergency reaction, the context-aware module can make an intelligent judgment that may jeopardize patient confidentiality. These and other difficulties must be addressed successfully by the Cloud Portal (Shown in Fig. 4).

Cloud computing is frequently linked to failures. In the distributed computing life cycle, a hazard of disappointment is characterized as the chance of misfortune or openness. Computer hazards are decreasing cloud functionality, so application accuracy has been decreasing. Any combination of policies, tools, and processes used to defend data, infrastructure, and services against cyber-attacks is included under the umbrella term "cloud security," which is still rather wide. Prior research concentrated on supplying security technology rather than service reliability, continuity, and availability; this is a significant shift. In addition, the cloud bank concept is an economic resource management approach [14]. Its deposit and loan operations are pretty similar to those of commercial banks. Organizations that use cloud infrastructure to deliver SaaS have several possibilities. IT can decide towards utilizing their private cloud to alleviate chance and keep up with control, utilize public cloud framework, stage, or examination administrations to additional upgrade adaptability, or carry out a mixed-race model that consolidates private and public cloud resources and services by weighing workload, cost, security, and data interoperability [15]. Cloud computing stores a large amount of data to retrieve quickly for later use. Cloud computing is capable of a wide range of security features in addition to storage. In recent years, cloud storage has grown in popularity owing to several advantages, including decreased storage management difficulties, open access with geographical independence, and the avoidance of capital expenditures on hardware, software, and personal maintenance, to mention a few. Cloud computing is gaining traction in the public sector [16]. However, security is always a concern [17]. This research will highlight the most critical cloud concerns and problems for banking institutions [4].

For predicting the tumor category, an artificial Neural Network model was proposed. The model was trained using the feedforward backpropagation algorithm. The model's factors were derived from a data set representing patient test results. The model was put to the test, with a total score of 76.67%. This study demonstrated the artificial neural network's ability to determine tumor kind based on a body test. Artificial Neural Networks (ANN) are computer components that simulate how the human mind analyses and measures data. They remain the premise of Artificial Intelligence (AI). Also, they handle what would be unthinkable or hard to answer utilizing human or factual strategies. As more information opens, ANN can self-learn and convey better outcomes [18]. Artificial Neural Networks (ANN) remain opening the way to forever-changing advances in all areas of the economy to be created. The old way of doing things is being disturbed by AI stages based on ANN. Computer-based intelligence stages improve exchanges and make administrations open to everyone at nominal costs, from understanding destinations into various lingos to having a modest assistant shop staple merchandise online to bantering with chatbots to handle issues [19].

ANNs are expected to take after the human psyche, with neuron centers interconnected in a web-like model. A significant number of neurons make up the human frontal cortex. Each neuron has a cell body responsible for storing and transporting information to and from the mind (sources and yields). Preparing units, coupled by hubs, contain hundreds or thousands of artificial neurons in an ANN. Info and yield units make up these preparing units. The information units get various structures and designs of data due to an inward weighing instrument. The neural organization learns about the data presented to create one yield report. Backpropagation, which is short for reverse engendering of error, is a set of learning standards used by ANNs to complete their yield outcomes in the same way that people go through rules and rules to accompany an outcome or yield. The ANN model goes through a stage of preparation in which it figures out how to perceive designs in information, regardless of whether outwardly, perceptually, or abstractly. During this managed stage, the association analyzes its absolute respect for its delivery, like the best yield. To change the mistake between the two yields, backpropagation is utilized. This infers that the affiliation works in reverse from the yield unit to the information unit, expanding the meaning of its connection between the units until the distinction between the natural and organized result is considered the littlest measure of blunder [20].

3.1 Cloud Computing Modeling Concepts for Banking Organizations

A cloud-based security service paradigm was used instead. Virtualization, multi-tenant, and data protection in service management methods were all modeled differently. It is necessary to have a general model of quantitative risk management for cloud computing, even though distinct security controls and methods are still in place for each component of cloud computing. The platform model offered risk assessment methodologies for determining cloud computing threats. Cloud users and suppliers can utilize linear, iterative, and incremental techniques to handle and explain cloud dangers. According to prior research, the cloud computing framework may be divided into five stages: mobility and financial apps, cloud services, cloud deployment, cloud risk management, and cloud security:

3.2 Cloud Security Issues

"On-demand" compute is possible with all four types of cloud computing. If you're looking to get your hands-on cloud banking services (BPAAS), then you'll need to go no farther than Amazon Web Services, Microsoft Azure, and Google Cloud Platform. However, in this section [21], the description of fundamental security problems in cloud banking should be highlighted: Policies and 3rd Parties (Providers) Security Concerns: Standards, Service Level Agreements (SLAs), Governance, Legality, and Regulation are all issues that need to be addressed. Cloud service providers should maintain standards, service, and risk protection; those are the top cloud security issues for better access. As a result, diverse types of resource pricing exist. In this sense, several irrational pricing strategies can cause some resources to be overloaded, whereas others appear to be idle. These circumstances prevent the capital from being used to its full potential (Fig. 5).

Meanwhile, an irrational price policy would make sure resource owners make big gains whilst others lose money. As a fair lever, the price would lose its ability to change capital allocation in the above scenario. The leading technology in Cloud Computing is resource pricing. Furthermore, resource pricing may have a significant

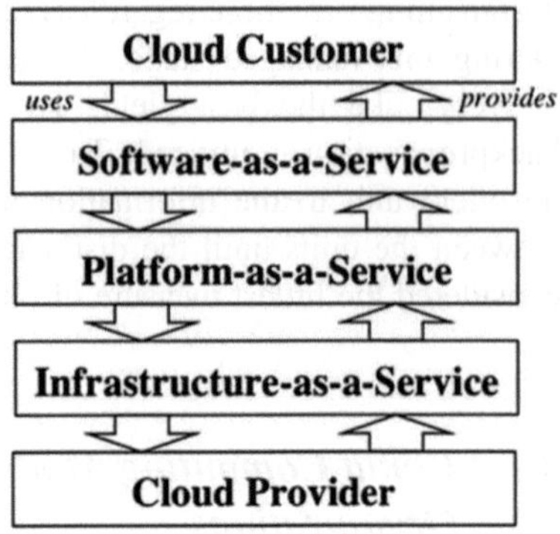

Fig. 5 Cloud risk and issues

impact on resource distribution. As a result, this chapter introduces a Cloud Bank model to aid in resource pricing analysis. Cloud Bank is an example of an IaaS programmer. The Cloud Bank approves the RC's resource-renting applications and provides an interest rate, after which it enters a deal with the RC and makes the services available. The cloud provider interface layer acts as the gateway to the cloud service. Mobile terminals and cloud-based healthcare portals need access to this network tier to interface with back-end cloud computing services. If the ID of a high-priority data request matches one in the service repository, it can be handled ahead of time. The resource manager then executes the job by allocating unique virtual execution services in the virtual resource layer. These virtual execution resources are typically discrete ecosystems where underlying physical resources perform, manage, and provide consumer applications.

4 Methodology (Materials and Methods)

Managers and cloud developers in banking organizations, on the other hand, are supplying the data for this study, which will be incorporated into the modeling. Artificial Neural Networks are recommended for predicting cloud protection issues in banking organizations (ANNs). Cloud computing security standards may be monitored and forecasted using artificial neural networks.

- Using the Cloud Delphi Technique, collect and prepare data for cloud protection problems.
- Using protection templates, assign a chance of incidence and magnitude to cloud security problems.
- Build a network overview.
- Train the neural network: The neural network is trained using a Cloud Delphi dataset with known output data instances.

- Bring the network to the test: A learned neural network is put to the test to see how accurately it predicts known and unknown performance values.
- Evaluate the performance effects of CSI using artificial neural networks to predict cloud protection problems. To predict an undefined performance value, a qualified neural network is used.

It contains several parameters thought to influence tumor classification. These elements were carefully examined and coordinated into a manageable quantity suitable for computer coding within the ANN modeling framework. These elements have been labeled as input variables. The output variables represent the projected tumor classification based on those inputs. Several characteristics that affect customer response were defined by looking thoroughly into the car kinds and soliciting the experience of human specialists on car execution. Inside the Just Neural Network (JNN) climate, these boundaries were painstakingly explored and adjusted into a helpful number reasonable for PC coding. The automobile data set contains 1728 instances. The data was then separated into two groups: training and validation. The data set was utilized for training the ANN model, then the validation data set was used to validate it. Furthermore, the factors' importance was examined, and the most influential element was identified. Non-linear models such as neural networks may be utilized to understand the relationship between inputs and outputs. They may be utilized in classification, function approximation, forecasting, clustering, and optimization, just to name a few. Static and dynamic neural organizations are the two kinds of neural organizations. In this examination, 768 informational collections are utilized to prepare static neural organizations to connect factors like relative conservativeness, rooftop region, general tallness, surface region, coating region, divider region, coating region dissemination of a structure, direction, and the structure's warming and cooling loads. It is done with the assistance of the NN Tool. It picks Heating Load and Cooling Load as yield factors (multi-yield) for preparing. To anticipate Heating and Cooling Load, it utilized eight info factors, three secret layers, and one yield.

4.1 Neural Network

Neural networks can efficiently operate cloud risk analysis in every field with intelligent operations. These are made up of trillions of neurons (nerve cells) exchanging action potentials and short electrical pulses. As seen in Fig. 6, the system is a multilayer perceptron neural network with a linear sigmoid function.

PC calculations that mimic these organic constructions are officially alluded to as fake neural organizations to isolate them from the soft things inside creatures. The majority of academics and architects, on the other hand, are less formal and use the term brain organization to refer to both biological and nonbiological systems

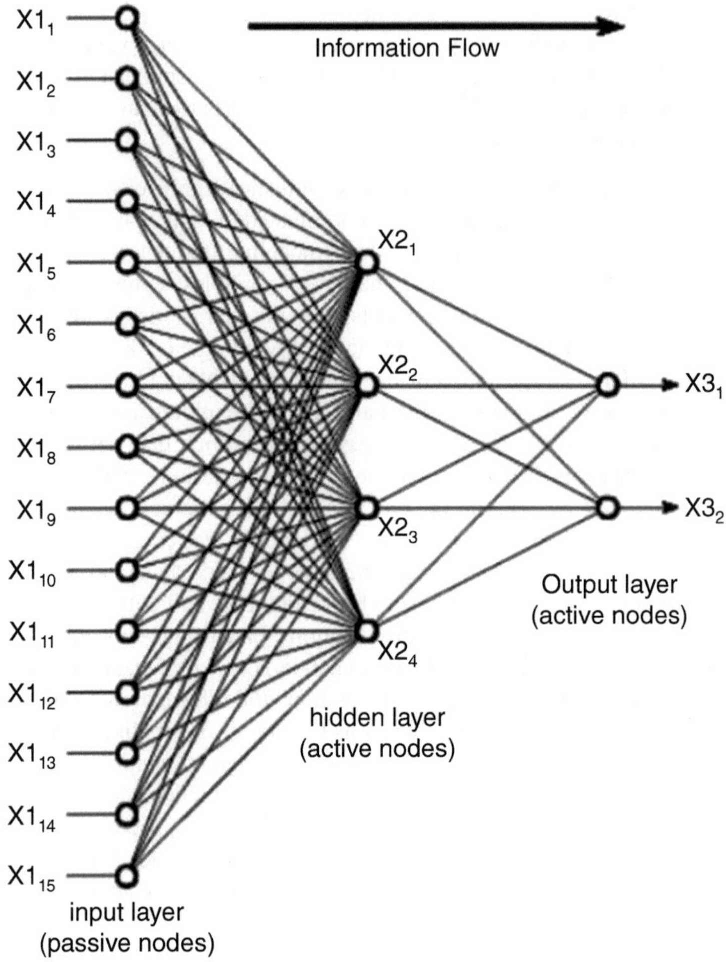

Fig. 6 The architecture of an Artificial Neural System

[22]. Two goals drive neural network research: a deeper comprehension of the human mind and improved PCs that adapt to extract and inadequately characterize issues. Ordinary PCs, for instance, experience issues getting discourse and recognizing individuals' appearances [23]. On the other hand, humans excel at these activities [24].

Table 1 MSE and Correlation results for the three forms are seen

Forms	Models	Training data (input) %	MSE	*R*
Preparation	29	72	4.94162 × e-7	9.95215 × e-1
Authentication	7	17	8.75809 × e-6	9.79264 × e-1
Challenging	7	17	1.95370 × e-5	9.49603 × e-1

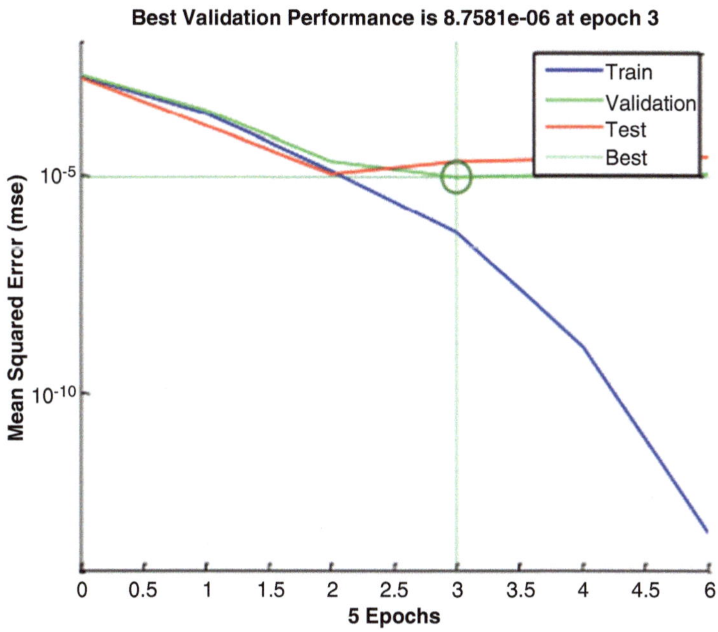

Fig. 7 The design and equations of the ANN scheme, as well as its development

5 Outcomes and Discussion

The Levenberg–Marquardt-based Back Propagation (LMBP) Systems, which are non-linear optimizations, were utilized to foresee the implications of the changes. Because of this, the MSE and regression (*R*) principles are listed in Table 1 for Training, Validation, and Testing purposes, respectively [25–31].

Table 1 demonstrates the cumulative MSE, which shows the proportion square root among the output information and targets information, and Regression (*R*), which tests similarity among the actual output's information to targets information for study planning, measurement, and assessment. The measurement accurateness is observed when *R* values are equal to 1. Consequently, utilizing (LMBP) algorithms to condition the dataset, the findings were obtained in three epochs with 10 concealed neurons harvests [32–37]. The outcomes revealed that the LMBP systems are good at calculating and training networks, as seen in Fig. 7.

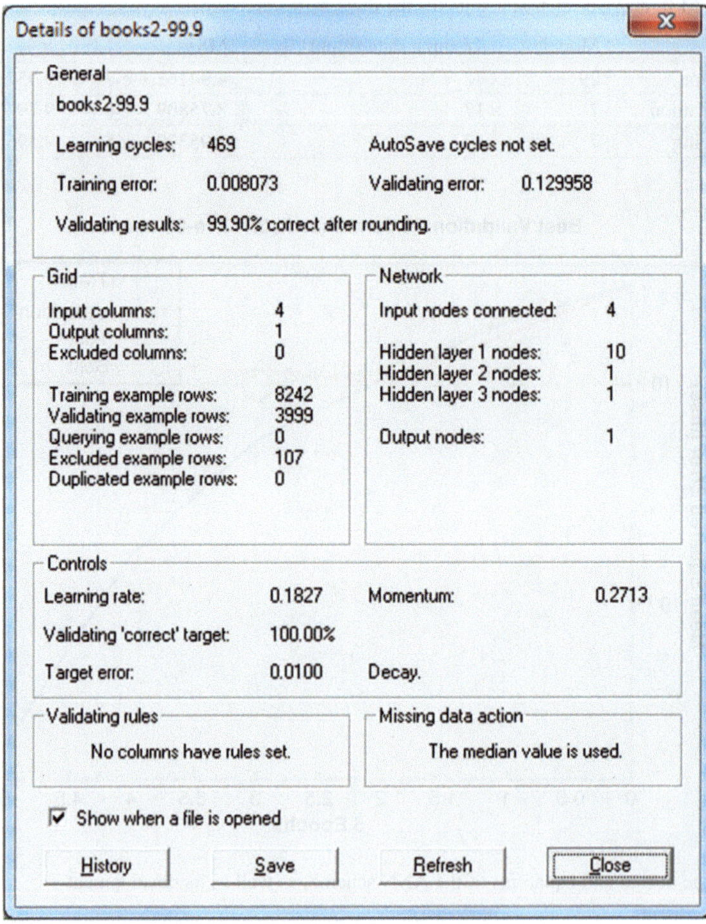

Fig. 8 Performance of LMBP Algorithm (MSE vs. Epochs)

Indeed, it has been learned to calculate network output using MATLAB R2013b's LMBP algorithms [38–41]. In addition, Fig. 8 shows the highest validation score of 0.0000087581 at epoch. Figure 9 shows the error histogram of 20 bins. As a result, the association between outputs and goals is calculated using regression *R* values. As a result, as seen in Fig. 8, the outputs and priorities are perfectly aligned in the regression analysis map. Moreover, a value of 1 indicates a close association between outputs and priorities, while a zero indicates a random correlation. The utility of the LMBP, Non-linear optimum models are used in order to evaluate the prediction method's accuracy, is calculated using the Mean Square Error (MSE). The performance is good if the MSE is bad [42–45]. Since cloud technology allows clients to dynamically scale up and scale down assets while in implementation or

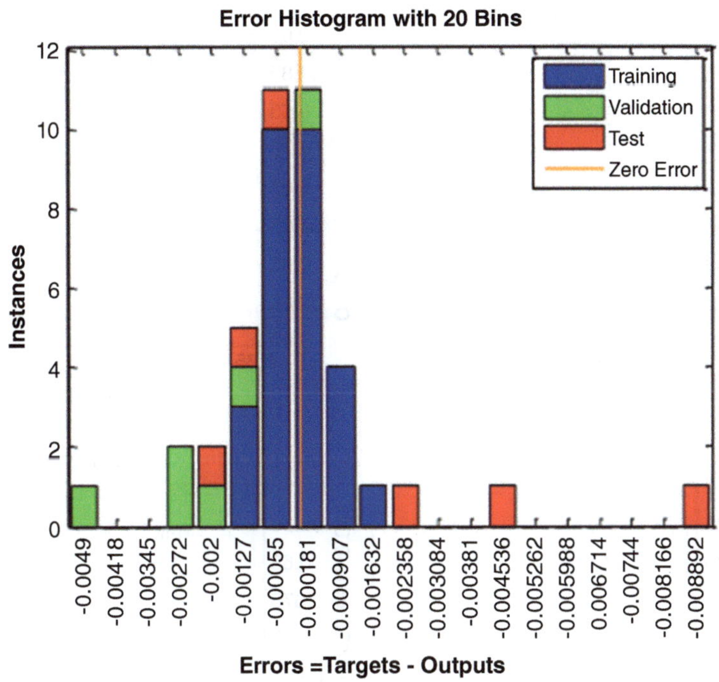

Fig. 9 LMBP-based error histogram of 20 bins

completely customize mobile apps by obtaining administrator rights without interrupting processes, it is currently the most promising implementation of utility registering in the corporate world [46–49]. It spread multiple computational activities through many computers in a pool resource. In cloud infrastructure, the delivery modes may be used to distribute services. The cloud infrastructure technology method is currently delivering support.

Figure 10 clearly explains target vs. range analysis; in this, at different levels, training, testing, validations, and ranging had been getting more improvement. The data, Fitness function, and Y-T curves differentiate the methodology.

6 Conclusion

This study uses Artificial Neural Network (ANN) algorithms to forecast important cloud computing security issues. However, Back Propagation (BP) Equations that are Levenberg–Marquardt based are presented to forecast cloud security level performance. The LMBP algorithm is also used to measure and assess the accuracy of cloud protection level prediction. Artificial neural networks (ANNs) are more

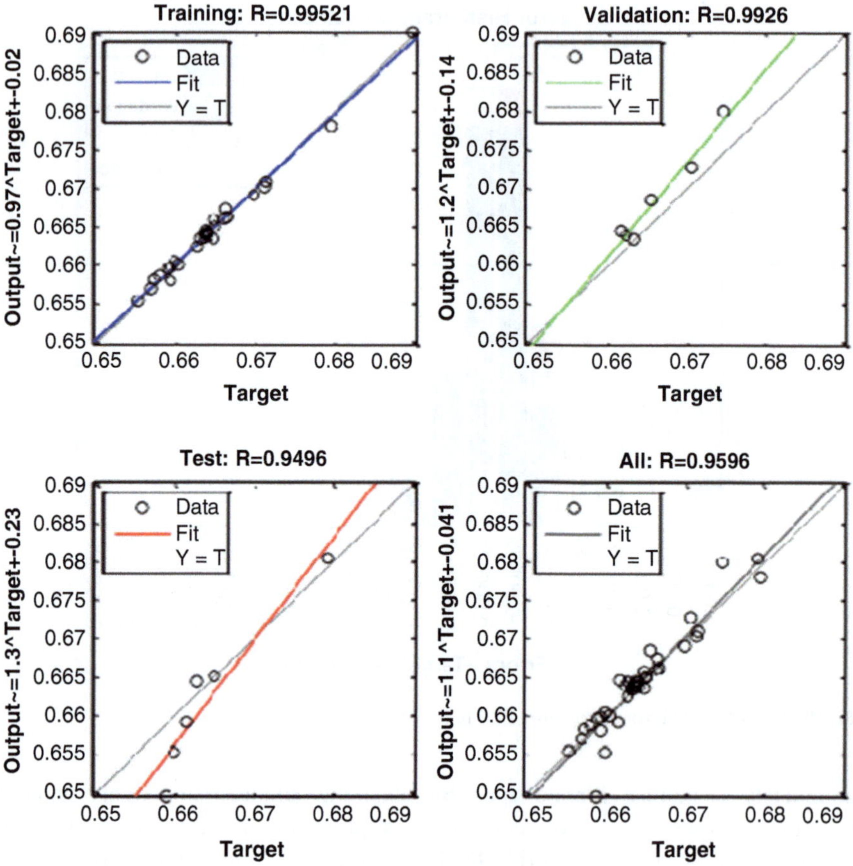

Fig. 10 Regression study plot-Levenberg-Marquardt backpropagation system

effective to improve efficiency and learning neural membership functions. Indeed, LMBP is used to assess the efficiency of cloud protection to get the best results in the forecasting models. Data collection and analysis used the cloud Delphi methodology in this chapter. Based on their experience with cloud computing in the banking industry, 40 bankers' data were designated from both inside and outside Malaysian banking organizations for this study. The performance measures like accuracy 98.76%, sensitivity 97.34%, Recall 94.53%, and F measure 97.82% had been attained. These results outperform the methodology and compete with current techniques.

References

1. Hoang, D. B., & Chen, L. Mobile cloud for assistive healthcare (MoCAsH). In 2010 IEEE Asia Pacific Services Computing Conference, pp. 325–332. IEEE (2010).
2. J. Miler and J. Górski, "Supporting Team Risk Management in Software Procurement and Development Projects," in 4th National Conference on Software Engineering, pp. 1–15 (2002).
3. Mounzer, J., Alpcan, T., & Bambos, N. Integrated security risk management for IT-intensive organizations. In 2010 Sixth International Conference on Information Assurance and Security, pp. 329–334. IEEE (2010).
4. IEEE. Li, H., Pu, Y., & Lu, J. A cloud computing resource pricing strategy research-based on resource swarm algorithm. In 2012 International Conference on Computer Science and Service System, pp. 2217–2222 (2012).
5. Gao, Z., Li, Y., Tang, H., & Zhu, Z. Management process based cloud service security model (2013).
6. Alemu, M., & Omer, A. Cloud computing conceptual security framework for banking industry. Journal of Emerging Trends in Computing and Information Sciences, 5(12), 921–930 (2014).
7. Alzahrani, A., Alalwan, N., & Sarrab, M. Mobile cloud computing: advantage, disadvantage and open challenge. In Proceedings of the 7th Euro American Conference on Telematics and Information Systems, pp. 1–4, (2014).
8. Aruna, E., Shri, A. A., & Lakkshmanan, A. Security concerns and risk at different levels in Cloud Computing. In 2013 International Conference on Green Computing, Communication and Conservation of Energy, pp. 743–746). IEEE (2013).
9. Beckers, K., Schmidt, H., Kuster, J. C., & Faßbender, S. Pattern-based support for context establishment and asset identification of the ISO 27000 in the field of cloud computing. In 2011 Sixth International Conference on Availability, Reliability and Security (pp. 327–333). IEEE (2011).
10. Goyal, S. Public vs private vs hybrid vs community-cloud computing: a critical review. International Journal of Computer Network and Information Security, 6(3), 20 (2014).
11. Khrisna, A. Risk management framework with COBIT 5 and risk management framework for cloud computing integration. In 2014 International Conference of Advanced Informatics: Concept, Theory and Application, pp. 103–108). IEEE (2014).
12. Kiran, M., Jiang, M., Armstrong, D. J., & Djemame, K. Towards a service lifecycle based methodology for risk assessment in cloud computing. In 2011 IEEE Ninth International Conference on Dependable, Autonomic and Secure Computing (pp. 449–456). IEEE (2011).
13. Ahmadalinejad, M., & Hashemi, S. M. A national model to supervise virtual banking systems through the Bank 2.0 approach. Advances in Computer Science: An International Journal, 4(1), 83–93 (2015).
14. Al-Anzi, F. S., Yadav, S. K., & Soni, J. Cloud computing: Security model comprising governance, risk management and compliance. In 2014 International Conference on Data Mining and Intelligent Computing, pp. 1–6). IEEE (2014).
15. Saikumar, K., & Rajesh, V. Coronary blockage of artery for Heart diagnosis with DT Artificial Intelligence Algorithm. International Journal of Research in Pharmaceutical Sciences, 11(1), 471–479 (2020).
16. Saikumar, K., Rajesh, V. A novel implementation heart diagnosis system based on random forest machine learning technique International Journal of Pharmaceutical Research 12, pp. 3904–3916 (2020)
17. Elzamly, A., Hussin, B., Abu Naser, S., Khanfar, K., Doheir, M., Selamat, A., & Rashed, A. A new conceptual framework modelling for cloud computing risk management in banking organizations. International Journal of Grid and Distributed Computing, 9(9), 137–154 (2016).
18. Elzamly, A., & Hussin, B. Classification of Critical Cloud Computing Security Issues for Banking Organizations: A Cloud Delphi Study. International Journal of Grid and Distributed Computing, 9(8), 137–158 (2016).

19. B. Ibrahim and A. Shanavas, "An Approach to Predict SOA Security Vulnerabilities using Feed Forward Artificial Neural Networks," SIJ Trans. Comput. Networks Commun. Eng., vol. 3, no. 4, pp. 54–58 (2015).
20. Ramaiah, V. S., Singh, B., Raju, A. R., Reddy, G. N., Saikumar, K., & Ratnayake, D. Teaching and learning based 5G cognitive radio application for future application. In 2021 International Conference on Computational Intelligence and Knowledge Economy, pp. 31–36). IEEE (2021).
21. Mohammad, M. N., Kumari, C. U., Murthy, A. S. D., Jagan, B. O. L., & Saikumar, K. Implementation of online and offline product selection system using FCNN deep learning: Product analysis. Materials Today: Proceedings, 45, 2171–2178 (2021).
22. K. Raju, A. Sampath Dakshina Murthy, B. Chinna Rao, Sindhura Bhargavi, G. Jagga Rao, K. Madhu, K. Saikumar. A Robust and Accurate Video Watermarking System Based on SVD Hybridation For Performance Assessment International Journal of Engineering Trends and Technology, 68(7), 19–24 (2020).
23. Abu-Naser, S. S. Predicting learners performance using artificial neural networks in linear programming intelligent tutoring system (2012).
24. Abu-Naser, S. S., Zaqout, I. S., Abu Ghosh, M., Atallah, R. R., & Alajrami, E. Predicting student performance using artificial neural network: In the faculty of engineering and information technology (2015).
25. Padmini, G. R., Rajesh, O., Raghu, K., Sree, N. M., & Apurva, C. Design and analysis of 8-bit ripple Carry Adder using nine Transistor Full Adder. In 2021 7th International Conference on Advanced Computing and Communication Systems, Vol. 1, pp. 1982–1987. IEEE (2021).
26. U. Zulfiqar, S. Mohy-Ul-Din, A. Abu-Rumman, A. E. M. Al-Shraah, And I. Ahmed, "Insurance-Growth Nexus: Aggregation and Disaggregation," The Journal of Asian Finance, Economics and Business, vol. 7, no. 12, pp. 665–675, Dec. (2020).
27. Al-Shqairat, Z. I., Al Shraah, A. E. M., Abu-Rumman, A., "The role of critical success factors of knowledge stations in the development of local communities in Jordan: A managerial perspective," Journal of management Information and Decision Sciences, vol. 23, no. 5, pp. 510–526, (2020).
28. Abu-Rumman, Ayman. "Transformational leadership and human capital within the disruptive business environment of academia." World Journal on Educational Technology: Current Issues 13, no. 2: 178–187 (2021).
29. Almomani, Reham Zuhier Qasim, Lina Hamdan Mahmoud Al-Abbadi, Amani Rajab Abed Alhaleem Abu Rumman, Ayman Abu-Rumman, and Khaled Banyhamdan. "Organizational Memory, Knowledge Management, Marketing Innovation and Cost of Quality: Empirical Effects from Construction Industry in Jordan." Academy of Entrepreneurship Journal 25, no. 3: 1528–2686 (2019).
30. Alshawabkeh, Rawan, Amani Abu Rumman, Lina Al-Abbadi, and Ayman Abu-Rumman. "The intervening role of ambidexterity in the knowledge management project success connection." Problems and Perspectives in Management 18, no. 3: 56 (2020).
31. Surinder Singh and Hardeep Singh Saini "Security Techniques for Wormhole Attack in Wireless Sensor Network", International Journal of Engineering & Technology, Vol. 7, No. 2.23, 59–62 (2018).
32. Abu-Rumman, Ayman. "Gaining competitive advantage through intellectual capital and knowledge management: an exploration of inhibitors and enablers in Jordanian Universities." Problems and Perspectives in Management 16, no. 3: 259–268 (2018).
33. Surinder Singh and Hardeep Singh Saini "Security for Internet of Thing (IoT) based Wireless Sensor Networks", Journal of Advanced Research in Dynamical and Control Systems, 06-Special Issue, 1591–1596 (2018).
34. Surinder Singh and Hardeep Singh Saini "Security approaches for data aggregation in Wireless Sensor Networks against Sybil Attack," 2018 Second International Conference on Inventive Communication and Computational Technologies, pp. 190–193, Coimbatore, India (2018).

35. Abu-Rumman, A. Al Shraah, F. Al-Madi, T. Alfalah, "Entrepreneurial networks, entrepreneurial orientation, and performance of small and medium enterprises: are dynamic capabilities the missing link?" Journal of Innovation and Entrepreneurship. Vol 10 Issue 29, pp 1–16, (2021).
36. A.Al Shraah, A. Abu-Rumman, F. Al Madi, F.A. Alhammad, A.A. AlJboor, "The impact of quality management practices on knowledge management processes: a study of a social security corporation in Jordan" The TQM Journal. Vol. ahead-of-print No. Issue ahead-of- print, (2021).
37. Abu-Rumman, A. Al Shraah, F. Al-Madi, T. Alfalah, "The impact of quality framework application on patients' satisfaction", International Journal of Human Rights in Healthcare, Vol. ahead-of-print No. Issue ahead-of- print. (2021).
38. Zafar, S.Z., Zhilin, Q., Malik, H., Abu-Rumman, A., Al Shraah, A., Al-Madi, F. and Alfalah, T. F., "Spatial spillover effects of technological innovation on total factor energy efficiency: taking government environment regulations into account for three continents", Business Process Management Journal, Vol. 27 No. 6, pp. 1874–1891 (2021).
39. Hassan, M.I., Fouda, M.A., Hammad, K.M. and Hasaballah, A.I. Effects of midgut bacteria and two protease inhibitors on the transmission of Wuchereria bancrofti by the mosquito vector, Culex pipiens. Journal of the Egyptian Society of Parasitology. 43(2): 547–553 (2013).
40. F. J. John Joseph, R. T, and J. J. C, "Classification of correlated subspaces using HoVer representation of Census Data," in 2011 International Conference on Emerging Trends in Electrical and Computer Technology, pp. 906–911 (2011).
41. S. Bhoumik, S. Chatterjee, A. Sarkar, A. Kumar, and F. J. John Joseph, "Covid 19 Prediction from X Ray Images Using Fully Connected Convolutional Neural Network," in CSBio '20: Proceedings of the Eleventh International Conference on Computational Systems-Biology and Bioinformatics, pp. 106–107 (2020).
42. Fouda, M.A., Hassan, M.I., Hammad, K.M. and Hasaballah, A.I. Effects of midgut bacteria and two protease inhibitors on the reproductive potential and midgut enzymes of Culex pipiens infected with Wuchereria bancrofti. Journal of the Egyptian Society of Parasitology. 43(2): 537–546 (2013).
43. J. Kubiczek and B. Hadasik, "Challenges in Reporting the COVID-19 Spread and its Presentation to the Society," J. Data and Information Quality, vol. 13, no. 4, pp. 1–7, (2021).
44. Hasaballah, A.I. Toxicity of some plant extracts against vector of lymphatic filariasis, Culex pipiens. Journal of the Egyptian Society of Parasitology. 45(1): 183–192 (2015).
45. Thowfeek MH, Samsudeen, SN, Sanjeetha, MBF. Drivers of Artificial Intelligence in Banking Service Sectors, Solid State Technology; 63(5): 6400 – 6411 (2020).
46. Samsudeen SN, Thowfeek MH, Rashida, MF. School Teachers' Intention to Use E-Learning Systems in Sri Lanka: A Modified TAM Approach, International Journal of Information and Knowledge Management; 5(4), 55–59 (2015).
47. G. S. Sajja, K. P. Rane, K. Phasinam, T. Kassanuk, E. Okoronkwo, and P. Prabhu, "Towards applicability of blockchain in agriculture sector," Materials Today: Proceedings, (2021).
48. H. Pallathadka, M. Mustafa, D. T. Sanchez, G. Sekhar Sajja, S. Gour, and M. Naved, "Impact of machine learning on management, healthcare and agriculture," Materials Today: Proceedings, (2021).
49. Guna Sekhar Sajja, Malik Mustafa, R. Ponnusamy, Shokhjakhon Abdufattokhov, Murugesan G., Dr. P. Prabhu, "Machine Learning Algorithms in Intrusion Detection and Classification", Annals of RSCB, vol. 25, no. 6, pp. 12211–12219, (2021).

A Solution to Pose Change Challenge: Real-Time, Robust, and Adaptive Human Tracking Systems Using SURF

Anshul Pareek and Poonam Kadian

1 Vision-Based Tracking

How do we feel about the world we live in? It is by looking and seeing. There are countless objects present in our surrounding environment with their impressions. Vision can be better explained as a way to understand the environment that surrounds us. Even after decades, the exact working of the visual system is a mystery for the scientist involved in its investigation. When eye based vision in living creatures is replaced by computational instruments it is defined as computer vision. In other words, computer vision is artificial mimicry of vision in living creatures, where digital images and videos which are captured by cameras are further analyzed by computers obtaining an optimum level of understanding from it.

Human/object tracking when done on an array of frames is an operation of tracking any mobile target object over a span of time with the help of any mobile or immobile camera. It has been a critical issue in the arena of computer vision as it is used in a number of application fields like security, surveillance, human–computer interaction, augmented reality, video communication and compression, medical imaging, traffic control, video editing, and assistive robotics [1–3]. This is a highly studied problem and remains to be a complex problem to solve. In object tracking in any given video, the major task is to trace the target object in upcoming video frames. To track the object efficiently a complete knowledge of the target is needed, also the tracking parameters are required and the type of video is being analyzed is to be known [13].

Object tracking is a principal segment of human–computer interaction in a real-time environment, where the computer obtains a finer model of a real-time world.

A. Pareek · P. Kadian (✉)
ECE Department, Maharaja Surajmal Institute of Technology, New Delhi, India
e-mail: er.anshulpareek@msit.in; poonam.dahiya@msit.in

P. Agarwal et al. (eds.), *Artificial Intelligence for Smart Healthcare*,
EAI/Springer Innovations in Communication and Computing,
https://doi.org/10.1007/978-3-031-23602-0_7

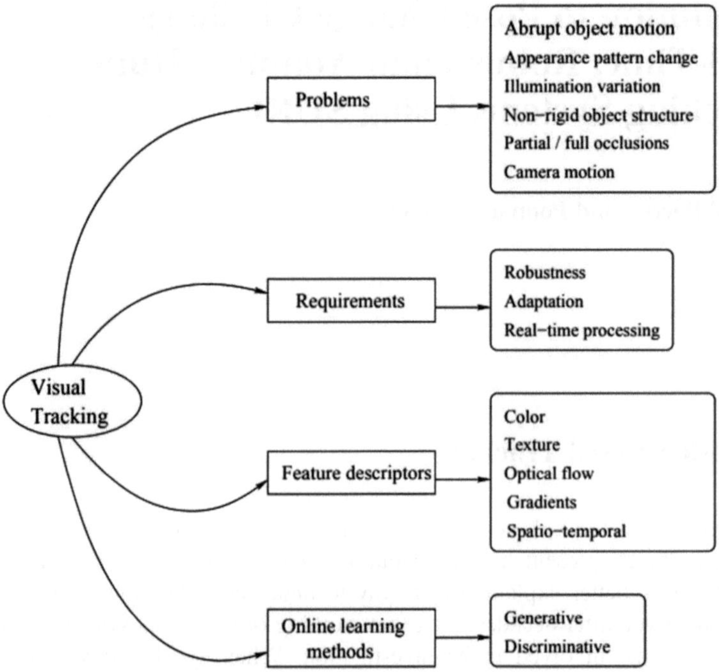

Fig. 1 Visual tracking at a glance

For example, when autonomous vehicles are talked about, a human being cannot transmit the exact state of surroundings precisely and speedily enough.

The wide-ranging scope of the application review the significance of dependable, exact, and efficacious object tracking. To obtain an effective tracking the two most important parameters to be included are first, the selection of the model and secondly, the tracking method worthy for the task.

The fundamental necessities of any tracking structure are first, a robust system, secondly, an adaptive system, and lastly, real-time processing requirement [3, 4]. The famous state-of-art tracking strategies are interest point-based tracking [10], multiple hypothesis tracking [5, 6], kernel-based tracking [7, 8], and optical flow-based tracking [9]. This area has observed a remarkable elevation due to available low cost, advanced technology cameras, and low computing complexity, corresponding to the inclination of ingenious approaches for image and video processing. Excellent reviews on the state-of-art techniques in this area have been provided in [11, 12]. An overview of vision-based tracking is provided in Fig. 1.

1.1 Difficulties in Visual Tracking

Regardless of the achievements acquired in the tracking field, it still faces challenges that may crop up because of any reasons stated below.

- Unanticipated object motion.
- Partial/ full occlusion
- Illumination variation.
- Non-rigid object structure.
- Pose change.
- Camera motion

1.2 Required Features of Visual Tracking

To develop a robust visual tracking system, these difficulties should be addressed properly along with some basic requirements of visual tracking.

- Robustness: The tracking algorithm should be able to follow the target object even in adverse conditions.
- Adaptation: The tracking algorithm should be adaptive to the changes in the environment as well as to the changes in the target itself.
- Real-time processing: The algorithm should be computationally least intensive to enable it to be implementable in real time. This is one of the primary concerns as the work is related to the navigation of the robot while tracking a target human.

1.3 Feature Descriptors for Visual Tracking

In visual tracking, image feature selection is a critical task. The basic entity required for feature points selected is its onliest property which differentiates it in the feature space. The visual features often used are described as mentioned below:

Colour – Two physical factors influence the appearance of colour, one is the spectral power distribution of the illuminant and the other is the surface reflectance properties of the object. RGB which is a non-uniform colour space is commonly used to define colour in image processing. Whereas HSV is defined to be one of the uniform spaces.

Recent advances divide the colour descriptors into two categories that are histogram and SIFT-based in [3], it is declared that when the hue samples are weighted by their saturation it results in a robust hue histogram. The authors also proposed a link of hue with SIFT. RG histogram based on RGB colour model is used by Gevers et al. [4]

Texture – Texture computes the variation of illumination on any surface by finding its levelness [5, 6]. The most common feature is the Gabor wavelet [7]. In recent years, the focus is laid on attaining superior detection by finding local patterns of the given image. Ojala et al. [8] proposed a gray-scale invariant texture measure that exhibits high tolerance against intensity variation and low computation time.

Optical Flow – Optical flow can be defined as an intense area containing the displacement vectors of pixel translation. The luster constancy is assumed of the proximate pixels in successive frames [9]. Lucas and Kanade tracker are one such popular example of optical flow [10].

Gradient – The gradient features are mainly divided into two categories. The first is to define the contours [11] and in the second statistical summary of gradients is used. Lowe [12] proposed SIFT for detection. Bay et al. introduced SURF [13], which is three times speedier than SIFT. Dalal and Triggs [14] gave the most robust algorithm ever based on the Histogram of Oriented Gradient (HOG) descriptor to train the SVM classifier.

Spatio-temporal features – Local space-time features are very useful in extracting motion patterns by providing spatio-temporal shifts [15].

Selecting a feature for an initial object model description is a crucial task, there is a linear relationship between the qualities of the description to the success of the tracking. Even after having a high-quality object description given a priori, continual adaptation to appearance change is necessary to achieve robust tracking. The important task is to manage the appearance changes of the target object. The appearance variations can be divided into two categories (i) intrinsic and (ii) extrinsic. When intrinsic variation is stated it includes targets pose change and shape malformation. Whereas any changes occurring due to full/partial occlusion, illumination variation, and unanticipated camera motion count under the extrinsic category. These variations can only be handled with adaptive methods that can incrementally update their representations. Thus, there is a need for online algorithms that can learn continuously. A brief description of the online learning algorithms is presented in the following subsection.

1.4 Online Learning Algorithms

There are two categories for online algorithms: generative and discriminative. In the former, the model is generally updated in online mode, whereas in the latter, offline training using datasets is used.

1.5 Applications

There are a lot of applications that require object tracking by a robust tracker. Object tracking is applied to various fields from electron microscopy images [75] to understanding trajectories [76] and many others. A few of these applications are recorded below.

- Visual surveillance: When surveillance videos are talked about, they have immense data to be monitored. As a result, it requires some platform to automatically analyze any unusual or abnormal behaviour. These behaviours are predicted based on the object's actions and the trajectories associated [77]. And these are obtained by the exact location of the target and later tracking them.
- Human–Computer Interface (HCI): To make HCI more real and intelligent, visual information is an important parameter. Visual information is defined by the appearance and gesture, visual tracking is an important technique to obtain them. Hence tracking becomes a crucial step in HCI.
- Virtual and Augmented Reality: In virtual reality, a relationship is generated between the human and virtual environment, and this is where tracking becomes an integral part of building a natural relationship. Whereas in the case of augmented reality the virtual objects are located in a real-time scenario, it is important to know the exact position, the pose, and the trajectory of the object. These parameters are best presented by tracking.
- Robotics: Visual trackers are an integral part of the robotics segment. In medical fields the robot is equipped with a tracker to enhance its performance; the most common example of it is robot-assisted surgery. Rehabilitation robots keep a record of patient's movements and their interaction in their neighbourhood which helps in providing better therapeutic training [78].
- Sports Analysis: In today's sports automatic tracking is of prime importance for the players, coaches, audience, and referees. Not all sports allow the use of GPS sensors; in sports like basketball, soccer, and hockey it is completely prohibited. Manual scouting is a tedious job. Here object tracking comes into the picture, trackers track the players and the ball and record their interactions. The game statistics are calculated by the trajectories attained during tracking. This also helps in training players by improving their performance [79].
- Customer Analysis: In the present scenario analysis of customer behaviour in supermarkets, shopping malls, and carnivals is done to increase sales. Trajectories of the customer are recorded and analyzed to offer better deals to them [80]. Their interaction with goods is studied and accordingly assistance and recommendations are prepared for them.
- Biomedical Analysis: Today tracking has become a crucial study in the medical field. During diagnosis, a lot of data in the form of images are obtained. Manual labelling and tracking become almost impossible. As a result, visual tracking is applied to all such fields [81]. This speeds up the process multi-fold.

2 Object Detection and Tracking

In computer vision, detection and tracking are crucial challenges to meet to date. When we say object detection, it means locating and detecting the target object in all the frames of the given video sequence. Whereas, tracking means keeping a record of all the detected images concerning time. In other words, the trajectory of the target is computed in the image plane. Researchers are showing immense interest in this field because of the wide area of applications, increase in computational power, and last but not least low-cost cameras with high picture quality. The video analysis involves three major steps:

- Detection of target among other moving objects.
- Tracking of the target in real-time scenario facing all challenges.
- Understanding the behaviour, an analysis of the trajectory is done.

2.1 Object Representation

Object tracking is implemented in a number of applications. The target in each case is different depending on the application, like in the medical field it can be human or the cluster of cells in the body. The same way the traffic is dealt with; the target is either car or human. When satellites are talked about, planets are the targets. Animals in zoo applications, missiles in defence, humans in the supermarket, etc. are a few of the many examples where tracking is implemented. The target object can be defined by its shape and appearance. Object representation comes into the picture when it is decided how it is to be presented by the tracker. Some of the state-of-art methods are discussed below.

- Point: The target is represented by a single point or multiple points. When single point representation is considered it is generally the centroid of the target. This representation is used when the surroundings are small or the target is small in itself.
- Geometric shapes: In this case, the target is represented by shapes such as square, circle, rectangle, or ellipse. This is commonly used for rigid objects, also successful when simple non-rigid objects are being tracked.
- Silhouette and and contour: This technique is used for complex non-rigid objects. Boundary drawn over the target is termed as its contour whereas silhouette is the region that is around this contour.
- Articulated shape models: Articulated shapes are the segments in the body that are held by joints like hands, legs, and torso. These segments are represented by geometric shapes like rectangle ellipse etc. The relationship among the body parts is established by using some kinetic motion model.

- Skeletal models: To represent the target objects its skeleton is created inside its silhouette or its boundary. It represents the shape of the target. Successfully used for rigid and non-rigid structures.
- Templates: The template is generated from the basic structure of the target i.e. its geometry or the silhouette. It contains the appearance as well as any special information regarding the target, which is the major advantage. The demerit associated with it is that it is not effective in case of pose change during tracking as the template has only one view of the object.

So, we can conclude that there's a strong bonding between target representation and target tracking. Point representation is perfect for the cases where the target is present in a small frame. The geometric shape is suitable for cases where the target is easily fitted in rectangles, circles, or ellipse. When the target is complex in structure, for example human body, contour or silhouette representation is the best.

2.2 *Object Detection*

It is a process of detecting or locating the target in each frame of any video sequence. It is important to avoid false detection while tracking. There are some techniques for object detection stated below:

- Point Detectors: Here, the feature extraction technique provides the interest points over the targets. These points are stored from the frame where the target is located. Later, in all the frames the same points are looked for and the target is detected where the points are found. Literature study shows many such detectors like SURF, SIFT, HARRIS, and KLT detectors.
- Background Subtraction: It is a technique that allows foreground extraction, which can be used for tracking the object. The word foreground is used for the target in the scene and background for the surroundings of the target. Feature extractor finds the key points for foreground and all other key points are treated as background. This technique is commonly used for the static background.
- Segmentation: It is a technique that partitions any digital image into a number of segments. The main aim of segmentation is to transform the image into something more purposeful. The common methods of segmentation are thresholding, clustering, motion and interactive segmentation, compression-based, graph-based, histogram-based, etc.

2.3 *Object Tracking*

It is a technique that traces the movement of a single object or multiple objects in a sequence of frames captured by a single or multiple cameras. The main aim of tracking is to associate target in all the video frames. It estimates the trajectory of the

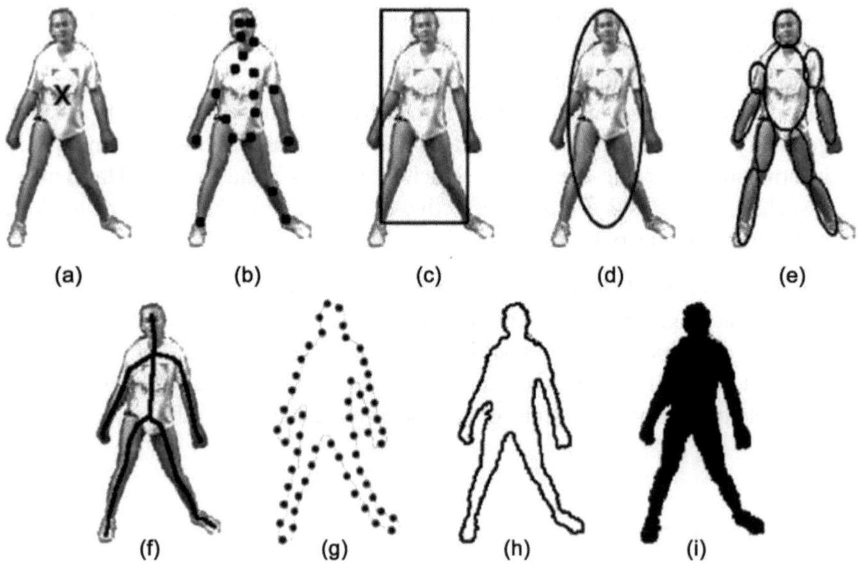

Fig. 2 Representations of targets (**a**) single point, (**b**) multiple points, (**c**) rectangular shape, (**d**) elliptical shape, (**e**) part-based multiple geometric shape, (**f**) skeleton of object, (**g**) contour of object, (**h**) targets contour, (**i**) silhouette of target

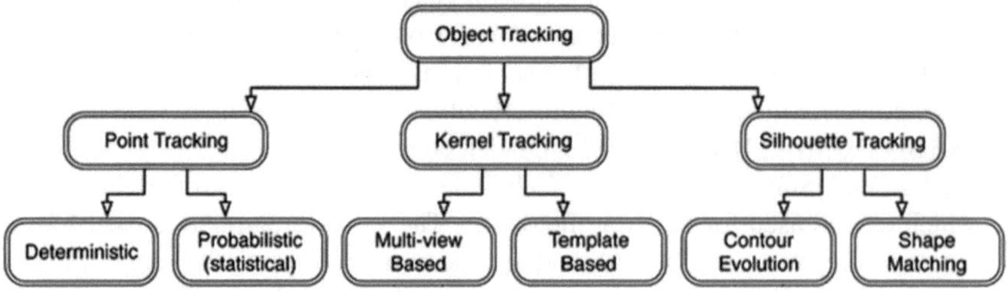

Fig. 3 Object tracking methods

moving target in any scene over an image plane. Figure 3 shows various tracking methods.

- Point tracking: This technique is used when targets are represented as points. This technique associates points over different frames. This association is termed correspondence. This in itself is a complicated problem. The complexity increases when real-time challenges like occlusion or pose change are encountered. This approach is further divided into two categories: statistical and deterministic. The difference between the two is in their approach how to reduce correspondence cost. Correspondence cost is defined as a process of matching all objects present in frame *t*-1 to that of the object in frame t.

- Kernel tracking: This technique involves the usage of the motion model in the tracking process. The motion model helps in computing the motion of the target from one frame to the next and also predicting the position of the target. They are sub-categorized into two parts: one is template based and the other is multi-view based. The objects are represented by geometrical shapes
- Silhouette tracking: This is a region-based tracking overcoming the limitations of geometrical shape-based tracking. It provides the exact shape of the target structure. During tracking object models in form of object contour or shape or colour histogram is generated, once they are obtained they are matched with regions on current frames that match the model. They are of two types: contour evolution and shape matching.

2.4 Prediction Methods

An important part of a tracking system is the ability to predict where an object will be in the next frame. This is needed to aid the matching of the tracks to detect objects and to predict the position during occlusion. There are four common approaches to predict the objects' positions:

- Block matching
- Kalman filters
- Motion models
- Particle filter

3 Literature Review

This chapter mainly concerns vision-based human tracking, therefore, a detailed survey of vision-based human tracking algorithms for mobile robotic platforms is provided in the next subsection but before discussing it a survey of feature extraction and image matching algorithms is initially discussed.

Feature extraction and image matching are used in a number of vision-based applications like object detection and tracking, biometric applications image registration, classification and retrieval, and scene reconstruction.

Richard [82] gave a detailed insight to point, edges, and line-based features and their vivid applications. A detailed survey on feature detection-description and image matching was presented by M. Hassaballah et al. [83]. Here the image features were divided into two categories: global and local. Later detectors were discussed under three headings: single-scale detectors, multi-scale detectors, and affine transformation. Once the key point detectors which are based on key point location, content, scale, and orientation were found, their descriptors are allocated. The descriptors are figured based on binary pixels or vectors. The next step is feature matching using Brute-force, KNN, and FLANN for vector descriptors, and for binary ones, Hamming distance is used. Chris Harris and Mike Stephenes [84] proposed a combination of corner and edge detector based on auto-correlation function. This combination gave more clarity to natural scenarios which include urban buildings, trees, bushes, and roads. The solution was to detect both the corners and edges of any image.

David.G. Lowe [12] proposed one of the most robust images matching algorithms SIFT (Scale Invariant Feature Transform). This algorithm came up with scale and rotation invariant features. Scale-space extremes are detected using the Difference of Gaussian (DOG) and compared to its eight neighbors, thus detecting its local maxima and minima.

E. Rosten and T. Drummond came up with one more effective feature detector algorithm which is FAST (Feature from Accelerate Segment Test) [85]. It proved to be efficient in real-time processing as it is faster than the pre-existing corner detection algorithm. The disadvantage it suffers is that it is not effective for high noise levels also it needs a threshold.

M. Calonder et al. [86] proposed an algorithm BRIEF (Binary Robust Invariant Scalable Keypoints) to overcome the demerits of SIFT and SURF which uses high memory when it has to manage large datasets. BRIEF algorithm is implemented on image patches, which works as binary strings making it use low memory. When compared to SIFT, it is faster than it and comparable to SURF and U-SURF.

S. Leutenegger et al. [87] introduced a FAST-based algorithm along with a bit string descriptor. It was able to extract quality features even in real-time implementations.

E. Rublee et al. [88] proposed a novel algorithm ORB. It was a combination of oFAST (FAST key point orientation) and rBRIEF (Rotated BRIEF). The results showed that it is computationally inexpensive as compared to SURF and SIFT. Hence proved to be successful in real-time tracking and object detection based on texture. Alcantarilla, P.F et al. [89] put forward KAZE features that are two dimensional in non-linear scale-spaces. When compared to SIFT and SURF, effective results were obtained for transformation and distortion like noise, blurring, and rotations, which also, proved to be computationally inexpensive than SIFT.

In this section, survey of vision-based human tracking is discussed. Human tracking is widely explored in computer vision for video surveillance applications [16–20]. The state-of-the-art survey of human tracking for video surveillance can be found in [21, 22]. Despite several human tracking algorithms available for video surveillance applications, vision-based human tracking with mobile robots is a challenging task as the background is dynamic. Vision-based human tracking has become an attractive area of research in the past decade, the reason being its capability in the application areas like application in military areas, site surveillance [23], medical institutes rehabilitation centres [24, 25], guided trips in galleries/museums/libraries [26], and work station assistance [27]. In such real-time applications, it's not sufficient to locate the target object but continuous tracking in a superficially changing environment is required. Not in all situations background segmentation can be sufficient.

The human visual system differentiates different objects based on colour and depth information extracted from stereo vision [28]. Therefore, in the course of the development of machine vision, object tracking started with the colour feature. Colour is a basic but very valuable feature of an image. The colour feature has the following limitations:

- Sensitive to illumination.
- Objects having similar colour distribution cannot be differentiated by colour features.

In spite of these limitations, a number of tracking algorithms based on colour features have been proposed. Here, basically, the target human is detected by feature extraction like face [29, 30], skin [31–33], clothing texture, and it's colour [34]. For the above-mentioned techniques which normally use vision sensors, the major requirement is that target should be facing the camera [29, 33, 35]. In human tracking applications such as elderly care, the robot may see neither the face nor the skin. For instance, in [35] human tracking fails when face detection is used. The cloth-colour-based detection methods [34] fail to differentiate between the human and other objects having the same colour distribution. The most popular colour histogram-based tracking algorithms, such as mean-shift [36, 37], CAMShift [38, 39], and hybrid CAMshift [40] algorithm track the human as an object. Specifically, human features such as shape and aspect ratio are not considered in these algorithms, so these algorithms cannot differentiate between other objects and the human. All such algorithms which use a single feature like cloth colour, skin colour, or face to track object are computationally inexpensive but show low success rate in a real-time environment. This leads to multiple combinations of various features in one algorithm to make it robust and useful in a real-time environment. Schlegal et al. [34] have combined a cloth-colour-based approach with a contour-based approach to differentiate between the human and non-human objects having the same colour distribution. Normalized colour components (NCC) colour space is used for image representation and a 2-D histogram is used for the colour model. The internal representation is a combination of contour and colour distribution of the target object. Here edge-based technique is used to match the contour, and colour-distribution pattern. Segments the images in a line. The contour matching is restricted to colour-based pre-selections, and thus, requires less computation power and real-time performance can be achieved. The object model is continuously updated to overcome any changes in contour resulting from out-of-plane rotation and non-rigidness of the target object. Also, the illumination variations are taken care of.

Grest and Koch [41] proposed a single object tracking algorithm using stereo vision. Face detection by Viola and Jones [42] is used here for detecting the human target. As soon as the target is detected two-colour histograms of face and chest are generated. They further are used by particle filter to predict the location of the target in the next frame. The stereo vision helps in providing details of the target in a closed room, later this information is used to compute the exact location of the target in the virtual environment. The main limitation posed by this approach is that it is successful until the face of the target is visible in the frame while tracking else drift is encountered.

Dixit and Venkatesh [43] have proposed a human tracking algorithm that combines the colour and edge information. This algorithm is an example of the implementation of locating the target in parts. The entire body is divided into three parts, head, torso, and legs, and are tracked in all the successive frames. In this part-based tracking the non-parametric colour probability density estimates of the three parts are used to track them independently using mean-shift. To authenticate and clarify, on the mean shift estimates of the three parts edge matching algorithm is implemented.

In [44], Gaverila implemented an algorithm by combining four modules and they are (i) stereo-based region of interest (ROI) generation, (ii) shape-based detection, (iii) texture-based classification and (iv) stereo-based verification. It is used for the detection and tracking of pedestrians in a real-time environment from a mobile van.

Darrell et al. [45] came up with collective visual methods for human tracking in real-time scenarios. A dense stereo technique in real-time is used to extort base knowledge of the target treated as foreground and later sector it from background environment. The subtracted region algorithm based on face detection and skin colour is implemented. The major drawback is the use of pre-specified skin colour which leads to inaccurate tracking when exposed to light variations that are different from the training sets [46]. The solution to this problem is resolved by [47] where a dynamic skin colour prototype is implemented.

In, Jia et al. came forward with human detection and tracking structure using stereo vision. The target disparity appearance is extracted from a stereo camera, and later using image processing the detectable model of the human is extracted. Hu moment [48] is used to detect humans and robust tracking is performed with an extended Kalman filter.

Zhang et al. [49] used the colour-depth camera for human tracking in a real-time environment. Initially, they worked on 3-D point clouds by getting rid of the ground as well as roof planes. This helped in extracting the target point clusters. The candidate is identified for detection using the notion of Depth of Interest (DOI). To differentiate the target human from the rest and other objects in the background a series of detectors is applied.

Hirai and Mizoguchi have used template matching to detect the shoulder and back part of the human. Yoshimi et al. [50] detect humans through the colour and textures of the attire using a stereo camera system. In [51], the mobile robot tracks the human through a 3D mean-shift algorithm, which uses RGBD information.

Researchers have also explored gradient features for robust human tracking. Optical flow has been used as a short-term tracker in a large number of tracking algorithms, as in Kalal's TMD model [52], active appearance models (AAM) [53], and with SURF [54], etc. Motokucho and Oda [55] have proposed a power-aided wheelchair-using optical flow field for human trailing control.

Dalal and Triggs [14] proposed an algorithm using Histograms of Oriented Gradient (HOG) descriptors and a support vector machine (SVM) classifier for human tracking. This algorithm is considered to be amongst the top robust algorithms to date. Later, Li et al. [56] used the same technique along with sequential mean shift, occlusion reasoning, and a stereo-vision system for multi-target tracking. The major drawback of using HOG-based detection is that it requires offline training, which makes it computationally expensive to be used in real time.

Angelov et al. [57] have proposed a consolidation of recursive density estimation (RDE) strategy and the scale-invariant feature transformation (SIFT) for tracking an immobile target by a non-stationary camera. Here RDE builds a model of the background, this approach involves building a model of the background using RDE and its output is a foreground descriptor representing the target object. After the object of interest is located, this cluster of descriptors is confined in a rectangular region of interest (ROI). Later these ROI details are used by the algorithm to detect the target in consecutive frames by matching SIFT key-points. If failed tracking is encountered, the RDE algorithm reinstates.

In [58], Lien et al. have proposed a human tracking based on SURF-badge. The blob-based object detection and verification are used to initialize the object tracking scheme. A moving object region is segmented into three portions for locating the SURF feature points as the badge of the moving object. The dynamic updating of the SURF feature points is applied for the purpose of robust target tracking. Most of the existing work on human tracking with the mobile robotic platform only deals with colour, texture, and shape features. Other visual features are not investigated thoroughly due to the real-time processing requirement of mobile robots. Thus, the challenge lies in exploring these features for robust human tracking in dynamic environments with real-time computation power.

In [59], Garg and Kumar proposed an algorithm based on SURF and Mean-Shift. When mean-shift is directly applied to the SURF algorithm the major drawbacks are firstly it is computationally expensive and secondly unavailability of the satisfactory number of key-points over frames. To overcome these issues, re-projection technique is implemented by the authors. But this algorithm was not successful for cases that include tracking of non-rigid objects, as there's no accountability of algorithm for pose change due to non-rigid motion, scale, and illumination variations.

In [60], Gupta et al. have used mean shift with SURF features with online updation of template pool. This algorithm is prone to drifting error and does not consider a case of pose change. Also, the time taken is not suitable for real-time processing.

4 Motivation

In present times, the fast pace technology has contributed a lot to low-cost sensors and devices making visual tracking better. This led to large research in this field and the development of vision-based applications in a wide area using digital videos. Digital video is a sequence of images commonly called frames at a uniformly distributed time gap. This video gives detailed information about the target and the dynamic background containing it. After a thorough study of literature, successful human tracking remains to be a big challenge for the researchers in a real-time environment where the major challenges are faced. These challenges are change in light intensity, sudden pose change, the abrupt motion of the camera, scaling of the target, and most important of all partial and full occlusion. Since a large number of frames are accounted for successful tracking, it becomes a time-consuming affair. Developing a successful tracking algorithm that can be used in the real-time scenario is still a big challenge.

The application area is wide in today's world like robotics, augmented reality, the medical field, defence, and surveillance. There's a large possibility of research observed in this field as human tracking involves feature extraction of notable parameters like motion analysis, foreground segmentation, object detection and classification, and behavioural analysis of human interaction with the background. With so much of an area to be explored, human tracking offers a wide research perspective.

5 Terminology

The major terminologies referred to in this chapter are discussed in this section.

- Detection: The process of identifying the target during tracking is the first and foremost task. This is usually done by the user through the manual selection and later detected in all other frames using feature extraction techniques. For example, in the first frame, the target is located manually. This becomes the reference and feature key points for it are looked for in the rest of the sequence.
- Tracking: It is a process of detecting a moving target in due course of time by a stationary or dynamic camera. This process is done for all the frames of any video sequence. In other words, it is a process of linking trajectories. For example, in this chapter a human is manually selected in a frame later it is tracked in real-time conditions. If tracking is lost due to challenges as discussed before a motion model using estimators and predictors is used to predict the location of the target in consecutive frames.

So, the main objective of this chapter is the detection and tracking of the target. In the next Sect. 5.1, a general categorization of a standard visual tracking system is discussed.

5.1 Categorization

To provide a clear picture of what actual tracking is about the entire process is divided into four major categories and then reveal the state of this chapter based on this.

Based on the number of targets to be tracked the tracking process is categorized as:

- Single target tracking: As the name suggests the target is one in the real-time scenario [61–63]. If the target is the only moving object in the background the tracking is comparatively easy. At the same time if the background is dynamic in nature and other than the target there are other moving objects, the complexity increases.
- Multiple target tracking: Here during tracking more than one target to chase and tracked [64–66]. This is a more complex process as compared to single tracking. Also, in such cases initially, the number of targets is undisclosed. This makes it a little more complex problem to tackle because the tracker needs to figure out the exact number of targets and their associated trajectories.

After the target the next important subject is the number of cameras used while tracking:

- Single Camera: Such tracking is also defined as monocular tracking [67–69]. In such cases, there's no surety about calibration variables details given a priori. If in such case the variables are pre-specified, it is image space-based tracking. So, the trajectories obtained are in 2D and not in 3D.
- Stereo vision or multiple cameras: In this set up multiple cameras are used to give 3D trajectories [70–72]. It gives a more accurate location of the target when compared to a single camera set up. Also, it is very helpful in occlusion cases because the target is captured by different cameras at different angles. But it makes it a more complex and computationally expensive setup.

The next category that comes into the picture is the movement of the camera whether moving or steady.

- Steady Camera: A steady camera has all the calibration variables constant in the entire course of tracking.
- Dynamic Camera: The cameras are mobile during the video capturing process. So the calibration variables change and have to be re-estimated time and again.

The last and the most important category of tracking is based on detection or motion model evolution.

- By detection: The targets are detected by implementing detectors on each frame. Later the entire tracking process is treated as a data association process. The aim is to generate trajectories with these detections over the period taken. This is a successful technique when multiple targets are taken into account. It is more robust as compared to the other technique stated below [74].
- By motion model evolution: this technique is more successful for single target based tracking. It is based on Bayes formulation where probability density function is estimated depending on the monitoring. The most common types of approach are Kalman filter [73] and particle filter [60].

The focus of the chapter involves single target tracking using a single steady/dynamic camera. The motion model evolution is used based on the interest point technique.

6 Evaluation Metrics

- Overlap Percentage: Overlapping area of tracker window on ground truth window [10].
  - Overlap % = [area ($W_g \cap W_t$)/area ($W_g \cup W_t$)] × 100
  - W_t = Tracker window
  - W_g = Ground truth window
  - It should be high, above 50% for successful tracking.
  - Overlap percentage is a measure of the accuracy of tracking which in turn affects the success rate.
- Success Rate: The ratio of successful tracking frames (n) to the total number of frames (N) [8].
  - Success Rate = (n/N) × 100
  - It should be high during tracking.
  - The success rate is an integral measure of the robustness of the entire tracking process.
- Average Time: Overall average time required for computation while tracking in msec. For efficient tracking, it should be low. Less average time signifies the compatibility of real-time tracking.

7 SURF-Based Algorithm to Deal with Pose Change Challenge

Computer vision-based algorithm helps us attain robust and accurate human tracking that combats the growing need in wide applications. This research proposes an inventive approach to steer the crucial real-time challenges. The two aforesaid issues are still a challenge to be conquered. Here a SURF-based human tracker is proposed that hunts the target object in an expanded rectangular area around the target location in the last frame. Fresh templates are selected for online updation of the object model timely resulting in robust tracking. Descriptor points from the last frames are superimposed to the current frame by affine transformation. Affine transformation is used to confirm pose change by computing the aspect ratio of the target enclosed region. An auto-tuned classifier is used to discriminate pose change from occlusion and affirm tracking abortion. The success rate and computational time prove the accomplishment of the proposed algorithm.

One of the major challenges faced while tracking non-rigid objects is the pose change. It is expected from any human to turn when and where required, tracking failure is confronted in such condition by most of the pre-existing algorithms. To overrule this challenge while tracking, SURF-based dynamic object model is proposed in this chapter. The steps involved are a selection of new frames whenever pose change is affirmed, besides this a motion predictor the Unscented Kalman Filter [UKF]. Whenever the target undergoes occlusion, predictor searches for the new location and re-initiate the tracking. Each time the predictor is updated in accordance to overcome a similar situation in the future [75, 76]. After predictor, a classifier is also used that is useful in discriminating the pose change from occlusion. In this study, an auto-tuned classifier is used in our research [77]. Autotuned classifier [78] automatically works as a selector, which selects the needful index type (linear, kmeans, kd-tree) to provide optimal performance. Once pose change is confirmed scaling and repositioning are implemented. Also, an expanded rectangular region search is conducted when the target is missing during or after occlusion.

8 Problem Statement

Assume the set of frames from a recorded/live stream video be F_i, where $i = 0$, 1, 2...N. In the first frame F_0 of the video, a rectangular polygon B_0 is encased over the target. SURF descriptors are computed over the target in the box B_i for frame sequence F_i and is stated as given below

$$L\left(B_i\right) = \{(k_1, l_1, w_1), (k_2, l_2, w_2) \ldots\ldots (k_n, l_n, w_n)\} \tag{1}$$

x_i – feature point location in 2D of 64-dimensional SURF features L_i.
w_i are the weights allocated to SURF descriptors L_i.
l_k is a set of feature point locations in a given frame within a window
l_y is the corresponding set of descriptors to l_k.
B_s and B_t are the source and target window.

The set of good matching points between B_s and B_t are as follows

$$L(B_s \sim B_t) = \begin{matrix} \{(k_1, l_1, w_1)^s, (k_2, l_2, w_2)^s \ldots\ldots (k_m, l_m, w_m)^s, (k_1, l_1, w_1)^t, (k_2, \\ l_2, w_2)^t \ldots\ldots (k_m, l_m, w_m)^t\} \end{matrix} \tag{2}$$

Where $(k_m, l_m, w_m)^t$ are SURF descriptors for the target window and $(k_m, l_m, w_m)^s$ are SURF descriptors for the source window. The tracking window B has parameters center (c), width (w), and height (h) and is represented as

$$B = (c, w, h) \tag{3}$$

The aim is now to find the parameters of tracking window $B_i = (c_i, w_i, h_i)$ for the rest of the frames in the video.

Descriptors from the foreground (FG) as well as background (BG) surface in this rectangular region of interest. The presence of SURF descriptors from background progress to model drifting over time. The remedy to it is to minimize the background from the region of interest and this is done by fitting an elliptical region [E_0] inside a rectangular box encasing the target object in it. The set of SURF descriptors present in this area for frame F_o is stated

$$L\left(E_0\right) = \{(k_i, l_i, w_i) \mid (k_i, l_i, w_i) \in L(B_n) \land k_i \in E_0\} \tag{4}$$

where $w_i = 20$ and $i = 1, 2, 3...m$

The object model derived from the above conditions is stated as

$$O_t = \{(k_i, l_i, w_i) \mid (k_i, l_i, w_i) \in L(B_n) \land k_i \in E_0 \land k_n \notin BG_R) \tag{5}$$

BG_R is the segmented background region. O_t (object template) initializes the object model O_m. The initial weight assigned to O_m here is 20.

9 Tracking Algorithm

The tracking algorithm is shown in Fig. 4. The steps of execution are explained point-wise and stated below:

- Initialization of algorithm is done by the selection of the first frame of the video that consists of target present in it.
- Our region of interest is one that has the target in it. A rectangular box is manually drawn over the target for its selection.
- To track this target on all the coming frames, SURF descriptors are extracted on the target. But in the rectangular region, both FG and BG are present. To avoid any drifting of the model it's important to rectify background descriptors as much as possible, for this ellipse is fitted in this rectangular region. This discards more portion of background from the desired region but not all background is removed. Further, the GRAB-CUT algorithm [79] is implemented on the first frame which removes the entire background leaving behind only SURF descriptors from the foreground. GRAB-CUT is a region growing algorithm based on graph cuts and uses a Gaussian mixture model to predict the target object's colour distribution and that of background also. SURF correspondences are obtained between two frames using image matching. Due to the displacement of the target in two frames, scaling is observed. If the limit of scaling exceeds 10% RANSAC is used to remove the outliers.
- To calculate the success of tracking, the tracked window is compared with the ground truth image and their overlap is computed [80]. When the overlap of the tracking window on ground truth is greater than 50%, the target is successfully tracked on the frame processed.

The overlapping is computed by

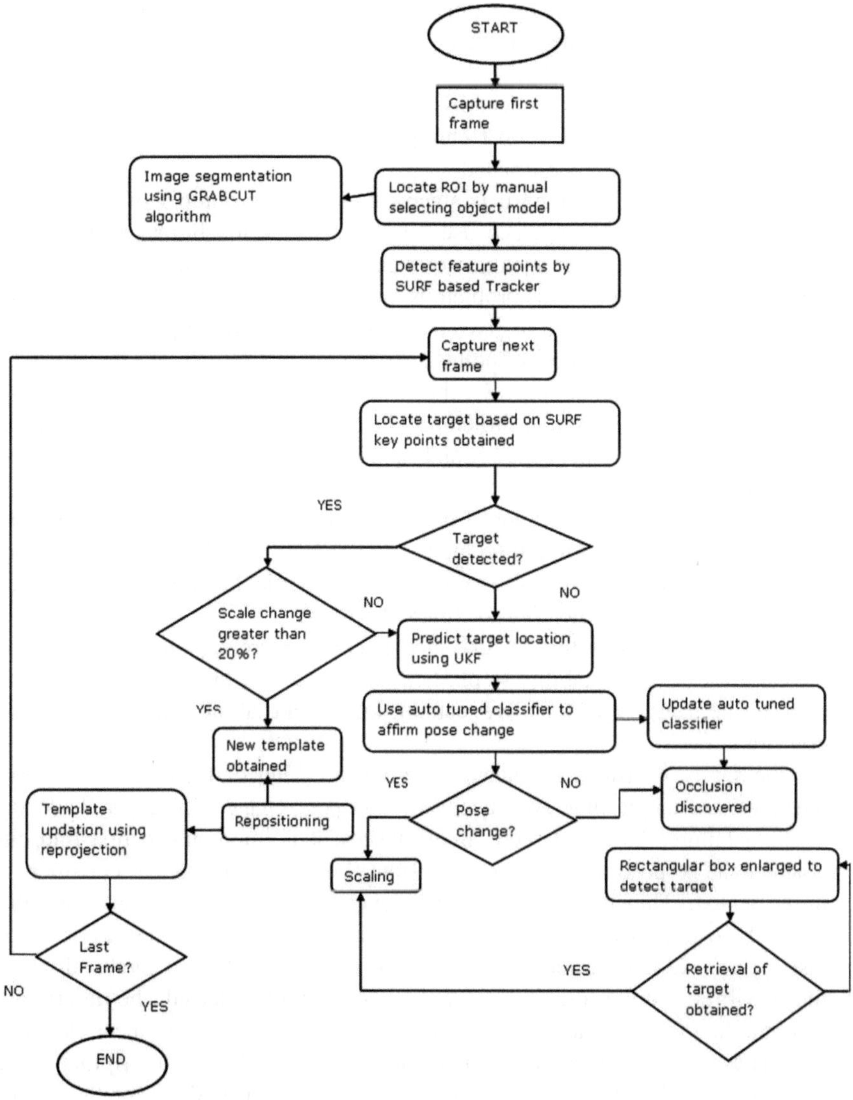

Fig. 4 Tracking Algorithm

$$\text{OVERLAP\%} = (S_m/S_c)^* \ 100 \qquad (6)$$

where S_m is the number of SURF key points from the last selected template and S_c is the number of SURF key points obtained through correspondences.

- After this image segmentation, the object model is initialized and its template is generated for tracking. During tracking, there's the tendency of fading of the number of matching points over time. To make them stay for few more frames weights are assigned to them, initially, the value is 20 and increases every time a new template is allotted. If the descriptor is a matching point, the weight is increased by 2, if not it is reduced by 1.

- By using tracking by detection technique on object template selected, target's location on each frame is estimated
- As we proceed with tracking it is always seen that the number of background descriptors keeps on rising, because it's not possible to eliminate each background descriptor. Even if a single point gets trespassed, it will tend to multiply for each tracking frame. This problem is handled by scaling.
- Not the entire human structure gives the same amount of descriptors. It is always observed that a good number of points are obtained on the torso of a human and a very few on the head and legs. So, the scaling is computed for the human torso instead of on the entire human structure. The centre of the human body is allotted to the torso only. This centre point is moved as per the body ratio and repositioning is attained.
- Since the target undergoes a lot of transitions during tracking, it's important to update the object model in online mode from time to time. So, whenever during tracking, more than 20% limit is observed, that particular frame is selected as template and stored in the pool for future references.
- Scaling is not the sole reason for failed tracking, there are other reasons also behind it for example stability vs plasticity dilemma. The human torso is considered to be rigid object as we cannot implement affine transformation to non-rigid ones.
- All the safety measures are taken to avoid any kind of tracking failure. But whenever the target undergoes occlusion and pose change, there's a chance of tracking failure. To avoid such circumstances, it is important to first find out whether it is pose change or occlusion. For this auto-tuned classifier is implemented. This is a classifier that generates an index and automatically channels to tune between randomized kd-tree, hierarchical K-means, or linear fast search. Kd-tree searches in parallel, k means searches hierarchically and linear will do a brute-force search. In any of the three selected, the descriptors from the first template are used for creating kd-tree, k-means, or linear classifier data. These descriptors are loaded in the template pool. All the descriptors of the new template chosen are pushed in this pool. This step is done for the reconstruction and updation of the classifier.
- If failed tracking is encountered, the new location of the target is predicted by UKF. This uses the nearest neighbour search to detect the closest match. Here the calculation of FG descriptor (FGD) and BG descriptor (BGD) is done. If the FGD number is 1.5 less than the BGD count, this is a case of occlusion encountered else the pose change is affirmed. For occlusion, UKF does the recovery of target by window expansion till the target is recovered. If not tracking is declared to be failed.

10 Results

The performance evaluation of the algorithm is done by implementing it on a number of data sets. The targets in the datasets face various real-time challenges. Six sets of videos are used, 1 set is from the pedestrian data-set of Pedestrian, 1 set is from the IIT-k dataset, and the 2 self-shot sets. In all the datasets, the target undergoes various real-time challenges.

The results of the experiment are discussed in this section for the above-mentioned datasets. The evaluation of the efficiency of the algorithm is done by implementing it on the datasets. Figure 5 shows how the target is selected and the application of region growing algorithm i.e. grab cut on the target. In Fig. 5a the manual selection of target enclosed in a rectangular box is shown. Later ellipse is fitted in a box, the entire human body is divided into head, torso, and legs. SURF descriptors extracted on the target are shown in red colour blobs for all four datasets. Later implementation of grab cut on the first frame is shown in Fig. 5b. Projection points on target are shown in Fig. 6a–c for various poses. Projection points that are bounded inside the ellipse are shown in Fig. 6d–f for all four data. These images show how a number of projection points vary with the pose. Whenever there is a pose change the number of points lie in a line. How pose change is confirmed and a new template is selected is shown in Fig. 7? As can be seen in Fig. 7a the distribution of projection points is distributed over the entire human structure. In the next frame, the target is subjected to pose change. In this case, all the projection points lie in a line due to affine transformation as shown in Fig. 7b. This case can be compared to a transparent ball where all the points lie on the ball's periphery. If the ball is observed from a distance and the ball is rotated continuously, the points appear to come close to each other.

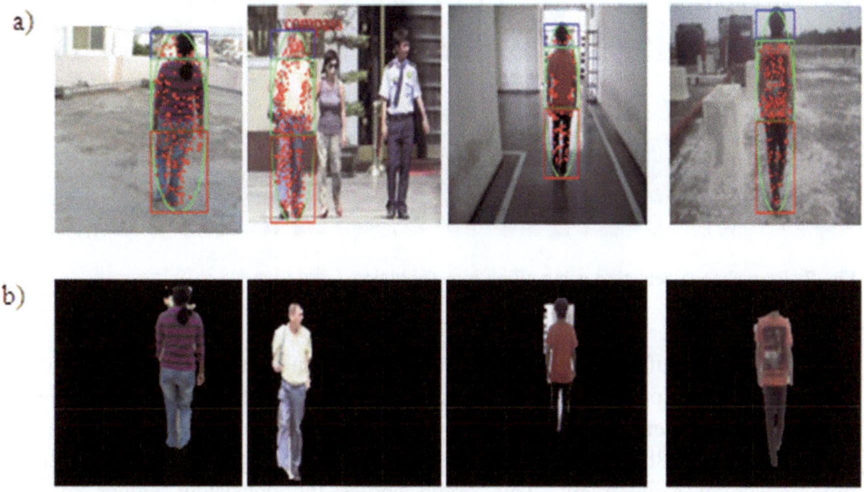

Fig. 5 (**a**) Selection of target. (**b**) Grab Cut segmented image

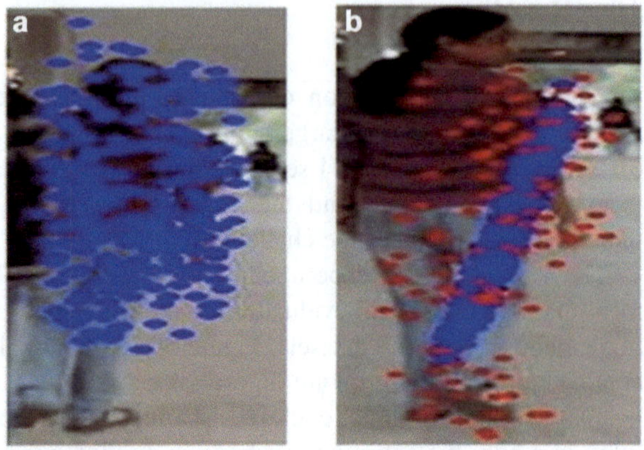

Fig. 6 Projection points under various poses

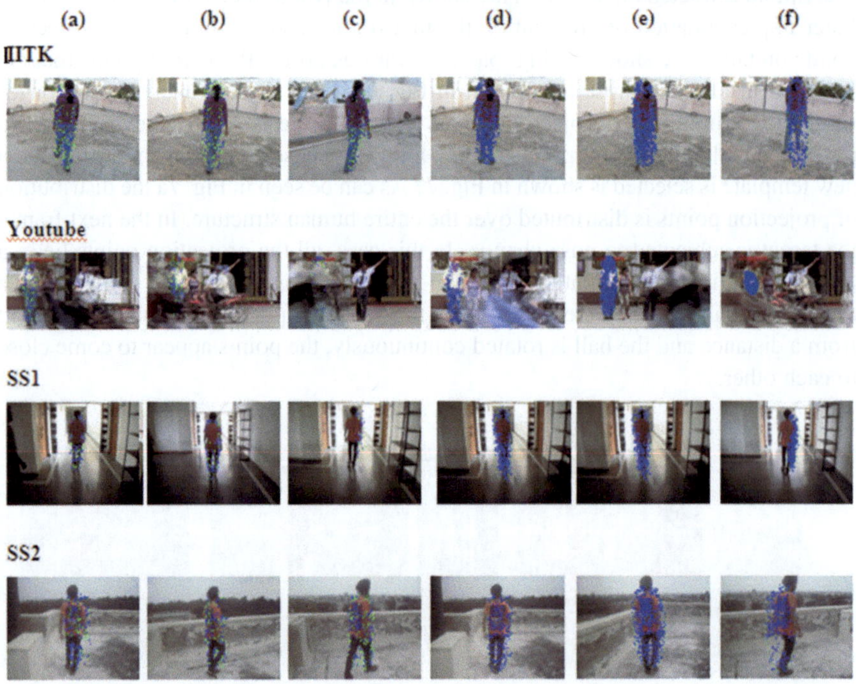

Fig. 7 Pose change detection using affine transformation

When the ball suffers a displacement of 90°, one can see that all the points lie in a line. This is how pose change is confirmed in any frame. Further, this plane is selected as a new template.

In Figs. 8a and 8b statistical data of the number of descriptors and computational time is shown respectively. This graph shows the consistent values of both

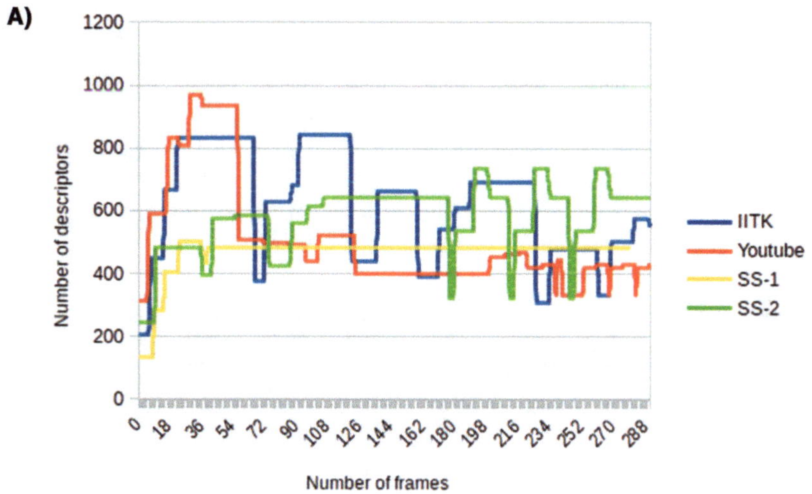

Fig. 8a Average number of descriptors

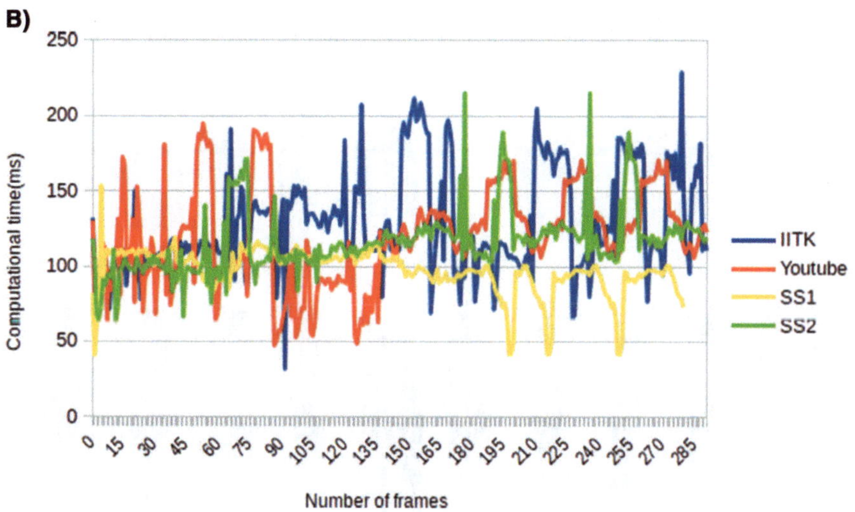

Fig. 8b Average computational time

parameters giving consistent average data throughout the tracking process. This shows the robustness of the algorithm.

Each dataset during execution generates and selects fresh templates for online updation of the object model. The templates for each dataset are shown in Fig. 9. Each template is selected when pose change is encountered and this is prominently visible in Fig. 9. The original video of tracking is available online for inspection and viewing [82–84]. Tracking snapshots for various frames are shown in Fig. 10 for all four data sets.

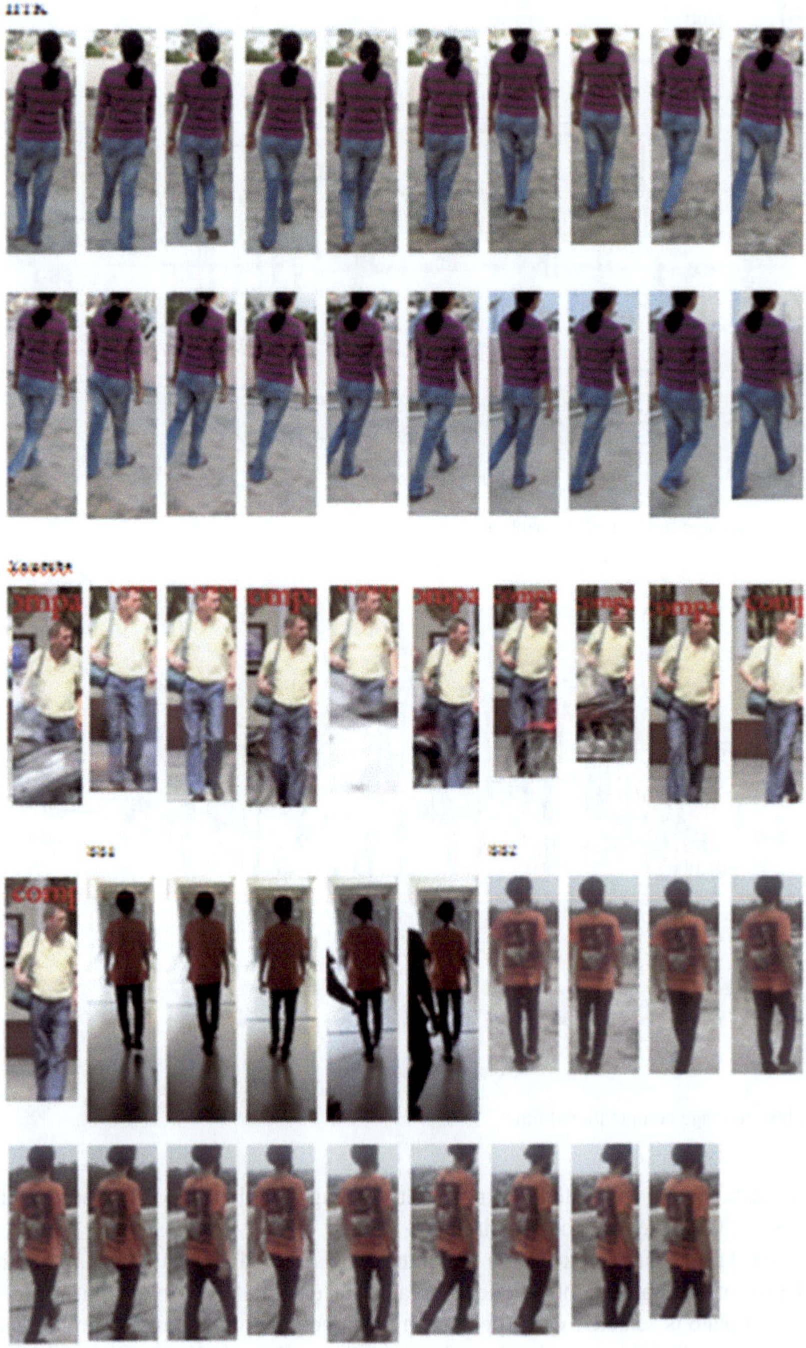

Fig. 9 Templates selected for each dataset

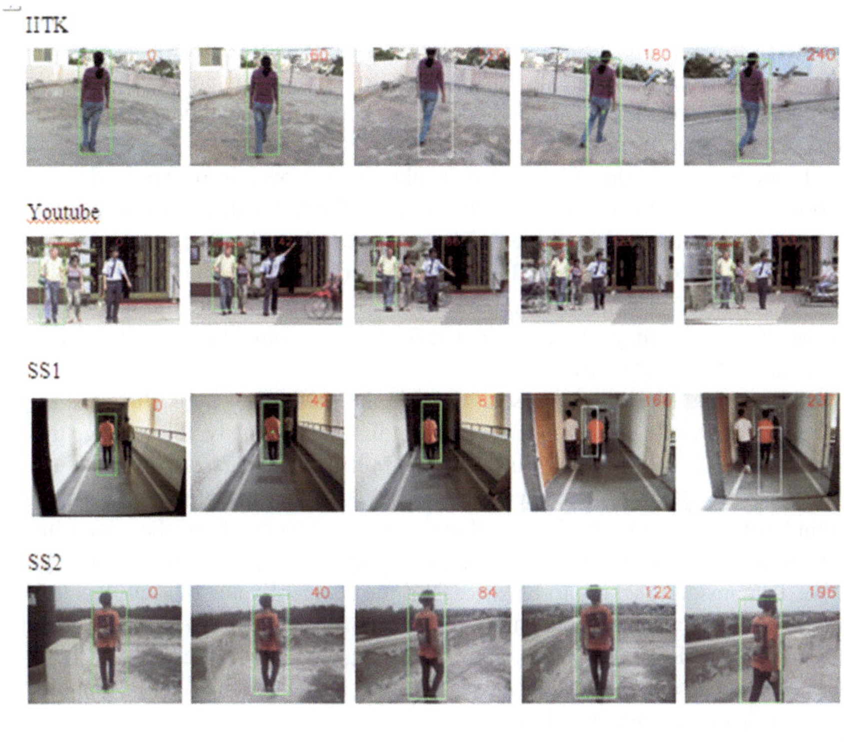

Fig. 10 Tracking results

Table 1 Result analysis

Dataset	Total no. of frames	Camera motion and pose change	Scaling up to	No. of descriptors	No. of templates generated	Average time (ms)	Success rate
IITK	290	Abrupt, Yes	18%	200–900	20	129	96.78
YouTube	290	Smooth, Yes	51%	300–1000	11	120	82.56
SS1	280	Abrupt, No	2%	100–500	5	97	86.23
SS2	290	Abrupt, Yes	20%	200–800	13	117	98.74

The performance analysis of the proposed algorithm for all four datasets is shown in Table 1. Three out of four datasets exhibit abrupt camera motion and pose change, and target undergoes scaling between 2% and 51%, still the success rate achieved is in between 82% and 98%. This proves the robustness and accuracy of the proposed algorithm. The maximum limit of descriptor is 1000, this limit is suitable for real-time implementation as it requires low memory consumption for template storage. Also, this value is quite less than other approaches discussed in previous chapter.

The analysis states the efficiency of the algorithm. Now it is to be proved how this algorithm is better than other pre-existing algorithms. To attain this, a transparent comparison is presented in Table 2. The proposed algorithm is compared with the reprojection-based Mean-Shift-SURF algorithm (61) and SURF Mean-Shift-based object model (62). The evaluation parameters for comparison are the standard open CV parameters and they are success rate (SR), average computational time (AT), and Percentage of Overlap (AOL).

The analysis states the efficiency of the algorithm. Now it is to be proved how this algorithm is better than other pre-existing algorithms. To attain this, a transparent comparison is presented in Table 2. The proposed algorithm is compared with the reprojection-based Mean-Shift-SURF algorithm (61) and SURF Mean-Shift-based object model (62). The evaluation parameters for comparison are the standard open CV parameters and they are success rate (SR), average computational time (AT), and percentage of overlap (AOL).

AT is computed in msec or sec, and this the time taken by each frame to get processed, and in the end average is taken for all frames. Finally, this average time is compared for all the three algorithms when applied to the datasets.

The next evaluation parameter is AOL. To compute it, for each frame manual ground truth is extracted. The tracking window generated by the algorithm is compared with this ground truth, the percentage overlap of two windows gives AOL. To consider tracking to be successful the standard value of AOL has to be a minimum of 50% else tracking on a particular frame is treated as a failure. The factor that computes SR is also AOL. The success rate is simply the ratio of the total number of successfully tracked frames (n) to that of the total number of frames (N). Mathematically it is presented as

$$\mathrm{SR} = (n/N) \times 100 \tag{7}$$

To design a robust and accurate tracking algorithm the algorithm must exhibit low AT.

The comparison analysis as shown in Table 2 suggests that the highest success rate for all the datasets is delivered by the proposed algorithm. Reprojection-based Mean-Shift-SURF algorithm shows good results for IITK and SS2 datasets because the target faces no occlusion and also the colour of the foreground is quite different from the background. But at the same time, it is quite unsuccessful while tracking Youtube and SS2 datasets because there are a number of occlusions, and colour intensity is dark in respective datasets. But it takes less time than the proposed algorithm in all the cases. The proposed algorithm surpasses the performances of the SURF Mean-Shift-based object model in all the datasets and parameters.

11 Conclusion

The proposed algorithm puts forward the scheme of online update of an object model from time to time. This enhances the robustness of the algorithm.

Table 2 Comparative analysis

Dataset	Parameters	Algorithms comparative analysis		
		Reprojection-based Mean-Shift	SURF Mean Shift based object model	Proposed algorithm
IITK	SR	88.29	46.56	96.78
	AOL	68.9%	60.32%	65.34%
	AT	126 ms	582 ms	129 ms
YouTube	SR	0	6.25	82.56
	AOL	8.34%	24.24%	63.23%
	AT	102 ms	431 ms	120 ms
SS1	SR	14.67	38.45	86.23
	AOL	29.64%	40.23%	47.24%
	AT	88 ms	320 ms	97 ms
SS2	SR	92.45	62.47	98.74
	AOL	71.9%	64.34%	76.2%
	AT	110 ms	576 ms	117 ms

The most stable matching points are superimposed on the current frame using affine transformation. The template selected from this process shows temporal and stable data information.

- The proposed algorithm has tremendous potential to overcome the real-time challenges. Besides pose change, other challenges are also successfully handled like, considerable scaling factor, intensity variation, abrupt camera motion, and partial or full occlusion.
- Implementation of auto-tuned classifier discriminates pose change from occlusion, making it a new contribution to track.

References

1. Yilmaz, A., Javed, O., & Shah, M. (2006). Object tracking: A survey. *Acm computing surveys (CSUR)*, *38*(4), 13-es.
2. Yang, H., Shao, L., Zheng, F., Wang, L., & Song, Z. (2011). Recent advances and trends in visual tracking: A review. *Neurocomputing*, *74*(18), 3823–3831.
3. Van de Weijer, J., Gevers, T., & Bagdanov, A. D. (2005). Boosting color saliency in image feature detection. *IEEE transactions on pattern analysis and machine intelligence*, *28*(1), 150–156.
4. Lukac, R., & Plataniotis, K. N. (Eds.). (2018). *Color image processing: methods and applications*. CRC press.
5. Shotton, J., Winn, J., Rother, C., & Criminisi, A. (2009). Textonboost for image understanding: Multi-class object recognition and segmentation by jointly modeling texture, layout, and context. *International journal of computer vision*, *81*(1), 2–23.
6. Winn, J., Criminisi, A., & Minka, T. (2005, October). Object categorization by learned universal visual dictionary. In *Tenth IEEE International Conference on Computer Vision (ICCV'05) Volume 1* (Vol. 2, pp. 1800–1807). IEEE.

7. Manjunath, B. S., & Ma, W. Y. (1996). Texture features for browsing and retrieval of image data. *IEEE Transactions on pattern analysis and machine intelligence*, *18*(8), 837–842.
8. Ojala, T., Pietikainen, M., & Maenpaa, T. (2002). Multiresolution gray-scale and rotation invariant texture classification with local binary patterns. *IEEE Transactions on pattern analysis and machine intelligence*, *24*(7), 971–987.
9. Horn, B. K., & Schunck, B. G. (1981). Determining optical flow. *Artificial intelligence*, *17*(1–3), 185–203.
10. Lucas, B. D., & Kanade, T. (1981, April). An iterative image registration technique with an application to stereo vision.
11. Sabzmeydani, P., & Mori, G. (2007, June). Detecting pedestrians by learning shapelet features. In *2007 IEEE Conference on Computer Vision and Pattern Recognition* (pp. 1–8). IEEE.
12. Lowe, D. G. (2004). Distinctive image features from scale-invariant keypoints. *International journal of computer vision*, *60*(2), 91–110.
13. Bay, H., Ess, A., Tuytelaars, T., & Van Gool, L. (2008). Speeded-up robust features (SURF). *Computer vision and image understanding*, *110*(3), 346–359.
14. Dalal, N., & Triggs, B. (2005, June). Histograms of oriented gradients for human detection. In *2005 IEEE computer society conference on computer vision and pattern recognition (CVPR'05)* (Vol. 1, pp. 886–893). IEEE.
15. Feichtenhofer, C., & Pinz, A. (2013). Spatio-temporal good features to track. In *Proceedings of the IEEE International Conference on Computer Vision Workshops* (pp. 246–253).
16. Sanoj, C. S., Vijayaraj, N., & Rajalakshmi, D. (2013, February). Vision approach of human detection and tracking using focus tracing analysis. In *2013 International Conference on Information Communication and Embedded Systems (ICICES)* (pp. 64–68). IEEE.
17. Puri, N. V., & Devale, P. R. (2012). Development of human tracking in video surveillance system for activity analysis. *IOSR J. Comput. Eng*, *4*(2), 26–30.
18. Xu, Y., Qin, L., Jiang, S., & Huang, Q. (2011, September). Human tracking by structured body parts. In *2011 18th IEEE International Conference on Image Processing* (pp. 2305–2308). IEEE.
19. Zhao, T., Nevatia, R., & Wu, B. (2008). Segmentation and tracking of multiple humans in crowded environments. *IEEE transactions on pattern analysis and machine intelligence*, *30*(7), 1198–1211.
20. Ramanan, D., Forsyth, D. A., & Zisserman, A. (2006). Tracking people by learning their appearance. *IEEE transactions on pattern analysis and machine intelligence*, *29*(1), 65–81.
21. Ogale, N. A. (2006). A survey of techniques for human detection from video. *Survey, University of Maryland*, *125*(133)
22. Howlett, R. J., & Jain, L. C. (2005). *Knowledge-based intelligent information and engineering systems*. Springer Berlin/Heidelberg.
23. Luo, R. C., Lin, T. Y., & Su, K. L. (2009). Multisensor based security robot system for intelligent building. *Robotics and autonomous systems*, *57*(3), 330–338.
24. Matarić, M. J., Eriksson, J., Feil-Seifer, D. J., & Winstein, C. J. (2007). Socially assistive robotics for post-stroke rehabilitation. *Journal of NeuroEngineering and Rehabilitation*, *4*(1), 1–9.
25. Napper, S. A., & Seaman, R. L. (1989). Applications of robots in rehabilitation. *Robotics and Autonomous Systems*, *5*(3), 227–239.
26. Burgard, W., Cremers, A. B., Fox, D., Hähnel, D., Lakemeyer, G., Schulz, D., ... & Thrun, S. (1999). Experiences with an interactive museum tour-guide robot. *Artificial intelligence*, *114*(1–2), 3–55.
27. Asoh, H., Motomura, Y., Asano, F., Hara, I., Hayamizu, S., Itou, K., ... & Krose, B. (2001). Jijo-2: An office robot that communicates and learns. *IEEE Intelligent Systems*, *16*(5), 46–55.
28. Batchelor, B. G. (Ed.). (2012). *Machine vision handbook* (pp. 801–870). London, UK:: Springer.

29. Suzuki, S., Mitsukura, Y., Takimoto, H., Tanabata, T., Kimura, N., & Moriya, T. (2009, November). A human tracking mobile-robot with face detection. In *2009 35th Annual Conference of IEEE Industrial Electronics* (pp. 4217–4222). IEEE.
30. Luo, R. C., Tsai, A. C., & Liao, C. T. (2007, November). Face detection and tracking for human robot interaction through service robot. In *IECON 2007-33rd Annual Conference of the IEEE Industrial Electronics Society* (pp. 2818–2823). IEEE.
31. Sidenbladh, H., Kragic, D., & Christensen, H. I. (1999, May). A person following behaviour for a mobile robot. In *Proceedings 1999 IEEE International Conference on Robotics and Automation (Cat. No. 99CH36288C)* (Vol. 1, pp. 670–675). IEEE.
32. Wu, Y., & Huang, T. S. (2002). Nonstationary color tracking for vision-based human-computer interaction. *IEEE transactions on neural networks*, *13*(4), 948–960.
33. Wu, T., Zou, Y., & Wang, W. (2008, September). Skin-color based particle filtering for human face tracking. In *2008 IEEE Conference on Cybernetics and Intelligent Systems* (pp. 728–733). IEEE.
34. Schlegel, C., Illmann, J., Jaberg, H., Schuster, M., & Wörz, R. (1998, September). Vision based person tracking with a mobile robot. In *BMVC* (pp. 1–10).
35. Vadakkepat, P., Lim, P., De Silva, L. C., Jing, L., & Ling, L. L. (2008). Multimodal approach to human-face detection and tracking. *IEEE transactions on industrial electronics*, *55*(3), 1385–1393.
36. Dorin Comaniciu, Visvanathan Ramesh, and Peter Meer, "Real-time tracking of non-rigid objects using mean-shift," in Proceedings of International Conference on Computer Vision and Pattern Recognition (CVPR), Hilton Head Island, CS, 2000, pp. 142–149, vol. 2, IEEE.
37. Aras Dargazany, Ali Soleimani, Alireza Ahmadyfard, "Multibandwidth Kernel-Based Object Tracking", Advances in Artificial Intelligence, vol. 2010, Article ID 175603, 15 pages, 2010. https://doi.org/10.1155/2010/175603
38. Gary R. Bradski, "Computer vision face tracking for use in a perceptual user interface," Intel Technology Journal, 1998, 2nd Quarter.
39. Allen, J. G., Xu, R. Y., & Jin, J. S. (2004, June). Object tracking using camshift algorithm and multiple quantized feature spaces. In *ACM International Conference Proceeding Series* (Vol. 100, pp. 3–7).
40. Gupta, M., Uggirala, B., & Behera, L. (2008). Visual navigation of a mobile robot in a cluttered environment. *IFAC Proceedings Volumes*, *41*(2), 14816–14821.
41. Grest, D., & Koch, R. (2004, September). Realtime multi-camera person tracking for immersive environments. In *IEEE 6th Workshop on Multimedia Signal Processing, 2004.* (pp. 387–390). IEEE.
42. Viola, P., & Jones, M. (2001, December). Rapid object detection using a boosted cascade of simple features. In *Proceedings of the 2001 IEEE computer society conference on computer vision and pattern recognition. CVPR 2001* (Vol. 1, pp. I-I). IEEE.
43. Dixit, M., & Venkatesh, K. S. (2009, September). Combining edge and color features for tracking partially occluded humans. In *Asian Conference on Computer Vision* (pp. 140–149). Springer, Berlin, Heidelberg.
44. Gavrila, D. M., & Munder, S. (2007). Multi-cue pedestrian detection and tracking from a moving vehicle. *International journal of computer vision*, *73*(1), 41–59.
45. Darrell, T., Gordon, G., Harville, M., & Woodfill, J. (2000). Integrated person tracking using stereo, color, and pattern detection. *International Journal of Computer Vision*, *37*(2), 175–185.
46. Martinkauppi, B., Soriano, M., & Pietikainen, M. (2003, September). Detection of skin color under changing illumination: a comparative study. In *12th International Conference on Image Analysis and Processing, 2003. Proceedings.* (pp. 652–657). IEEE.
47. Sigal, L., Sclaroff, S., & Athitsos, V. (2004). Skin color-based video segmentation under time-varying illumination. *IEEE Transactions on Pattern Analysis and Machine Intelligence*, *26*(7), 862–877.
48. Mercimek, M., Gulez, K., & Mumcu, T. V. (2005). Real object recognition using moment invariants. *sadhana*, *30*(6), 765–775.

49. Zhang, H., Reardon, C., & Parker, L. E. (2013). Real-time multiple human perception with color-depth cameras on a mobile robot. *IEEE Transactions on Cybernetics*, *43*(5), 1429–1441.
50. Yoshimi, T., Nishiyama, M., Sonoura, T., Nakamoto, H., Tokura, S., Sato, H., ... & Mizoguchi, H. (2006, October). Development of a person following robot with vision based target detection. In *2006 IEEE/RSJ International Conference on Intelligent Robots and Systems* (pp. 5286–5291). IEEE.
51. Hu, J. S., Wang, J. J., & Ho, D. M. (2013). Design of sensing system and anticipative behavior for human following of mobile robots. *IEEE Transactions on Industrial Electronics*, *61*(4), 1916–1927.
52. Kalal, Z., Matas, J., & Mikolajczyk, K. (2009, September). Online learning of robust object detectors during unstable tracking. In *2009 IEEE 12th International Conference on Computer Vision Workshops, ICCV Workshops* (pp. 1417–1424). IEEE.
53. Matthews, I., & Baker, S. (2004). Active appearance models revisited. *International journal of computer vision*, *60*(2), 135–164.
54. Li, J., Wang, Y., & Wang, Y. (2012). Visual tracking and learning using speeded up robust features. *Pattern Recognition Letters*, *33*(16), 2094–2101.
55. Motokucho, T., & Oda, N. (2014, March). Vision-based human-following control using optical flow field for power assisted wheelchair. In *2014 IEEE 13th International Workshop on Advanced Motion Control (AMC)* (pp. 266–271). IEEE.
56. Li, L., Yan, S., Yu, X., Tan, Y. K., & Li, H. (2012). Robust multiperson detection and tracking for mobile service and social robots. *IEEE Transactions on Systems, Man, and Cybernetics, Part B (Cybernetics)*, *42*(5), 1398–1412.
57. Angelov, P., Gude, C., Sadeghi-Tehran, P., & Ivanov, T. (2012, September). ARTOT: Autonomous real-time object detection and tracking by a moving camera. In *2012 6th IEEE International Conference Intelligent Systems* (pp. 446–452). IEEE.
58. Lien, C. C., Lin, S. J., Ma, C. Y., & Lin, Y. W. (2013). SURF-badge-based target tracking. *World Academy of Science, Engineering and Technology*, *77*, 877–883.
59. Garg, S., & Kumar, S. (2013). Mean-shift based object tracking algorithm using SURF features. In *Recent Advances in Circuits, Communications and Signal Processing Conference* (pp. 187–194).
60. Gupta, A. M., Garg, B. S., Kumar, C. S., & Behera, D. L. (2013, September). An on-line visual human tracking algorithm using SURF-based dynamic object model. In *2013 IEEE International Conference on Image Processing* (pp. 3875–3879). IEEE.
61. Isard, M., & Blake, A. (1998). Condensation—conditional density propagation for visual tracking. *International journal of computer vision*, *29*(1), 5–28.
62. D. Comaniciu, V. Ramesh, and P. Meer, “Kernel-Based Object Tracking,” *IEEE Transactions on Pattern Analysis and Machine Intelligence*, vol. 25, no. 5, pp. 564–575, 2003.
63. Kalal, Z., Mikolajczyk, K., & Matas, J. (2011). Tracking-learning-detection. *IEEE transactions on pattern analysis and machine intelligence*, *34*(7), 1409–1422.
64. Koller, D., Weber, J., & Malik, J. (1993). Robust Multiple Car Tracking with Occlusion Reasoning, Report No. UCB/CSD 93/780. *Computer Science Division (EECS) UC-Berkeley*, *22*.
65. Zhao, T., & Nevatia, R. (2004). Tracking multiple humans in complex situations. *IEEE transactions on pattern analysis and machine intelligence*, *26*(9), 1208–1221.
66. Nillius, P., Sullivan, J., & Carlsson, S. (2006, June). Multi-target tracking-linking identities using Bayesian network inference. In *2006 IEEE Computer Society Conference on Computer Vision and Pattern Recognition (CVPR'06)* (Vol. 2, pp. 2187–2194). IEEE.
67. Koller, D., Daniilidis, K., & Nagel, H. H. (1993). Model-based object tracking in monocular image sequences of road traffic scenes. *International Journal of Computer 11263on*, *10*(3), 257–281.
68. Andriluka, M., Roth, S., & Schiele, B. (2008, June). People-tracking-by-detection and people-detection-by-tracking. In *2008 IEEE Conference on computer vision and pattern recognition* (pp. 1–8). IEEE.

69. Fossati, A., Dimitrijevic, M., Lepetit, V., & Fua, P. (2007, June). Bridging the gap between detection and tracking for 3D monocular video-based motion capture. In *2007 IEEE Conference on Computer Vision and Pattern Recognition* (pp. 1–8). IEEE.
70. Fleuret, F., Berclaz, J., Lengagne, R., & Fua, P. (2007). Multicamera people tracking with a probabilistic occupancy map. *IEEE transactions on pattern analysis and machine intelligence, 30*(2), 267–282.
71. Khan, S. M., & Shah, M. (2008). Tracking multiple occluding people by localizing on multiple scene planes. *IEEE transactions on pattern analysis and machine intelligence, 31*(3), 505–519.
72. Berclaz, J., Fleuret, F., Turetken, E., & Fua, P. (2011). Multiple object tracking using k-shortest paths optimization. *IEEE transactions on pattern analysis and machine intelligence, 33*(9), 1806–1819.
73. Kalman, R. E. (1960). A new approach to linear filtering and prediction problems.
74. Ellis, A., Shahrokni, A., & Ferryman, J. M. (2009, December). Pets 2009 and winter-pets 2009 results: A combined evaluation. In *2009 Twelfth IEEE International Workshop on Performance Evaluation of Tracking and Surveillance* (pp. 1–8). IEEE.
75. Chen, X., Wang, W., Meng, W., & Zhang, Z. (2010, June). A novel UKF based scheme for GPS signal tracking in high dynamic environment. In *2010 3rd International Symposium on Systems and Control in Aeronautics and Astronautics* (pp. 202–206). IEEE.
76. Kiruluta, A., Eizenman, M., & Pasupathy, S. (1997). Predictive head movement tracking using a Kalman filter. *IEEE Transactions on Systems, Man, and Cybernetics, Part B (Cybernetics), 27*(2), 326–331.
77. Song, T. L., & Speyer, J. L. (1986). The modified gain extended Kalman filter and parameter identification in linear systems. *Automatica, 22*(1), 59–75.
78. Wan, L., Liu, Y. C., & Pi, Y. M. (2007). Comparing of Target-Tracking Performances of EKF, UKF and PF [J]. *Radar science and technology, 1*, 003.
79. Kalal, Z., Matas, J., & Mikolajczyk, K. (2010, June). Pn learning: Bootstrapping binary classifiers by structural constraints. In *2010 IEEE Computer Society Conference on Computer Vision and Pattern Recognition* (pp. 49–56). IEEE.
80. Rother, C., Kolmogorov, V., & Blake, A. (2004). " GrabCut" interactive foreground extraction using iterated graph cuts. *ACM transactions on graphics (TOG), 23*(3), 309–314.
81. Bashir, F., & Porikli, F. (2006, June). Performance evaluation of object detection and tracking systems. In *Proceedings 9th IEEE International Workshop on PETS* (pp. 7–14).
82. *AnshulPareek-Human Tracking* https://youtu.be/T9mTClv4RZA
83. *AnshulPareek Human Tracking* https://youtu.be/gdLrWOIgFzA
84. *AnshulPareek-Human Tracking* https://youtu.be/mMhuW0697yI
85. Rosten, E., & Drummond, T. (2006, May). Machine learning for high-speed corner detection. In European conference on computer vision (pp. 430-443). Springer, Berlin, Heidelberg.
86. Calonder, M., Lepetit, V., Strecha, C., & Fua, P. (2010, September). Brief: Binary robust independent elementary features. In European conference on computer vision (pp. 778-792). Springer, Berlin, Heidelberg.
87. Leutenegger, S., Chli, M., & Siegwart, R. Y. (2011, November). BRISK: Binary robust invariant scalable keypoints. In 2011 International conference on computer vision (pp. 2548-2555). Ieee
88. Rublee, E., Rabaud, V., Konolige, K., & Bradski, G. (2011, November). ORB: An efficient alternative to SIFT or SURF. In 2011 International conference on computer vision (pp. 2564-2571). Ieee.
89. Alcantarilla, P.F., Bartoli, A. and Davison, A.J., 2012, October. KAZE features. In European Conference on Computer Vision (pp. 214-227). Springer, Berlin, Heidelberg

Analysis on Identification and Detection of Forgery in Handwritten Signature Using CNN

T. Vasudeva Reddy, D. Harikrishna, V. Hindumathi, P. Asha Rani, and T. Keerthi

1 Introduction

The need for signature detection is incredibly vital because, in contrast to passwords, signatures cannot be modified or forgotten due to their distinctiveness, and it's considered because of the vital technique for detection. The techniques and systems accustomed to solving signature detection are divided into offline signature and online signature ways. In the offline signature detection technique, a lot of hardware modules weren't used, and pictures were captured using the camera. In contrast, many hardware modules were used in the online detection technique, and the hardware modules were directly connected to the PC [1]. The options used for offline detection square measure are less complicated. The signatures from the info are preprocessed using varied preprocessing techniques; then, the preprocessed info features are extracted [2]. The automatic offline signature detection solutions may be classified into two categories: handcrafted feature extraction algorithms and profound learning ways. The deep learning methods are measured, particularly thought of as the foremost promising approach for their excellent image recognition and detection capability. Though profound learning studies with small-scale data are gaining substantial attention in recent years, most deep learning ways still would like an extensive range of samples to train their system. In alternative words, most of the studies still need many (more than one) signature samples to accomplish their

T. Vasudeva Reddy (✉) · D. Harikrishna · P. Asha Rani · T. Keerthi
Department of ECE, B. V. Raju Institute of Technology, Medak, Telangana, India
e-mail: vasu.tatiparthi@bvrit.ac.in; harikrishna.dodde@bvrit.ac.in; asharani.p@bvrit.ac.in; keerthi.t@bvrit.ac.in

V. Hindumathi
Department of ECE, B V R I T College of Engineering for Women, Medak, Telangana, India
e-mail: hindumathi.v@bvrithyderabad.edu.in

P. Agarwal et al. (eds.), *Artificial Intelligence for Smart Healthcare*,
EAI/Springer Innovations in Communication and Computing,
https://doi.org/10.1007/978-3-031-23602-0_8

coaching method. This chapter proposes an offline handwritten signature detection technique exploitation convolution neural network (CNN).

Signature forgery detection finds its application within the field of internet banking, passport verification system, master card transactions, and bank checks. Therefore, with the growing demand for the protection of individual identity, the look of an automatic signature system is required [3]. Within the sight of master fabrications, where a falsifier approaches an individual's mark and intentionally endeavours to copy it, it is troublesome to confirm its distinguishing proof utilising manually written marks. The robust data of the mark composing measure is lost in independent (static) signature confirmation, making it trying to build excellent component extractors that can recognise genuine marks from skillful phonies [4, 5]. This is reflected in the generally horrible showing of the best frameworks in writing, which have check blunders of generally 7%. We propose utilising Convolutional Neural Networks to take in portrayals from signature photographs in a writer-independent way to resolve the issue of gathering good highlights and expanding framework execution. We present another definition of the issue that joins data of able frauds from a subset of clients in the component learning measure, fully intent on catching viewable signals that distinguish genuine marks from falsifications paying little mind to the client. Comprehensive testing was completed on four datasets: the GPDS, MCYT, CEDAR, and Brazilian PUC-PR datasets [11, 12]. On the GPDS-160, we accomplished a massive improvement in best-in-class execution, with an Equal Error Rate of 1.72% contrasted with 6.97% in writing. We likewise affirmed that the highlights sum up past the GPDS dataset, beating cutting-edge execution in extra datasets without calibrating each dataset's portrayal [6].

Mark confirmation frameworks work by distinguishing an individual's manually written mark to approve their recognisable proof. To distinguish an individual, they depend on perceiving a particular, very much educated motion. This varies from frameworks that depend on the responsibility for the object (e.g., a key, a smartcard) or the information on something (e.g., a secret word), just as other biometric frameworks, like fingerprints, because the mark stays the most socially and legitimately acknowledged technique for distinguishing [7, 8]. The disconnected (static) signature check includes filtering a record containing the mark and depicting it as an advanced picture after the creative cycle is finished. Subsequently, dynamic data concerning the mark creation measure (e.g., pen area and speed over the long run) is lost, making the issue incredibly hard to settle [9, 10].

2 Literature Review

Alarood, A. A et al. [13] have planned a technique to compensate for the shortage of dynamic info from static signature pictures through the employment of separate argon on transform (DRT), principal part analysis (PCA) & probabilistic neural network (PNN). A median filter and gray scaling of pictures are completed to eliminate noise and minimise database storage of pictures. A two-dimensional signature image has been placed on an editable line to adjust the similarity scale. PCA is employed towards compress feature information in this case. This chapter uses a Probabilistic neural network (PNN) rather than a similarity matching idea. Al-Khasawneh, M. A et al. [14] explain signature importance and usage on different platforms such as banks, post offices, and financial organizations. This chapter discusses offline identity verification and verification systems, and mistreatment neural networks. This method permits the client to confirm whether a mark is unique or a pretend.

Rani, R et al. [15] have worked a signature verification system mistreatment Error Back Propagation Coaching Algorithm designed mistreatment Neural Network tool chest of MATLAB to verify the signatures. The digital and natural signatures have been affected when any unauthorized person tries to change content. A two-step methodology is planned to identify the signature within the commencement, followed by individual verification. Each step is done by Neural Networks trained exploitation Error Back-Propagation Training algorithmic program. Al-Khasawneh, M. A et al. [16] explain biometric features and their essential applications in the current economy. One among the foremost necessary and standard biometrics is signature. Vargas-Bonilla et al. [6] have proposed a technique for directing disconnected composed mark confirmation. It works at the world picture level and measures the faint level assortments inside the picture's applied mathematical surface choices.

Author	Technique	Keynote	Advanced model
Chai Quek et.al [1]	Fuzzy-based fake sign detection	This model cannot identify the faults in stress point	RFO model
Hanmandlu, M et al. [2]	Unconstrained fuzzy logic	In this model, an advanced fuzzy-based fake signature model is analysed	SVM
Bin Xiao et al. [3]	Reconstructive CNN	In this model rCNN based fake sing detection is implemented, but this model is not that efficient	ResNet CNN model
Hong et al. [5]	Optimized KNN	This model predicts fake and forgery signatures easily but cannot identify stress points.	Adaptive SVM

3 Methodology

For developing the system, specific methodologies are used. The methodology utilised in this work is image classification using CNN.

3.1 Convolution Neural Network (CNN)

A CNN is mutli-level neural organisation with a profound regulated learning plan that has the symbolic capacity to extricate highlights for arrangement all alone [17]. CNN comprises two parts: a self-ruling element extractor and a teachable classifier. A multi-facet neural organisation with a profound managed learning plan that has the symbolic capacity to separate highlights for order all alone [18, 19]. CNN comprises two parts: an independent element extractor and a teachable classifier. The feature extractor uses two procedures to extract features from incoming data: convolution filtering and downsampling.

3.1.1 Convolution Filtering

K area unit, which is usually 3 by 3 or 5 by 5 inches in size. A picture is represented by matrix *I*, where *I*(*x*, *y*) is the brightness of the component at the specified coordinates (*x*, *y*). A convolution product is calculated between matrix *I* and the kernel matrix *K*, which indicates the filter type. The end consequence of this product is the component's improved brightness (*x*, *y*).

The convolution product of product * for a kernel of size three × three is defined by: -

$$I^{*}K = \begin{pmatrix} I(1,1) & I(1,2) & \cdots & I(1,n) \\ \vdots & & I(x,y) & \vdots \\ I(m,1) & I(m,2) & \cdots & I(m,n) \end{pmatrix} * \begin{pmatrix} K(1,1) & K(1,2) & K(1,3) \\ K(2,1) & K(2,2) & K(2,3) \\ K(3,1) & K(3,2) & K(3,3) \end{pmatrix} \tag{1}$$

Where

$$I^{*}K_{x,y} = \sum_{i=-1}^{1} \sum_{j=-1}^{1} I(x+i, y+j)^{*} K(2+i, 2+j) \tag{2}$$

The choice of filter depends on the worth of *K*.

The back-propagation rule appearance for the minimum error value performs in weight space using a technique known as the delta rule or gradient descent. The weights that minimise the error performed answer the training drawback (Shown in Fig. 1). Working of Back-propagation algorithm:

(a) We first initialised some random worth to 'W' and propagated forward.
(b) Then, we tend to notice that there's some error. To scale back that error, we tend to propagate backwards and increase the value of 'W'.
(c) After that, we tend to notice that the error has increased. We tend to understand that we can't increase the 'W' value.
(d) So, we tend to propagate backwards once more, decreasing the 'W' value. Now, we tend to notice that the error has reduced.

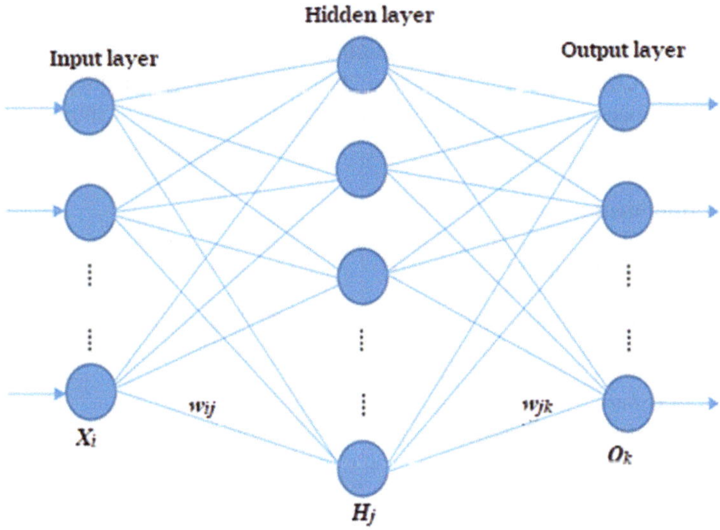

Fig. 1 Multilayer feed-forward neural network

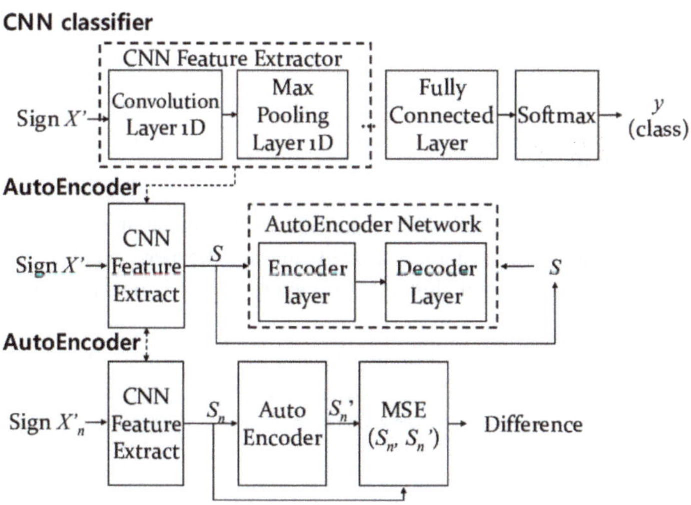

Fig. 2 CNN classifier with Auto Encoder

A CNN is used as both a feature extractor and a classifier in the suggested method. The proposed CNN-AE model is depicted below (Shown in Fig. 2). In CNN, the extraction method is recording equipment, just like in other deep neural networks, and the actual properties of the options remain unknown.

An autoencoder remains an unsupervised artificial neural network that learns efficient knowledge codings [20]. By training the network to disregard signal "noise," an autoencoder can find a representation (encoding) for a collection of knowledge, usually for spatial property reduction [21, 22]. The output of ci is fed into the ReLU (Rectified Linear Activation function) activation function, as shown in the equation below [23, 24]. A convolution map is created from the activation results. The processes for the convolution layer are listed below: (Shown in Fig. 3).

3.1.2 Implementation

The steps involved to build this model:

(a) Data Acquisition
(b) Preprocessing

Gray to Binary
Noise Removal and Resizing

(c) Adding CNN Layers
(d) Feature Extraction
(e) Training with Tensor Flow model
(f) Testing and Predicting the output

3.1.3 Flow Diagram

3.1.4 Data Acquisition

To build a knowledge base for every user, handwritten signatures are gathered, and some unique features are extracted. For evaluating the performance of signature detection, a standard dataset of signatures for every person is needed. So, the dataset

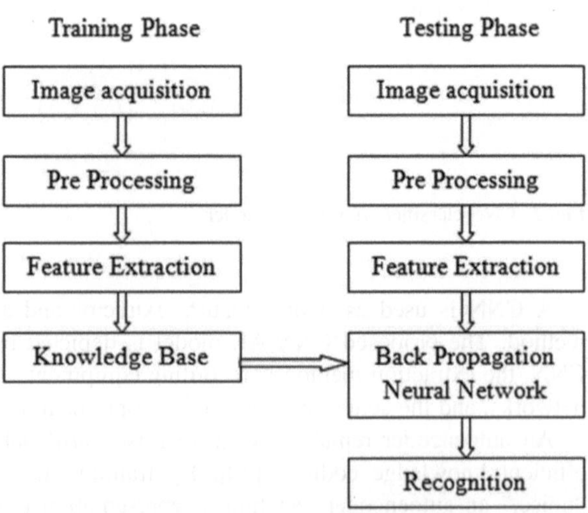

Fig. 3 Flow model

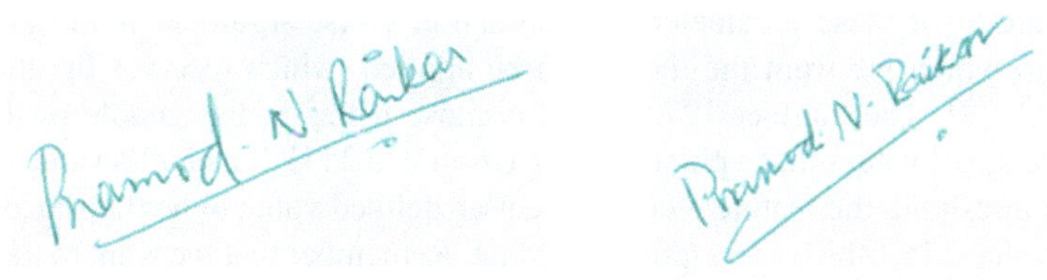

(a) (b)

Fig. 4 (**a**) Real signature image, (**b**) Forged signature image

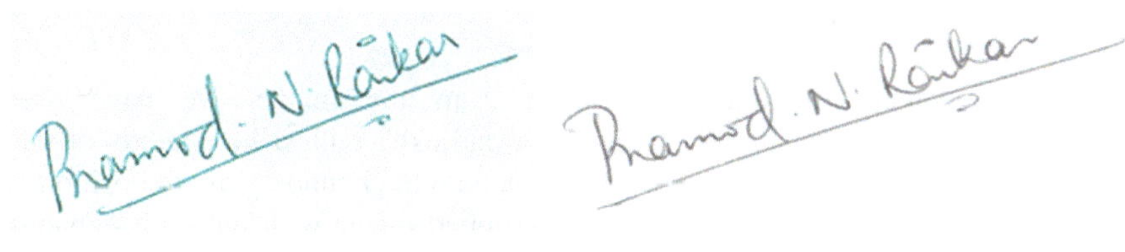

(a) (b)

Fig. 5 (**a**) RGB image, (**b**) Gray scale image

we collected from Kaggle is a selection of nearly 2000 images of genuine and forged signatures of a person [25, 26]. This is the dataset that has been used in our work. As it is a massive set of images, we have taken a sample of images for 30 persons, with authentic and forged images for each individual [27–32]. The dataset is divided into a genuine and forged set of images. All the images are in RGB format, collected for this work (Shown in Fig. 4).

3.1.5 Preprocessing

The Genuine and Forged Images have been pre-processed through the histogram equalization method. Any RGB image is represented in layman's terms as a matrix of X, Y, and a depth of three planes where the plane consists of red, green, and blue values ranging from 0 to 225. Whereas in a gray image, only one plane is represented as a Matrix of X, Y, and depth. We have used SK image libraries to convert an RGB signature into gray in this work (Shown in Fig. 5).

3.1.6 Gray to Binary

To convert our Gray image to Binary, we need to "import from skimage. filters import threshold_otsu". As we work with a grayscale image, pixel values range from 0 to 255. When the image resolution value exceeds 255, convert the source image into RBG -to-Gray for better perceptions. The threshold function, of course, aids in the definition of these parameters. The function's first argument is the grayscale picture to which we want the method to be applied, which receives the threshold value [33–38]. The number 127 is used because it lies in the middle of the gray scale's range of values that a pixel can take (from 0 to 255). If a pixel's value is larger than the threshold, the feature receives the user-defined value to be translated. We'll use the value 255, which corresponds to white. Remember that we want to transform the image to black and white, which means we want an image with pixels that are either 0 or 255 at the end [39–42].

3.1.7 Noise Removal and Resizing

To remove small components or noise from the image, we have used "img = ndimage. gaussian_filter (IMG, blur_radius)", with a blur radius of 0.8. And next to that, we will make a bounding box with the boundary as the position of pixels on the extreme. Thus, we will get a cropped image with only the signature part [43].

3.1.8 Adding CNN Layers

First, import the required Packages. Keras could be a framework for building deep neural networks using Python [44–48]. To avoid quality, it is designed to create a deep neural network by several lines of code. Keras provides a straightforward front-end layer towards creating a deep neural network utilising Tensor Flow at the back end. It allows quick experimentation with deep neural networks [49–52].

3.1.9 Pooling Layer

When the photos become too huge, the pooling layers section would reduce the number of parameters [53]. Spatial pooling, also known as subsampling or downsampling, is a technique for reducing the spatial property while keeping the necessary data. There are many different types of spatial pooling:

1. Max Pooling
2. Average Pooling
3. Sum Pooling

Max pooling extracts the most information from the rectified feature map. The most significant portion may also entail common pooling (Shown in Fig. 6). Sum pooling is the sum of all components within the feature map choice.

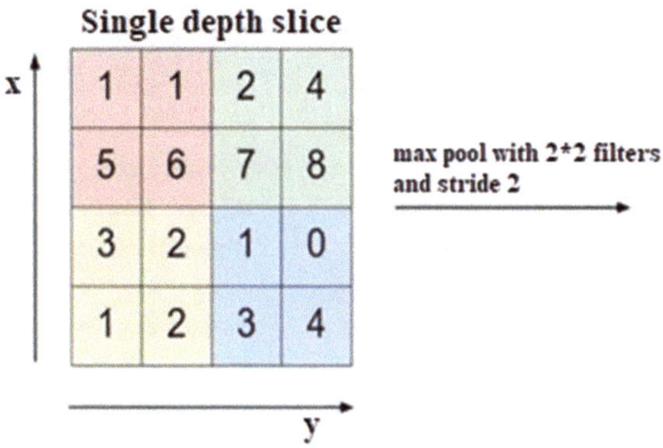

Fig. 6 Max pooling

3.1.10 Flatten

Flattening is needed to convert multi-dimensional data into usable knowledge for the fully connected layers. The fully convolutional layer output has been converted into a 1D vector for better classification, which is shown in Fig. 6. Our convolution layers use 2D images (images). Before it is fed into the classifier, it needs to be reshaped, or planar, to one dimension.

3.1.11 Dense- Softmax

Our final fully connected layer can use the softmax function. The proposed work concentrates on original image authentication and forged image features i.e., two classes. The forged image is a binary classification problem wherever softmax can be accustomed to changing the classes for every image.

3.1.12 Feature Extraction

We are going to extract some features from each image. The pre-processing stage has been adjusting the images like resizing, scaling, RGB to Gray, etc. Features like ratio, centroid, eccentricity, solidity, skewness, and kurtosis are extracted from each signature image and are saved into Comma Separated Format files for each individual.

Training with Tensor Flow Model: We build use of CNN during this work. A CNN (or ConvNet) may be a deep, feed-forward artificial neural network category that has been with success applied to imaginary visual analysis (Shown in Fig. 7). Biological processes motivated CNN in that the communication pattern between neurons parallels the organisation of the visual cortex of animals. Our study used the Keras library to implement CNN with the "Tensor Flow" backend. The preprocessed

Name	Date modified	Type	Size
testing_001	6/22/2021 1:54 PM	Microsoft Excel Co...	1 KB
testing_002	6/22/2021 1:54 PM	Microsoft Excel Co...	1 KB
testing_003	6/22/2021 1:54 PM	Microsoft Excel Co...	1 KB
testing_004	6/22/2021 1:55 PM	Microsoft Excel Co...	1 KB
testing_005	6/22/2021 1:55 PM	Microsoft Excel Co...	1 KB
testing_006	6/22/2021 1:55 PM	Microsoft Excel Co...	1 KB
testing_007	6/22/2021 1:55 PM	Microsoft Excel Co...	1 KB
testing_008	6/22/2021 1:55 PM	Microsoft Excel Co...	1 KB
testing_009	6/22/2021 1:55 PM	Microsoft Excel Co...	1 KB
testing_010	6/22/2021 1:57 PM	Microsoft Excel Co...	1 KB
testing_011	6/22/2021 1:57 PM	Microsoft Excel Co...	1 KB
testing_012	6/22/2021 1:57 PM	Microsoft Excel Co...	1 KB

Fig. 7 Saving features in the training set

image directory is loaded, and we then train the model to predict the performance. In this work, we have created a model called logits, three input layers with different weights and biases and three hidden layers with a set of neurons and an output layer to show the final output (Genuine or Forged). We have also defined loss and optimiser to minimise the loss and applied softmax to calculate the accuracy. Testing and Predicting the output: The model is first tested with the test set of images in the Jupyter notebook before running it with the user interface. After training with Tensor Flow, it is tested by giving input images. The testing can be done by entering the person's ID and image path. Finally, after evaluating the model, we will receive output on whether the image is Genuine or Forged. Our model predicts the output with an accuracy of 85%.

Prediction of Forged image

```
Enter person's id : 001
Enter path of signature image : C:\Users\Sneha\Desktop\Main Project\Project\forged\021001_000.png
This Signature belongs to Fake Person
Out[22]: False
```

Prediction of Forged image

```
Enter person's id : 001
Enter path of signature image : C:\Users\Sneha\Desktop\Main Project\Project\real\001001_002.png
This Signature belongs to Genuine Person
Accuracy: 0.8333333
Out[23]: True
```

4 Results

The Detection of Handwritten Signature Forgery model using CNN is built using the Convolution Neural Network technique. In this model, a total of 1500 signature images are taken. But due to the huge dataset, we consider a sample of 30 person images. We have trained and tested the model, which predicts whether the image is genuine or forged. The model achieved an accuracy of 86% on the scale. The user interface is built with Flask API to ensure the interactive UI for the user. The output is seen through the user interface, consisting of the button to upload the image. It shows the output by considering the input as an uploaded image. If we give the image, then it predicts the respective output of an image as Genuine or Forged.

5 Discussions

CNN is an image classification algorithm that is commonly utilised. CNN is a reasonably robust technique for various image and object identification applications because of its hierarchical structure and extensive feature extraction capabilities from a picture. The depth-wise separable convolutional neural network model created in this study is especially suited for mobile devices since it has low latency, uses less computational power while at the same time maintains high accuracy. Finally, the developed system included a signature forgery detection map feature. CNN is an exceptionally robust method for image and object recognition applications because of its hierarchical structure and excellent feature extraction capabilities from an image. The advantage of CNN is that it automatically detects the essential features. CNN gives the best accuracy for image classification among all the algorithms (Shown in Figs. 8 and 9).

The figures explain the deep signature analysis of original vs. forgery sign analysis, using our proposed CNN model to identify the fake sign. Moreover, easily, our model presents accurate outcomes compared to existing models.

Table 1 clearly explains different users' signatures like Saikumar, Anil Kumar, Ravi Kumar, Swathi, Vamsi. All five users' signatures are forged by other sources using various image processing models. Therefore the CNN mechanism is necessary to cover this problem. Table 2 explains the comparison of results with various methodologies like GA (Genetic Algorithm), SVM(support vector machine), RFO (random forest optimisation), X boost, and Convolutional neural networks. Compared to all models, the proposed CNN technique achieves more improvement and provides accurate experimental outcomes.

Figure 10 clearly explains the comparison of outcomes using various approaches such as the genetic algorithm, support vector machine, random forest optimisation, X boost, and convolutional neural networks. Compared to all other models, the suggested CNN approach achieves a higher level of improvement and provides more accurate experimental results.

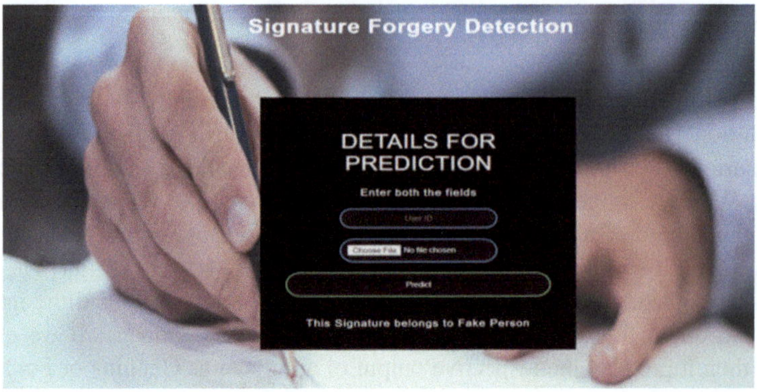

Fig. 8 The output of Forged Image

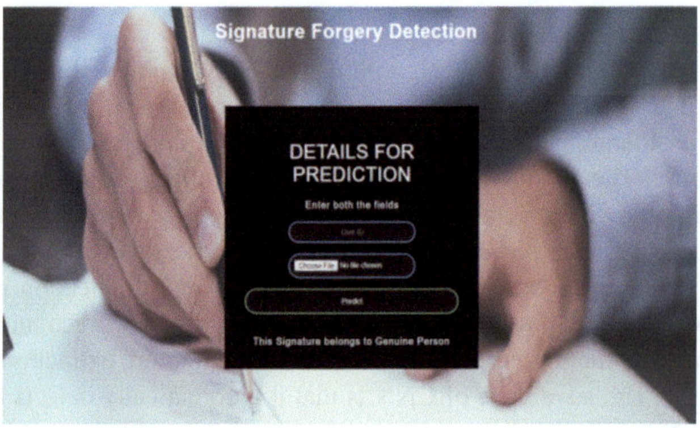

Fig. 9 The output of Genuine Image

6 Conclusion

This framework helps to identify the signatures of a person, whether the signature is from a genuine or fake person. This device can be utilised in various government offices that require handwritten signatures for approval or validation. Although CNN is used in this strategy, it may be considered severe. In the model established in this work, two classes are created for each user (genuine and forgery). If 500 people's natural and forged signatures are provided, the model will have 500 classes to forecast, lengthening the learning process. Extensive research on loss functions and the development of custom loss functions (ideally two) that can forecast the user to whom the signature belongs and whether it is a forgery or not is a possible development. Such implementation can be deemed severe. Two classes are created

Table 1 Different signatures original vs. forgery

S no	Name of user	Original sign	Forgery sign
1	K Saikumar	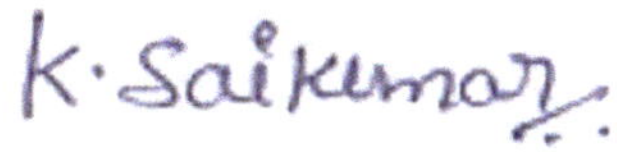	K saikumar
2	K Vamsi	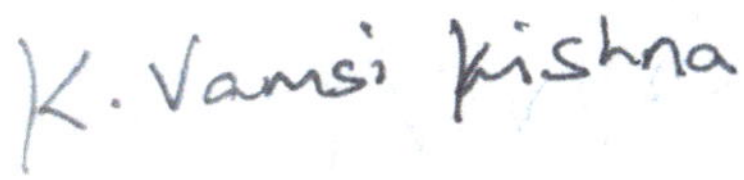	K vamsi krishna
3	K Swathi	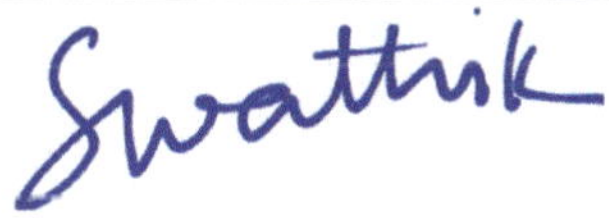	Swathi k
4	A.Ravi Kumar	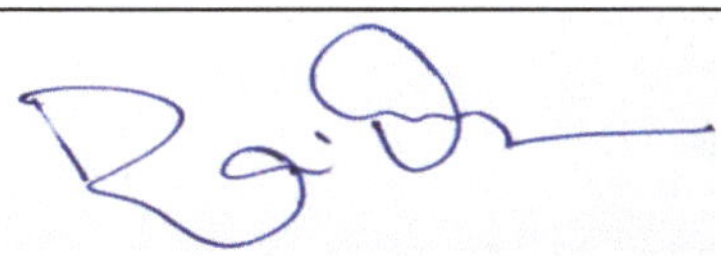	A.Ravi Kumar
5	G.Anil Kumar	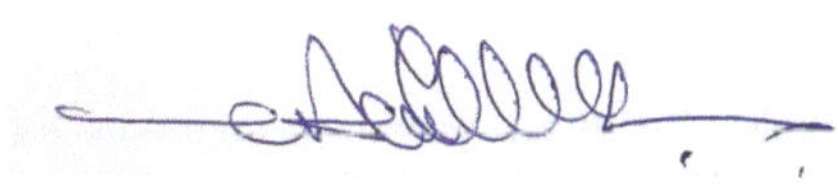	G.Anil Kumar

Table 2 Comparison of results

Model	Accuracy	Sensitivity	Recall	F Score	Throughput
GA	77.23	76.32	79.23	81.23	82.45
SVM	89.34	91.38	72.34	77.28	83.78
RFO	91.28	92.29	89.27	91.38	91.37
Xboost	94.78	95.71	91.28	89.18	93.45
CNN proposed	98.27	99.21	98.24	97.23	98.91

for each user in the model created in this work (Real and forgery). We have 30 users, so we have a model that can estimate 150 groups. The highest accuracy we got was 94.78%. The average accuracy is about 83.3%, sensitivity 99.2, recall 98.24, F score 97.23, and throughput 98.91 had been attained; those improved results were more accurate than earlier models.

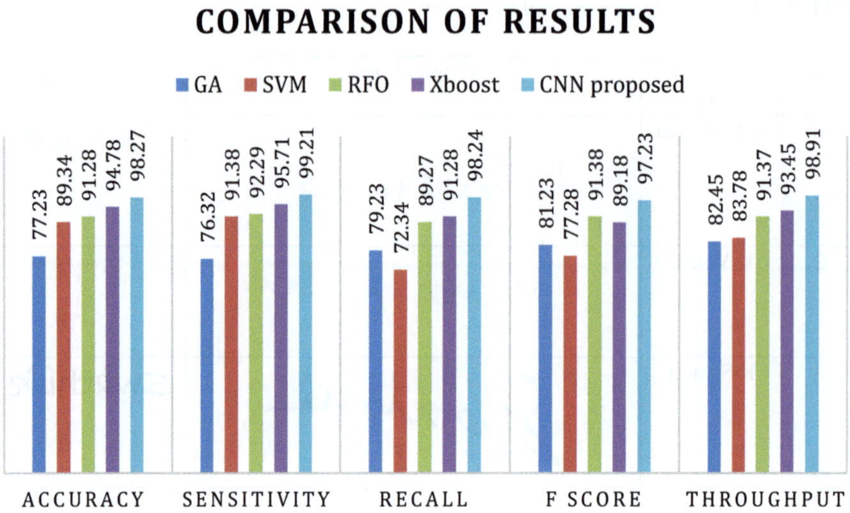

Fig. 10 Comparison results

6.1 *Future Scope*

This work is most suitable for future level fake signature forgery detection applications. Using an advanced CNN model, this functionality gets very easy compared to earlier models. Moreover, this framework helps to identify the signatures of a person, whether it is correct or not.

References

1. Chai Quek & R.W. Zhou.: Antiforgery: A novel pseudo-outer product based fuzzy neural network driven signature verification system. *Pattern Recognition Letters*. 23(14): 1795–1816 (2002).
2. Hanmandlu, M., Mohan, K. M., Chakraborty, S., Goyal, S., & Choudhury, D. R.: Unconstrained handwritten character recognition based on fuzzy logic. *Pattern Recognition*, 36(3), 603–623 (2003).
3. Bin Xiao, Yang Wei, Xiuli Bi and Weisheng Li.: Image Splicing Forgery Detection Combining Coarse to Refined Convolutional Neural Network and Adaptive Clustering. *Information Sciences*. 511:172–191 (2020).
4. Ruiz, V., Linares, I., Sanchez, A., and Velez, J. F.: Offline Handwritten Signature Verification Using Compositional Synthetic Generation of Signatures and Siamese Neural Networks. *Neurocomputing*. 374:30–41 (2020).
5. Hong, Yan.: Handwritten digit recognition using an optimised nearest neighbor classifier. *Pattern Recognition Letters*. 15(2):207–211 (1994).
6. Vargas-Bonilla, J. Ferrer-Ballester, Miguel Travieso, Carlos Alonso and Jesús.: Offline signature verification based on grey level information using texture features. *Pattern Recognition*. 44(2):375–385 (2011).

7. Saeid Fazli & Shima Pouyan.: High Performance Offline Signature Verification and Recognition Method using Neural Network. *International Journal of advanced studies in Computer Science and Engineering*. 4(6):9–13 (2015).
8. Bin Xiao, Yang Wei, Xiuli Bi and Weisheng Li.: Image Splicing Forgery Detection Combining Coarse to Refined Convolutional Neural Network and Adaptive Clustering. *Information Sciences*. 511:172–191 (2020).
9. Ruiz, V., Linares, I., Sanchez, A., and Velez, J. F.: Offline Handwritten Signature Verification Using Compositional Synthetic Generation of Signatures and Siamese Neural Networks. *Neuro computing*. 374:30–41 (2020).
10. IS. I Abuhaiba and Pervez Ahmed.: A fuzzy graph theoretic approach to recognise the unconstrained handwritten numerals. *Pattern Recognition*. 26(9):1335–1350 (1993).
11. C. L. Walker, M. Brown and Temple H. Fay.: Handprinted symbol recognition system. *Pattern Recognition*. 21(2):91–118 (1988).
12. Blanco-Gonzalo R., Sanchez-Reillo R., Liu-Jimenez, J. and Miguel-Hurtado O. (2014). Performance Evaluation of Handwritten Signature Recognition In Mobile Environments. *IET Biometrics*. 3(3):139–146 (2014).
13. A. A. Alarood, E. Alsolami, M. A. Al-Khasawneh, N. Ababneh, and W. Elmedany, "IES: Hyper-chaotic plain image encryption scheme using improved shuffled confusion-diffusion," Ain Shams Eng. J., vol. 13, no. 3, p. 101583, 2022.
14. M. A. Al-Khasawneh, I. Uddin, S. A. A. Shah, A. M. Khasawneh, L. Abualigah, and M. Mahmoud, "An improved chaotic image encryption algorithm using Hadoop-based MapReduce framework for massive remote sensed images in parallel IoT applications," Cluster Comput., vol. 25, no. 2, pp. 999–1013, 2022.
15. R. Rani, S. Kumar, O. Kaiwartya, A.M. Khasawneh, J. Lloret, M.A. Al-Khasawneh, M. Mahmoud, A.A. Alarood, "Towards green computing oriented security: A Lightweight Postquantum signature for IoE," Sensors (Basel), vol. 21, no. 5, p. 1883, 2021.
16. M. A. Al-Khasawneh, S. M. Shamsuddin, S. Hasan, and A. A. Bakar, "An improved chaotic image encryption algorithm," in 2018 International Conference on Smart Computing and Electronic Enterprise (ICSCEE), 2018.
17. Ramaiah, V. S., Singh, B., Raju, A. R., Reddy, G. N., Saikumar, K., & Ratnayake, D.: Teaching and Learning based 5G cognitive radio application for future application. In 2021 International Conference on Computational Intelligence and Knowledge Economy, (pp. 31–36). IEEE (2021).
18. Mohammad, M. N., Kumari, C. U., Murthy, A. S. D., Jagan, B. O. L., & Saikumar, K.: Implementation of online and offline product selection system using FCNN deep learning: Product analysis. Materials Today: Proceedings, 45, 2171–2178 (2021).
19. Padmini, G. R., Rajesh, O., Raghu, K., Sree, N. M., & Apurva, C.: Design and analysis of 8-bit ripple Carry Adder using nine Transistor Full Adder. In 2021 7th International Conference on Advanced Computing and Communication Systems, Vol. 1, (pp. 1982–1987). IEEE (2021).
20. K. Raju, A. Sampath Dakshina Murthy, B. Chinna Rao, Sindhura Bhargavi, G. Jagga Rao, K. Madhu, K. Saikumar. A Robust And Accurate Video Watermarking System Based On SVD Hybridation For Performance Assessment International Journal of Engineering Trends and Technology, 68(7),19–24 (2020).
21. Saba, S. S., Sreelakshmi, D., Kumar, P. S., Kumar, K. S., & Saba, S. R.: Logistic regression machine learning algorithm on MRI brain image for fast and accurate diagnosis. *International Journal of Scientific and Technology Research*, 9(3), 7076–7081 (2020).
22. Saikumar, K.: Rajesh V. Coronary blockage of artery for Heart diagnosis with DT Artificial Intelligence Algorithm. *Int J Res Pharma Sci,* 11(1), 471–479 (2020).
23. Saikumar, K., Rajesh, V.: A novel implementation heart diagnosis system based on random forest machine learning technique *International Journal of Pharmaceutical Research,* Vol. 12, pp. 3904–3916 (2020).
24. Raju K., Chinna Rao B., Saikumar K., Lakshman Pratap N.: An Optimal Hybrid Solution to Local and Global Facial Recognition Through Machine Learning. In: Kumar P., Obaid AJ, Cengiz K., Khanna A., Balas V.E. (eds) A Fusion of Artificial Intelligence and Internet of

Things for Emerging Cyber Systems. Intelligent Systems Reference Library, vol 210. Springer, Cham (2021). doi:https://doi.org/10.1007/978-3-030-76653-5_11
25. Sankara Babu B., Nalajala S., Sarada K., Muniraju Naidu V., Yamsani N., Saikumar K.: Machine Learning Based Online Handwritten Telugu Letters Recognition for Different Domains. In: Kumar P., Obaid AJ, Cengiz K., Khanna A., Balas V.E. (eds) A Fusion of Artificial Intelligence and Internet of Things for Emerging Cyber Systems. Intelligent Systems Reference Library, vol 210. Springer, Cham (2022). doi:https://doi.org/10.1007/978-3-030-76653-5_12
26. Kiran Kumar M., Kranthi Kumar S., Kalpana E., Srikanth D., Saikumar K.: A Novel Implementation of Linux Based Android Platform for Client and Server. In: Kumar P., Obaid AJ, Cengiz K., Khanna A., Balas V.E. (eds) A Fusion of Artificial Intelligence and Internet of Things for Emerging Cyber Systems. Intelligent Systems Reference Library, vol 210. Springer, Cham (2022). doi:https://doi.org/10.1007/978-3-030-76653-5_8
27. S. Sharma and A. J. Obaid.: Mathematical modelling, analysis and design of fuzzy logic controller for the control of ventilation systems using MATLAB fuzzy logic toolbox, *Journal of Interdisciplinary Mathematics*, vol. 23, no. 4, pp. 843–849, (2020).
28. T. A. Al-asadi, A. J. Obaid, R. Hidayat and A. A. Ramli.: A survey on web mining techniques and applications, International Journal on Advanced Science Engineering and Information Technology, vol. 7, no. 4, pp. 1178–1184, (2017).
29. S. Sharma and A. J. Obaid.: Contact-mechanics and dynamics analysis of three-different ellipsoidal raceway geometries for deep Groove ball bearing using Abaqus 6.13 version FEA simulation for high load-bearing as well as speed-rotating applications," International Research Journal of Multidisciplinary Science and Technology, vol. 3, no. 5, pp. 36–43, (2020).
30. Pandya, S., Wandra, K., Shah, J., A Hybrid Based Recommendation System to overcome the problem of sparcity, International Conference on emerging trends in scientific research, December, (2015).
31. Mehta, P., Pandya, S., A review on sentiment analysis methodologies, practices and applications, International Journal of Scientific and Technology Research, 9(2), pp. 601–609 (2020).
32. A.K. Gupta, Y. K. Chauhan, and T Maity.: Experimental investigations and comparison of various MPPT techniques for photovoltaic system. Sādhanā, Vol. 43, no. 8, pp. 1–15, (2018).
33. Sadiq, S., Umer, M., Ullah, S., Mirjalili, S., Rupapara, V., & NAPPI, M. Discrepancy detection between actual user reviews and numeric ratings of Google App store using deep learning. Expert Systems with Applications, 115111 (2021).
34. Rupapara, V., Narra, M., Gonda, N. K., Thipparthy, K., & Gandhi, S. Auto-Encoders for Content-based Image Retrieval with its Implementation Using Handwritten Dataset. 2020 5th International Conference on Communication and Electronics Systems, 289–294 (2020).
35. A.K. Gupta, Y.K Chauhan, and T Maity and R Nanda.: Study of Solar PV Panel Under Partial Vacuum Conditions: A Step Towards Performance Improvement. IETE Journal of Research, pp. 1–8, (2020).
36. A. Jain, A. Kumar, and S. Sharma, “Comparative Design and Analysis of Mesh, Torus and Ring NoC,” Procedia Comput. Sci., vol. 48, pp. 330–337, (2015).
37. A. Jain, R. Dwivedi, A. Kumar, and S. Sharma, “Scalable design and synthesis of 3D mesh network on chip,” in Proceeding of International Conference on Intelligent Communication, Control and Devices, pp. 661–666 (2017).
38. A. Jain, A. K. Gahlot, R. Dwivedi, A. Kumar, and S. K. Sharma.: Fat Tree NoC Design and Synthesis. in Intelligent Communication, Control and Devices, Springer, pp. 1749–1756 (2018).
39. A. Jain, A. Kumar, and S. Sharma. Comparative Design and Analysis of Mesh, Torus and Ring NoC. Procedia Comput. Sci., vol. 48, pp. 330–337, (2015).
40. A. Jain, R. Dwivedi, A. Kumar, and S. Sharma.: Scalable design and synthesis of 3D mesh network on chip.: in Proceeding of International Conference on Intelligent Communication, Control and Devices.: pp. 661–666 (2017).

41. A. Jain, A. K. Gahlot, R. Dwivedi, A. Kumar, and S. K. Sharma.: Fat Tree NoC Design and Synthesis. in Intelligent Communication, Control and Devices, Springer, pp. 1749–1756 (2018).
42. A. Jain, A. K. AlokGahlot, and S. K. S. RakeshDwivedi, "Design and FPGA Performance Analysis of 2D and 3D Router in Mesh NoC," *Int. J. Control Theory Appl.*, pp. 0974–5572, (2017).
43. N. Gupta and A. K. Agarwal.: "Object Identification using Super Sonic Sensor: Arduino Object Radar," 2018 International Conference on System Modeling & Advancement in Research Trends, 2018, pp. 92–96.
44. S. Shukla, A. Lakhmani and A. K. Agarwal, "A review on integrating ICT based education system in rural areas in India," 2016 International Conference System Modeling & Advancement in Research Trends, pp. 256–259 (2016).
45. Agarwal A.K., Rani L., Tiwari R.G., Sharma T., Sarangi P.K.: Honey Encryption: Fortification Beyond the Brute-Force Impediment. In: Manik G., Kalia S., Sahoo S.K., Sharma T.K., Verma O.P. (eds) Advances in Mechanical Engineering. Lecture Notes in Mechanical Engineering. Springer, Singapore (2021). doi:https://doi.org/10.1007/978-981-16-0942-8_64
46. Khullar V, Singh HP, Agarwal AK. Spoken buddy for individuals with autism spectrum disorder. Asian J Psychiatr. 62 102712 (2021).
47. A.K. Agarwal, A. Jain, Synthesis of 2D and 3D NoC Mesh Router Architecture in HDL Environment, Jour of Adv Research in Dynamical & Control Systems, Vol. 11, 04-Special Issue, (2019).
48. Hasaballah, A.I. Impact of paternal transmission of gamma radiation on reproduction, oogenesis, and spermatogenesis of the housefly, Musca domestica L. (Diptera: Muscidae). International Journal of Radiation Biology. 97(3): 376–385 (2021).
49. Mohan, V., Rani, A., & Singh, V. Robust adaptive fuzzy controller applied to double inverted pendulum. Journal of Intelligent & Fuzzy Systems, 32(5), 3669–3687 (2017).
50. Panjwani, B., Mohan, V., Rani, A., & Singh, V.: Optimal drug scheduling for cancer chemotherapy using two degree of freedom fractional order PID scheme. Journal of Intelligent & Fuzzy Systems, 36(3), 2273–2284 (2019).
51. Surinder Singh and Hardeep Singh Saini "Security approaches for data aggregation in Wireless Sensor Networks against Sybil Attack," 2018 Second International Conference on Inventive Communication and Computational Technologies, pp. 190–193, Coimbatore, India (2018).
52. H. Pallathadka, M. Mustafa, D. T. Sanchez, G. Sekhar Sajja, S. Gour, and M. Naved.: "Impact of machine learning on management, healthcare and agriculture," Materials Today: Proceedings, (2021).
53. B. Prabhu kavin, S. Ganapathy, P. Suthanthiramani, and A. Kannan, "A modified digital signature algorithm to improve the biomedical image integrity in cloud environment," Advances in Computational Techniques for Biomedical Image Analysis, pp. 253–271, (2020).

Experimental Analysis of Internet of Technology-Enabled Smart Irrigation System

Ramachandran Veerachamy, R. Ramalakshmi, C. Mageshkumar, and Rajasekar Rangasamy

1 Introduction

Sustainable technology changes are required to improve the performance and productivity over the agricultural field, which will improve the lifestyle of farmers and encourage them to do farming. The advancements of the latest technologies support the agricultural area and farmers in many ways; however, the level of trustworthiness, prediction strategies, and accuracy level of predictions are again an issue that needs to be resolved. Generally, India is one of the traditional agricultural countries in which the level of productivity and the growth of farmers are in leading range in the past few decades. However, nowadays, Indian farmers are committing suicide and relieving themselves from agriculture due to economic problems, climate conditions problems, and lack of productivity. These scenarios raise a question to introduce a new methodology to keep farming and agriculture to the next level. In this chapter, all the above-quoted problems are getting resolved. The Cloud Enabled Smart Agri-Handling Strategy, as proposed in this approach, introduces new methodologies that can significantly enhance farming practices to a higher level. IoT is a cutting-edge innovation for checking and controlling smart gadgets at any place globally. IoT can connect and interface gadgets with remote servers [1]. IoT is utilised not only in agriculture, but it also imprints in various other fields enabling remote monitoring and control over anything that need not have computational

R. Veerachamy · C. Mageshkumar · R. Rangasamy
Department of Computer Science and Engineering, GITAM – School of Technology, GITAM Deemed to be University, Bengaluru Campus, Bengaluru, India

R. Ramalakshmi (✉)
Department of Computer Science and Engineering, Kalasalingam Academy of Research and Education, Krishnankoil, Srivilliputhur, Tamil Nadu, India
e-mail: rama@klu.ac.in

P. Agarwal et al. (eds.), *Artificial Intelligence for Smart Healthcare*, EAI/Springer Innovations in Communication and Computing,
https://doi.org/10.1007/978-3-031-23602-0_9

features. The recent technologies like cloud, Fog computing, and machine learning can be converged comfortably with IoT for proposing new solutions for modern-day problems. These days, the versatile idea of the IoT has changed, in which a standard client can use it. The IoT has created a few strategies that have made day-to-day human activities simpler and agreeable, like keen schooling, urban communities, innovative health regions, and automation [2]. Aside from man's solaces, these systems should be actualised on essential requirements like food, which can be accomplished from the agricultural fields. World Bank has assessed that excess could be created before 2050 if the populace pattern is at the current rate.

In any case, the current atmosphere changes would not support such immense harvest creation, so field-based sensors, drones, progressed work vehicles, and aquaculture cultivating may assist future agricultural belonging persons with yielding more harvest, at less expense. Subsequently, the need for exquisite cultivating is developing dramatically, and a colossal measure of the water supplies is happening for cultivating. In this way, more safeguards and conversations should be made in the cultivation zone. Undoubtedly, the farming benefit is a significant piece of the course of action, and India is a country that is notable for its agriculture. Regarding developing yields, its water framework needs should be taken into notice, and agriculture requires a simple water system framework at legitimate time breaks for them to develop well [3]. Agriculture is where there is an appeal for the work, and the explanation behind the reduction in work power was deficient since youths were not energetic about cultivating part. They did not find a ton of changes in it. Along these lines, farming people who dedicate their occasions to creating crops in colossal locales are expected to go through their whole day outside to ensure that the harvests are appropriately grown [4].

Farming peoples now and again had great controls on yields and experienced staggering adversities in light of unforeseen and troublesome atmosphere conditions. Improving the farming procedures and agricultural growth in next level of technological development employing adding latest technologies such as IoT and Cloud Surface Monitoring with this environment will change the present level of agriculture system and make the farmers richer and provide complete safeguard to the crops as well [5]. One of the leading agricultural analysis organizations informed in the year 2050, all the crops, vegetables, and fruits rate will be ten times higher than the present level. The significant agricultural source of India will depend on other countries for feeding its population. This case will happen due to the lack of farming people and people's economy in the farming and agricultural field. The level of farmers and agriculture needs to be changed. It will happen by adapting the latest technologies to the agricultural field and changing the productivity ratio and performance of the environment, which automatically turns the level of farmers [6]. So, a new generation of people can easily enter into the agricultural field, grow based on the environmental nature, and produce good agricultural products at a low cost. The primary concern of agriculture is the source of water, which is the backbone of agriculture [7].

The main question in this field is how to preserve the water wastages and save water in a good way. Because water wastages are high in agricultural fields, many innovations are coming to solve such issues. However, all are a failure at a certain level. For example, the Global System for Mobile Communications (GSM)-based automatic agriculture management system was introduced. However, the service and support level of GSM is slow because of 2G-enabled communication services. A new methodology is introduced to resolve all the classical problems in the agricultural field. The proposed chapter adapts most of the latest technologies. It provides efficient support to farmers and agriculture, in which the adaptable technologies are IoT, Smart Irrigation System (SIS), Cloud Optimization Strategy (COS), and Systematic Monitoring. A most crucial smart gadget is placed in the Agricultural farming land for monitoring the crops and controlling the smart device via the IoT. The intelligent device comprises many intelligent sensors such as pH sensor, SMS, RS, temperature, and humidity sensors. The pH sensor is used to identify the acidity or alkalinity of the water passed to the agricultural land. The SMS is used to identify the soil conditions. An RS is used to identify the rain situations and operate the motor pumps accordingly, and the DHT 11 sensor monitors the temperature and humidity. The DHT-11 sensor effectively monitors the temperature and the humidity of the environment. These will help yield more agriculture yield, making the farmer's life beautiful. All these technologies and their associated functions are clearly described in other sections. The chapter is organised correctly such that the related study is described in Sect. 2, illustration of the proposed system methodologies is discussed in Sect. 3, the implementation results and its discussions were described in Sect. 4, and the conclusion of the proposed work and scope of future enhancements is discussed in Sect. 5. The forthcoming sections will explain the pre-mentioned details.

2 Related Study

In this chapter [8], the authors illustrated that the power of associating the IoT with the SIS helps achieve good agricultural yields. Such IoT-enabled devices make the farmer's life simpler than past farming methodologies. Agriculture gives a rich wellspring of boundaries for information analysis, which helps in better yielding of harvests. IoT gadgets in the field of agriculture help modernise data and correspondence in brilliant cultivating. The essential boundaries that can be considered for better development of yields are based on soil types and soil dampness, supplements, temperature, light, oxygen level, etc. The boundaries are detected using various sensors, and the collected data is then transmitted to the cloud. This chapter analyses some boundaries for information researches that help in proposing the clients to make better agricultural choices utilising the IoT. The proposed framework performed better and is actualised at the 'ThingSpeak' IoT cloud environment. The primary issue identified in this paper is the utilization of ThinkSpeak cloud associations. It is not suitable for commercials with customised options because this is a third-party association. So a customisable IoT environment is required to improve the proposed approach better. Timely alerts in the agriculture process, especially irrigation, help the farmers reduce water resource utilisation and improve crop quality due to the appropriate amount of irrigation [9].

Veerachamy.R. & Ramar. R proposed a paper related to Machine Learning-based Smart Agricultural Environment maintenance concerning the IoT norms. In this chapter [10], the authors illustrate that agriculture adjusts food necessity for humankind and supplies key crude materials for numerous businesses. It is the most critical and essential Indian occupation source. The progression in innovative cultivating methods is continuously improving the yield in the agriculture process, turning it more beneficial and lessening water consumption. The implemented system envisages the water prerequisite required during harvest, utilising artificial intelligence and machine learning-based estimations. Dampness, temperature, moistness, and humidity are the most fundamental boundaries to decide the amount of water needed in any agriculture field. An exciting machine learning principle is applied to the information detected from the field to foresee results proficiently [11]. The major drawback identified in this chapter is that it utilises all the IoT-based associations concerning Raspberry PI interfacing. The cost of such IoT devices is enormous, as well as the Raspberry PI device is a smart and nano computer. However, the concept of IoT is quite different because the Raspberry PI board is not intended to provide internet connectivity alone. It is considered as a PC for a Linux environment [12].

In this chapter [13], the creators represented that an agribusiness region is establishing India's economy, and its security issues should be considered. Security worries over agricultural fields are not in regards to resources just yet; instead also cultivating things that need security and protection at an early phase, like affirmation from attacks of rodents or bugs, in fields or grain stores. Such challenges ought to be mulled over, and the connected security structures used nowadays are not sharp enough to give steady notification in the wake of distinguishing the issue. The compromise of regular methodology with latest developments as the IoT and WSNs can incite country modernisation and keeping the present circumstance in thought in regards to the built model, attempted and inspected an IoT-based contraption which is suitable for analysing the identified information and a while later imparting it to the customer. This smart device can be controlled and seen from the distant region, and it will, in general, be executed in country fields, crop/grain stockpiles, and cold stockpiles for security reasons. The major drawback identified over these works [14, 15] is that the pooled analysis of security and crop monitoring and third-party IoT support creates privacy issues and performance degradation problems in the future.

Evapotranspiration is a significant element not only in irrigation management but also in many other applications. Evapotranspiration (ET) estimation depends on several models, and the Penman-Monteith is the highly followed standard across the globe among many researchers for estimation of ET [16]. Mohammadrezapour et al. in 2019 estimated the ET by comparing and contrasting the three models, namely the support vector machine (SVM), Adaptive neuro-fuzzy inference system (ANFIS), and Gene expression programming (GEP). All three models estimated the potential evapotranspiration for semi-arid land [17]. The simulation of ET is done for the data ranging from the year 1970 to 2010, with inputs of five different combinations in south-eastern Iran. Among the three models, ANFIS is a neural network model, SVM is a machine learning model, and GEP is an evolutionary computing technique. The SVM-based model performed better than the other two models, with sunshine hours, humidity, relative humidity, air temperature average, and wind speed as the input parameters for the model.

3 Methodologies

The proposed scheme called cloud-enabled Smart Agri-Handling Strategy (CSAHS) adapts several innovative technologies to provide ultimate support to the farmers to improve their lives in an exemplary manner. The associated technologies of CSAHS are listed as follows: IoT, SIS, COS, and Systematic Monitoring. These technologies are associated together and work for a smart agricultural management and automation system. The associated sensors are pH sensor, SMS, RS, and THS. All these sensor details are clearly explained further, and Fig. 1 elucidates the architecture of the proposed model.

3.1 pH Sensor

A pH sensor concept measures the acidity and alkalinity level of the input water to the range between 0 and 14. The ranges are deviated according to the consistency of water, and the ranges indicate several measures, such as the range of pH sensor lower than 7 means the respective water is considered to be more acidic. When the range crosses 7, it means the water is considered more alkaline. The level of 8.5 is considered more challenging, and the level of 7 is considered an average, and it is suitable for regular farming and agricultural usages. Figure 2 elucidates the view of a model pH sensor and the associated analogue board for serially providing the controller's values.

3.2 Soil Moisture Sensor

The purpose of using an SMS is to identify the moisture level inland, which is helpful to the crops to monitor the soil moisture level. Accordingly, the smart system can control the motor pumps and provide sufficient water to the respective crops. Once the soil moisture level attains the wet range, the sensor triggers the relay to turn off the motor pump. The SMS analyses the soil between the range of 0 to 70%, and from this sensor, the user can attain the accuracy range between plus or minus 3% actual variations. Figure 3 shows the model view of the SMS.

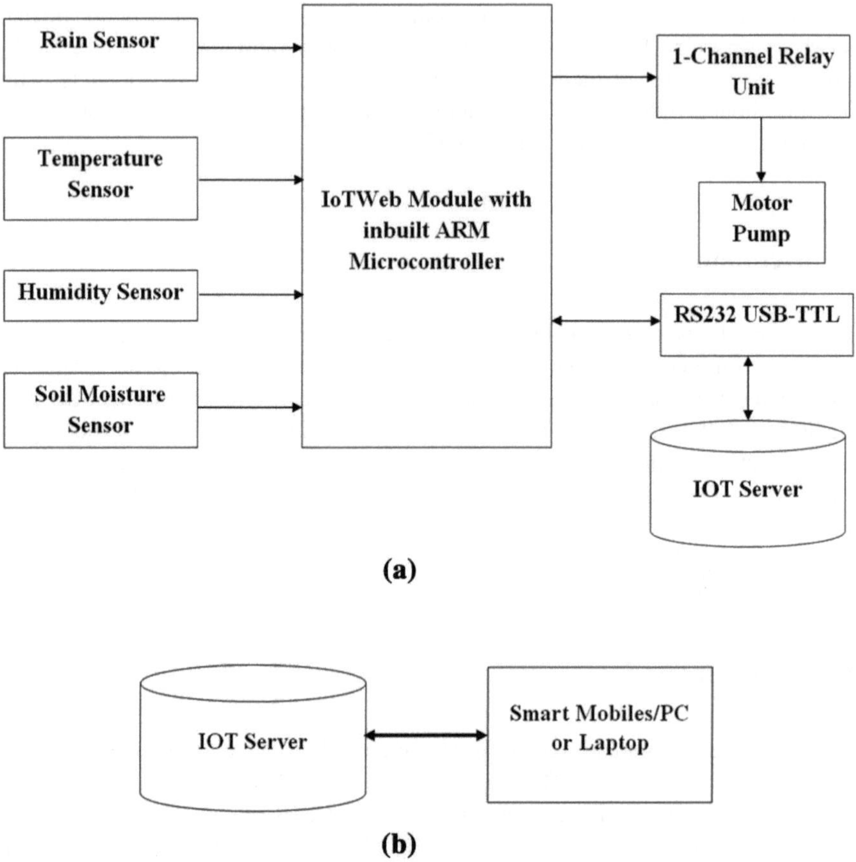

Fig. 1 Proposed architectural system block view. (**a**) Transmission and master smart gadget block unit (**b**) Receiver end monitoring and controlling block

3.3 Rain Sensor

An RS is considered a switch device, in which it switches the trigger based on the identification of rainfall. This sensor is most important to the SIS. For example, the SMS gives the soil dry trigger to the IoT-Web module and switches the pump on to provide water to the respective crops. If it rains under the same conditions, the rain detection sensor detects it and activates the motor pump to switch accordingly. This Rain Detection Sensor has the placement of infrared radiation beams with a 45-degree angle with a clear spread ratio to identify the raindrops immediately without any delay. Figure 4 shows the model view of the Rain Detection Sensor.

Fig. 2 pH sensor

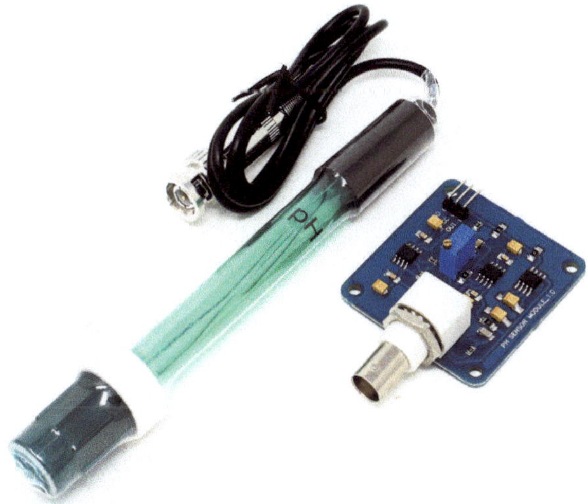

Fig. 3 SMS

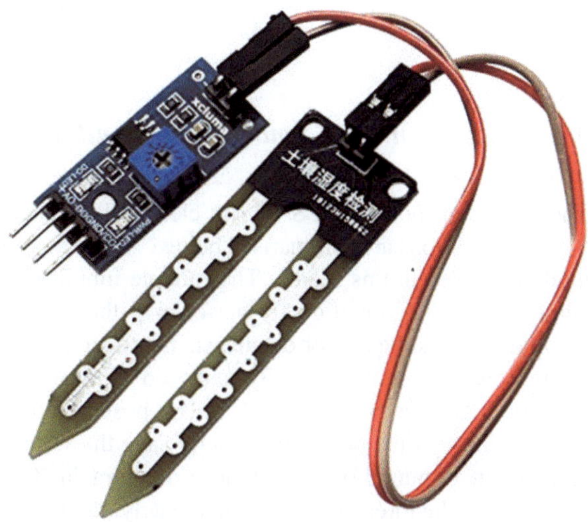

3.4 Temperature and Humidity Sensor

A well-known and commonly used sensor to identify the temperature and humidity level is the DHT11 sensor, which identifies the surrounding temperature and humidity level. This sensor is handy for monitoring the climate conditions properly and instantly providing an appropriate alert to the respective farmers. The measuring range of the DHT11 sensor ranges from −40 degrees Celsius to +125 degrees Celsius to plus or minus 0.5 degrees of actual accuracy. Figure 5 depicts the DHT-11(digital humidity and temperature) sensor.

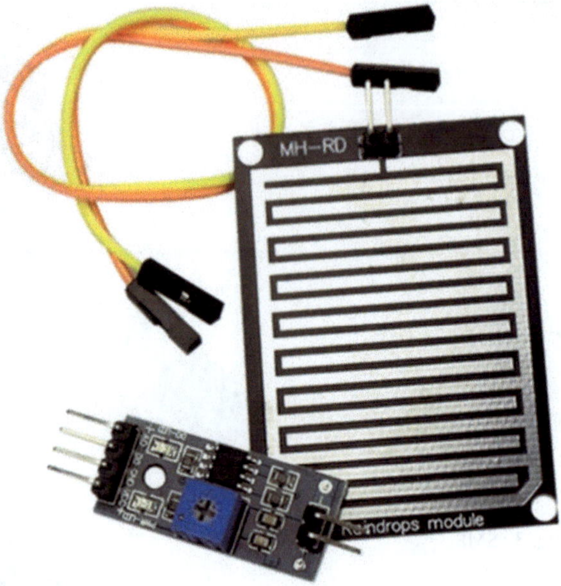

Fig. 4 Rain detection sensor

3.5 Cloud-Enabled Smart Agri-Handling Strategy (CSAHS)

The proposed model of CSAHS is clearly illustrated in Fig. 1, and the complete block descriptions are summarised below. A new innovative IoT Web interfaced IoT module is used in this model. The module inbuilt contains an ARM-based microcontroller unit for intelligently performing the required tasks. The connected IoT module receives the sensor details, such as accumulating the RS details. The motor pump condition is immediately analysed if the raindrops are identified over the module. If the pump state is ON, the proposed module immediately trips the relay and switches off the pump to instantly save the water. The THS senses the current temperature or humidity level of the agricultural land, and if the temperature exceeds much above the threshold level immediately, the information will be grasped by the IoT module and passed to the respective farmer as a message format and the associated details will be stored into the cloud server for future references. The connected SMS provides the analogue values to the IoT module, in which the value of the sensor crosses the threshold level immediately. The IoT module triggers the relay to the ON state, and the motor pump gets on to provide water to the crops in the agricultural land without any human intervention. Similarly, once the land gets wet immediately, the SMS analyses that and sends an associated trigger to the IoT module. It turns off the relay and stops watering the crops. So, a massive water level is preserved with this proposed methodology, and the innovative system helps maintain all the data into the server end for analysing purposes. The cloud server utilised in this chapter is the ThingSpeak server. It is an open-source server with certain limitations. The integration of the cloud server is quite simple as it facilitates

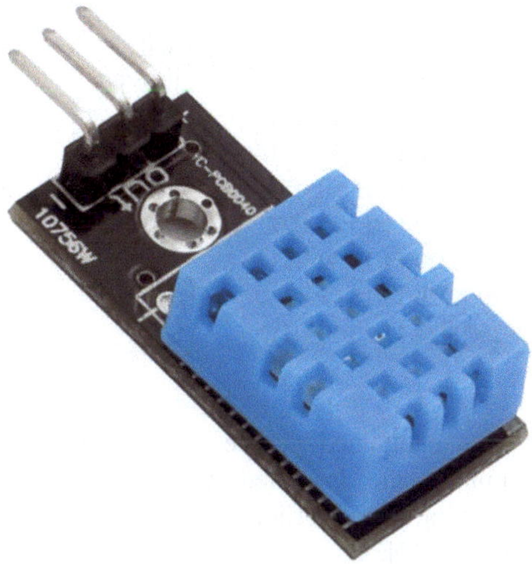

Fig. 5 Digital humidity and temperature (DHT) 11 sensor

the user with separate read and writes API keys. The server also enables the creation of separate channels for storing separate data. Each channel has separate read and write keys to classify data stored. The server also features MATLAB analysis as a part of the platform. Visualisations as charts and graphs are embedded as a feature in the platform that can be utilised by the user directly with developer tools and codes available in the ThingSpeak platform.

3.6 *Cloud Optimization Strategy*

The cloud server maintains the periodical agricultural data from the smart device with associated sensors over the farmland. This kind of cloud server storage allows the user to instantly monitor the details of crops, and the server's analysis is easy with the help of date-wise analysis options [18]. The data collected from the sensors are accumulated by the IoT device and passed to the remote cloud server, in which the data will be processed and stored into the server with proper identities to date and time considerations [19–21]. The Cloud Server mentioned in this chapter is a customised cloud server. The user can change the attributes and levels of sensors and the display dashboard according to their convenience. Once the smart agriculture data is entered into the server, the data can be visible to the respective farmers or individuals from anywhere without any range considerations. The proposed approach of CSAHS associates the optimisation strategy to avoid the accumulation of duplicate contents stored into the server. Duplicate contents lead to the data overhead and searching delay problems raised into the server end. This is achieved by verifying the incoming data from the sensors to already stored records for the last few hours; once the current record is not matched with the already recorded data, it

Table 1 Maintained into server in data samples

Date and time	Soil moisture	Rain status	pH Level	DHT11 values
2020/12/20 11:15:20 UTC	286	NIL	7.23	21 °C, 30 °F
2020/12/20 11:15:25 UTC	290	NIL	7.35	22 °C, 31 °F
2020/12/20 11:15:30 UTC	285	NIL	7.24	21 °C, 29 °F
2020/12/20 11:15:35 UTC	300	NIL	7.85	20 °C, 28 °F
2020/12/20 11:15:40 UTC	305	NIL	7.00	20 °C, 34 °F
2020/12/20 11:15:45 UTC	356	NIL	7.53	21 °C, 30 °F
2020/12/20 11:15:50 UTC	302	NIL	7.15	20 °C, 35 °F

will be maintained into the server for processing [22–24]. This optimisation strategy eliminates the unwanted storage burden and data repetitions on the server end, improving timing efficiency. Table 1 shows the view of accumulated agricultural data [25–32].

The following formulation (Table 1) is used to analyse the harvesting duration. This will allow the farmer to maintain the crops safely for the coming years.

$$H^x = 1 + \frac{W_1}{T_1} + \frac{W_2}{T_2} + \frac{W_3}{T_3} + \ldots, \quad -T\infty < \beta < \infty \tag{1}$$

Where W indicates the weight factor, T indicates the temperature level of the atmosphere, and β indicates the soil type.

The limitations of rainfall measurements are estimated with the help of the following function.

$$_{in} \leq r_T \leq R_{\text{Max}} \ ¥ \ € \{ T + \triangle R_1 + \triangle R_2 + \triangle R_3 + \ldots + \triangle R_n \} \tag{2}$$

Where $_{in}$ and R_{Max} indicates the maximum and minimum values of rain quantity during the harvesting period, and the top limit of the irrigation level is formulated using:

$$\sum_{t=1+\triangle}^{T+t\triangle} \left(\frac{Q}{T}\right) \triangle a \leq R^{n-k} \tag{3}$$

$$\sum_{R=1+\triangle r}^{R+T\triangle} \left(\frac{Q}{R}\right) \triangle a \leq T^{n-k} \tag{4}$$

Additionally, the rainfall rate and the soil moisture level, water flow rate, and drain level are all positive real-values, and this is indicated as:

$$R_T; S_T; D_T; Q_T \geq 1 \tag{5}$$

4 Discussion

In this summary, the performance ratio of the proposed approach Cloud-enabled Smart Agri-Handling Strategy (CSAHS) is analysed clearly [33–37]. The performance ratio of the approach is estimated to be cost-efficiency, server processing time, and data maintenance accuracy. The proposed model is implemented, and the sensed data is collected over the cloud server; the sensors were placed into the agricultural land for more than 1 month and tested clearly [38–41]. The positioning of the Smart device is placed in several atmospheric conditions [42–46]. Figure 6 illustrates an empirical evaluation of systematic irrigation control cost efficiency as a classic human intervention model with the proposed approach [47].

Figure 7 illustrates the time efficiency achieved in the proposed approach, in comparison with CSAHS [48–53]. The analysts' research is based on several constraints with numerous optimisation algorithms such as NP-Hard and Network Neural Scheme. Nevertheless, all are inevitable delays over data processing speed accumulated from the smart devices placed into the agricultural land. The same concern needs to get clarity regarding the reverse control [54–58]. In the same way, the smart device needs to be controlled from the IoT module, in which it accumulates the trigger coming from the server end and processes the total smart device according to the received trigger. For example, the IoT Web module senses the low moisture level on soil; in this case, two types of operations are required to process immediately. One is to inform the respective detail to the farmer accordingly, and the other is to store the data into the server instantly without any delay. Based on the timing efficiency consideration, these processes are estimated and provided below.

Figure 8, illustrates the irrigation data maintenance accuracy levels with proper semantics. The data maintenance accuracy ratio is estimated by analysing the

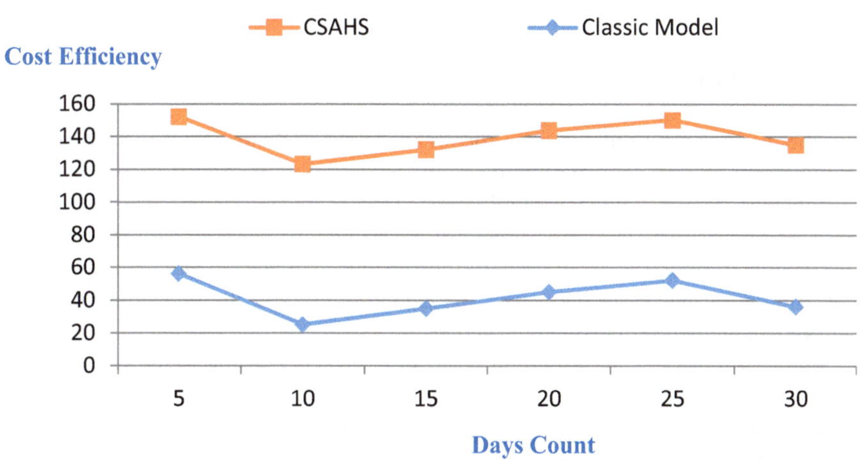

Fig. 6 Cost-efficiency

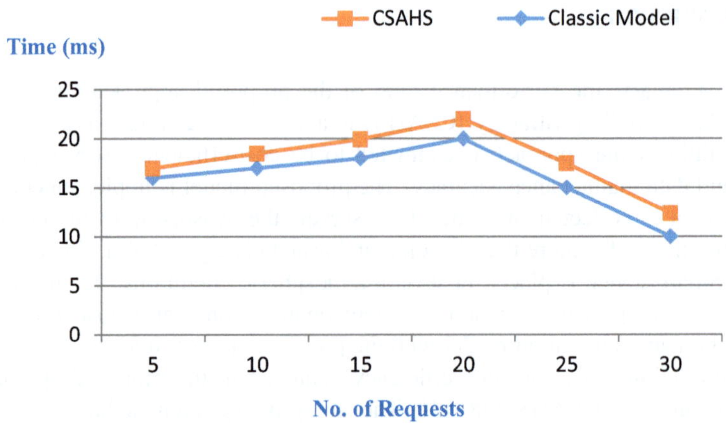

Fig. 7 Time-efficiency

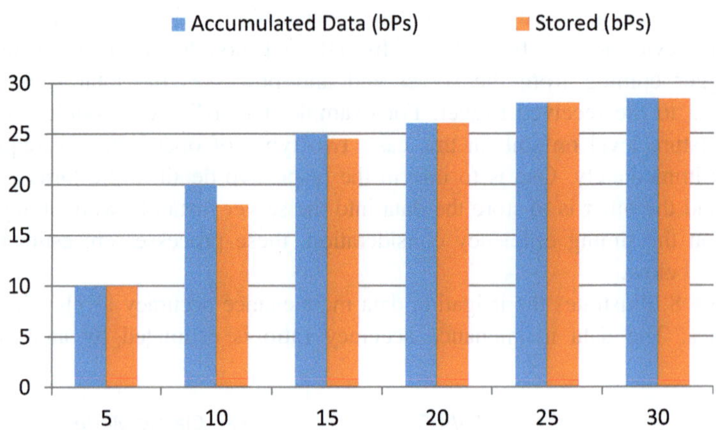

Fig. 8 Data maintenance accuracy

number of data accumulated from the smart device and stored adequately into the cloud server. To improve our approach, the focus should be on a different standard, specifically data redundancy elimination. This is necessary because the Cloud-enabled Smart Agri-Handling Strategy (CSAHS) we propose already takes care of eliminating duplicated data in the cloud and ensures that there is only one copy of the data stored on the server. However, the data coming after the threshold time limit will be maintained properly on the server.

Figure 9 illustrates the irrigation water flow level according to the soil moisture levels of the implementation period over the agricultural land. During 1 month, the ratios of soil moisture are accumulated properly and maintained into the server end. It is easy to estimate the water flow level to the crops concerning that. Figure 9 shows the details clearly with proper mentioning of the X-axis as soil irrigation level and the Y-axis as the water flow level.

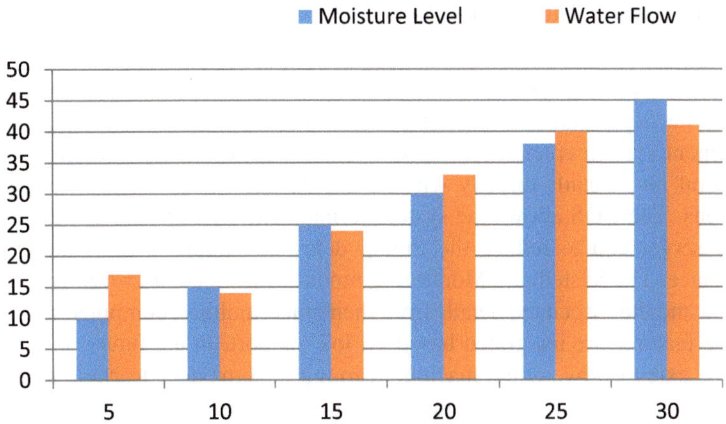

Fig. 9 Water flow ratio analysis

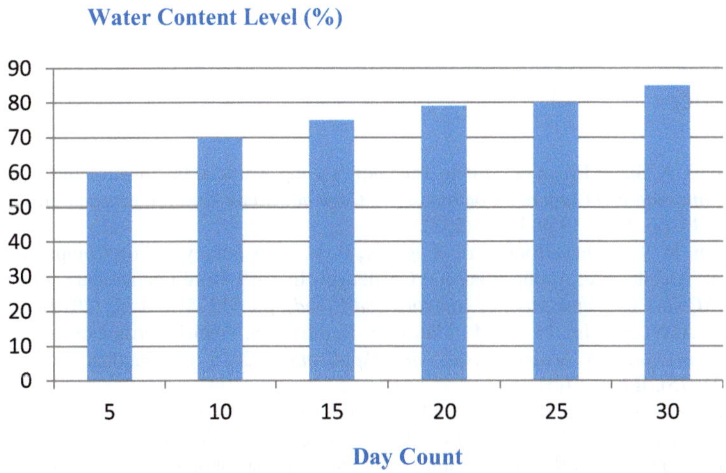

Fig. 10 Moisture level measurement w.r.t water content

Figure 10 illustrates the Moisture Level Measurement analysis for the water content level on the agricultural land following Fig. 10, in which it shows the details clearly with proper mentioning of the X-axis as the day of the month to identify in which day the level of moisture is mentioned, and the Y-axis indicates the water content level in %.

5 Conclusion and Future Scope

This paper introduces a new Smart agriculture management scheme methodology based on the cloud with IoT associations. This IoT-based cloud-enabled agricultural management system enhances the power of farmers to monitor the crops and the agricultural land details directly without any human interventions and any range restrictions. The COS allows the system to maintain the flaw-free agricultural data into the server end to reduce the timing delay and improve the entire system's performance. The Systematic Monitoring module allows the user/farmer to monitor their land and the associated details from their smart mobiles, computer, and laptops. All these features are integrated based on IoT support. In the future, the work can further be extended by adding machine learning or some deep learning strategies to classify the stored agricultural data and identify the required and unwanted details. Once the machine learning principle classifies the required data, which will be sufficient to maintain, the other details can be eliminated from the server instead of storing that unwantedly into the server and releasing the space on it.

References

1. Blessy, J. A. Smart Irrigation System Techniques using Artificial Intelligence and IoT. In *2021 Third International Conference on Intelligent Communication Technologies and Virtual Mobile Networks*, pp. 1355–1359. IEEE (2021).
2. Sanketh, R. S., MohanaRoopa, Y., & Reddy, P. V. N. A Survey of Fog Computing: Fundamental, Architecture, Applications and Challenges. In 2019 Third International conference on I-SMAC (*IoT in Social, Mobile, Analytics and Cloud*), pp. 512–516. IEEE (2019).
3. Harun, A. N., Kassim, M. R. M., Mat, I., & Ramli, S. S. Precision irrigation using wireless sensor network. *In Smart Sensors and Application*, 2015 International Conference on (pp. 71–75). IEEE (2015).
4. Kalathas, J., Bandekas, D. V., Kosmidis, A., & Kanakaris, V. Seedbed based on IoT: A Case Study. *Journal of Engineering Science & Technology Review*, 9(2) (2016).
5. V.Ramachandran and R. Ramalakshmi, "Suitable crop plantation recommendation system for profitable harvest using deep learning". *International Journal of Grid and Distributed Computing* 8, no. 2 (2015): 331–331 (2020).
6. Ramachandran, V., Ramalakshmi, R., & Srinivasan, S. An automated irrigation system for smart agriculture using the Internet of Things. In 2018 15th International Conference on Control, *Automation, Robotics and Vision*, pp. 210–215. IEEE (2018).
7. Ryu, M., Yun, J., Miao, T., Ahn, I. Y., Choi, S. C., & Kim, J. IEEE. Design and implementation of a connected farm for smart farming system. *In Sensors*, 2015 IEEE pp. 1–4 (2015).
8. Bhanu K.N., Mahadevaswamy H.S. and Jasmine H.J., "IoT based Smart System for Enhanced Irrigation in Agriculture", *IEEE*, (2020).
9. Dhamal, P., & Mehrotra, S. Automation Soil Irrigation System Based on Soil Moisture Detection Using Internet of Things. *In Machine Intelligence and Smart Systems* (pp. 665–673). Springer, Singapore (2021).
10. Veerachamy, R., & Ramar, R. Agricultural Irrigation Recommendation and Alert (AIRA) system using optimisation and machine learning in Hadoop for sustainable agriculture. *Environmental Science and Pollution Research*, 1–20 (2021).

11. Kasara Sai Pratyush Reddy, Y Mohana Roopa, Kovvada Rajeev L N and Narra Sai Nandan, "*IoT based Smart Agriculture using Machine Learning*", IEEE, (2020).
12. Lee, M., Hwang, J., & Yoe, H. Agricultural production system based on IoT. In *Computational Science and Engineering (CSE),* 2013 IEEE 16th International Conference on, pp. 833–837. IEEE (2013).
13. Baranwal, T., & Pateriya, P. K. Development of IoT based smart security and monitoring devices for agriculture. In *Cloud System and Big Data Engineering* (Confluence), 2016 6th International Conference (pp. 597–602) (2016). IEEE.
14. Wenting, H., Zhiping, X., Yang, Z., Pei, C., Xiangwei, C., & Ooi, S. K. Real-time remote monitoring system for crop water requirement information. *International Journal of Agricultural and Biological Engineering,* 7(6), 37–46 (2014).
15. Deksnys, V., et al. "Remote agriculture automation using wireless link and IoT gateway infrastructure." *Database and Expert Systems Applications*, 2015 26th International Workshop on. IEEE, (2015).
16. Jing, W., Yaseen, Z. M., Shahid, S., Saggi, M. K., Tao, H., Kisi, O., & Chau, K. W. Implementation of evolutionary computing models for reference evapotranspiration modeling: short review, assessment and possible future research directions. *Engineering applications of computational fluid mechanics*, 13(1), 811–823 (2019).
17. Mohammadrezapour, O., Piri, J., & Kisi, O. Comparison of SVM, ANFIS and GEP in modeling monthly potential evapotranspiration in an arid region (Case study: Sistan and Baluchestan Province, Iran). *Water Supply*, 19(2), 392–403 (2019).
18. Patil, N., & Khairnar, V. D. Smart Farming System Using IoT and Cloud. In Computer *Networks and Inventive Communication Technologies*, pp. 215–232. Springer, Singapore (2022).
19. Sindhwani, Nidhi, Vijay Prakash Maurya, Amit Patel, Roopesh Kumar Yadav, Sheetanshu Krishna, and Rohit Anand. "Implementation of Intelligent Plantation System Using Virtual IoT." In *Internet of Things and Its Applications*, pp. 305–322. Springer, Cham, (2022).
20. S. Sudhakar and S. Chenthur Pandian "Secure packet encryption and key exchange system in mobile ad hoc network", *Journal of Computer Science*, vol. 8, no. 6, pp. 908–912, (2012).
21. S. Sudhakar and S. Chenthur Pandian, "Hybrid cluster-based geographical routing protocol to mitigate malicious nodes in mobile ad hoc network", *International Journal of Ad Hoc and Ubiquitous Computing*, vol. 21 no. 4, pp. 224–236, (2016).
22. A. U. Priyadarshni and S. Sudhakar, "Cluster-based certificate revocation by cluster head in mobile ad-hoc network", *International Journal of Applied Engineering Research*, vol. 10, no. 20, pp. 16014–16018, (2015).
23. S. Sudhakar and S. Chenthur Pandian, "Investigation of attribute aided data aggregation over dynamic routing in wireless sensor," *Journal of Engineering Science and Technology*, vol. 10, no. 11, pp. 1465–1476, (2015).
24. S. Sudhakar and S. Chenthur Pandian, "Authorised node detection and accuracy in position-based information for MANET", *European Journal of Scientific Research*, vol. 70, no. 2, pp. 253–265, (2012).
25. Dilip Kumar Sharma, "Some Generalized Information Measures: Their characterization and Applications", *Lambert Academic Publishing,* Germany. ISBN: 978-3838386041 (2010).
26. D. K. Sharma, B. Singh, R. Regin, R. Steffi and M. K. Chakravarthi, "Efficient Classification for Neural Machines Interpretations based on Mathematical models," 2021 7th *International Conference on Advanced Computing and Communication Systems,* pp. 2015–2020 (2021).
27. F. Arslan, B. Singh, D. K. Sharma, R. Regin, R. Steffi and S. Suman Rajest, "Optimization Technique Approach to Resolve Food Sustainability Problems," 2021 *International Conference on Computational Intelligence and Knowledge Economy*, pp. 25–30 (2021).
28. G. A. Ogunmola, B. Singh, D. K. Sharma, R. Regin, S. S. Rajest and N. Singh, "Involvement of Distance Measure in Assessing and Resolving Efficiency Environmental Obstacles," 2021 *International Conference on Computational Intelligence and Knowledge Economy*, pp. 13–18 (2021).

29. D. K. Sharma, B. Singh, M. Raja, R. Regin and S. S. Rajest, "An Efficient Python Approach for Simulation of Poisson Distribution," 2021 7th *International Conference on Advanced Computing and Communication Systems,* pp. 2011–2014 (2021).
30. A.K. Gupta, Y.K Chauhan, and T Maity and R Nanda, "Study of Solar PV Panel Under Partial Vacuum Conditions: A Step Towards Performance Improvement," *IETE Journal of Research,* pp. 1–8, (2020).
31. Rustam, F., Khalid, M., Aslam, W., Rupapara, V., Mehmood, A., & Choi, G. S. A performance comparison of supervised machine learning models for Covid-19 tweets sentiment analysis. *PLOS ONE*, 16(2), e0245909 (2021).
32. D. K. Sharma, B. Singh, E. Herman, R. Regine, S. S. Rajest and V. P. Mishra, "Maximum Information Measure Policies in Reinforcement Learning with Deep Energy-Based Model," 2021 *International Conference on Computational Intelligence and Knowledge Economy,* pp. 19–24 (2021).
33. A.K. Gupta, Y. K. Chauhan, and T Maity, "Experimental investigations and comparison of various MPPT techniques for photovoltaic system," *Sādhanā*, Vol. 43, no. 8, pp. 1–15, (2018).
34. D. K. Sharma, N. A. Jalil, R. Regin, S. S. Rajest, R. K. Tummala and T. N, "Predicting Network Congestion with Machine Learning," 2021 *2nd International Conference on Smart Electronics and Communication,* pp. 1574–1579 (2021).
35. A. Jain, A. K. Gahlot, R. Dwivedi, A. Kumar, and S. K. Sharma, "Fat Tree NoC Design and Synthesis," in *Intelligent Communication, Control and Devices*, Springer, pp. 1749–1756 (2018).
36. D. Ghai, H. K. Gianey, A. Jain, and R. S. Uppal, "Quantum and dual-tree complex wavelet transform-based image watermarking," *Int. J. Mod. Phys.* B, vol. 34, no. 04, p. 2050009, (2020).
37. A. Jain and A. Kumar, "Desmogging of still smoggy images using a novel channel prior," *J. Ambient Intell. Humaniz. Comput.,* vol. 12, no. 1, pp. 1161–1177,(2021).
38. S. Kumar et al., "A Comparative Analysis of Machine Learning Algorithms for Detection of Organic and Nonorganic Cotton Diseases," *Math. Probl. Eng.,* vol. 2021, (2021).
39. Yousaf, A., Umer, M., Sadiq, S., Ullah, S., Mirjalili, S., Rupapara, V., & Nappi, M. Emotion Recognition by Textual Tweets Classification Using Voting Classifier. *IEEE Access,* 9, 6286–6295 (2021b).
40. A.K. Gupta, "Sun Irradiance Trappers for Solar PV Module to Operate on Maximum Power: An Experimental Study," *Turkish Journal of Computer and Mathematics Education,* Vol. 12, no. 5, pp. 1112–1121, (2021).
41. J. Kubiczek and B. Hadasik, "Challenges in Reporting the COVID-19 Spread and its Presentation to the Society," *J. Data and Information Quality*, vol. 13, no. 4, pp. 1–7, Dec. (2021).
42. Agarwal, A.K., Jain, A, Synthesis of 2D and 3D NoC Mesh Router Architecture in HDL Environment, *Jour of Adv Research in Dynamical & Control Systems*, 11(04) (2019).
43. N. R. Misra, S. Kumar, and A. Jain, "A Review on E-waste: Fostering the Need for Green Electronics," in 2021 *International Conference on Computing, Communication, and Intelligent Systems*, 2021, pp. 1032–1036 (2021).
44. Hassan, M.I., Fouda, M.A., Hammad, K.M. and Hasaballah, A.I. Effects of midgut bacteria and two protease inhibitors on the transmission of Wuchereria bancrofti by the mosquito vector, Culex pipiens. *Journal of the Egyptian Society of Parasitology*. 43(2): 547–553 (2013).
45. G. S. Sajja, K. P. Rane, K. Phasinam, T. Kassanuk, E. Okoronkwo, and P. Prabhu, "Towards applicability of blockchain in agriculture sector," *Materials Today: Proceedings,* (2021).
46. H. Pallathadka, M. Mustafa, D. T. Sanchez, G. Sekhar Sajja, S. Gour, and M. Naved, "Impact of machine learning on management, healthcare and agriculture," *Materials Today: Proceedings,* (2021).
47. Guna Sekhar Sajja, Malik Mustafa, R. Ponnusamy, Shokhjakhon Abdufattokhov, Murugesan G., P. Prabhu, "Machine Learning Algorithms in Intrusion Detection and Classification", *Annals of RSCB*, vol. 25, no. 6, pp. 12211–12219, (2021).

48. Fouda, M.A., Hassan, M.I., Hammad, K.M. and Hasaballah, A.I. Effects of midgut bacteria and two protease inhibitors on the reproductive potential and midgut enzymes of Culex pipiens infected with Wuchereria bancrofti. *Journal of the Egyptian Society of Parasitology.* 43(2): 537–546 (2013).
49. Surinder Singh and Hardeep Singh Saini, "Detection Techniques for Selective Forwarding Attack in Wireless Sensor Networks", *International Journal of Recent Technology and Engineering,* Vol. 7, Issue-6S, 380–383 (2019).
50. Hasaballah, A.I. Toxicity of some plant extracts against vector of lymphatic filariasis, Culex pipiens. *Journal of the Egyptian Society of Parasitology.* 45(1): 183–192 (2015).
51. O. M. Abo-Seida, N. T. M. El-dabe, A. Refaie Ali and G. A. Shalaby, "Cherenkov FEL Reaction with Plasma-Filled Cylindrical Waveguide in Fractional D-Dimensional Space," in *IEEE Transactions on Plasma Science*, vol. 49, no. 7, pp. 2070–2079, (2021).
52. Osama M. Abo-Seida, N.T.M.Eldabe, Ahmed Refaie Ali, & Gamil.Ali Shalaby. Far-Field, Radiation Resistance and temperature of Hertzian Dipole Antenna in Lossless Medium with Momentum and Energy Flow in the Far- Zone. *Journal of Advances in Physics,* 18, 20–28 (2020).
53. N.T.M. El-Dabe, A.Refaie Ali, A.A. El-shekhipy, Influence of Thermophoresis on Unsteady MHD Flow of Radiation Absorbing Kuvshinski Fluid with Non-Linear Heat and Mass Transfer, *American Journal of Heat and Mass Transfer* (2017).
54. Osama M. Abo-Seida, N.T.M.Eldabe, M. Abu-Shady, A.Refaie Ali, " Electromagnetic non-Darcy Forchheimer flow and heat transfer over a nonlinearly stretching sheet of non-Newtonian fluid in the presence of a non-uniform heat source", *Solid State Technology,* Vol. 63 No. 6 (2020).
55. N.T. El-dabel; A.Refaie Ali; A. El-shekhipy, A.; and A. Shalaby, G. "Non-Linear Heat and Mass Transfer of Second Grade Fluid Flow with Hall Currents and Thermophoresis Effects," *Applied Mathematics & Information Sciences*: Vol. 11: Iss. 1, Article 73 (2017).
56. Sadiq, S., Umer, M., Ullah, S., Mirjalili, S., Rupapara, V., & NAPPI, M. Discrepancy detection between actual user reviews and numeric ratings of Google App store using deep learning. *Expert Systems with Applications*, 115111 (2021).
57. N. Gupta and A. K. Agarwal, "Object Identification using Super Sonic Sensor: Arduino Object Radar," 2018 *International Conference on System Modeling & Advancement in Research Trends,* 2018, pp. 92–96 (2018).
58. S. Shukla, A. Lakhmani and A. K. Agarwal, "A review on integrating ICT based education system in rural areas in India," 2016 *International Conference System Modeling & Advancement in Research Trends,* pp. 256–259 (2016).

Analysis on Exposition of Speech Type Video Using SSD and CNN Techniques for Face Detection

Y. M. Manu, Chetana Prakash, S. Santhosh, Shaik Shafi, and K. Shruthi

1 Introduction

There is a lot of interest in facial analysis in computer vision (CV) and affective computing (AC). Research in the field constantly produces cutting-edge results for various face-related analysis and classification tasks such as facial recognition, facial expression identification, emotion estimation, action unit detection, face attribute recognition, and age estimation. On the other hand, recent research has focused on developing specialised architectures for various face analysis tasks. Nowadays many researchers are using earlier models, as they face high computational task issues. In order to overcome the above-described issues, we offer Face-SSD through the CNN network that performs concurrently face detection and one or more face analysis tasks in a single architecture. Conference recordings, video addressing, video journals, video messaging on social media platforms, and recordings in various places are beginning to supplant older forms of data exchange. Since 2019, there

Y. M. Manu (✉)
Department of CSE, BGS Institute of Technology-Adichunchanagiri University, Javarana Hally, Karnataka, India
e-mail: manuym@bgsit.ac.in

C. Prakash
Department of CSE, Bapuji Institute of Engineering and Technology, Davangere, Karnataka, India

S. Santhosh
Department of CSE, Kalpataru Institute of Technology, Tiptur, Karnataka, India

S. Shafi
Department of ECE, B V Raju Institute of Technology, Narsapur, Medak, Telangana, India

K. Shruthi
Department of ECE, KSRM College of Engineering, Kadapa, Andra Pradesh, India

P. Agarwal et al. (eds.), *Artificial Intelligence for Smart Healthcare*,
EAI/Springer Innovations in Communication and Computing,
https://doi.org/10.1007/978-3-031-23602-0_10

are video accounts for 80% of worldwide internet activity, excluding P2P channels, according to Cisco Visual networking index: projection and methodology by 2016–2021. As a result, much-improved video administration tactics are necessary, such as video exposition. A perfect video exposition can give clients the most extreme target video data in the briefest time. Its objective is to deliver a compact, however comprehensive, outline to empower a productive browsing encounter. The video rundown has to pass on most key data enclosed within the unique video. Video exposition could be an assignment where a video arrangement is diminished to a few still pictures known as keyframes, now and then known as storyboard or thumbnails extraction, or a shorter video arrangement composed of key shots, too known as video skim or dynamic rundowns. Most of the important information in the unique film was conveyed via key-frames or images [20–23]. The structure's square might represent a video frame compared to lossy video compression. The pre-processing stage consists of short video clips training along with features extraction. In a common video exposition framework, picture highlights of video outlines are extracted, and after that, the foremost agent outlines are chosen while analysing the visual varieties amongst visual features. Moreover, the earlier models cannot solve ToC (Time of Conversion) and accuracy of quality, by means of the proposed model, the limitations are overcome and less complex operations are required. Those endeavours depend on worldwide highlights such as colour, surface, and movement data.

Clustering methods are also utilised for exposition. An improved frame-synchronisation approach has been presented based on convolutional neural networks (CNNs) [24–28]. In most cases, the receiver uses a correlator to determine how long it will be until the actual delivery of the package. The conventional edge synchronisation strategy searches for a relationship top inside a given time stretch. The proposed technique, again, uses a CNN to decide the bundle appearance time. In the recommended technique, the yield of a 1D correlator is reshaped into a 2D network, and then the subsequent sign remains taken care of into the proposed 4-layer CNN classifier. At that point, the CNN gauges when the bundle will show up [29]. PC reproductions for two-channel models: added substance white Gaussian clamour and blurring channels are utilised to check outline synchronisation execution. The recommended CNN-based synchronisation technique outperforms the standard connection-based procedure by 2 dB, as indicated by reenactment information.

Figuring out the bundle appearance time or casing synchronisation at the beneficiary remains an essential advance that should be finished before information gathering can start. A parcel is sent at a foreordained time in synchronised correspondence organisations, for example, time division multiple access (TDMA) and synchronised carrier sense multiple access (CSMA) frameworks [30–33]. In internet-of-things (IoT) interchanges, these frameworks are habitually utilised. The transmission (Tx) and receiver (Rx) perform data transfer operations with the proposed algorithm. The bundle's appearance [34]. The transmitter normally sends a unique word before the packet to help frame synchronisation (or preamble). The packet arrival time is determined by the receiver identifying the got introduction. It is possible to use an introduction to synchronise edge synchronisation plans for binary phase-shift keying (BPSK) frameworks, M-ary PSK frameworks, continuous phase modulation (CPM) frameworks, and orthogonal frequency division multiple access (OFDM) frameworks [35–37]. The greatest likelihood (ML) technique achieves optimal frame synchronisation. The ML approach necessitates a thorough examination of all probable packet arrival timings. It is challenging to deal with such a large amount of data [39, 40]. As a result, there has been a lot of study into effective frame synchronisation systems. Regardless of modulation systems, feasible frame synchronisation solutions depend on connection top inquiry. In other words, conventional edge synchronization frameworks decide the parcel appearance time by contrasting the got signal with the introduction. In more detail, when the correlator's yield surpasses a particular limit, the parcel appearance time is resolved to be the occasion [41–44]. As a rule, the best limit is controlled by the sign-to-commotion proportion (SNR). Accordingly, before outline synchronisation, the SNR of the got sign ought to be determined to set up the best limit. Since outline synchronisation execution relies on SNR gauge precision, top identification of the correlator yield inside the time window is normally utilised as quite possibly the most natural way [45–48]. Although outline synchronisation through top pursuit at the correlator yield has a long history, it remains the most widely utilised procedure in current correspondence frameworks [49].

2 Related Work

The standard video rundown algorithm was designed for recordings handled by experienced editors [50–52]. The earlier camera-based videos have been facing blur and less accurate media, so an efficient algorithm is required to solve this limitation. As a result, the standard algorithms for determining the hazy shot boundaries also determine the essential frames in a shot that speak to the shot. For example, Omidyeganeh et al. [1] developed a keyframe extraction technique that used highlights taken from each frame's wavelet change sub-bands to divide the whole film into sub-shots and choose the final keyframes. The scene discovery was formulated as a keyframe arrangement by Chas anis et al. [2], who utilised shot boundary detection and the unearthly clustering technique in their calculation. Though there are too numerous strategies that don't distinguish shot boundaries [3] [4], isolating the full video into sub-shots contributes to stabilising the keyframe extraction results.

In any case, as expressed within the presentation, the above-expressed strategies don't work well for unstructured recordings (beginner and shopper recordings) since they are ineffectively shot and altered [5]. These recordings have numerous vague shot boundaries, and then they moreover have good for nothing, repetitive, or low-quality outlines. Subsequently, cantering on unstructured recordings has been picking up consideration, centred on inactive or energetic rundowns of the customer and/or self-cantered recordings. Cong et al. [6] treated video exposition as a dictionary selection issue. Important frames that speak to the complete video substance shape the word reference for a few examples of passive exposition methodologies we investigate in this study. However, because a word reference doesn't well speak to the long substance, this method isn't suited for long and complex recordings. Ejaz et al. [7] suggested a formula based on the assumption that visual examination would reveal the relevance of each outline in common recordings. They prioritised movement data and then used spatial and temporary consideration values. Regardless, these methods are limited by a few criteria, such as the development and prominence of outlines of the capturers or objects and the amount of time spent creating a scene. In the meanwhile, there are a few computations that concentrate on self-cantered recordings [8]. They execute transient division and grade the outlines based on specified criteria, similar to those used for regular customer recordings. However, they use data limited to first-individual perspectives and require high computational burdens, making them inadmissible for accounts not recorded by first-individual cameras or potentially long chronicles. There are an excessive number of strategies that emphasise the global division of customer recordings, where "temporal segmentation" can serve as "shot boundary detection" for well-edited recordings and is also linked towards video explanation calculations [9].

The difficulty of recognising a person from an image or video is automatic face recognition. Face recognition may be separated into face identification and face verification. Face recognition, alignment, representation, and classification are the four phases in the usual technique for training a CNN to solve these challenges. The task of giving an identity to a picture from a list of IDs is known as identification. Another way to look at it is similar to finding the best matching face in a gallery for a particular probing picture. On the other hand, face verification entails determining if two face photos belong to the same individual. This is commonly done by calculating the similarity between the two faces' feature representations. Developments in deep learning algorithms and more powerful CNN have greatly aided identification and verification. Multi-tracking of generic objects and individual faces is a hot issue in the science of computer vision, with applications in biometrics, security, and other fields. The fast development of deep neural networks has resulted in significant improvements in face recognition and object detection difficulties, which aids in advancing multiple-face tracking approaches based on the detection method. Face recognition trained on a head dataset is used in our suggested technique to overcome the face distortion issue in the tracking phase. Furthermore, we apply the Hungarian matching approach to match tracks with tracking faces utilising robust face characteristics collected from the deep face recognition network. We got encouraging results using deep facial features and head detection in a face tracking benchmark.

In computer vision, one of the most difficult problems is facial identification. Artefacts like noise and deterioration taint images in the actual world. The robustness of SSD and Faster R-CNN networks against salt and pepper noise, gaussian blur, and JPEG compression is examined in this study. Our study was built on the Wider Face dataset. In these experiments, the Faster R-CNN outperformed the SSD in terms of resistance to Gaussian blur. On the other hand, JPEG compressed photographs of inferior quality are more resistant to SSD. Faster R-sensitivity CNNs to the texture of the objects should be the reason for this. Furthermore, our studies discovered that both networks were equally resilient to salt and pepper noise. Due to differences in appearance, occlusions, and complicated backdrops, detecting faces and heads in video streams is difficult in real-world video surveillance applications. Numerous CNN designs have been created lately to enhance detector accuracy, albeit their computational cost may be an impediment, especially in real-time applications requiring the identification of faces and heads in real-time using high-resolution cameras. The accuracy and complexity of contemporary CNN architectures for face and head recognition are compared in this work. Single-pass and region-based designs are evaluated and compared to baseline procedures regarding accuracy, speed, and memory complexity on a range of hard datasets. Several systems are examined for their usefulness with real-time applications in mind. According to the research results, even while CNN architectures may achieve exceptionally high degrees of precision, their computational expense may impede many real-time applications.

3 Approach

In this work, we use deep learning techniques for keyframe taking out and video skimming for the exposition of a video. The single shot multi box detector (SSD) and Convolutional neural networks (CNN) have been imported to conversion mechanism which was better than earlier methods for video enhancement. The step-by-step procedure of the Flow Diagram of our approach is in Fig. 1.

In our work, there are following steps to be followed:

(a) Frame Extraction: Video is broken down into frames, and 1 frame is taken from every second.
(b) Face and Emotion Detection: Faces identify in the entire take out frames. The emotion of the takeout faces is then detected to determine the emotional score of every frame.
(c) Frame Ranking and Selection: Frames having strong emotions are collected and then ranked.
(d) Extraction: Video subtitles are prepared to represent the text and the timestamps. From the subtitles, the sentences corresponding to these selected frames are extracted along with the starting and ending times of the sentence. The summary is prepared by merging the video corresponding to all these intervals.

In this process, we extract a single frame per second. Emotions of the extracted frames are detected to determine the emotional value of every frame. The extracted frames are passed on to the deep learning model to detect the emotions. The deep learning model is implemented in two stages, one is Face Detection and the other is Emotion Classification. Face Detection is done using SSD (Single Shot Multi-box Detector). The bounding box obtained from SSD is passed on to a CNN-based

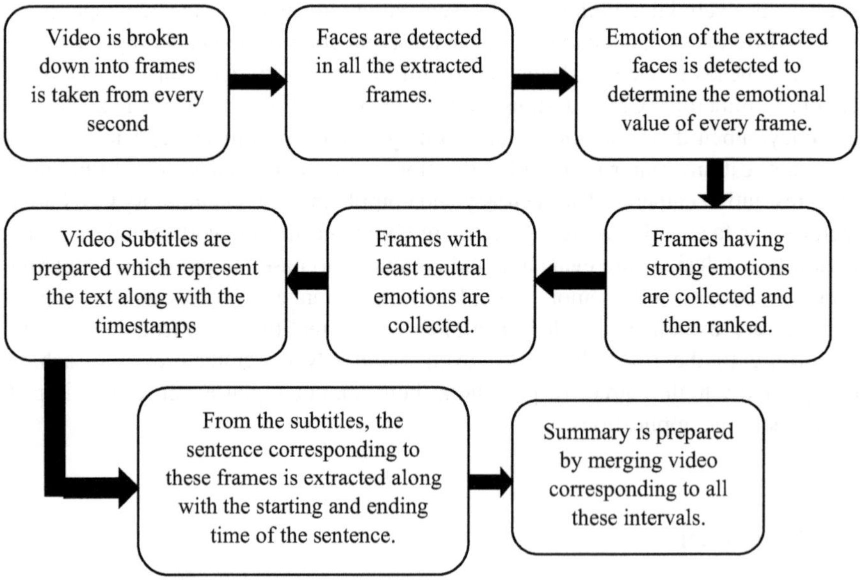

Fig. 1 Flow diagram of our approach

emotion classifier. We execute a clustering on the surround to classify them into motivating and unexciting frames utilising the techniques.

3.1 Single Shot Multi-box Detector (SSD)

The SSD object detection is composed of two parts: Extract features maps and relate convolutional filters to notice objects. The SSD based VGG16 deep learning model were map video frames acceleration with less ToC. The following process can helps the Region of interest improvement for better quality. At that point, it recognises objects utilising the Conv4_3 layer. Each expectation comprises a boundary box and 21 scores for each lesson, and we choose the most noteworthy score as the lesson for the bounded object. The bounding box obtained from SSD is passed on to a CNN-based architecture. This architecture of emotion classification is trained on the FER2013 dataset. It gives the prospect allocation of seven dissimilar emotions as follows: repulsion, happiness, fear, sadness, surprise, and neutrality.

3.2 Convolution Neural Network (CNN)

A Convolution neural network (CNN) [10] is a neural arrangement with one or more convolution layers and is utilised basically for picture preparing, classification, and division conjointly for other auto-related information. A convolution is sliding a channel over the input. We use the Convolution Neural Network (CNN) to detect emotion in every frame after face detection [11].

3.3 Frame Selection

After the emotion score for each frame is estimated, the frames are then sorted based on the neutral emotion score [12, 13]. Once this is done, the first k frames are chosen at random (*k* depending on the desired length of the video). If multiple faces are there in the frame, then for every face, we find the emotion score and average it with the emotion score of the rest of them.

Figure 2 shows two frames along with emotion probability distribution. F1 is selected because the neutral value is less than other emotions [14]. And F2 is discarded since the surprise emotion has the lowest value, as shown in Fig. 2.

From Fig. 3, we can infer that the neutral value for both frames is low. Since the value of emotion in the frame F1 (Angry) is more than the frame F2 (Sad), the frame F1 will be hierarchically above F2 in the sequence [15]. The selected frames will be processed for the exposition of the video depicted in Fig. 3.

Figure 4 shows the frame extraction from the video and Fig. 5 shows the summarised images for video exposition, which contains important data.

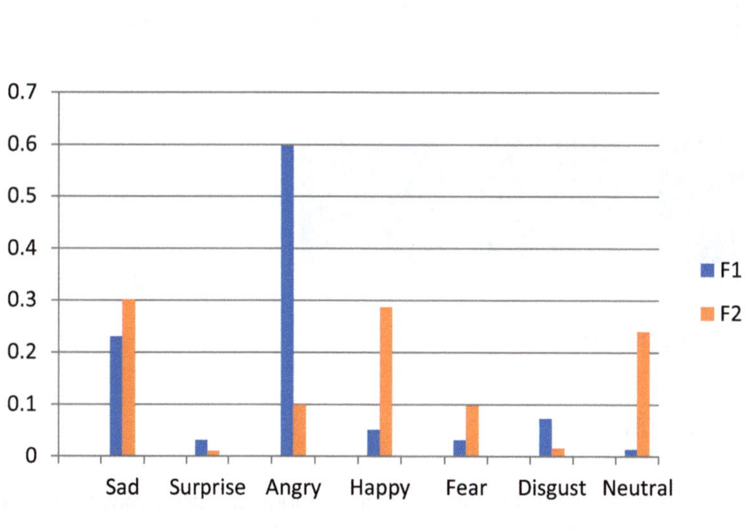

Fig. 2 Average probability table

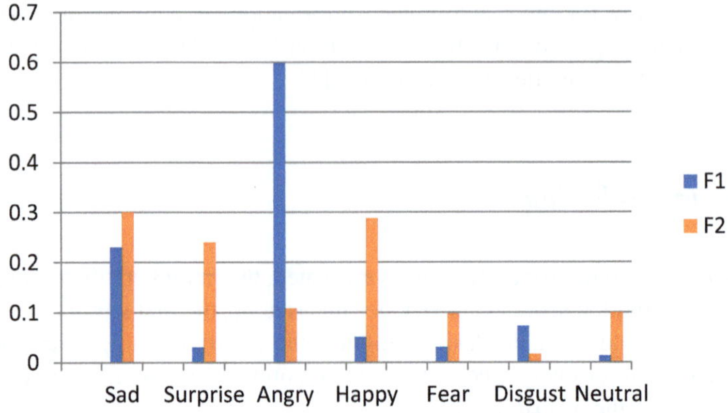

Fig. 3 Frame ranking table

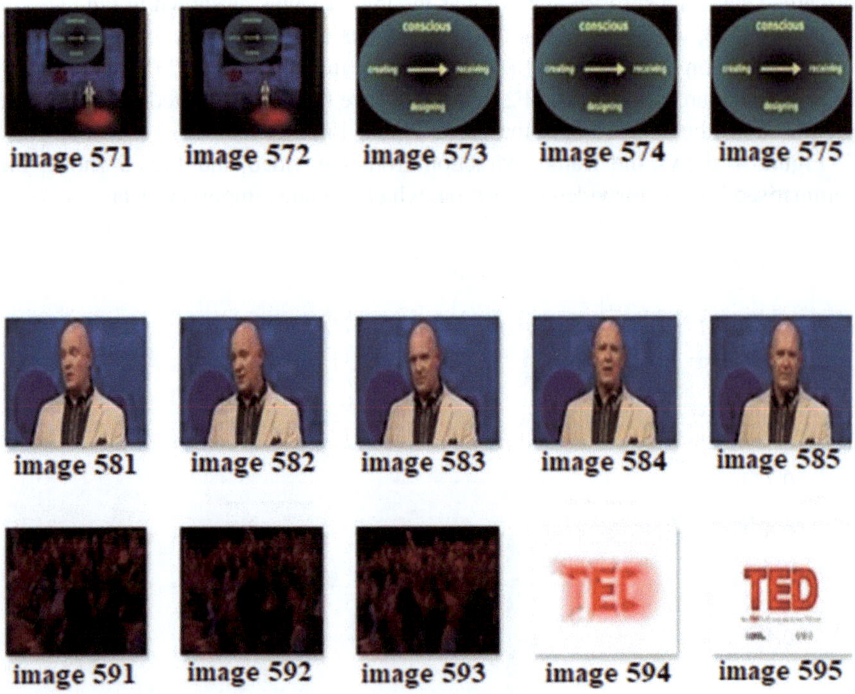

Fig. 4 Dividing the keyframe

3.4 VSUMM

This tactic has been one of the foundational methods in video exposition within the unsupervised setup. The calculation uses the usual K-means calculation to cluster

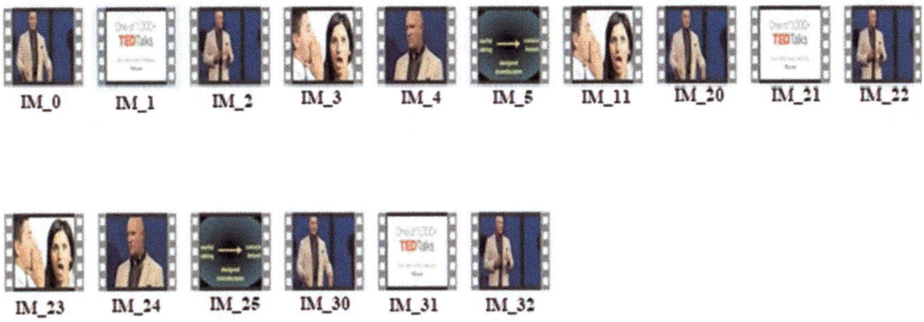

Fig. 5 Selecting the frame

highlights extracted from each outline. In [8], shading histograms are proposed to be utilised. Shading histograms are three-dimensional tensors in which the value of each pixel in the RGB channels determines which container it belongs in. Because each channel's value ranges from 0 to 255, 16 canisters are often used for each channel, resulting in a 16×16×16 tensor. A reorganised version of this histogram was generated for computational reasons, in which each channel was addressed independently, resulting in highlight vectors for each outline with a spot in R 48. Clustering's recommended settle step is minimally diverse. On the other hand, the rearranged colour histograms allow for comparable execution to the original colour histograms. At the second entirely associated layer [9], the highlights extracted from VGG16 were attempted.

3.5 *Video Exposition*

The VSUMM strategy [10] impacts our video presentation strategy. To begin, SSD is used to extract important frames containing critical data. The outlines were divided to reduce the video division's computation time. Suppose the arrangement of outlines is undeniably connected, the contrast between one outline and the following is amazingly evident when investigated at high frequencies, for example, 30 frameworks each second. Instep's utilisation of a moo repeat pace of 5 blueprints each second had little impact on the results, yet it sped up by a critical degree [11]. We used a testing rate of 5 outlines per second for our tests and discarded the extra outlines. Following the extraction of all relevant frames, we cluster the outlines to categorise them into intriguing and uninteresting outlines, using the methodologies described in area III-C. The video's breakdown was created using the cluster with the oddly outlined objects. However the proposed model can workout on irregular frames count, which were send to VGG16 deep learning model, so that human can visible video in clarity manner. Using a 1.8 s skim from the oddly extricated outline, this problem was solved. As a result, the outline is nonstop and easy to follow [12]. The CNN based deep learning model can check video frames quality continually if any blurred frame came again it send to SSD mechanism. The total accuracy of the work is 71%, and the existing system accuracy is 69%.

4 Results and Discussion

The popularity of online videos has exploded. It is becoming more necessary to assist human users effectively browsing videos [13]. Video summarising may assist in digesting movie data by automatically shortening a video by identifying key shots from the raw video. A modern supervised video summarising algorithm learns directly from humanly written summaries to imitate humans' keyframe/key-shot selection criteria [14]. Humans often produce a summary after watching and comprehending the whole movie, and the global attention mechanism, which captures information from all video frames, is critical to the summarising process. On the other hand, previous supervised methods disregarded temporal relationships or merely described local interdependencies across frames [16]. We suggested a memory-enhanced extractive video summariser resulting from this discovery, which uses external memory to store high-capacity visual information from the whole film. The video summariser forecasts the relevance score of a video taken using external memory based on a global comprehension of the video frames. The suggested technique outperforms state-of-the-art methods on the public SumMe and TVSum datasets. More crucially, we show that global attention modelling has two distinct advantages: excellent data transmission and strong tolerance to noisy videos.

After executing the code, it provides an IP address, copied and pasted in the web browser. So, the above page is displayed after pressing the enter button [17]. When user enter the summarised step then application can provide video length, Id and quality rate which were shown in below Fig. 6. and complete process has been explained in [18].

Figure 7 shows the input video, and Fig. 8 shows the summarised video [19]. When compared between these two videos, the time between the video is reduced and meaningless information has been removed, giving accurate results.

5 Conclusion

This chapter presents a novel Face-SSD, a face detecting model through the convolutional neural networks (CNN). These models can extract the particular face emotions through the detection and classification of even a running video. Especially these proposed models can summarise a speech type video in a continuous trailer like format without any gap or breakthroughs. The model can provide a space and information efficient summary. SSD is used for face detection, and CNN is

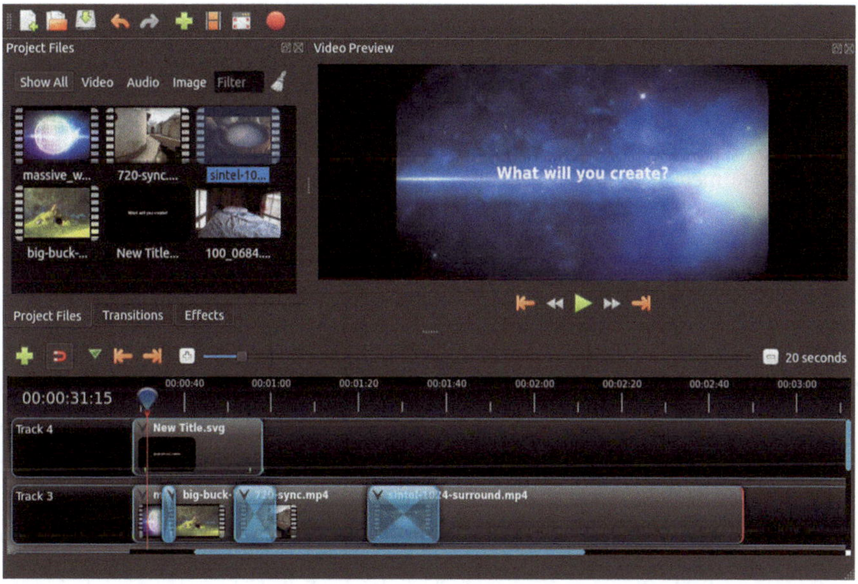

Fig. 6 Video summarizer

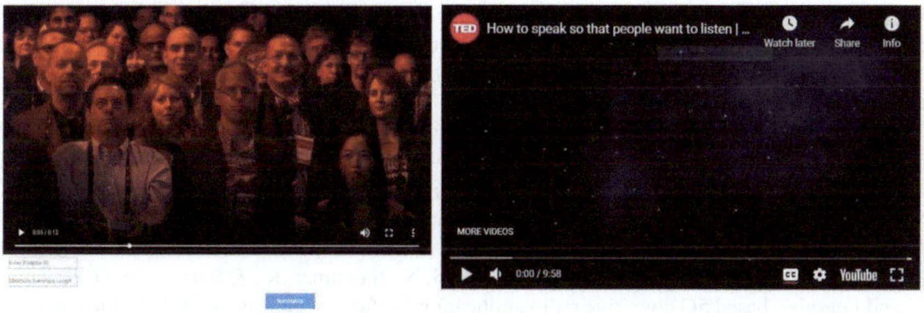

Fig. 7 The input videos

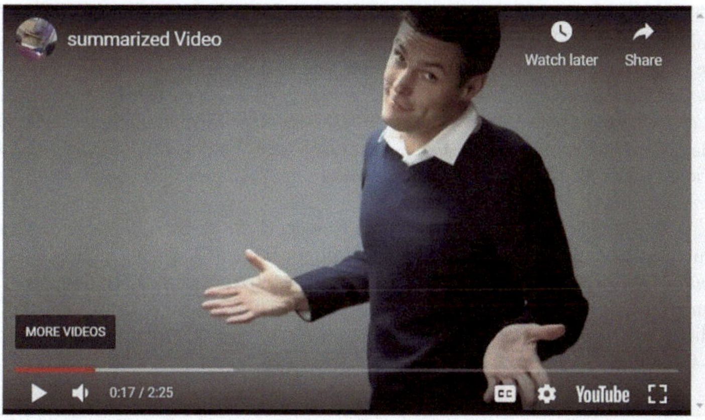

Fig. 8 The summarised video

used for emotional crises. VSUMM is a method used for video exposition. The earlier techniques like RFO, GA, DT, and X-Boosting cannot solve face detection in dynamic video. Hence, the proposed techniques outperform the past models. Finally, performance measures have been estimated to have an accuracy of 98.45%. Sensitivity 97.34%, recall 94.23%, and throughput. Further research can be performed on the topic by adding more algorithms to each routine.

References

1. Ejaz, N., Tariq, T. B., & Baik, S. W.: Adaptive key frame extraction for video summarisation using an aggregation mechanism. *Journal of Visual Communication and Image Representation*, 23(7), 1031–1040 (2012).
2. De Avila, S. E. F., Lopes, A. P. B., da Luz Jr, A., & de Albuquerque Araújo, A.: VSUMM: A mechanism designed to produce static video summaries and a novel evaluation method. *Pattern Recognition Letters,* 32(1), 56–68 (2011).
3. Omidyeganeh, M., Ghaemmaghami, S., & Shirmohammadi, S.: Video keyframe analysis using a segment-based statistical metric in a visually sensitive parametric space. IEEE *Transactions on image processing,* 20(10), 2730–2737 (2011).
4. Chasanis, V. T., Likas, A. C., & Galatsanos, N. P. Scene detection in videos using shot clustering and sequence alignment. *IEEE transactions on multimedia,* 11(1), 89–100 (2008).
5. Furini, M., Geraci, F., Montangero, M., & Pellegrini, M.: STIMO: STIll and MOving video storyboard for the web scenario. *Multimedia Tools and Applications,* 46(1), 47–69 (2010).
6. Cong, Y., Yuan, J., & Luo, J. Towards scalable summarisation of consumer videos via sparse dictionary selection. *IEEE Transactions on Multimedia,* 14(1), 66–75 (2011).
7. Ejaz, N., Mehmood, I., & Baik, S. W.: Efficient visual attention based framework for extracting key frames from videos. *Signal Processing: Image Communication,* 28(1), 34–44 (2013).
8. Jadon, S.: Introduction to different activation functions for deep learning. Medium, *Augmenting Humanity*, 16 (2018).
9. Ramaiah, V. S., Singh, B., Raju, A. R., Reddy, G. N., Saikumar, K., & Ratnayake, D. Teaching and Learning based 5G cognitive radio application for future application. In 2021 *International Conference on Computational Intelligence and Knowledge Economy*, (pp. 31–36). IEEE (2021).
10. Mohammad, M. N., Kumari, C. U., Murthy, A. S. D., Jagan, B. O. L., & Saikumar, K.: Implementation of online and offline product selection system using FCNN deep learning: Product analysis. *Materials Today: Proceedings,* 45, 2171–2178 (2021).
11. Padmini, G. R., Rajesh, O., Raghu, K., Sree, N. M., & Apurva, C.: Design and analysis of 8-bit ripple Carry Adder using nine Transistor Full Adder. In 2021 *7th International Conference on Advanced Computing and Communication Systems*, Vol. 1, pp. 1982–1987. IEEE (2021).
12. K. Raju, A. Sampath Dakshina Murthy, B. Chinna Rao, Sindhura Bhargavi, G. Jagga Rao, K. Madhu, K. Saikumar. A Robust And Accurate Video Watermarking System Based On SVD Hybridation For Performance Assessment *International Journal of Engineering Trends and Technology*, 68(7), 19–24 (2020).
13. Saba, S. S., Sreelakshmi, D., Kumar, P. S., Kumar, K. S., & Saba, S. R. Logistic regression machine learning algorithm on MRI brain image for fast and accurate diagnosis. *International Journal of Scientific and Technology Research,* 9(3), 7076–7081 (2020).
14. Saikumar, K., & Rajesh, V.: Coronary blockage of artery for Heart diagnosis with DT Artificial Intelligence Algorithm. *International Journal of Research in Pharmaceutical Sciences*, 11(1), 471–479 (2020).

15. Saikumar, K., Rajesh, V.: A novel implementation heart diagnosis system based on random forest machine learning technique International *Journal of Pharmaceutical Research* 12, pp. 3904–3916 (2020).
16. Jang, Y., Gunes, H., & Patras, I.: Registration-free face-ssd: Single shot analysis of smiles, facial attributes, and affect in the wild. *Computer Vision and Image Understanding,* 182, 17–29 (2019).
17. Ranjan, R., Bansal, A., Zheng, J., Xu, H., Gleason, J., Lu, B., ... & Chellappa, R.: A fast and accurate system for face detection, identification, and verification. *IEEE Transactions on Biometrics, Behavior, and Identity Science*, 1(2), 82–96 (2019).
18. Xie, R., Zhang, Q., Yang, E., & Zhu, Q.: A method of small face detection based on CNN. In *2019 4th International Conference on Computational Intelligence and Applications,* (pp. 78–82). IEEE (2019).
19. Rehman, B., Ong, W. H., Tan, A. C. H., & Ngo, T. D.: Face detection and tracking using hybrid margin-based ROI techniques. *The Visual Computer,* 36(3), 633–647 (2020).
20. Agarwal A.K., Rani L., Tiwari R.G., Sharma T., Sarangi P.K.: Honey Encryption: Fortification Beyond the Brute-Force Impediment. In: Manik G., Kalia S., Sahoo S.K., Sharma T.K., Verma O.P. (eds) Advances in Mechanical Engineering. *Lecture Notes in Mechanical Engineering. Springer, Singapore* (2021).
21. Khullar V, Singh HP, Agarwal AK. Spoken buddy for individuals with autism spectrum disorder. *Asian J Psychiatr.* Aug;62 102712 (2021).
22. N. R. Misra, S. Kumar, and A. Jain, "A Review on E-waste: Fostering the Need for Green Electronics," in 2021 *International Conference on Computing, Communication, and Intelligent Systems*, pp. 1032–1036 (2021).
23. S. Shukla, A. Lakhmani and A. K. Agarwal, "A review on integrating ICT based education system in rural areas in India," *2016 International Conference System Modeling & Advancement in Research Trends*, pp. 256–259 (2016).
24. Joshi M., Agarwal A.K., Gupta B.: Fractal Image Compression and Its Techniques: A Review. In: Ray K., Sharma T., Rawat S., Saini R., Bandyopadhyay A. (eds) Soft Computing: Theories and Applications. *Advances in Intelligent Systems and Computing, vol 742. Springer, Singapore* (2019).
25. Saleem A., Agarwal A.K.: Analysis and Design of Secure Web Services. In: Pant M., Deep K., Bansal J., Nagar A., Das K. (eds) Proceedings of Fifth International Conference on Soft Computing for Problem Solving. *Advances in Intelligent Systems and Computing*, vol 437. Springer, Singapore (2016).
26. A. Jain, A. K. AlokGahlot, and S. K. S. RakeshDwivedi, "Design and FPGA Performance Analysis of 2D and 3D Router in Mesh NoC," *Int. J. Control Theory Appl. IJCTA* ISSN, pp. 0974–5572, (2017).
27. Pandya S, Wakchaure MA, Shankar R, Annam JR.: Analysis of NOMA-OFDM 5G wireless system using deep neural network. *The Journal of Defense Modeling and Simulation.* (2021).
28. Awais, M.; Ghayvat, H.; Krishnan Pandarathodiyil, A.; Nabillah Ghani, W.M.; Ramanathan, A.; Pandya, S.; Walter, N.; Saad, M.N.; Zain, R.B.; Faye, I.: Healthcare Professional in the Loop (HPIL): Classification of Standard and Oral Cancer-Causing Anomalous Regions of Oral Cavity Using Textural Analysis Technique in Autofluorescence Imaging. *Sensors*, 20, 5780 (2020).
29. Patel, C.I.; Labana, D.; Pandya, S.; Modi, K.; Ghayvat, H.; Awais, M. Histogram of Oriented Gradient-Based Fusion of Features for Human Action Recognition in Action Video Sequences. *Sensors*, 20, 7299 (2020).
30. Ghayvat, H.; Awais, M.; Pandya, S.; Ren, H.; Akbarzadeh, S.; Chandra Mukhopadhyay, S.; Chen, C.; Gope, P.; Chouhan, A.; Chen, W. Smart Aging System: Uncovering the Hidden Wellness Parameter for Well-Being Monitoring and Anomaly Detection. *Sensors,* 19, 766 (2019).

31. Barot, V., Kapadia, V., & Pandya, S., QoS Enabled IoT Based Low Cost Air Quality Monitoring System with Power Consumption Optimization, *Cybernetics and Information Technologies*, 20(2), 122–140 (2020).
32. Sur, A., Sah, R., Pandya, S., Milk storage system for remote areas using solar thermal energy and adsorption cooling, *Materials Today*, Volume 28, Part 3, Elsevier, Pages 1764–1770, (2020).
33. H. Ghayvat, Pandya, S., and A. Patel, "Deep Learning Model for Acoustics Signal Based Preventive Healthcare Monitoring and Activity of Daily Living," 2nd International Conference on Data, *Engineering and Applications (IDEA),* Bhopal, India, pp. 1–7, (2020).
34. Pandya, S., Shah, J., Joshi, N., Ghayvat, H., Mukhopadhyay, S.C. and Yap, M.H. A novel hybrid based recommendation system based on clustering and association mining. In *Sensing Technology (ICST),* 2016 10th International Conference on (pp. 1–6). IEEE (2016).
35. Rupapara, V., Narra, M., Gonda, N. K., & Thipparthy, K. Relevant Data Node Extraction:A Web Data Extraction Method for Non Contagious Data. 2020 5th International Conference on Communication and Electronics Systems, 500–505 (2020).
36. Renuka J Bathi, Sameena Parveen, Neeraj Taneja, Oral Tuberculous Ulcer-A Report of Two Cases, Journal of Indian Academy of Oral Medicine and Radiology, Volume 15, Issue 2, Pages 62–65 (2003).
37. Sameena Parveen, Impact of Calorie Restriction and Intermittent Fasting on Periodontal Health, Periodontology, Volume 87, Issue 1, Pages 315–324 (2021).
38. T. Radhika K Mohideen, C Krithika, N Jeddy, S Parveen, A Meta-Analysis in Assessing Oxidative Stress Using Malondialdehyde in Oral Submucous Fibrosis, European Journal of Dentistry, (2021).
39. Ishaq, A., Sadiq, S., Umer, M., Ullah, S., Mirjalili, S., Rupapara, V., & Nappi, M. Improving the Prediction of Heart Failure Patients' Survival Using SMOTE and Effective Data Mining Techniques. *IEEE Access*, 9, 39707–39716 (2021).
40. Rustam, F., Khalid, M., Aslam, W., Rupapara, V., Mehmood, A., & Choi, G. S. A performance comparison of supervised machine learning models for Covid-19 tweets sentiment analysis. *PLOS ONE*, 16(2), e0245909 (2021).
41. Yousaf, A., Umer, M., Sadiq, S., Ullah, S., Mirjalili, S., Rupapara, V., & Nappi, M. Emotion Recognition by Textual Tweets Classification Using Voting Classifier. *IEEE Access*, 9, 6286–6295 (2021).
42. Sadiq, S., Umer, M., Ullah, S., Mirjalili, S., Rupapara, V., & NAPPI, M. Discrepancy detection between actual user reviews and numeric ratings of Google App store using deep learning. *Expert Systems with Applications,* 115111 (2021).
43. Thowfeek MH, Samsudeen, SN, Sanjeetha, MBF. Drivers of Artificial Intelligence in Banking Service Sectors, Solid State Technology; 63(5): 6400 – 6411 (2020).
44. Samsudeen SN, Thowfeek MH, Rashida, MF. School Teachers' Intention to Use E-Learning Systems in Sri Lanka: A Modified TAM Approach, *International Journal of Information and Knowledge Management*; 5(4), 55–59 (2015).
45. Samsudeen, SN, Thowfeek, MH. Small Medium Entrepreneurs' Intension to Use Cloud Computing: Reference to Eastern Province of Sri Lanka, *Journal of Management*;11(1), 1–10 (2014).
46. Thowfeek, MH. Salam, MNA. Students' Assessment on the Usability of E-learning Websites. *Procedia-Social and Behavioral Sciences*;141; 916–922 (2014).
47. Tawfiq A. Al-Asadi, Ahmed J. Obaid, Ahmed A. Alkhayat. Proposed Method for Web Pages Clustering Using Latent Semantic Analysis, *Journal of Engineering and Applied Science*, Vol. 12, No. 8: 8270–8277 (2017).
48. Nora Omran Alkaam, Ahmed J. Obaid, Mohammed Q. Mohammed, 2018. A Hybrid Technique for Object Detection and Recognition Using Local Features Algorithms, *Journal of Advanced Research in Dynamical and Control Systems,* Vol. 10, No. 2: 2330–2344 (2018).

49. K. Balachander, S. Ramesh, Ahmed J. Obaid. Simulation Of 1KW Multi-Level Switch Mode Power Amplifier, *International Journal of Innovations in Scientific and Engineering Research*, Vol. 5, No. 9: 85–92 (2018).
50. Samsudeen, S. N. Acceptance of cloud of things by small and medium enterprises in Sri Lanka, *Journal of Advanced Research in Dynamical and Control Systems*;12(2), 2276–2285 (2020).
51. Thowfeek, MH, Samsudeen SN. Readiness of Resources for Flipped Classroom. In Proceedings of the 2019 8th International Conference on Educational and Information Technology; (pp. 92–96) (2019).
52. Rupapara, V., Rustam, F., Shahzad, H. F., Mehmood, A., Ashraf, I., & Choi, G. S. Impact of SMOTE on Imbalanced Text Features for Toxic Comments Classification using RVVC Model. *IEEE Access*, 1–1 (2021).

Part II
AI-Enabled Innovations in the Health Sector

Depressive Disorder Prediction Using Machine Learning-Based Electroencephalographic Signal

Govinda Rajulu Ganiga, Kalvikkarasi Subramani, Dilip Kumar Sharma, Sudhakar Sengan, Kalaiyarasi Anbalagan, and Priyadarsini Seenivasan

1 Introduction

EEG measures the electric motion of the human brain. It explains why the brain's functions change over time. Doctors use the EEG, and scientists study the process of the EEG to diagnose neurological disorders. EEG recording was used to identify nervous illnesses such as epilepsy, brain tumors, head injuries, sleep illnesses, and dementia and monitor general anesthesia's profundity throughout the surgical procedure [1]. EEG recordings are used to identify anomalies, behavior problems, learning difficulties, attention deficit disorder, and speech problems, among other things. Hans Berger was the first to incorporate the EEG machine in 1929. Berger

G. R. Ganiga (✉)
Department of Computer Science and Engineering, St. Martin's Engineering College, Secunderabad, Telangana, India

K. Subramani
Department of Electronics and Communication Engineering, Podhigai College of Engineering and Technology, Tirupattur, Tamil Nadu, India

D. K. Sharma
Department of Mathematics, Jaypee University of Engineering and Technology, Guna, Madhya Pradesh, India

S. Sengan
Department of Computer Science and Engineering, PSN College of Engineering and Technology, Tirunelveli, Tamil Nadu, India

K. Anbalagan
Department of Information Technology, Muthayammal Engineering College, Rasipuram, Tamil Nadu, India

P. Seenivasan
Department of Computer Science and Engineering, P.S.R Engineering College, Sivakasi, Tamil Nadu, India

P. Agarwal et al. (eds.), *Artificial Intelligence for Smart Healthcare*, EAI/Springer Innovations in Communication and Computing, https://doi.org/10.1007/978-3-031-23602-0_11

studied neuropsychiatry at Jena University in Germany. Electroencephalogram is a graphical analysis that measures electrical activity in the brain. According to him, brain's electrical activity varies depending on the brain's function. This concept has created a new branch of medicine known as neurophysiology [2]. The EEG signal was created by Hans Berger first. He realized that EEG documents change depending on the person's consciousness. First, temporary glues keep various small electrodes in different scalp surfaces. After that, each electrode and the EEG recording machine are linked to the amplifier. The brain's digital data are converted into wavy lines on a computer—up to 25 electrodes placed in parallel in the multichannel EEG recording to record the results [3].

In EEG recording, the channel is formed by one pair of electrodes and generates a signal. EEG recordings are classified as scalp or intracranial EEG based on the signal obtained from the head. EEG was placed on the scalp with significant electrical and powered interaction for the scalp. A specific electrode type is transplanted from the brain during surgery in intracranial EEG [4]. The electrocardiogram consists of EEG recordings taken from the cortical exterior using subdural conductors. An EEG recording amplitude for an average adult is between 1 and 100 V, and it is between 10 and 20 mV when measured with subdural electrodes. The electrodes' placement is critical because various activities are processed in many lobes of the cerebral cortex. The global 10–20-electrode system is the standard technique for locating scalp electrodes [5]. The actual distance among neighboring electrodes in this system is determined by the numbers 10 and 20. In this method, the letters F, T, C, P, and O stand for frontal, temporal, central, parietal, and occipital. The electrodes intended to keep in the midline are denoted by the letter Z. In the traditional process, an even number indicates the electrode's location on the right hemisphere. In contrast, an odd number implies the electrode's location on the left hemisphere [6]. The voltage signal indicates the voltage differences between the two electrodes. The EEG device is used in a few different ways. The electrode placement for reading EEG is referred to as the montage, and it is tracked by several montages, as shown below:

Bipolar Montage comprises three channels connected in series, each referring to two electrodes. Channel Fp1-F3 emphasizes the variance in power between Fp1 and F3. The next channel determines the voltage difference among F3 and C3, F3-C3, repeated for all electrodes [7].

Referential Montage: This montage's corresponding circuit emphasizes the contrast between that specific electrode and a defined reference electrode [8]. Since it did not amplify the signal, this method selected the midpoint.

Average Reference Montage: The description method is followed to all amplifier outputs and the avg signal in this montage. The intermediate accuracy signal is often used as a standard reference signal [9].

Laplacian Montage: Every channel in this montage calculates the total average variance between the electrode and the surrounding electrodes. All signals are then converted to electronic form and deposited in a specific montage using electronic EEG. Ultimately, EEG can be observed using an EEG device and viewed using any montage [10].

EEG Signal Rhythms: The signal strength determines the functional behavior of the EEG signal. The ability to identify the irregularity in the EEG signal is critical in clinical research [11].

EEG signals contain many bands, including the following:

- δ is 0.5–4 Hz.
- θ is 4–8 Hz.
- (α) is 8–13 Hz.
- (β) is 13–30 Hz.
- (γ) is >30 Hz.

- *Delta Wave:* This wave has the highest amplitude and is the most minor in shape, ranging from 0.5 to 4 Hz. Hypnotherapy, extreme mental illnesses, and the walkable state are all represented by this wave's severe mental diseases, representing the walkable state.
- *Theta Wave:* A wave with a frequency between 4 and 8 Hz and amplitude more significant than 20 V. This wave represents mental illness, impatience or frustration, unconscious components, creativity, and deep meditation.
- *Alpha Wave:* A wave with a frequency of 8–13 Hz and an amplitude of 30–50 V is known as an alpha wave. Anxiety, mental activity, and tension are all associated with this wave. Alpha activity, also known as mu action, is measured in the brain's sensory-motor areas [12].
- *Beat Wave:* The frequency of a beat wave is between 13 and 30 Hz. It consists of low-frequency and varying-frequency sounds in both sides' frontal areas. The beta wave is produced during brain processing and when a strong mentality engages the brain. Beta wave is associated with active attention, valuable things, and focusing on the outside world.
- *Gamma Wave:* The frequency range of the gamma wave is more significant than 30 Hz. This wave or rhythm can have the highest speed of 80–100 Hz at times. This wave represents the motor functions [13].

The organization of this article is proposed ML is an effective method to analyze enormous information sets precisely, particularly those with recognized designs. Section 2 describes related works. Section 3 proposes a detailed assessment of the EEG signal.

2 Related Works

In 1958, the 10–20-electrode system, which Jasper proposed, defined the name of the electrode and later became the international standard EEG layout system. As sensor technology was invented, the electrode was relatively small than the traditional method, with the electrodes measuring a comprehensive EEG. In 1985, additional electrodes were added to variable sites between the existing 10–20-electrode system and gradually expanded into a 64-electrode system. Because of the complexity of the 28-electrode system of complete human brain system and the 256-electrode system, researchers strictly limited their mobile and everyday use. Tus also gradually developed 8-electrode and 16-electrode devices with small sizes, with the innovation of universal and overall technological advancement [14].

Machine learning (ML) [15] is an excellent tool for the accurate evaluation of massive datasets, primarily those with identifiable designs, which has also been proven to be helpful for the analysis of EEG signals due to lower bias frequency and high sensitivity to a pattern. More recently, the EEG, a test that monitors brain wave activity, has been observed in indications other than classic neurodegenerative ones. Thatcher and colleagues revealed that EEG had more than 90% diagnostic performance in classifying people with high and low IQ. A study conducted in rural Pakistan found that children with improved cognitive abilities and executive function showed a more significant rise in gamma frequency bands than children with weaker cognitive abilities. According to the author, EEG can reveal changes in a child's brain maturity and decision-making system at a younger age compared to conventional testing. EEG can be more objective in screening since it is less motivated than psychological testing. EEG is relatively inexpensive in high-income countries. Due to the flexible approach of collecting, evaluating, and storing data, experts have indicated that quantitative EEG could be one of the ways to address EEG needs in inefficient healthcare classifications [16].

3 Scope of the Work

The EEG signal substantially contributes to bioengineering; a detailed assessment of the EEG signal is required since it provides a complete picture of the patient's history. The classification of the time-varying EEG signal into usual or disorder is challenging in medical research. Many other categorization methodologies have been introduced using a standard EEG signal sequence to determine EEG signal illnesses and recognize a person's various states of disability, such as a depressed signal [48]. Electroencephalographers with perception assess the EEG signal by visually scanning many EEG records [17]. Visually checking an EEG signal is not an effective mechanism since it is not evaluated using standard methods. It also takes a long time to estimate the signal's details, resulting in inaccuracy. As a result, a fully automated framework is designed to categorize the EEG signal. It is not easy to develop a high-efficiency classification scheme because electroencephalography (EEG) encompasses so many different subjects and classes (Fig. 1 and Table 1).

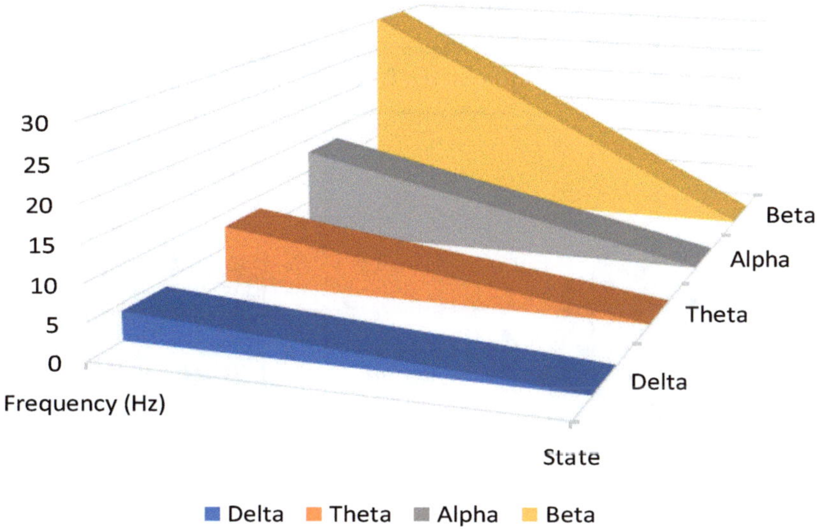

Fig. 1 Varying frequencies of the brain (EEG)

Table 1 Brain wave frequency range

Band	Frequency (Hz)	State
δ	0.51–4.01	Sleep
θ	4.1–8.10	Mental imagery
α	8.10–13.19	Sensory and motor activity, as well as relaxation
α	13.25–30.34	Motor idling and active concentration

3.1 The Research Objective

The following is the study work's objective [18]:

- The power spectral density is computed using the Welch approach to find the low voltage complexity algorithm and architectural design.
- The appropriate frequency band as delta (δ), theta (θ), alpha (α), and beta (β) using wavelet transforms is obtained.
- Merged filters minimize the error in the EEG signal.

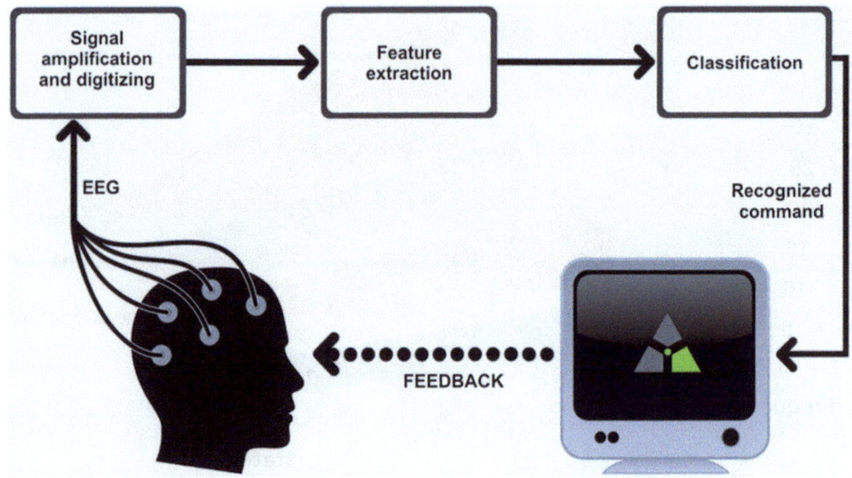

Fig. 2 EEG activity flow

4 Proposed Block Diagram

4.1 Overall Working Principle of EEG Signal

The flow of activities throughout this research work is demonstrated in Fig. 2. The first step is to conduct a research study to gather all relevant details about the survey. Numerous facts and concepts, especially about the analysis and testing of EEG signals, are examined in pertinent technical papers and articles. The research is introduced by acquiring raw EEG signal data processing parameters. Experimental studies with a variety of subjects are achieved for this aim. Each event is requested to move their left or right hand for 30 s with their eyes open in the current physical activity investigation and imagine activity and their left or right hand with their eyes closed in the imaginary movement investigation. The exercises during the testing sessions are associated with the physical or imaginary activities [19].

In this research, two phases are created to recognize or identify the EEG signal as an average or depressed EEG signal. Figure 3 demonstrates a new structure in the block diagram. The two stages are as follows [20]:

- Based on the Welch method, an effective customized VLSI architectural design for computing power spectral density
- Effective EEG analyzer hardware architectural style for diagnosing mental illness

The European Data Format (EDF) is an accessible, multiplatform, and global viewer and toolkit for time storage files such as EEG, EMG, and ECG. An EEG is an assessment used to identify the brain's electrical activity anomalies. The input EEG

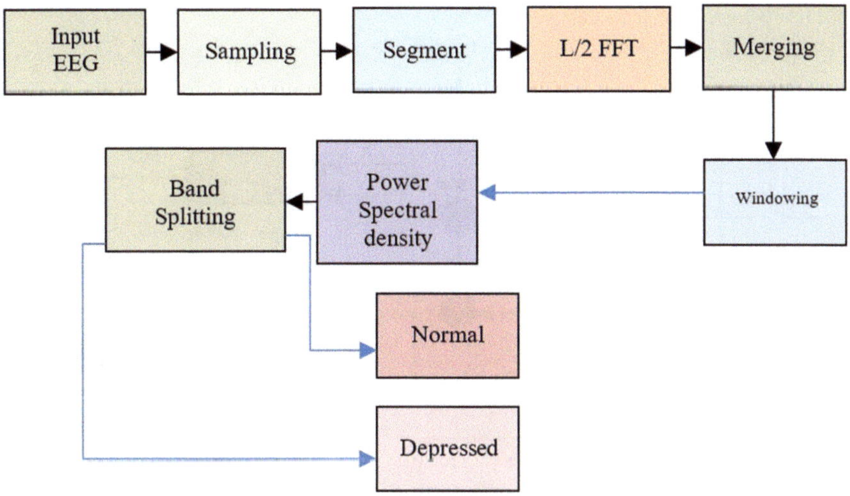

Fig. 3 Block diagram

signal is received from public databases. A tiny metal disc with a fine wire is positioned on the slab, and a signal is sent to a pc to record the outcome. The brain's electrical activity follows a predictable pattern. The wavelet packet transform breaks down the input signal's high- and low-frequency elements into any decomposition level [21].

4.2 *Procedure for PSD Calculation*

In Fig. 4, the proposed diagram shows segmentation, windowing function, FFT process, period grams process, and obtained PSD processing. Figure 5 shows the architectural design for PSD estimation using the Welch algorithm with lower power consumption. Our analysis's primary goal is to achieve the hardware's computation time, energy, and size [22].

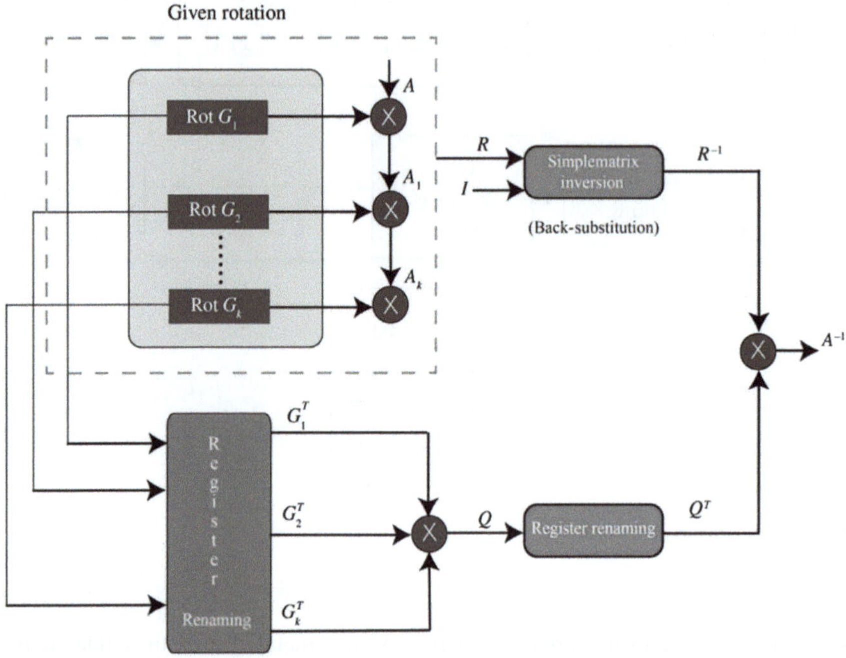

Fig. 4 Flowchart PSD computation

4.3 Algorithm for Feature Extraction by ML Method

```
procedure
  Take a set of n EEG signal epochs; i = 0;
  Extract a multi – dimensional feature vector FV;
  while termination condition is not satisfied do
    apply Discrete wavelet transformation;   //get decomposed signal sub-bands
    for each decomposed signal of EEG do
      perform time – domain analysis;   //extract temporal features
      perform frequency – domain analysis;   //extract spectral features
    end for
    performance – based comparative analysis of extracted features;
    i++;
  end while
  return the most discriminating feature vector FV from EEG signals;
end procedure
```

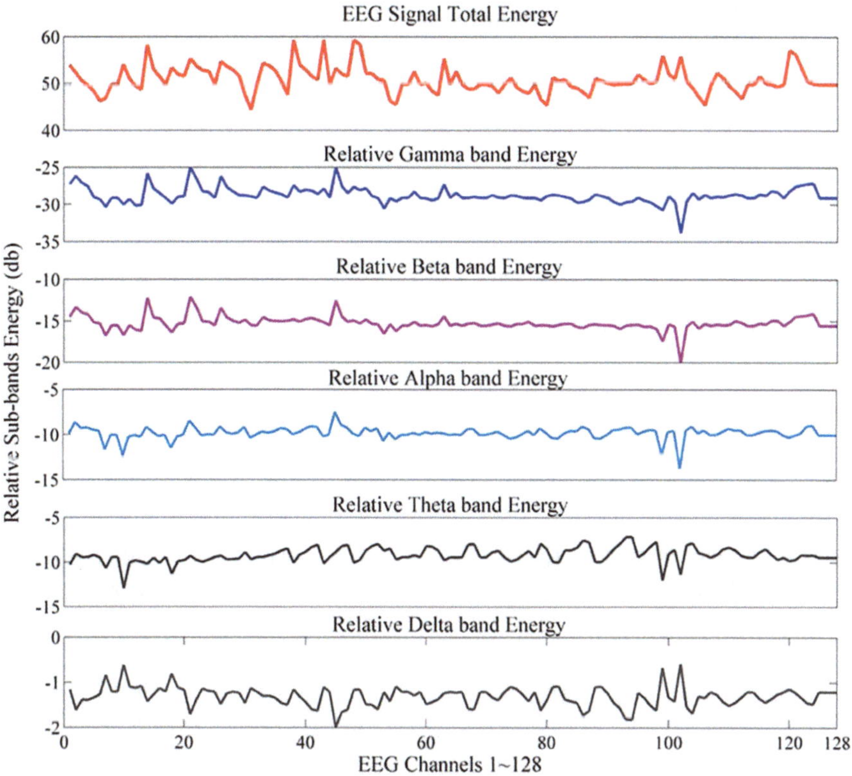

Fig. 5 Classification of EEG

5 Results and Discussion

EEG signal and PSD are used to obtain waves such as delta, theta, alpha, beta, and gamma waves. The data collected from these sources is fed into a MATLAB that classifies the patients' illnesses as shown in Fig. 6. The outcomes of the ANN classification are provided and explained in this section, based on the three datasets: (a) physical and (b) imaginary activities and (c) the combination of physical and imaginary activities. The classification of the ML algorithm also contains two ECG signals as inputs: PSD and ESD power ratio (dB). Three distinct classification analysis methods are conducted in this research, each based on a different type of database [23]. To begin, the classification of ML analysis is defined as the physical dataset, which captures EEG statistical information on the subjects' actual physical activities of lifting either the right or left hand [24–29]. The classification analysis is executed using the imaginary activity set of data. The research study findings will be assessed by comparing it to the research results of the first physical activities of

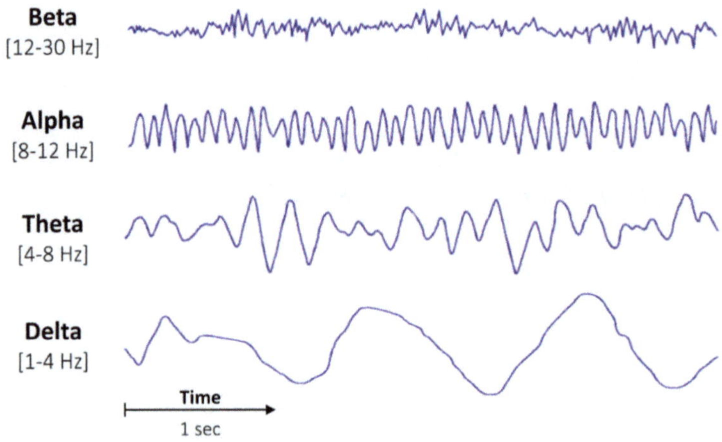

Fig. 6 Power concerning frequency

Table 2 Classification of the physical activity dataset

Hidden neurons	PSD	ESD power ratio
10	94.56	77.8
20	89.19	78.19
30	82.34	79.19
40	85.29	82.19
50	91.10	83.49

multi-label classification [30–35]. Finally, the combined physical and imaginary activity metrics are used in the third multi-label classification [36]. The primary goal of this investigation is to evaluate whether there is a significant correlation between the physical and fictitious large datasets when exercising either left or right motion [37].

With ESD-dB features as inputs, the classification analysis shows the highest accuracy of 85.15% for both elements, specifically for 50 hidden units [38–42]. Based on the physical activity dataset, it can be determined that PSD is the best EEG feature to be feed as input to the ML classifier because it produces the highest accuracy value of 94.56% with the fewest hidden neurons (Table 2 and Fig. 7).

The results of the classification research analysis on the imaginary activity dataset are summarized in Table 3 and Fig. 8. According to the research findings, the best prediction value is obtained when the PSD feature is used as input, with a value of 78.19%, or 60 hidden units [43–47]. When ESD power ratio features are used as input variables, the classification accuracy results drop to 66.71% and 76.17% for 50 hidden units. Compared to the physical dataset, the patterns encoded in the imaginary dataset are much more difficult to classify and clearly distinguish based on the accuracy parameters determined.

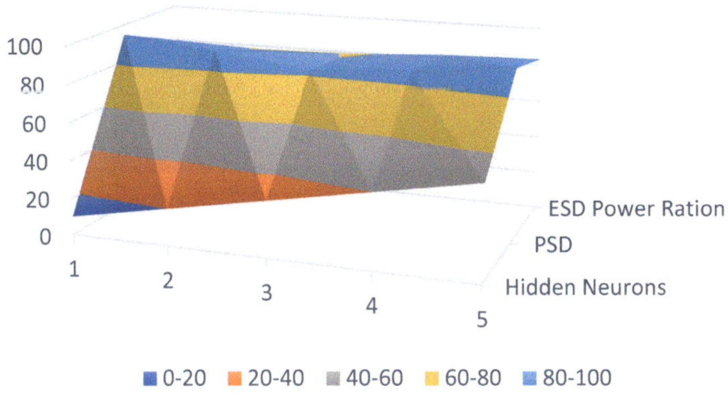

Fig. 7 Physical activity

Table 3 Classification of imaginary activity dataset

Hidden neurons	PSD	ESD power ratio
10	67.18	56.88
20	68.19	57.18
30	71.298	60.19
40	73.487	61.24
50	78.9	63.4

Fig. 8 Imaginary activity

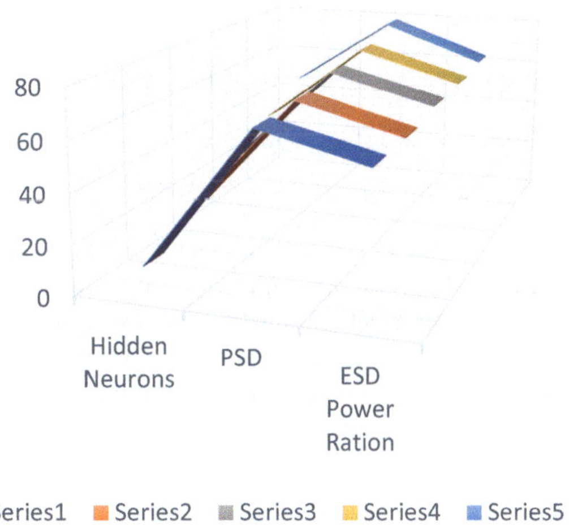

The classification of ML research analysis outcome on the imaginary activity dataset is summarized in Table 4 and Fig. 9. According to the research findings, the highest accuracy matrix is determined when the PSD feature is used as input, with a value of 79.12% for 50 hidden units. When ESD-dB features were used as inputs, the classification factor analysis revealed highly lower accurate results of 67.15% and 78.17% for 50 hidden units. Compared to the physical dataset, the patterns encoded

Table 4 Performance analysis of physical vs imaginary activity dataset

Hidden neurons	PSD	ESD power ratio
10	81.239	65.68
20	82.39	67.87
30	84.239	68.29
40	86.79	69.19
50	89.19	73.40

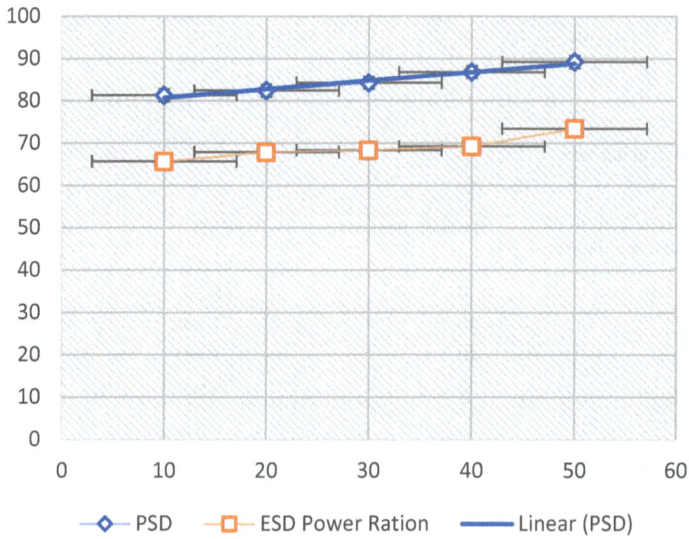

Fig. 9 Physical vs imaginary activity

in the imaginary dataset are much more difficult to classify and distinguish between, based on the accuracy parameters determined. According to the result obtained from the three different classification analyses, PSD performs effectively with ML classifier, mainly when dealing with physical datasets, with a high accuracy value of 95.116%, compared to lower prediction performance when ESD-dB is used as the classification inputs.

6 Conclusion and Future Work

The EEG signal samples are collected from publicly available datasets. The EEG signal was read with EDF Browser Software and then loaded into MATLAB to acquire spectral density bands. EEG signal will be transmitted as a standard or depressive disorder, depending on power spectral density (PSD), which is more significant than the best NPR tool classification. PSD outperforms ESD-dB when using an ML classifier, mainly when dealing with physical datasets, with a high accuracy value of 95.116%, compared to lower prediction accuracy when using ESD-dB as the ML classification variables. Bipolar disorder is a significant issue, and thus prognostication contributes to preventing it. This research could be enhanced to include a more incredible amount of EEG tests, making the indicator more accurate. Real-time-based EEG signals will be interfaced in the future research work.

References

1. Duan L, Duan H, Qiao Y, Sha S, Qi S, Zhang X, Huang J, Huang X, and Wang C.: Machine learning approaches for MDD detection and emotion decoding using EEG signals, Frontiers Hum. Neurosci., 14, 284, (2020).
2. Fisch, B, J.: EEG Premier: Basic principles of digital and analog EEG (3rd Edition), Elsevier publication, (1999).
3. Harris, F.J.: On the use of windows for harmonic analysis with discrete Fourier transform, Proceedings of the IEEE, 66 (1), 51–83, (1978).
4. Hazarika, N., Chen, J.Z., Tsoi, A.C., Sergejew, A.: Classification of EEG Signals Using the Wavelet Transform, Signal Process, 59 (1), 61–72, (1997).
5. Jasper, H.H.: The ten-twenty electrode system of the International Federation, Electroencephalogram. Clinical. Neurophysiology, 10, 367–380, (1958).
6. Khan, N.A., Jönsson, P., Sandsten, M., Performance comparison of time-frequency distributions for estimation of instantaneous frequency of heart rate variability signals. Appl. Sci. 7 (3), 221 (2017).
7. Knott, Verner., Mahoney, Colleen., Kennedy, Sidney, Evans, Kenneth: EEG power, frequency, asymmetry and coherence in male depression. Psych. Res. Neuroimaging Sect. 106, 123–140 (2001).
8. S. Sudhakar and S. Chenthur Pandian "Secure packet encryption and key exchange system in mobile ad hoc network", *Journal of Computer Science*, vol. 8, no. 6, pp. 908–912, (2012).
9. S. Sudhakar and S. Chenthur Pandian, "Hybrid cluster-based geographical routing protocol to mitigate malicious nodes in mobile ad hoc network", *International Journal of Ad Hoc and Ubiquitous Computing*, vol. 21 no. 4, pp. 224–236, (2016).
10. A. U. Priyadarshni and S. Sudhakar, "Cluster-based certificate revocation by cluster head in mobile ad-hoc network", *International Journal of Applied Engineering Research*, vol. 10, no. 20, pp. 16014–16018, (2015).
11. S. Sudhakar and S. Chenthur Pandian, "Investigation of attribute aided data aggregation over dynamic routing in wireless sensor," *Journal of Engineering Science and Technology*, vol. 10, no. 11, pp. 1465–1476, (2015).
12. S. Sudhakar and S. Chenthur Pandian, "Trustworthy position-based routing to mitigate against the malicious attacks to signifies secured data packet using geographic routing protocol in MANET", *WSEAS Transactions on Communications*, vol. 12, no. 11, pp. 584–603, (2013).
13. S. Sudhakar and S. Chenthur Pandian, "A Trust and co-operative nodes with affects of malicious attacks and measure the performance degradation on geographic aided routing in mobile ad hoc network", Life *Science Journal*, vol. 10, no. 4s, pp. 158–163, (2013).
14. S. Sudhakar and S. Chenthur Pandian, "An efficient agent-based intrusion detection system for detecting malicious nodes in MANET routing", *International Review on Computers and Software (I.RE.CO.S.)*, vol. 7, no. 6, pp. 3037–304, (2012).

15. S. Sudhakar and S. Chenthur Pandian, "Authorized node detection and accuracy in position-based information for MANET", *European Journal of Scientific Research*, vol. 70, no. 2, pp. 253–265, (2012).
16. Li X, La R, Wang Y, Hu B and Zhang X, A deep learning approach for mild depression recognition based on functional connectivity using electroencephalography, Frontiers Neurosci., 14, 192, (2020).
17. Mohanty N.P., Dash S.S., Sobhan S., Swarnkar T. Prediction of Depression Using EEG: A Comparative Study. In: Panigrahi C.R., Pati B., Mohapatra P., Buyya R., Li KC. (eds) Progress in Advanced Computing and Intelligent Engineering. Advances in Intelligent Systems and Computing, 199. Springer, Singapore (2021).
18. Muthuswamy, J., Sherman, D., Thakor, N.: Higher-order spectral analysis of burst patterns in EEG, IEEE Transactions on Biomedical Engineering, 46 (1), 92–99, (1999).
19. Niedermeyer, E., Lopes da Silva, F.: Electroencephalography: basic principles, clinical applications, and related fields, Lippincott Williams & Wilkins, ISBN 0781751268, 5th Edition, (2005).
20. Palaniappan, P.: Identifying Individuality Using Mental Task-Based Brain-Computer Interface, in 3rd International Conference on Intelligent Sensing and Information Processing, ICISIP, 238–242, (2005).
21. Sri, K.S., Rajapakse, J.C.: Extracting EEG rhythms using ICA-R. In: IEEE International Joint Conference on Neural Networks, IJCNN 2008. (IEEE World Congress on Computational Intelligence), 2133–2138 (2008).
22. WHO-World Health Organization, website: http://www.who.int, (2011).
23. Xie Y, Yang B, Lu X, Zheng M, Fan C, Bi X, Zhou S and Li Y, Anxiety and depression diagnosis method based on brain networks and convolutional neural networks, in Proc. 42nd Annu. Int. Conf. IEEE Eng. Med. Biol. Soc. (EMBC), 1503–1506, (2020).
24. A. Jain, A. Kumar, and S. Sharma, "Comparative Design and Analysis of Mesh, Torus and Ring NoC," Procedia Comput. Sci., vol. 48, pp. 330–337, (2015).
25. A. Jain, R. Dwivedi, A. Kumar, and S. Sharma, "Scalable design and synthesis of 3D mesh network on chip," in Proceeding of International Conference on Intelligent Communication, Control and Devices, pp. 661–666 (2017).
26. A. Jain, A. K. Gahlot, R. Dwivedi, A. Kumar, and S. K. Sharma, "Fat Tree NoC Design and Synthesis," in Intelligent Communication, Control and Devices, Springer, pp. 1749–1756, (2018).
27. S. K. Sharma, A. Jain, K. Gupta, D. Prasad, and V. Singh, "An internal schematic view and simulation of major diagonal mesh network-on-chip," J. Comput. Theor. Nanosci., vol. 16, no. 10, pp. 4412–4417, (2019).
28. D. Ghai, H. K. Gianey, A. Jain, and R. S. Uppal, "Quantum and dual-tree complex wavelet transform-based image watermarking," Int. J. Mod. Phys. B, vol. 34, no. 04, p. 2050009, (2020).
29. A. Jain and A. Kumar, "Desmogging of still smoggy images using a novel channel prior," J. Ambient Intell. Humaniz. Comput., vol. 12, no. 1, pp. 1161–1177, (2021).
30. S. Kumar et al., "A Comparative Analysis of Machine Learning Algorithms for Detection of Organic and Nonorganic Cotton Diseases," Math. Probl. Eng., vol. 2021, (2021).
31. N. R. Misra, S. Kumar, and A. Jain, "A Review on E-waste: Fostering the Need for Green Electronics," in 2021 International Conference on Computing, Communication, and Intelligent Systems, pp. 1032–1036 (2021).
32. A. Jain, R. Dwivedi, A. Kumar, and S. Sharma, "Network on chip router for 2D mesh design," Int. J. Comput. Sci. Inf. Secur., vol. 14, no. 9, p. 1092, (2016).
33. A. Jain, A. K. AlokGahlot, and S. K. S. RakeshDwivedi, "Design and FPGA Performance Analysis of 2D and 3D Router in Mesh NoC," Int. J. Control Theory Appl. IJCTA ISSN, pp. 0974–5572, (2017).
34. D. S. Gupta and G. P. Biswas, "On securing bi-and tri-partite session key agreement protocol using IBE framework," Wireless Pers. Commun., vol. 96, no. 3, pp. 4505–4524, (2017).

35. Agarwal A.K., Rani L., Tiwari R.G., Sharma T., Sarangi P.K. Honey Encryption: Fortification Beyond the Brute-Force Impediment. In: Manik G., Kalia S., Sahoo S.K., Sharma T.K., Verma O.P. (eds) Advances in Mechanical Engineering. Lecture Notes in Mechanical Engineering. Springer, Singapore. https://doi.org/10.1007/978-981-16-0942-8_64 (2021).
36. Khullar V, Singh HP, Agarwal AK. Spoken buddy for individuals with autism spectrum disorder. Asian J Psychiatr. Aug; 62 102712. https://doi.org/10.1016/j.ajp.2021.102712. PMID: 34091205 (2021).
37. Agarwal, A.K., Jain, A., Synthesis of 2D and 3D NoC Mesh Router Architecture in HDL Environment, Jour of Adv Research in Dynamical & Control Systems, 11(04) (2019).
38. Mathivanan, S., & Jayagopal, P. A big data virtualization role in agriculture: a comprehensive review. Walailak Journal of Science and Technology (WJST), 16(2), 55–70 (2019).
39. D. S. Gupta and G. P. Biswas, "An ECC-based authenticated group key exchange protocol in IBE framework," International Journal of Communication Systems, vol. 30, no. 18, p. e3363, (2017).
40. Kumar, M. S., & Prabhu, J. Hybrid model for movie recommendation system using fireflies and fuzzy c-means. International Journal of Web Portals, 11(2), 1–13 (2019).
41. F. J. John Joseph, R. T, and J. J. C, "Classification of correlated subspaces using HoVer representation of Census Data," in 2011 International Conference on Emerging Trends in Electrical and Computer Technology, pp. 906–911, (2011).
42. S. Bhoumik, S. Chatterjee, A. Sarkar, A. Kumar, and F. J. John Joseph, "Covid 19 Prediction from X Ray Images Using Fully Connected Convolutional Neural Network," in CSBio '20: Proceedings of the Eleventh International Conference on Computational Systems-Biology and Bioinformatics, pp. 106–107, (2020).
43. Rajendran, S., Mathivanan, S. K., Jayagopal, P., Janaki, K. P., Bernard, B. A. M. M., Pandy, S., & Somanathan, M. S. Emphasizing privacy and security of edge intelligence with machine learning for healthcare. International Journal of Intelligent Computing and Cybernetics (2021).
44. Nora Omran Alkaam, Ahmed J. Obaid, Mohammed Q. Mohammed, 2018. A Hybrid Technique for Object Detection and Recognition Using Local Features Algorithms, Journal of Advanced Research in Dynamical and Control Systems, Vol. 10, No. 2: 2330–2344.
45. Ishaq, A., Sadiq, S., Umer, M., Ullah, S., Mirjalili, S., Rupapara, V., & Nappi, M. Improving the Prediction of Heart Failure Patients' Survival Using SMOTE and Effective Data Mining Techniques. IEEE Access, 9, 39707–39716 (2021).
46. Rajendran, S., Mathivanan, S. K., Jayagopal, P., Venkatasen, M., Pandi, T., Somanathan, M. S., ... & Mani, P. Language dialect based speech emotion recognition through deep learning techniques. International Journal of Speech Technology, 1–11 (2021).
47. D. S. Gupta and G. P. Biswas, "Design of lattice-based ELGamal encryption and signature schemes using SIS problem," Trans. Emerg. Telecommun.Technol., vol. 29, no. 6, Art. no. e3255 (2018).
48. Kumar, S., & Jayagopal, P. Delineation of field boundary from multispectral satellite images through U-Net segmentation and template matching. Ecological Informatics, 64, 101370 (2021).

Generation of Masks Using nnU-Net Framework for Brain Tumour Classification

G. Jaya Lakshmi, Mangesh Ghonge, Ahmed J. Obaid, and Muthmainnah

1 Introduction

A brain tumour is a bulge-like growth of abnormal cells within the brain or skull, either cancerous or non-cancerous. Some are benign; others are malignant tumours originating in brain tissue (number 1) or cancer, as other parts of the frame may be in the brain (metastasis). Treatment options depend on the type of tumour, its length, and its location. Therapeutics may be aware of signs of treatment or relief. Of the 120 types of brain tumours, many can be treated effectively. Symptoms of tumours can include regular migraines and headaches. It can also cause a long period of lack of imagination and prophecy. There is little known about its origins and the factors that contributed to this remarkable increase in other technical knowledge. Tumours are divided based on whether they are tumours or not, and their source is their neighbourhood. The non-tumour form of cancer is called benign. They have a high velocity and are easy to distinguish. Cancer tumours are called malignant. They are extremely aggressive and can endanger life while also being difficult to detect. In the

G. Jaya Lakshmi (✉)
Department of Information Technology, V R Siddhartha Engineering College, Vijayawada, India
e-mail: jaya1123@vrsiddhartha.ac.in

M. Ghonge
C and E Department, Sandip Institute of Technology and Research Center, Nashik, India

A. J. Obaid
Faculty of Computer Science and Mathematics, University of Kufa, Kufa, Iraq
e-mail: ahmedj.aljanaby@uokufa.edu.iq

Muthmainnah
Department of Language Education, Universitas Al Asyariah Mandar, Polewali Mandar, Indonesia

P. Agarwal et al. (eds.), *Artificial Intelligence for Smart Healthcare*, EAI/Springer Innovations in Communication and Computing,
https://doi.org/10.1007/978-3-031-23602-0_12

case of tumour detection, doctors can choose both X-rays and MRIs. MRIs are appropriate, but not all other tests provide enough information. An MRI experiment generates precise images by using radio and magnetism waves. Most neurosurgeons write MRIs, giving them enough records to detect even minor abnormalities.

1.1 Imaging Modalities

Pixel-based classification is the principal task for the U-Net model to delineate and separate different objects in an image, i.e. to classify various objects rather than the complete image. As the diagnosis of medical circumstances necessitates careful examination of local regions in an image, segmenting and classifying them is a critical task in the medical imaging society. Diagnosing brain tumours would necessitate separating the tumours from the remaining parts of the brain structures. The U-net design has found widespread application in medical imaging [1–4]. These health imaging modalities are implicated in every level of health concern. They are involved in public health, preventive medicine situations, and medical care, with a greater emphasis on analgesic care. The key point is to institute accurate diagnoses.

Furthermore, medical imaging helps extract exact information from an MRI image, as in the case of brain tumour MRI images. This procedure ensures the maximum amount of diagnostic information. The radiopharmaceuticals for planar imaging are more than radionuclides. Other nonradioactive types of imaging comprise ultrasound, elastography, and photoacoustic imaging. Magnetic resonance imaging (MRI) of the body uses dominant magnetic field radio waves and a computer to create detailed pictures of the inside of the body. It may diagnose and treat various chest, abdomen, and pelvis conditions [3, 5]. The diagnostic ultrasound (US) method exploits high-frequency sound waves to generate images of the body's inner organs next to flexible tissue. Many health imaging modalities make use of X-ray emission to allow for imaging on top of the body [5]. When these X-ray beams go by the person's body, several are absorbed, and the ensuing image is discovered on the additional part of the body (Fig. 1).

Magnetic resonance imaging (MRI) is the same experiment that utilises radio wave energy with magnet pulses to create frames and organ images. An exact body is inside the device with a strong magnetic field at the time of the MRI test. The

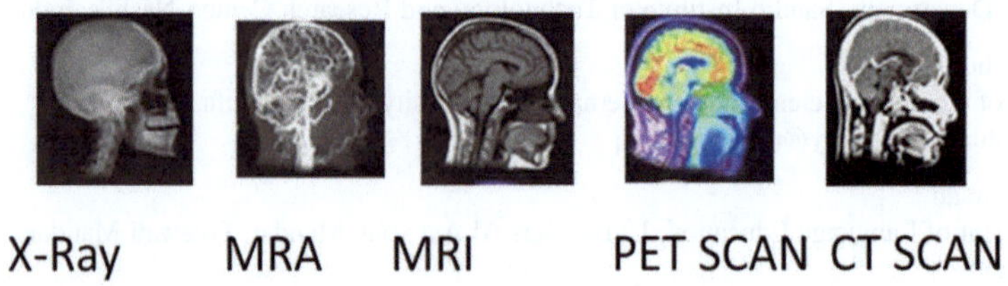

Fig. 1 Brain imaging modalities

received MRI test image is a virtual image stored on a laptop to study the elements. Brain tumours are the result of abnormal and uncontrolled cell proliferation. Some are born in the mind and are called “number one”. And the only thing that can develop from other metastases in the body through the brain is secondary. Both types are undoubtedly capable of neutralising the elements of the body and risking existence. Because the internal space in the skull is limited, their internal stress increases as they grow, and they cause Adam, which is a decrease in blood flow and transplantation resulting from healthy tissue [1]. Why do we use MRI in the treatment of brain tumours? Because MRI provides specific information about mobile devices’ structure, vascular transmission, and anatomy. In addition to treating and monitoring the disease, these items become an essential environmental tool for accurately diagnosing the disease [2].

1.2 General Analysis Objectives

Image segmentation and classification are the two most important mainstays of processing images. Several methods have been used for the segmentation and classification functions. Medical image segmentation is a process that uses automatic or semiautomatic identification of boundaries within a 2D or 3D image to locate the area of interest, otherwise separating the image interested in diverse areas or distinct foreground and organ pixels from the background in use in various modalities: MRI, microscopy, endoscopy, CT, and X-ray. Due to the dissimilar individual investigations and elevated inconsistency, medical image segmentation, or labelling data augmentation, is a key confrontation.

Medical imaging can be used for both analysis and treatment, making it one of the most common resources available to efficiently care for patients [3]. From well-premeditated studies, one can execute a statistical investigation to discover localised brain transforms that match the tasks done in the scanner. These analyses produce images that highlight statistically significant task-related transforms in neural action, whether predicted or not. A classification study stands to include a considerable amount of translational contact. For instance, one can use basic imaging and clinical data to produce maps predicting metabolic action in the brain of a 6-month follow-up Alzheimer’s disease patient [4]. The article intends to present a broad review of the entire analysis of brain images for tumour detection. Numerous statistical and analytical tools have been built to attend to these universal intents in brain imaging reviews.

The motivation for the proposed method is to make masks and predict the condition of a genetic biomarker significant for curing brain cancer using it. This involves a change in encoder-decoder architecture by increasing semantic information. The input image is straightaway fed into the encoder unit to omit connections that skip to an arrangement of incompatible feature maps. Decoder features are produced by multiplying the encoder features and then concatenating them with the equivalent decoder features [6, 7]. Furthermore, the key assessments for designing a thriving segmentation pipeline for the brain dataset with three cohorts for training, validation, and testing must be reduced and automated [8–10]. The novelty of our work is that pipelines developed on one type of dataset are intrinsically irreconcilable with further datasets in the area; we designed the process of making masks using nnU-Net to standardise baseline and 3D segmentation without the need for manual interference and a fast and efficient segmentation framework [11, 12].

2 Literature Review

Brain MRI image datasets are available from various data repositories. Incorporating recognised biological data into statistical and analytic models is frequently advantageous, but the brain's inherent complexity presents challenges. All image sets contain T1-weighted (T1w), fluid-attenuated inversion recovery (FLAIR), T2-weighted (T2w), Apparent Diffusion Coefficient aphasia quotient (ADC AQ) standardised cerebral blood flow, standardised relative cerebral blood level, and binary tumour masks created using T1w images. The perfusion images are created from dynamic vulnerability contrast GRadient Echo sequence-Echo-Planar Imaging-Dynamic Susceptibility-Contrast(GRE_EPI-DSC) imaging following a preload of dissimilarity agents. All sequences are co-registered with the T1+C images [13–17]. This type of dataset aims to assess how deep learning algorithms predict tumour development [18].

When a glioma is alleged or when dealing with a brain abrasion on MRI, radiologists still try to diagnose it as per the histological subtype. However, this diagnosis is a relatively subjective challenge [19–22]. The diagnostic accuracy of forecasting the histological subtype of glioma and the connection between molecular profiling and imaging are also challenges [23–29]. Another challenge is identifying and classifying patients in a definite category in brain tumour segmentation, from absolute response to partial response to constant disease in development, because the classification takes into account T1-weighted sequences with contrast supervision and, to a minor degree, features on T2 and FLAIR images [30–38]. As a result, there are numerous challenges in the accurate diagnosis and transcription of gliomas (Fig. 2).

Noise reduction and filtering are also possibilities for brain MRI image analysis as preprocessing steps [39–42]. The primary step in any data-motivated revision is preprocessing the unprocessed images. Preprocessing removes noise by ensuring uniformity amongst all the images, which, in a twist, formulates the segmentation along with attribute extraction steps further successfully [5, 43–49]. This engrosses performing processes to take out works of art, adjust image resolution, and deal with contrast differentiation under diverse attainment hardware and constraints. Bias fields are one type of general noise resource that originate from low-regularity signals produced by the MRI machine collectively through patient examination and eventually lead to homogeneities in the magnetic ground [6, 50]. Diverse methods have been used for predisposition field improvements, such as

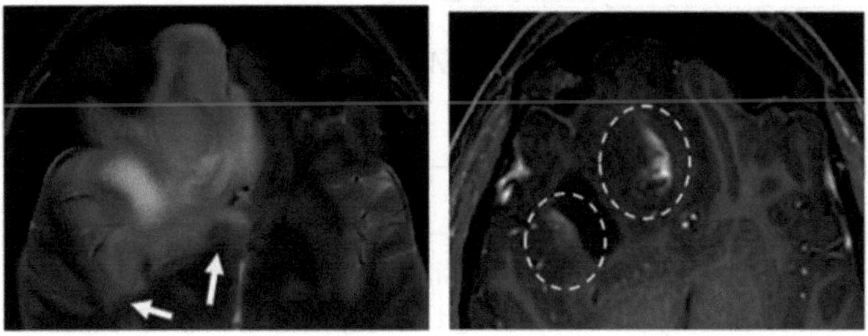

Fig. 2 An example of the difficulty of distinguishing oedema, a non-enhancing tumour or tumour nucleus, an enhancing tumour, and necrosis in a tumoural abrasion in the right anterior lobe

pre-scanned images, high-pass filtering, and homomorphism filtering [7, 51]. It is a multiplicative model with additive noise, as expressed below:

- $S(p,q) = I(p,q)\ B(p,q) + \eta(p,q)$.
- Where (p,q) index pixel in the image, and if an image has M rows and N columns, we have 16 × 6 M and 16by6 N. This noise η tracks a Gaussian probability distribution, specifically scanner noise.

De-noising the noisy image has thus become critical in the processing of medical MR images [52–56]. Many denoising methods performed on MR images include linear filters and nonlinear filters [57–59]. The methods are given in the following Fig. 3.

In general, full indication metrics such as PSNR (peak signal to noise ratio) and MSE (mean square error) are used to assess image quality. In addition to MSE and PSNR, two additional full indication metrics, FSIM (feature similarity indexing method) and SSIM (structured similarity indexing method), have recently been in use with the goal of comparing structural and characteristic similarity measures between reinstated and original objects based on observation.

For example, the signal-to-noise ratio SNR can be calculated using the ratio of the noisy image to the dissimilarity between the original and noisy images.

Signal-to-noise ratio:

$$\frac{\sum_{i=0}^{P-1}\sum_{j=0}^{Q-1} y(i,j)2}{\sum_{i=0}^{N-1}\sum_{j=0}^{M-1} [x(i.j) - y(i,j)2}$$

Different methods used in the region-based methods are watershed, region-based, and edge-based methods [8]. For region-based segmentation, it is complicated and almost unfeasible to change the edges into ridges by determining a superiority map of the image. The Mumford-Shah model [9] was one of the primary region-based routines where the image is approximated using an even task within the regions and not merely at their boundaries. Using region-based analysis, the image is continuously divided into various subregions in the hope that all brain pixels are assigned to

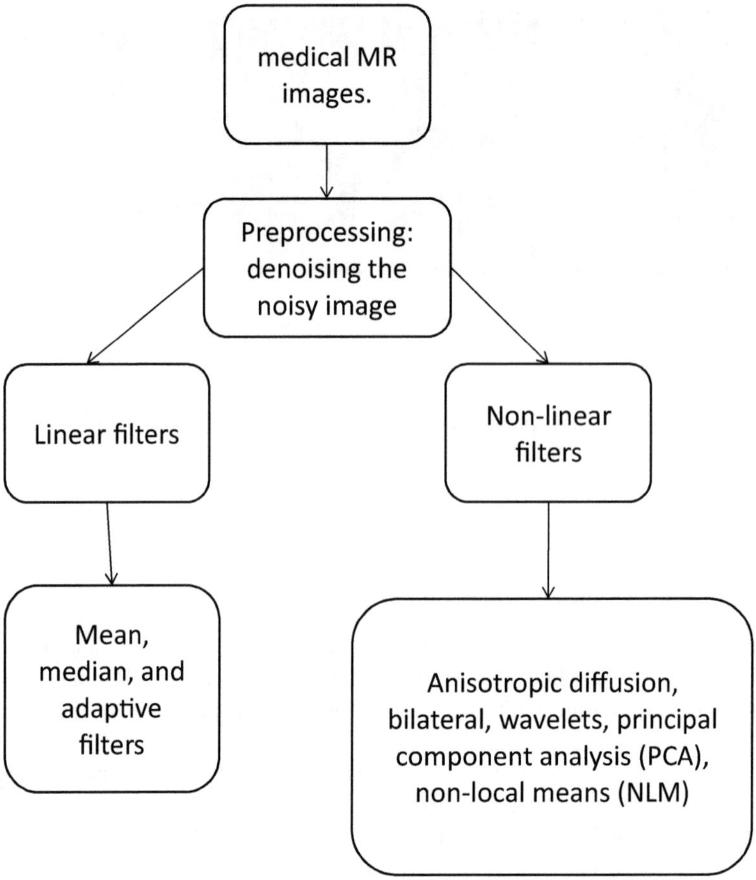

Fig. 3 Denoising techniques: linear filters and nonlinear filters for MR images

the appropriate areas [10]. To avoid dangerous over-segmentation, the watershed is generally managed by region growth based on markers. Morphological operations change the image, and attrition is applied to identify the tumour.

$$P \,\theta\, Q = \{P(i,j) : Q(i,j)\}$$

where $P =$ the binary image, $Q =$ the construction factor, and $(i, j) =$ the centre pixel of construction aspect.

The adaptive fuzzy K-means clustering algorithm differentiates those three regions, and, auxiliary, the results are distinguished through the fuzzy C-means clustering algorithm [11]. A competent image segmentation method using a K-means clustering system was incorporated using a fuzzy C-means algorithm [12].

Table 1 Development of research related to brain tumour detection

No	Year	Researchers	Usefulness	Definition
1	2019	Siar and Teshnehlab [51]	Identification of tumour detection from brain images	A convolutional neural network (CNN) was used to identify a tumour through brain MRI images. The accuracy of the Softmax Fully Connected layer is utilised to categorise images and has attained 98.67%. The accuracy of the CNN is 97.34% with the radial basis function (RBF) model and 94.24% with the decision tree (DT)
2	2020	Wentao et al. [57]	A deep convolutional neural network-fusion support vector machine (DCNN-F-SVM) approach	The classifier is largely composed of DCNN and incorporates SVMs associated with sequence. The execution of the representation is separated into various stages. The model's execution demonstrated the advantage and effectiveness of the projected model
3	2020	Bhandari et al. [58]	CNNs are used to segment brain tumours	Quantitative parameters of brain tumours, such as shape, texture, and signal strength, forecast medical outcomes such as survival and response to therapy
4	2020	Rammurthy and Mahesh [59]	Whale Harris Hawks optimisation (WHHO) for brain tumour recognition by MR images	A cellular automaton and rough set theory execute segmentation. In total, the aspects are mined from the segments, including tumour size, local optical oriented pattern (LOOP), mean, variance, and kurtosis

$$\mathcal{H}\mu = ((1:k) \times m)/((k+1))$$

where $\mathcal{H}\mu$ is the first means that can be calculated appropriately to k. k is the number of clusters, and m is described as:

$$m = \max\ (\text{MR image}) + 1$$

When principal component analysis was functional on GMM aspects, every feature vector of GBM and typical brain was extracted from numerous Gaussian distributions characterised by the standard deviation, average, and weight [50] (Table 1).

3 Proposed Methodology

3.1 *Materials and Methods*

We apply nnU-Net to the RSNA-MICCAI Brain Tumor Radiogenomic Classification dataset. Three cohorts provide the data: training, validation, and testing. The three cohorts are pre-configured as structural multiparametric MRI (mpMRI) scans in DICOM format. We proposed nnU-Net, a segmentation method that repeatedly iterates itself, including preprocessing, network design, training, and post-processing for any novel task.

3.2 *Experimental Setup*

As a first step, nnU-Net mines a dataset for dataset specific properties and is used to generate three U-Net configurations such as 2D U-Net and 3D U-Net that operate on full resolution images with 3D U-Net flow, where the first U-Net creates a crude segmentation plan in down sampled images, which the subsequent U-Net then refines (Fig. 4).

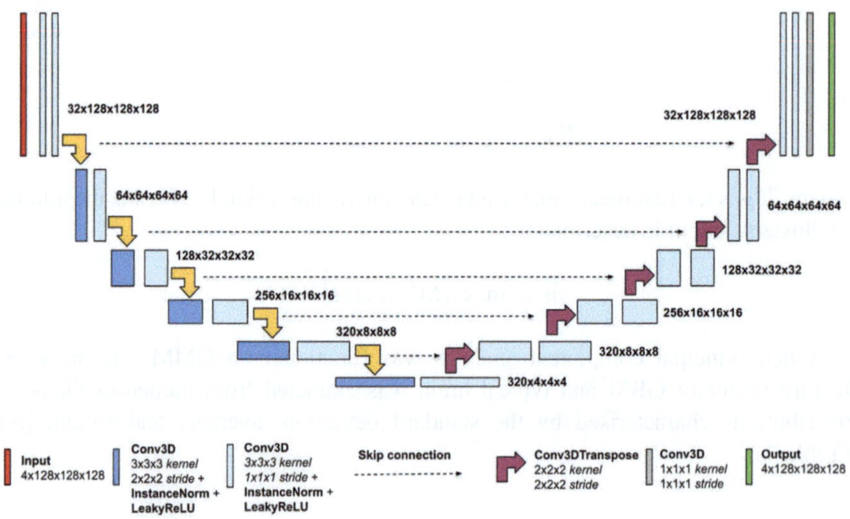

Fig. 4 nnU-Net for RSNA-MICCAI Brain Tumor Radiogenomic Classification

3.3 Model Training and Making Masks

nnU-Net trains every U-Net arrangement in a fivefold cross-validation. This allows nnU-Net to decide the post-processing and ensemble on the training dataset. By default, every U-Net must be run on a given dataset (Fig. 5).

The data is prepared according to nnU-Net's necessity, and masks are made and checked. Here, nnU-Net focuses on the adaptation process thoroughly. In this framework, the image is scanned and produces proposals, and through these proposals, bounding boxes and masks are generated (Fig. 6).

First, we have a constricting path using an encoder that progressively reduces the dimension of the image, and the number of filters is increased to generate blockage features. This is then fed into a decoder block, which gradually expands the

```
Cloning into 'nnUNet'...
remote: Enumerating objects: 5497, done.
remote: Counting objects: 100% (1754/1754), done.
remote: Compressing objects: 100% (257/257), done.
remote: Total 5497 (delta 1613), reused 1531 (delta 1497), pack-reused 3743
Receiving objects: 100% (5497/5497), 1.34 MiB | 3.18 MiB/s, done.
Resolving deltas: 100% (4353/4353), done.
Cloning into 'apex'...
remote: Enumerating objects: 8248, done.
remote: Counting objects: 100% (335/335), done.
remote: Compressing objects: 100% (180/180), done.
remote: Total 8248 (delta 199), reused 246 (delta 143), pack-reused 7913
Receiving objects: 100% (8248/8248), 14.20 MiB | 15.36 MiB/s, done.
Resolving deltas: 100% (5598/5598), done.
```

```
  Switched to a new branch 'bugfix/get_trace_graph'
  Branch 'bugfix/get_trace_graph' set up to track remote branch 'bugfix/get_trace_grap
h' from 'origin'.
Building wheels for collected packages: hiddenlayer
  Building wheel for hiddenlayer (setup.py) ... - done
  Created wheel for hiddenlayer: filename=hiddenlayer-0.2-py3-none-any.whl size=19741
sha256=cab5623cb1cbafa6c59b939c7a694deebe85a175bfd2e884cd0ac5e6b1a69018
  Stored in directory: /tmp/pip-ephem-wheel-cache-yrmuvmm4/wheels/0f/3c/46/3186246513d
3a9b8ac0784f551043ede398addafc2d15c2cd6
Successfully built hiddenlayer
Installing collected packages: hiddenlayer
Successfully installed hiddenlayer-0.2
WARNING: Running pip as root will break packages and permissions. You should install p
ackages reliably by using venv: https://pip.pypa.io/warnings/venv
```

Fig. 5 Git clone and setup of nnU-Net

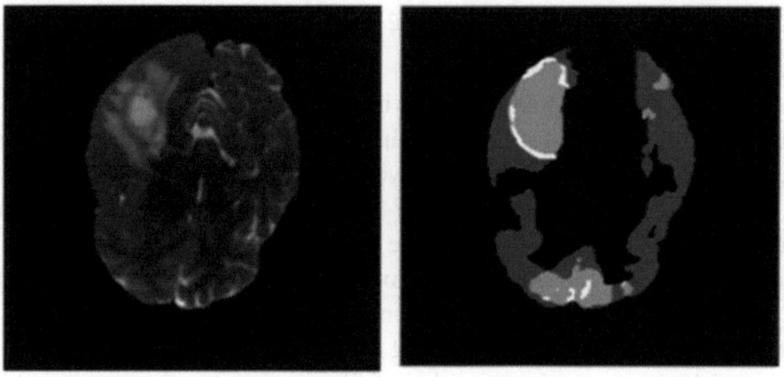

Fig. 6 Making of masks of nnU-Net framework

dimension to produce the desired forecasted output mask. The model is then trained with the Adam optimiser and dice loss as the loss function. The model will be predicting only the mask. To acquire the skull-stripped image, an overlay is needed on the raw image to acquire the skull-stripped image.

4 Conclusion

This paper describes the automatic segmentation and classification of glioblastoma from MRI images using a hybrid deep nnU-Net. The proposed work is implemented on the original U-Net by changing encoder construction to avoid low-level features. High-level features, including tumour region masks, are investigated, and middle layers are exploited for investigating the mid-level features by counting edges, curves, and points. At first, 3D U-Net is trained on the RSNA-MICCAI Brain Tumor Radiogenomic Classification dataset. Then the segmentation outcome is compared to and conceded to a subsequent 3D U-Net trained on areas. The nnU-Net baseline arrangement achieved a respectable result. Even though the proposed approach outperforms other recently published approaches in terms of feature extraction performance, our algorithm is still limited when the size of the tumour's predictable area increases. As a result, we intend to extend a proposed algorithm in the nnU-Net architecture for spatial information of volumetric medical image data in future work.

References

1. Medical Imaging and Technology Alliance 2018, Medical Imaging Modalities, MITA, Arlington, VA, viewed 12 January 2018, http://www.medicalimaging.org/about-mita/medical-imaging-primer/
2. NPS MedicineWise 2017, Imaging Explained, NPS MedicineWise, Surry Hills, NSW, viewed 11 January 2018, https://www.nps.org.au/medical-info/consumer-info/imaging-explained.

3. Hughes, Z. (2018). Medical Imaging Types and Modalities. Ausmed. Retrieved from https://www.ausmed.com/cpd/articles/medical-imaging-types-and-modalities
4. Bowman, F Dubois. "Brain Imaging Analysis." Annual review of statistics and its application vol. 1 (2014): 61 85.
5. Van Ginneken B, Schaefer-Prokop CM, Prokop M. Computer-aided diagnosis: how to move from the laboratory to the clinic. Radiology. 2011;261(3):719–732
6. Song S, Zheng Y, He Y. A review of methods for bias correction in medical images.
7. Biomed Eng Rev. 2017;3(1). https://doi.org/10.18103/bme.v3i1.1550
8. BH. Brinkmann et al. Optimized homomorphic unsharp masking for MR grayscale inhomogeneity correction. IEEE Trans. Med. Imag., (17):161–171, 1998.
9. D. Mumford and J. Shah, "Optimal approximations by piecewise smooth functions and associated variational problems," Communications on Pure and Applied Mathematics, vol. 42, no. 5, pp. 577–685, 1989.
10. Yazdani S, Yusof R, Karimian A, Mitsukira Y, Hematian A (2016) Automatic Region-Based Brain Classification of MRI-T1 Data. PLoS ONE 11(4): e0151326.
11. A. Naveen & T. Velmurugan. (2018). Clustering Techniques on Brain MRI. Indian Journal of Public Health Research & Development. 9. 430.
12. Man Abdel Maksoud, Mohammed Elmogy, Rashid Al-Awadi, Brain tumor segmentation based on a hybrid clustering technique, Egyptian Informatics Journal, Volume 16, Issue 1,2015, Pages 71–81, ISSN 1110-8665.
13. Agarwal, A. K., & Jain, A. (2019). Synthesis of 2D and 3D NoC mesh router architecture in HDL environment. Journal of Advanced Research in Dynamical and Control Systems, 11(4), 2573–2581.
14. Agrawal, N., Jain, A., & Agarwal, A. (2019). Simulation of Network on Chip for 3D Router Architecture. International Journal of Recent Technology and Engineering, 8, 58–62.
15. Anand, L., and S. P. Syed Ibrahim. "HANN: a hybrid model for liver syndrome classification by feature assortment optimization." Journal of medical systems 42, no. 11 (2018): p1–11.
16. Anand, L., and V. Neelanarayanan. "Enchanced multiclass intrusion detection using supervised learning methods." In AIP Conference Proceedings, vol. 2282, no. 1, p. 020044. AIP Publishing LLC, 2020.
17. Anand, L., MB Mukesh Krishnan, K. U. Senthil Kumar, and S. Jeeva. "AI multi agent shopping cart system based web development." In AIP Conference Proceedings, vol. 2282, no. 1, p. 020041. AIP Publishing LLC, 2020.
18. Anand, L., V. Nallarasan, MB Mukesh Krishnan, and S. Jeeva. "Driver profiling-based anti-theft system." In AIP Conference Proceedings, vol. 2282, no. 1, p. 020042. AIP Publishing LLC, 2020.
19. Dr. W. Vinu, Analysis of percent body fat among all India inter university hand ball players. International Journal of Advanced Educational Research, Vol.1, no.1, p.36–38, 2016.
20. Ghai, D., Gianey, H. K., Jain, A., & Uppal, R. S. (2020). Quantum and dual-tree complex wavelet transform-based image watermarking. International Journal of Modern Physics B, 34 (04), 2050009.
21. Gopal, V. Nanda, Fadi Al-Turjman, R. Kumar, L. Anand, and M. Rajesh. "Feature selection and classification in breast cancer prediction using IoT and machine learning." Measurement 178 (2021):p 109442.
22. Gupta, N., Jain, A., Vaisla, K. S., Kumar, A., & Kumar, R. (2021). Performance analysis of DSDV and OLSR wireless sensor network routing protocols using FPGA hardware and machine learning. Multimedia Tools and Applications, 80(14), 22301–22319.
23. Gupta, N., Vaisla, K. S., Jain, A., Kumar, A., & Kumar, R. (2021). Performance Analysis of AODV Routing for Wireless Sensor Network in FPGA Hardware. Computer Systems Science and Engineering, 39(2), 1–12.
24. J.-G. Han and S.-Y. Park, "The Difference in Job-seeking Stress between Perceived Parents' Parenting Style and Perfectionism of University Students", Int. J. Theory Appl. Elem. Second. Sch. Educ., vol. 1, no. 1, pp. 47–54, Apr. 2019.

25. Jain, A., & Kumar, A. (2021). Desmogging of still smoggy images using a novel channel prior. Journal of Ambient Intelligence and Humanized Computing, 12(1),1161–1177.
26. Jain, A., Dwivedi, R. K., Alshazly, H., Kumar, A., Bourouis, S., & Kaur, M. Design and Simulation of Ring Network-on-Chip for Different Configured Nodes Computers, Materials, & Continua; Henderson Vol. 71, Iss. 2, (2022): 4085–4100.
27. Jain, A., Dwivedi, R., Kumar, A., & Sharma, S. (2017). Scalable design and synthesis of 3D mesh network on chip. In Proceeding of International Conference on Intelligent Communication, Control and Devices (pp. 661–666). Springer, Singapore.
28. Jain, A., Gahlot, A. K., Dwivedi, R., Kumar, A., & Sharma, S. K. (2018). Fat Tree NoC Design and Synthesis. In Intelligent Communication, Control and Devices (pp. 1749–1756). Springer, Singapore.
29. Jain, A., Kumar, A., & Sharma, S. (2015). Comparative Design and Analysis of Mesh, Torus and Ring NoC. Procedia Computer Science, 48, 330–337.
30. Jothi, K.R., W. Vinu, & Eleckuvan, R.M., "Effect of Concurrent Strength and Plyometric Training on Selected Biomotor Abilities." Recent Research in Science and Technology, Vol. 2, no.5, p.124–126, 2010.
31. K. Balachander, S. Ramesh, Ahmed J. Obaid, 2018. Simulation Of 1KW Multi-Level Switch Mode Power Amplifier, International Journal of Innovations in Scientific and Engineering Research, Vol. 5, No. 9: 85–92.
32. Kumar, A., & Jain, A. (2021). Image smog restoration using oblique gradient profile prior and energy minimization. Frontiers of Computer Science, 15(6), 1–7.
33. Kumar, R., Fadi Al-Turjman, L. Anand, Abhishek Kumar, S. Magesh, K. Vengatesan, R. Sitharthan, and M. Rajesh. "Genomic sequence analysis of lung infections using artificial intelligence technique." Interdisciplinary Sciences: Computational Life Sciences 13, no. 2 (2021): p192–200.
34. Kumar, S., Jain, A., Kumar Agarwal, A., Rani, S., & Ghimire, A. (2021). Object-Based Image Retrieval Using the U-Net-Based Neural Network. Computational Intelligence and Neuroscience, 2021.
35. Kumar, S., Jain, A., Shukla, A. P., Singh, S., Raja, R., Rani, S., … & Masud, M. (2021). A Comparative Analysis of Machine Learning Algorithms for Detection of Organic and Nonorganic Cotton Diseases. Mathematical Problems in Engineering, 2021.
36. L. J. Capacio, "Improving Mathematics Achievement in the New Normal Education System Using Genyo E-Learning", Int. J. Theory Appl. Elem. Second. Sch. Educ., vol. 3, no. 2, pp. 07–21, Oct. 2021.
37. M. Efendi, A. Ambarita, and Pargito, "Improving Students' Creativity through Development of Teaching Material Lampung Local Wisdom Search, Draw, and Make-Based", Int. J. Theory Appl. Elem. Second. Sch. Educ., vol. 3, no. 1, pp. 35–43, Apr. 2021.
38. M. Emayavaramban, R. K. Kandasamy, S. Muthusamy, and M. Manickam, "India"., Int. J. Theory Appl. Elem. Second. Sch. Educ., vol. 2, no. 2, pp. 121–142, Oct. 2020.
39. M. N. Tahsildar, "Investigating Features Related to Chinese Linguistic Complexities among International Students Learning Chinese as a Foreign Language", Int. J. Theory Appl. Elem. Second. Sch. Educ., vol. 1, no. 1, pp. 63–78, Apr. 2019.
40. M. Silalahi, "Improving Students' Interest in Learning English by Using Games", Int. J. Theory Appl. Elem. Second. Sch. Educ., vol. 1, no. 1, pp. 55–62, Apr. 2019.
41. Misra, N. R., Kumar, S., & Jain, A. (2021, February). A Review on E-waste: Fostering the Need for Green Electronics. In 2021 International Conference on Computing, Communication, and Intelligent Systems, (pp. 1032–1036). IEEE.
42. Mozhi, A. A., & W. Vinu, "A comparative study of aggression between men and women kabaddi and kho-kho players." International Journal of Physiology, Nutrition and Physical Education, Vol. 4, no.1, p.380–382, 2019.
43. Mozhi, A. A., & W. Vinu, "A comparative study of competition anxiety between men and women boxers and fencers." International Journal of Yogic, Human Movement and Sports Sciences, Vol.4, no.1, p.203–205, 2019.

44. N. A. Wiyani, "Implementation of Character-Based Central Learning Program in Kindergarten al-Irsyad al-Islamiyyah Purwokerto", International Journal of Emerging Issues in Early Childhood Education, vol. 1, no. 2, pp. 79–93, Mar. 2020.
45. Nora Omran Alkaam, Ahmed J. Obaid, Mohammed Q. Mohammed, 2018. A Hybrid Technique for Object Detection and Recognition Using Local Features Algorithms, Journal of Advanced Research in Dynamical and Control Systems, Vol. 10, No. 2: 2330–2344.
46. O. Majebi and E. Oduolowu, "Correlational Study of Culturally-Based Instructional Strategy and Cognitive Competencies on Problem Solving, Speaking and Listening: An Evidence in Oyo State Nigeria", International Journal of Emerging Issues in Early Childhood Education, vol. 3, no. 2, pp. 28–41, Nov. 2021.
47. R. J. Sari, N. Nurhafizah, and Y. Yaswinda, "Portraits of Children's Autonomy in PAUD Alam Minangkabau", International Journal of Emerging Issues in Early Childhood Education, vol. 1, no. 2, pp. 142–148, Mar. 2020.
48. R. Subedi and M. Shrestha, "Enabling Environment for Early Childhood Development: A Narrative Study of Preschools in Nepal", International Journal of Emerging Issues in Early Childhood Education, vol. 2, no. 1, pp. 58–72, May 2020.
49. Ravi, R. A., & W. Vinu, "Effects of adapted physical exercise on development of reaction time among children with autism." International Journal of Yogic, Human Movement and Sports Sciences, Vol.4, no.1, p.1307–1309, 2019.
50. Ahmad Chaddad, "Automated Feature Extraction in Brain Tumor by Magnetic Resonance Imaging Using Gaussian Mixture Models", International Journal of Biomedical Imaging, vol. 2015, Article ID 868031, 11 pages, 2015.
51. M. Siar and M. Teshnehlab, "Brain Tumor Detection Using Deep Neural Network and Machine Learning Algorithm," 2019 9th International Conference on Computer and Knowledge Engineering, Mashhad, Iran, 2019, pp. 363–368.
52. S. Aisyah, "Development of Thinking Skills in Early Childhood", International Journal of Emerging Issues in Early Childhood Education, vol. 1, no. 1, pp. 51–67, Mar. 2020.
53. S. Dutta, "Swami Vivekananda's Introspection on Education: A Study based on 24 Parganas(s), West Bengal, India", International Journal of Emerging Issues in Early Childhood Education, vol. 1, no. 2, pp. 108–116, Mar. 2020.
54. Sharma, S. K., Jain, A., Gupta, K., Prasad, D., & Singh, V. (2019). An internal schematic view and simulation of major diagonal mesh network-on-chip. Journal of Computational and Theoretical Nanoscience, 16(10), 4412–4417.
55. Subramani, Prabu, Fadi Al-Turjman, Rajagopal Kumar, Anusha Kannan, and Anand Loganthan. "Improving medical communication process using recurrent networks and wearable antenna s11 variation with harmonic suppressions." Personal and Ubiquitous Computing (2021):p 1–13.
56. Tawfiq A. Al-Asadi, Ahmed J. Obaid, Ahmed A. Alkhayat, 2017. Proposed Method for Web Pages Clustering Using Latent Semantic Analysis, Journal of Engineering and Applied Science, Vol. 12, No. 8: 8270–8277.
57. Wentao Wu, Daning Li, Jiaoyang Du, Xiangyu Gao, Wen Gu, Fanfan Zhao, Xiaojie Feng, Hong Yan, "An Intelligent Diagnosis Method of Brain MRI Tumor Segmentation Using Deep Convolutional Neural Network and SVM Algorithm", Computational and Mathematical Methods in Medicine, vol. 2020, Article ID 6789306, 10 pages, 2020.
58. Bhandari, A., Koppen, J. & Agzarian, M. Convolutional neural networks for brain tumour segmentation. Insights Imaging 11, 77 (2020). https://doi.org/10.1186/s13244-020-00869-4
59. D. Ramamurthy, P.K. Mahesh, Whale Harris hawks optimization-based deep learning classifier for brain tumor detection using MRI images, Journal of King Saud University – Computer and Information Sciences, 2020, ISSN 1319-1578.

A Brain Seizure Diagnosing Remotely Based on EEG Signal Compression and Encryption: A Step for Telehealth

Shokhan M. Al-Barzinji, M. N. Saif Al-din, Azmi Shawkat Abdulbaqi, Bharat Bhushan, and Ahmed J. Obaid

1 Introduction

Medical issues develop daily because of several factors, such as unhealthy lifestyles and a patient's genetic heritage. These factors are involved in the development of chronic diseases, including cancer, diabetes and cardiovascular disorders. These diseases then contribute to the development of many other diseases. A World Health Organization survey has shown that chronic diseases [1] such as cardiovascular diseases, diabetes and cancer are the leading causes of death globally. Therefore, effective cardiovascular disease diagnostics has become a significant subject in the realm of biomedical research. EEG signals are seen as a potential non-inventive tool to assess the function, functionality, and functionality of neurological-related activities and provide structural brain information for neurological disorder [2] analysis. Figure 1 illustrates the brain waves as a sequence of waves called delta, gamma, beta, alpha and theta waves by displaying the EEG data. For medical analysis, there are various sorts of intervals. This time span gives a range of essential information that is useful for the study of the brain. EEG signals are frequently utilised with modern telemedical applications to remote health monitoring systems where patients may be

S. M. Al-Barzinji · M. N. S. Al-din · A. S. Abdulbaqi (✉)
Department of Computer Science, College of Computer Science and Information Technology, University of Anbar, Ramadi, Iraq
e-mail: shokhan.albarzinji@uoanbar.edu.iq; saifaddin.r@uoanbar.edu.iq; azmi_msc@uoanbar.edu.iq

B. Bhushan
Department of Computer Science and Engineering, School of Engineering and Technology, Sharda University, Greater Noida, India

A. J. Obaid
Faculty of Computer Science and Mathematics, University of Kufa, Kufa, Iraq
e-mail: ahmedj.aljanaby@uokufa.edu.iq

P. Agarwal et al. (eds.), *Artificial Intelligence for Smart Healthcare*, EAI/Springer Innovations in Communication and Computing,
https://doi.org/10.1007/978-3-031-23602-0_13

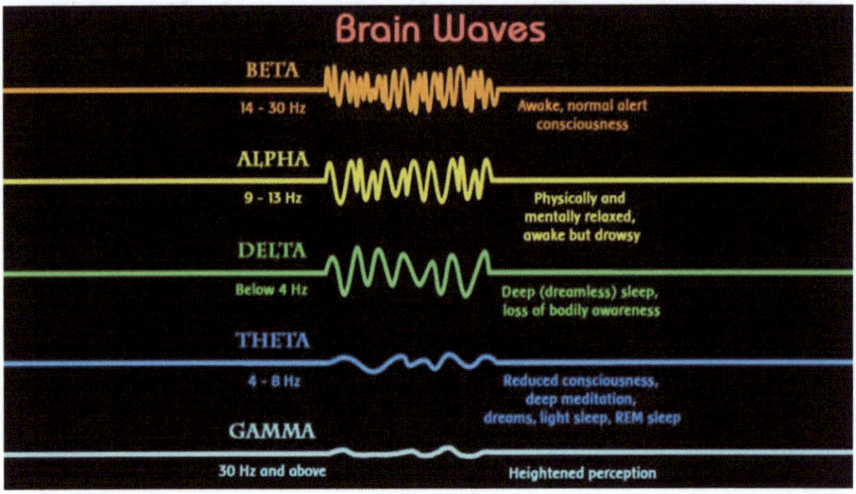

Fig. 1 The five standards of EEG waves [12]

diagnosed and treatment can be done remotely. The signals are relayed across a wireless communication channel, causing a genuine signal to be degraded (OrgSig) [3].

Furthermore, problems with the EEG signal require more data transfer for storage and bandwidth, so security also becomes essential to the research community through the unprotected channel [4]. To reduce data storage needs and increase security, EEG compression and encryption methods are used. Furthermore, the problem of privacy is unlimited in trade, preventing data collecting assaults and keeping transaction records open [5]. Channel circumstances impact the quality of the EEG signal through signal transmission for remote surveillance systems [6]. The main contribution of the manuscript is the safe, reliable and rapid real-time diagnosis of patients with brain disorders.

However, several complications arise because of the improper transmission rate or the inadequate channel capacity. Continuous signal flows can often cause increased volume of data [7]. Therefore, the dimensions of data on the communication channel significantly impact the inappropriate or low bandwidth transmission rate [8, 9]. The constant flows of an EEG signal typically findings in a packet decrease, thereby significantly losing information. However, data compression is vital to reduce data redundancies to maximise storage and minimise the time required for data transmission [10]. Moreover, the enhancement of the compression method depends on the assessment criterion of performance. However, the new suggested compression technique is of the greatest importance and generally requires a small root mean square difference (PRD). In addition, EEG biophysical signals provide sensitive private health information and patient distinction data, so that illegal access by opponents from cyber-attack must be pre-coded before public transmission [11].

2 Related Literature Works

Many researchers have recently been drawn to the conjunction between compression and encryption techniques. In this article [14], the idea of compressed sensing (CS) was presented [13, 14]. This was one of the newest signal processing techniques for compressing EEG signals with extremely low compression complexity for encrypting transmission data across unsafe channels. In addition, an emerging electroencephalogram (EEG) compression approach for e-health applications was reported in [15] adapting adaptive Fourier decomposition (AFD). The result is an average CR of 17.6 to 44.5 with a very linear and robust PRD-CR association of 0.8% to 2.0%. Another research [16] has proposed a system for compressing data and utilising a cryptographical strategy to protect secrecy from unwanted access without losing critical information. They utilise mobile computer devices to eliminate computer utilisation in their job. You do preparations like Gaussian and baseline noise removal, locate peaks, analyse the brain wave frequency and compress the EEG data. The wavelet transition (db04) is utilised for compression and threshold techniques. The next approach for compressing and encrypting the signal is Huffman coding (HuCd). They achieve the 97.72% compression rate, which is extremely suitable for any compression system. In addition, EEG data are forwarded for a specialist's evaluation through the TCP/IP telemedicine clinic. Otherwise, the existing compression and then encryption processing techniques suggested in [17] safeguard the confidentiality of data and deliver the revised signal with the same quality without losing compression efficiency. In addition, another research project [18] has suggested methods for the CHB-MIT Scalp EEG database compression-then-encryption. Their system comprises the sorting of beat, 2D EEG, normalisation time, Dc, complexity sorting, codec and JPEG2000 codec and the coupler change of the chaotic map. The wireless transmissions from EEG through OFDM (orthogonal frequency division multiplexing) across the Rayleigh fading channel of wireless communication are supposed to increase the correction of deteriorating samples via MMF (moving median filtering). They have a 2D compression technique to exhibit storage space reduction and paired it with a chaotic mutation system to randomise the EEG vector to ensure data security. The study, therefore, demonstrates that most efforts in the past focused more on wave-based signal quality but lacked security aspects. Though few works are discovered in the security model and compression techniques, the systems are not efficient enough to offer security by combining lossless compression or a hybrid encryption approach. A new method based on a lossless scheme like AdHuCd for compression is proposed to avoid a loss of information during reconstruction. Moreover, hybrid devices are utilised between symmetrical and asymmetric keys, including AES CBC, RSA and Diffie-Hellman algorithms to prevent data manipulation opportunities.

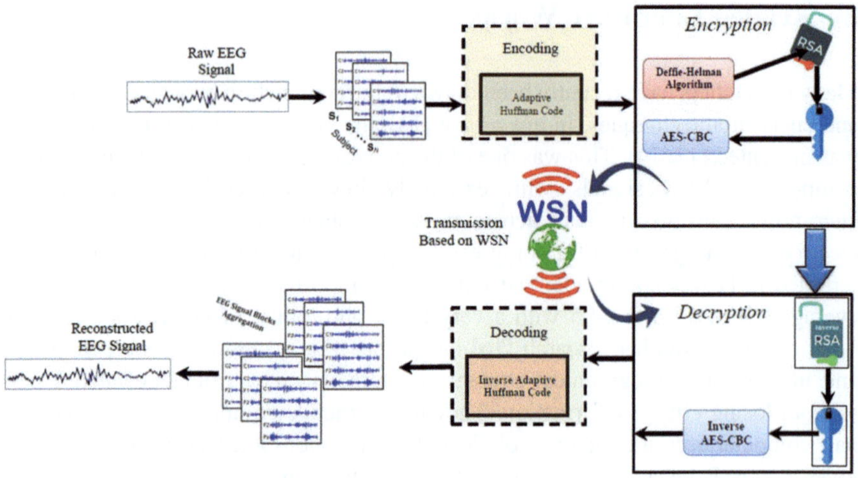

Fig. 2 The infrastructure of the proposed method

3 Methodology

This section shows suggested EEG encoding and decoding solution, combining the proposed AdHuCd weighted method to key generation with AES-CBC, RSA and EEG data encryption based on Diffie-Hellman key exchange. As indicated in Fig. 2, the procedure is separated into the next steps.

An EEG signal is taken out of the CHB-MIT Scalp EEG dataset that is freely available. In this signal, we believe that the EEG signal is split into four blocks of equal size to ensure processing times and safety – i.e. the full signal is processed and then merged at the end of the receiver. This technique helps maintain the signal's secrecy and avoids the external signal attack. In the following phase, however, we examine the compressed EEG data of each block and execute the weighted AdHuEn. The 256-bit key AES-CBC for Diffie-Hellman key swap encryption scheme for encrypting each compressed block with the RSA-key generation method was utilised. These data are ready to be sent over unsafe routes at this point. Later, we utilise AES-based decryption systems for deciphering the data in its compressed or encoded form on each received block. Therefore, we employ an adaptive Huffman decoding (AdHuDc) technique for data reconstructing in its original shape for every block during the coming phase. Finally, we assess compression and cryptography performance in PRD, compression ratio and security analysis.

4 Research Parameters

The parameters utilised in the proposed technique are described below.

4.1 Exchange of Diffie-Hellman Key

The exchange of Diffie-Hellman key protocol provides a safe mechanism to send and receive cryptographic keys over a public network. The Diffie-Hellman algorithm can be considered as elliptic curves. Therefore, this algorithm is still utilised today. The authentication is built on top of the Diffie-Hellman algorithm to prevent threats, as it is deemed safe against eavesdroppers if the finite cyclic group is suitably chosen. When an active attacker launches an attack, it can establish two distinct key exchanges, one with the sender and the other with the recipient, essentially posing as the sender to the receiver and vice versa, allowing her to decode and then re-encrypt communications sent between them.

4.2 Signal Block Creation

NS refers to a noisy signal, L refers to a signal length, and NB refers to a no. of blocks required:

$$\mathrm{BS} = \mathrm{L}/\mathrm{NB} \tag{1}$$

So, B(i) is $|\mathrm{NS}|_i$, which is calculated as:

$$\mathrm{B}(i) = |\mathrm{NS}|_i = \left(\mathrm{NS}_{((i-1)*\mathrm{BS})+1}\mathrm{NS}_{((i-1)*\mathrm{BS}+2}, \ldots .\mathrm{NS}_{\mathrm{BS}*i}\right. \tag{2}$$

where $\mathscr{B}$ is the block of EEG signal.

4.3 Adaptive Huffman Encoding (AdHuEn)

We utilise the AdHuEn scheme to compress the EEG data according to the suggested flow in this phase. HuCd is frequently utilised for compression or encoding; thus, preset codeword values are replaced with an optimum set of codewords according to this procedure [19]. HuCd recognises any data entered as an input stream and distributes the frequency. Later the data is compressed utilising this frequency distribution. Data are compressed utilising a dynamic bit reducing approach in the first phase and HuCd in the second phase to compress data further to create the final result. When the user submits text input data, the system will first detect the number of unique symbols in the input text string and then assign a numeric code to these unique symbols. To produce (compressed) binary output, the necessary binary codes are created dynamically for each number code. The binary output is then converted into an ASCII code, the input for the system's second stage. HuCd is utilised in the second stage to compress the data and improve the performance of the dynamic bit reduction method in the first stage's output [20, 21].

HuCd follows the top-down method to create the ideal outcome by building the binary tree from top to bottom. The data file characters in HuCd are converted to binary code; the shortest binary and the fewer common characters in the file will have the longest binary code. The decompression approach similarly works in the reverse sequence. The Huffman decoder decompresses the compressed data first, and the original data is then returned utilising a dynamic compression decoder [22, 23]. Then you have to utilise our recommended technique to compress the data. The suggested technique initially identifies the presence of single symbols and then gives the detected set of symbols a unique numeric code value. A binary codeword is created for each first allocated symbol in the following stage. The compressed data is the binary codeword. HuCd is based on the top-down calculation technique, which constructs a binary tree for optimum data compression. Under the Huffman coding concept, data transformed to binary code is considered when most of the common characters in the input stream are allocated as the shortest binary code and the least common characters. The opposite technique of HuCd is also utilised to decompress data [24, 25].

5 Hybrid Cryptography for EEG Signal

The cryptographic model to protect the EEG signal during transmission through the unsecured channel is presented in this section. The AES 256-bit encryption model uses the CBC (cipher block chaining) mechanism to produce the cypher to carry out this work. The AES method is a symmetric key technique that receives input data of 128-bit blocks at defined times [26]. EncDec modules utilise the same user-supplied keys in this method. We include in this study the RSA-based methodology of key creation that is explained below. An encryption-decryption key can be 128-bit, 192-bit and 256-bit in the 128-bit input block. The encryption module creates input EEG input cipher data block and reconstructs the input cipher blocks of EEG signals [27]. However, the encryption module is significant since it depends on the size of the key to carry out several rounds on the input block. "Add round key", in which the input EEG data are "XOR'ed" with RSA-keys, is carried out in the initial round AES encrypting technique. EncDec methods based on AES are shown in Fig. 3 [28].

We utilise CBC AES algorithm mode to achieve the encryption. The chaining of input data with preceding ciphertext blocks is applied by this scheme [30]. Achieving this requires a non-safe yet unexpected initialisation vector (IV). The first block of an input signal, according to CBC, is initially "XOR'ed", which is the first cipher block generated utilising an initialising vector. The encryption block created is "XOR'ed", utilising the following plain text or EEG input signals. Therefore, "XOR" is formed between the cipher block and the plaint text by performing the cipher blocks. Figure 4

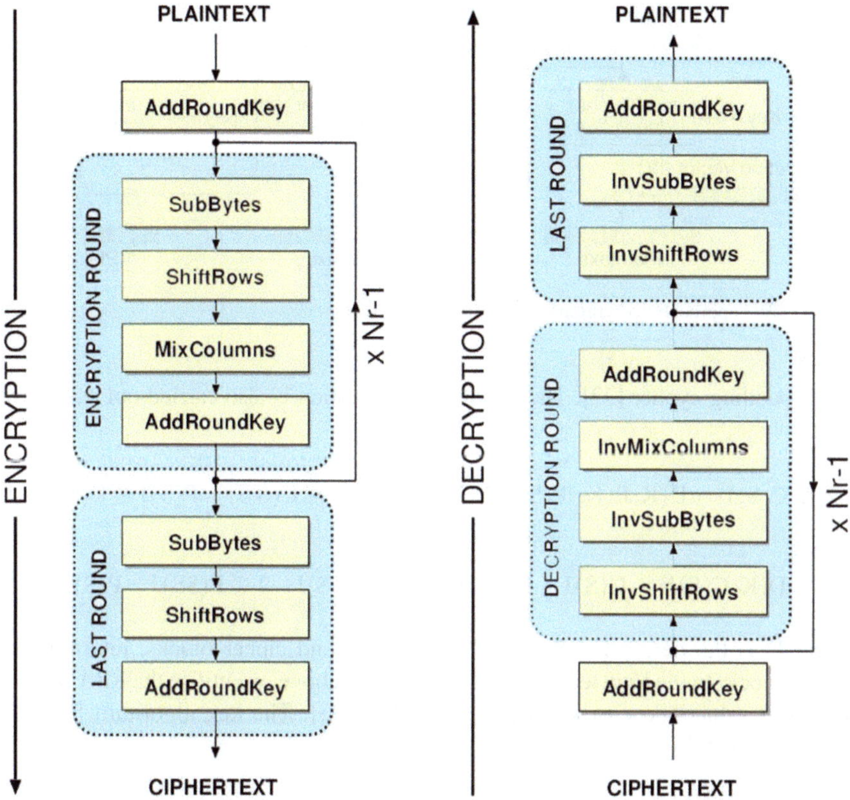

Fig. 3 Block diagrams of the AES algorithm [29]

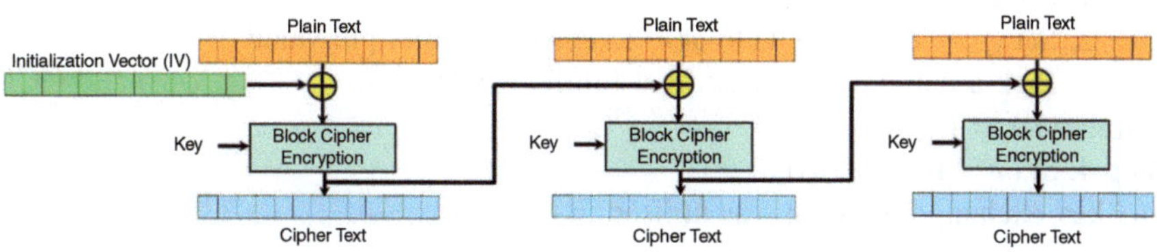

Fig. 4 CBC mode encryption

shows the encryption mode of the CBC. CBC mode decryption is shown in Fig. 5. The processing of encryption is shown as [31]:

$$C(S)j = \mathcal{E}(K, [P(S)\mathcal{J} \oplus C(S)\mathcal{J} - 1]), \mathcal{J} = 1, 2, .., N \tag{3}$$

This method is repeated for all blocks where $\mathcal{E}$ indicates a secret key encryption function "XOR" operation between the $P(S)\mathcal{J}$ single signal pad and the preceding

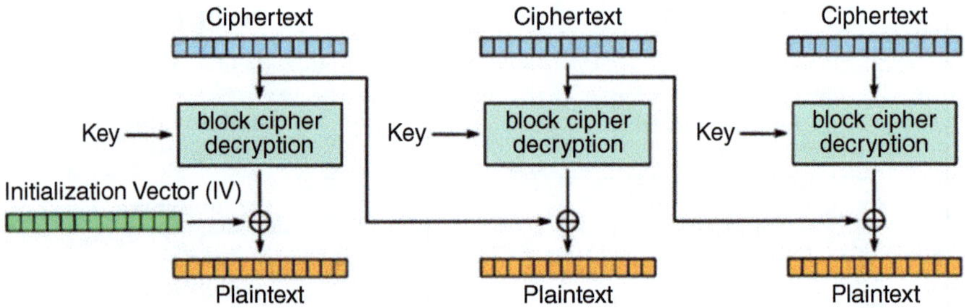

Fig. 5 CBC approach decryption

block padding cypher [22]. The method of decryption is also carried out as follows [32]:

$$\mathrm{D(K, C(S)J) = D(K, E(K, [P(S)J \oplus C(S)J - 1])D(K, C(S)J) = P(S)J \oplus C(S)J - 1} \tag{4}$$

$$\mathrm{D(K, C(S)J) \oplus C(S)J - 1 = C(S)J - 1 \oplus C(S)J - 1 \oplus P(SS)J = P(S)J} \tag{5}$$

where D is the decryption function's secret key and cipher blocks, returning the simple block. In the EncDec procedure mentioned above, we utilise the RSA method and the produced key to build the public key [33]. The key algorithm for RSA creation is as follows:

KeyGen of RSA ()
Insert: Add two big number primes, p and q, as input
Output: EncDec's public and private keys.
Step 1: calculate n as set $p * q$ to n to calculate n
Step 2: Set $(p - 1) * (q - 1)$ to $\varphi(n)$ to calculate Euler phi value
Step 3: Pick a number at random that fulfills the criterion. $1 < e < \varphi(n)$ and GCD $(e, \varphi(n)) = 1$
Step 4: Set e^{-1} mod $(\varphi(n))$ to d.
DH-key exchange protocol was utilised in that work.

Cryptography is essential for protecting IoT devices, but it necessitates utilising power resources when energy efficiency is already a flaw in IoT device design. To solve this difficulty, we convert the suggested system's cipher onto a microchip and utilise a public key cipher chip that consumes 99 percent less power and speeds up the process 500 times faster than existing approaches, i.e. in practice, combining cryptographic algorithms to boost security, improve efficiency and speed and tackle flaws with current algorithms.

The hybrid encryption steps are typically summarised as below:

1. The receiver generates an RSA-key pair. This key will endure for a long time.
2. The sender produces an AES256 key at random. This key can be utilised just once.
3. AES-key is utilised to encrypt the data.
4. RSA-key is utilised to encrypt the AES-key.
5. The encrypted data and key are transferred to the receiver.
6. The receiver decrypts the AES-key utilising their RSA-key.
7. The receiver decrypts the data utilising the AES-key.
8. The receiver deletes the encrypted data and AES-key.

6 Findings and Discussion

The experimental outcomes of the EEG signal filtering, compression and encryption are presented in this section. The entire investigation is conducted utilising the MATLAB program and verified using the CHB-MIT Scalp EEG database, which is accessible for all. This database comprises 48 (360 Hz) signals, every 30 min, of 47 distinct patients. The experimental performance utilizing 101, 102, 108, 202, 205, 209, 219, and 223 signals is provided for comparison with the techniques.

6.1 Compression Performance

The next goal is to obtain a higher compression rate without affecting the EEG data quality. It's time to modify the compression rate and other parameters to assess experimental findings for the reconstructed signal (RecSig) quality. Therefore, we have chosen the compression settings to validate compression dynamically and assess compression rate and PRD performance. The compression ratio (CR) is the compression metric produced by signals. It gives no information on the quality of a compressed signal but assesses the effectiveness of a storage area-reducing method [34]:

$$\mathrm{CR} = \frac{\sum_{n=1}^{N} \left(\mathrm{bit}(\dot{\overline{S[n]}})\right)}{\sum_{n=1}^{N} \left(\mathrm{bit}(\overline{S[n])}\right)} \tag{6}$$

The encoded signal ($S[n]$) and OrgSig $S[n]$ are then converted, with the encoded bits divided into bits with a CR value in the OrgSig length. Efficiency is enhanced when the CR is lower. The percentage of the root mean square difference (PRD) is presented in Eq. 7. However, a measurement is utilised to measure the error or variance among the OrgSig and the RecSig ($S[n^*]$), where N is the signal length S. The procedure can be specified as follows [35]:

$$\mathrm{PRD} = \sqrt{\frac{\sum_{n=1}^{N} (x(n) - x'(n))^2}{\sum_{n=1}^{N} x^2(n)}} \times 100 \tag{7}$$

As PRD depends heavily on the mean value of OrgSig, the measurement, as mentioned earlier, cannot be made accurately. Researchers have previously found that further efforts should be made to get rid of the baseline or lower the degree of DC. In order to solve this problem, the PRD equation in a modified and advanced form, regardless of mean value, is described [36]:

$$\mathrm{PRD\ New} = \mathrm{SQR}\left(\frac{\sum_{n=1}^{N} \overline{(S[n] - S'[n]))^2}}{\sum_{n=1}^{N} (S[n] - S'[n])^2} \times 100\right) \tag{8}$$

Here $S[n]$ shows the mean value for OrgSig $S[n]$. As the CR ratio increases, distortion should be increased by choosing the proper compression ratio for the service and the circumstances for the wireless communication channel. In order to improve the compression ratio, we have designed an adaptive Huffman method to signal to compress and signal to decompress. Any increase in CR might cause reduction in RecSig quality. The QS is utilised to evaluate compression efficiency while considering the faults of a faulty reconstruction [24]. The QS is described as [37, 38]:

$$\mathrm{QS} = \frac{\mathrm{CR}}{\mathrm{PRD}} \tag{9}$$

A higher QS is a higher compression quality in a loss compression technique. Table 1 illustrates CR, PRD, and QS parameters for various EEG database entries. All curves presented are comparable (since CR rises so does PRD), ensuring that the suggested procedure works with various EEG data [39, 40].

The suggested compression system delivers significant compression at a relatively low PRD rate. The average compression ratio for the AHC is 23.91. Therefore, the average PRD is equal to 0.2% for various datasets. Table 2 compares the state-of-the-art methods with various ones. Our compression method exceeds the state-of-the-art technology in terms of precision and efficiency.

We note, however, that between original and reconstructed signals, no substantial distortions are made. Compared with previous techniques, the EEG presented compression/decompression algorithm that is extremely minimal in complexity

Table 1 Findings achieved for eight records utilising the planned AHC

Dataset	CRs	PRDs (%)	QSs
100	24.39	0.25	98.67
111	35.9	0.13	198.49
109	16.31	0.19	77.30
127	30.22	0.24	201.61
119	20.18	0.19	171.31
231	21.91	0.21	121.76
255	19.88	0.17	119.97
217	26.41	0.19	165.66

Table 2 Performance of various EEG signals in # Rec. 100 [41, 42]

Algorithm	CRs	PRDs (%)	QSs
CS [25]	16.76	5.56	–
Lower coding static	36.13	0.0	–
Lower coding dynamic	40.82	0.49	–
Minimal window size dynamic [26]	42.13	0.0	
C.A.E [27]	31.39	1.44	–
S.V.D [17]	41.01	0.47	94.73
Q.L.V-Huffman skeleton [28]	16.91	0.43	29.36
Proposed algorithm	24.39	0.25	98.54

and highly effective. Moreover, enormous memory resources are not required [43–47].

6.2 *Analysing the Security of EEG Signals*

This part explains the many sorts of assaults that the proposed technique can mitigate [48]. Therefore, the safety of the data generated depends mostly on the key generator's security. In addition, attacks on privacy protection are the only offensive strategy that has a chance to be successfully applied to the suggested encryption system [49–52]. We also employ the DH-key exchange, AES encryption and division into four blocks of the full EEG signal by the security management element [53–55]. The proposed technique may thus be utilised to prevent attacks, such as user privacy, from being sent in plain-text form. We are not transmitting the data. The original data are encrypted utilising a 256-bit key through the AES-CBC method. Private information can therefore be secured. Before data is transmitted over an unprotected wireless communication channel, a DH-key is utilised to authenticate the receiver unit. This procedure helps prevent screeners. This process is called authentication. However, the mutual authentication procedure utilising DH-key exchanges helps against attacks by the person in the middle. In the key management session, we exchange DH-key, restricted for the current session, during data transmission. The wrong information is thus not transferable, i.e. the usage of the particular session key may only communicate user 1 information during the session. The phishing attack also helps protect the bogus recipient module from a phishing attack: this technique allows phishing assaults to be prevented. Therefore, by utilising a 256-bit key-based encryption approach, AES-CBC could secure data while transmitting data to enraptured form [21]. In addition, OrgSig is divided into many blocks, thereby ensuring privacy at various assaults. The technique additionally limits attacks by utilising an encrypted key exchange system.

7 Conclusion

This article focuses on designing a secure and effective EEG processing system, which provides significant challenges for EEG signal compression and encryption. However, the EEG signal compression is performed utilising an AHC technique and AES to encrypt data. We utilise the generation of RSA-key and exchange protocols of DH-key to improve security. PRD, CR and safety efficacy evaluate the effectiveness of the proposed technique. The findings are compared to the existing approaches, and the analysis reveals that the strategy provided achieves superior findings. The comparative analysis shows that the findings of this manuscript agree that the proposed approach, compression mechanism and cryptography methodology are applicable. This technique is considered a novel system concept for high compression with low irrelevant error and high security. There is a great possibility to provide such systems and protect important data (such as medical data via IoMT) through manufacturers converting the encryption system into a small chip with high encryption potential that will be an important supplement to the proposed system.

References

1. Jain D.K., Dubey S.B., et al., An approach for hyperspectral image classification by optimising SVM using self organising map, *Journal of Computational Science* (2017).
2. Zareapoor, M., Shamsolmoali, P. and Yang, J., Kernelized Support Vector Machine with Deep learning: an Efficient Approach for extreme multiclass dataset, *Pattern Recognition Letters* (2017).
3. K. Fu, J. Qu, Y. Chai, Y. Dong, Classification of seizure based on the time-frequency image of EEG signals using HHT and SVM, Biomed. *Signal Process. Control* 13, pp. 15–22 (2014).
4. S.-H. Lee, J.S. Lim, J.-K. Kim, J. Yang, Y. Lee, Classification of normal and epileptic seizure EEG signals using wavelet transform, phase-space reconstruction, and Euclidean distance, *Comput. Methods Programs Biomed.* 116, 10–25 (2014).
5. Shoeb, Ali H and Guttag, John V, Application of Machine Learning To Epileptic Seizure Detection, *Proceedings of the 27th International Conference on Machine Learning*, 975–982 (2010).

6. Zeng W, Li M, Yuan C, Wang Q, Liu F, Wang Y.: Classification of focal and non-focal EEG signals using empirical mode decomposition (EMD), phase space reconstruction (PSR) and neural networks. *Artif Intell Rev,* 52:625–647 (2019).
7. Abdulbaqi, A. S., Najim, S. A. D. M., & Mahdi, R. H.: Robust multichannel EEG signals compression model based on hybridisation technique. *International Journal of Engineering & Technology*, 7 (4), 3402–3405 (201).
8. Saini, N., Bhardwaj, S., & Agarwal, R.: Classification of EEG signals using hybrid combination of features for lie detection. *Neural Computing and Applications*, 1–11 (2019).
9. Lafuente V, Gorriz JM, Ramirez J, Gonzalez E.: P300 brainwave extraction from EEG signals: an unsupervised approach. *Expert Syst Appl* 74:1–10 (2017).
10. Bajaj V, Guo Y, Sengur A, Siuly S, Alcin OF.: A hybrid method based on time-frequency images for classification of alcohol and control EEG signals. *Neural Comput Appl* 28:3717–3723 (2017).
11. Riaz F, Hassan A, Rehman S, Niazi IK, Dremstrup K.: EMD based temporal and spectral features for the classification of EEG signals using supervised learning. *IEEE Trans Neural Syst Rehabil Eng* 24:28–35 (2016).
12. Lin, C. F., Shih, S. H., Zhu, J. D., & Lee, S. H.: Implementation of an offline chaos-based EEG encryption software. In *2012 14th International Conference on Advanced Communication Technology (ICACT)* (pp. 430–433). IEEE (2012).
13. Rajasekar, P., & Pushpalatha, M.: Huffman quantisation approach for optimised EEG signal compression with transformation technique. *Soft Computing*, 24 (19), 14545–14559 (2020).
14. G. Chen, Automatic EEG seizure detection using dual-tree complex wavelet-Fourier features, *Expert Syst. Appl.* 41, 2391–2394 (2014).
15. Y. Kumar, M. Dewal, R. Anand, Epileptic seizure detection using DWT based fuzzy approximate entropy and support vector machine, *Neurocomputing,*133, 271–279 (2014).
16. Sun L, Jin B, Yang H, Tong J, Liu C, Xiong H.: Unsupervised EEG feature extraction based on echo state network. *Inf Sci* 475:1–17 (2018).
17. Afrakhteh S, Mosavi MR, Khishe M, Ayatollahi A.: Accurate classification of EEG signals using neural networks trained by hybrid population-physic-based algorithm. Int J Autom Comput (2018). https://doi.org/10.1007/s11633-018-1158-3.
18. Michielli N, Acharya UR, Molinari F.: Cascaded LSTM recurrent neural network for automated sleep stage classification using single-channel EEG signals. *Comput Biol Med* 106:71–81 (2019).
19. Hussein R, Palangi H, Ward RK, Wang ZJ.: Optimised deep neural network architecture for robust detection of epileptic seizures using EEG signals. *Clin Neurophys* 130:25–37 (2018).
20. Doborjeh MG, Wang GY, Kasabov NK.: A spiking neural network methodology and system for learning and comparative analysis of EEG data from healthy versus addiction treated versus addiction not treated subjects. In: *IEEE transactions on biomedical engineering*, pp 0018–9294 (2015).
21. Doborjeh ZG, Doborjeh MG, Kasabov N.: Attentional bias pattern recognition in spiking neural networks from spatiotemporal EEG data. *Cognit Comput*. https://doi.org/10.1007/s12559-017-9517-x (2017).
22. Hadjileontiadis, L. J.: Biosignals and compression standards. In *M-Health* (pp. 277–292). Springer, Boston, MA (2006).
23. Lee, S., Kim, J., & Lee, M.: A real-time ECG data compression and transmission algorithm for an e-health device. *IEEE Transactions on Biomedical Engineering*, 58 (9), 2448–2455 (2011).
24. Sriraam, N., & Eswaran, C.: Performance evaluation of neural network and linear predictors for near-lossless compression of EEG signals. *IEEE Transactions on Information Technology in Biomedicine,* 12 (1), 87–93 (2008).
25. Sriraam, N., & Eswaran, C.: An adaptive error modeling scheme for the lossless compression of EEG signals. IEEE Transactions on Information Technology in Biomedicine, 12 (5), 587–594 (2008).

26. Banerjee, A., Basu, K., & Chakraborty, A.: Prediction of EEG signal by digital filtering. *In Proceedings of International Conference on Intelligent Systems & Networks, Jagadhri,* India (2007).
27. Abdulbaqi, A. S., Nejrs, S. M., Mahmood, S. D., & Panessai, I. Y.: A Tele Encephalopathy Diagnosis Based on EEG Signal Compression and Encryption. In *International Conference on Advances in Cyber Security* (pp. 148–166). Springer, Singapore (2020).
28. Dose, H., Møller, J. S., Iversen, H. K., & Puthusserypady, S.: An end-to-end deep learning approach to MI-EEG signal classification for BCIs. *Expert Systems with Applications*, 114, 532–542 (2018).
29. Salazar-Gomez, A. F., DelPreto, J., Gil, S., Guenther, F. H., & Rus, D.: Correcting robot mistakes in real time using EEG signals. In 2017 *IEEE International Conference on Robotics and Automation (ICRA)* (pp. 6570–6577). IEEE (2017).
30. Gao, J., Sultan, H., Hu, J., & Tung, W. W.: Denoising nonlinear time series by adaptive filtering and wavelet shrinkage: a comparison. *IEEE signal processing letters*, 17 (3), 237–240.(2009)
31. Sriraam, N.: Quality-on-demand compression of EEG signals for telemedicine applications using neural network predictors. *International Journal of telemedicine and applications*, (2011).
32. Sriraam, N.: Context-based near-lossless compression of EEG signals using neural network predictors. *AEU-International Journal of Electronics and Communications,* 63 (4), 311–320 (2009).
33. Ma, T., Shrestha, P. L., Hempel, M., Peng, D., Sharif, H., & Chen, H. H. (2012). Assurance of energy efficiency and data security for ECG transmission in BASNs. *IEEE Transactions on Biomedical Engineering,* 59 (4), 1041–1048 (2012).
34. Cetin, A. E., & Köymen, H.: Compression of digital biomedical signals. In The Biomedical engineering handbook: *Medical devices and systems* (pp. 3–1). CRC Press (2006).
35. Shamsollahi, M. B.: ECG denoising and compression using a modified, extended Kalman filter structure. *IEEE Transactions on Biomedical Engineering*, 55 (9), 2240–2248 (2008).
36. Akhila, V. A., Arunvinodh, C., Reshmi, K. C., & Sakthiprasad, K. M.: A new cryptographic key generation scheme using psychological signals. *Procedia technology*, 25, 286–292 (2016).
37. Roach, B. J., & Mathalon, D. H.: Event-related EEG time-frequency analysis: an overview of measures and an analysis of early gamma band phase locking in schizophrenia. *Schizophrenia Bulletin,* 34 (5), 907–926 (2008).
38. Pai, Y. T., Cheng, F. C., Lu, S. P., & Ruan, S. J.: Sub-trees modification of Huffman coding for stuffing bits reduction and efficient NRZI data transmission. *IEEE transactions on broadcasting,* 58 (2), 221–227 (2012).
39. Latré, B., Braem, B., Moerman, I., Blondia, C., & Demeester, P. A survey on wireless body area networks. *Wireless networks*, 17 (1), 1–18 (2011).
40. Somasundaram, M., & Sivakumar, R.: Security in wireless body area networks: A survey. *In International Conference on Advancements in Information Technology* (2011).
41. Elena H. Pereira, Veronica B. Canedo, et al.: A comparison of the performance of K-complex classification methods using feature selection in *Information Sciences* 328, 1–14 (2016).
42. Saadeh, W., Khan, F. H., & Altaf, M. A. B.: Design and implementation of a machine learning-based EEG processor for accurate estimation of the depth of anaesthesia. *IEEE transactions on biomedical circuits and systems,* 13 (4), 658–669 (2019).
43. Jain, A., Kumar, A., & Sharma, S.: Comparative Design and Analysis of Mesh, Torus and Ring NoC. *Procedia Computer Science*, 48, 330–337 (2015).
44. Jain, A., Dwivedi, R., Kumar, A., & Sharma, S.: Scalable design and synthesis of 3D mesh network on chip. In Proceeding of *International Conference on Intelligent Communication, Control and Devices*, pp. 661–666. Springer, Singapore (2017).
45. Jain, A., Gahlot, A. K., Dwivedi, R., Kumar, A., & Sharma, S. K.: Fat Tree NoC Design and Synthesis. *In Intelligent Communication, Control and Devices* (pp. 1749–1756). Springer, Singapore (2018).

46. Sharma, S. K., Jain, A., Gupta, K., Prasad, D., & Singh, V.: An internal schematic view and simulation of major diagonal mesh network-on-chip. *Journal of Computational and Theoretical Nanoscience,* 16 (10), 4412–4417 (2019).
47. Ghai, D., Gianey, H. K., Jain, A., & Uppal, R. S.: Quantum and dual-tree complex wavelet transform-based image watermarking. *International Journal of Modern Physics* B, 34 (04), 2050009 (2020).
48. Jain, A., & Kumar, A.: Desmogging of still smoggy images using a novel channel prior. *Journal of Ambient Intelligence and Humanized Computing*, 12 (1), 1161–1177 (2021).
49. Kumar, S., Jain, A., Shukla, A. P., Singh, S., Raja, R., Rani, S., ... & Masud, M.: A Comparative Analysis of Machine Learning Algorithms for Detection of Organic and Nonorganic Cotton Diseases. *Mathematical Problems in Engineering*, (2021).
50. Misra, N. R., Kumar, S., & Jain, A.: A Review on E-waste: Fostering the Need for Green Electronics. In 2021 *International Conference on Computing, Communication, and Intelligent Systems*, pp. 1032–1036. IEEE (2021).
51. K. Balachander, S. Ramesh, Ahmed J. Obaid.: Simulation Of 1KW Multi-Level Switch Mode Power Amplifier, *International Journal of Innovations in Scientific and Engineering Research,* Vol. 5, No. 9: 85–92 (2018).
52. Jain, A., AlokGahlot, A. K., & RakeshDwivedi, S. K. S.: Design and FPGA Performance Analysis of 2D and 3D Router in Mesh NoC. *International Journal of Control Theory and Applications*, ISSN, 0974–5572 (2017).
53. Agrawal, N., Jain, A., & Agarwal, A.: Simulation of Network on Chip for 3D Router Architecture. *International Journal of Recent Technology and Engineering*, 8, 58–62 (2019).
54. Tawfiq A. Al-Asadi, Ahmed J. Obaid, Ahmed A. Alkhayat.: Proposed Method for Web Pages Clustering Using Latent Semantic Analysis, *Journal of Engineering and Applied Science*, Vol. 12, No. 8: 8270–8277 (2017).
55. Nora Omran Alkaam, Ahmed J. Obaid, Mohammed Q. Mohammed.: A Hybrid Technique for Object Detection and Recognition Using Local Features Algorithms, *Journal of Advanced Research in Dynamical and Control Systems*, Vol. 10, No. 2: 2330–2344 (2018).

A Deep Convolutional Neural Network-Based Heart Diagnosis for Smart Healthcare Applications

K. Saikumar and V. Rajesh

1 Introduction

Predicting and diagnosing heart disorders is the most challenging task in the medical industry to save people from a sudden cardiac arrest. In the past, many heart diagnosis models were available which aid in diagnosing cardiac abnormalities, but these techniques could not give accurate solutions in less time. Several deep convolutional neural network (DCNN)-based approaches are available, but these are more complex to find abnormalities. Machine learning and artificial intelligence are technologies that help in diagnosing heart diseases [1]. According to the WHO, annually, 1.8 billion people are affected by heart-related health issues and are at increased risk of dying [2].

Table 1 shows a deep study on various heart disorder detection applications based on scan image type. The MRI/CT/SPECT/Echo scanned images are used to find hidden disorders based on the following models. Vendors like TCSS, Philips, CAD, etc. are implementing models to detect heart abnormalities, but necessary improvements are needed. Thus, a deep learning and machine learning-based heart disorder design is implemented in Python 3.6.7 software. Packages like TensorFlow, Keras, and NumPy are used to design mathematical modeling [3].

K. Saikumar (✉)
Department of ECE, Koneru Lakshmaiah Education Foundation, Guntur, Andhra Pradesh, India

School of Engineering, Department of AI-ML, Malla Reddy University, Research Scholar in Koneru Lakshmaiah Education Foundation, Hyderabad, India
e-mail: saikumarkayam4@ieee.org

V. Rajesh
Department of ECE, Koneru Lakshmaiah Education Foundation, Guntur, Andhra Pradesh, India
e-mail: rajesh4444@kluniversity.in

P. Agarwal et al. (eds.), *Artificial Intelligence for Smart Healthcare*,
EAI/Springer Innovations in Communication and Computing,
https://doi.org/10.1007/978-3-031-23602-0_14

Table 1 Heart abnormality detection using CAD (computer-aided design)

Method	Vendor	Model
CM_Tool	Cardiac image solution	MRI/CT
Heart_Suite	NEO Software	CTA/MRI
CVT56	Pyramid Cardiac image solution	MRI
Medi_suite	Medics	SPECT
Xilabs	CAD	MRI/CT
Q_LABS	Philips	Echo/CTA
TOMTECHS	Philips	MRI/SPECT
Z_HADD	Motorola	CT/MRI/SPECT/CTA
Dense_H	TCSS	SPECT
DCNN	Medics	MRI/SPECT

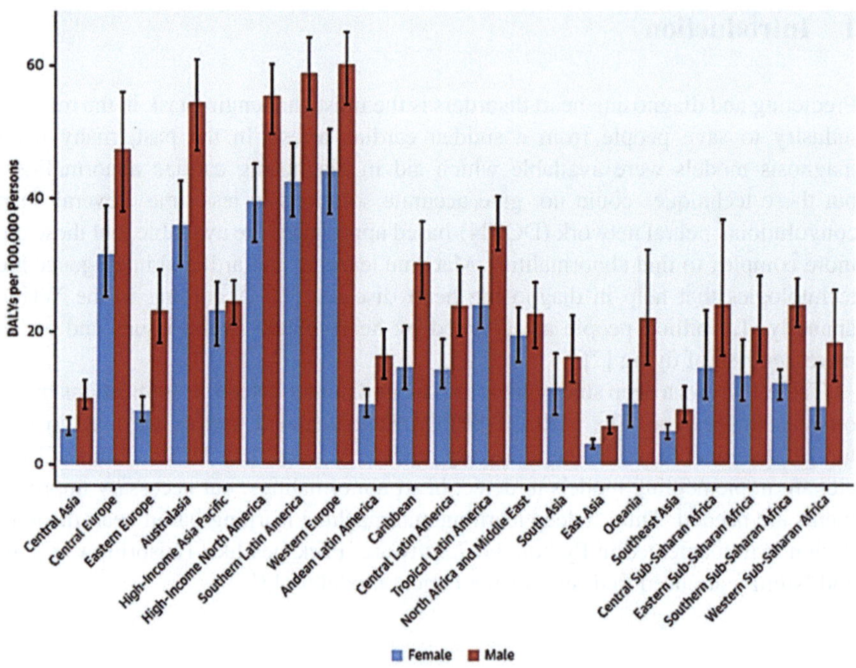

Fig. 1 Worldwide cardiovascular disease statistics

Using the LV and RV discharge part, RV and LV volume end-systole and end-diastole, myocardial mass, and the patients' stature and weight as information sources, an ANN (artificial neural network) was developed to analyze hypertrophic cardiomyopathy (HCM), myocardial infarction (MI), and strange RV (SRV) work. The specialists utilized a bunch of 32 qualities from clinical information to analyze enlarged cardiomyopathy, including launch portion, circulatory strain, sex, age, and another setup hazard factor (DCM). By coordinating discharge portions very still and stress with a pool of clinical factors, ML was utilized to predict CAD and cardiovascular disease location outcomes as shown in Fig. 1.

Heart disease detection is a major task for medical associates; in this context, the term "cardiovascular diseases" is defined as a group of disorders affecting the heart and blood vessels. According to a medical association's data [4], cardiac illnesses are now the leading cause of mortality worldwide, with 17.9 million deaths annually. High blood pressure, obesity, increased homocysteine levels, hypertension, and other harmful habits are all risk factors that led to the rise in cardiac diseases [5]. The American Diabetes Association [6] cites specific symptoms such as sleep disturbances; fluctuations of heartbeat, i.e., irregular heartbeat; swelling in legs; and fast weight gain, i.e., 1–2 kg per day [7]. These symptoms are similar to other conditions, such as those that affect the elderly, making it difficult to get an actual diagnosis, which could lead to death in the coming years. The computational complexity of data is a prevalent challenge in computer vision; the databases include large amounts of data and often 3D views. The dimensionality is a major concern [8]. As a result, when we execute operations on this data, we need a large amount of storage, and the data might expand rapidly, resulting in overfitting. The weighted features may be utilized to reduce the duplication in the information, which helps reduce the implementation's processing time [9]. A variety of feature design and feature selection methods may be used to reduce the dimension of a dataset by removing materials [10]. All the above discussion supports heart disease detection-related issues and their limitations.

2 Literature Survey

In this section, a brief discussion of heart-related disease detection is performed for image-based analysis. A machine learning model can be created to identify heart disorders easily, but the imaging inputs must be properly defined [11]. The unprocessed image information, i.e., pixel intensities and traditional heart index, and other modified measurable picture characteristics or region-based qualities generated as the picture can all be used as imaging inputs [12]. The distribution of input variables in the reviewed literature has been discussed about heart disease [13]. Traditional indices are the most common characteristics for training ML models, as seen in the pie chart, followed by region-based and deep learning techniques as shown in Fig. 2.

A list of popular input and output variables for machine learning (ML) algorithms for image-based diagnostics has been collected from the Kaggle database. Raw data, convolutional lists separated from an ROI or region based (cardiac anatomy definition is necessary in the last two cases), and planned yield are generally examples of heart imaging input features. Information is essential for an ML heart imaging application, and both structures shape it. Conventional imaging indices include ventricular elections and volumes in end-diastole/systole divisions, ordinarily utilized in clinical image investigation [14]. The endocardial and epicardial boundaries of the appropriate heart chambers must be contoured before these clinical indices can be calculated. Automated/semiautomated contouring techniques have been

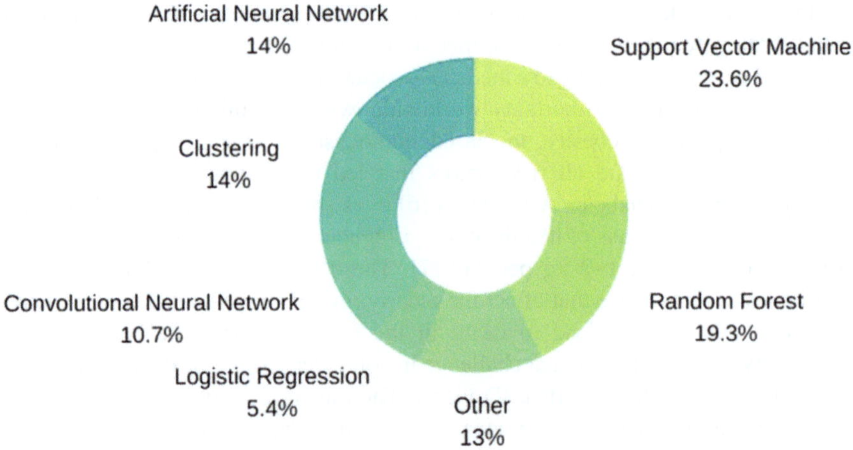

Fig. 2 Survey on different ML- and NN-based segmentation operations

developed using deep learning approaches designed for high-efficient and repeatable classification of heart volumes [15]. In motion, strain, and single intensity analyses, global spatiotemporal picture features are retrieved and fed into SVM (support vector machine) segmentation for heart LV valve motion evaluation. Pairwise solo force and different provincial varieties in SPECT perfusion examinations copy the medical method of subjectively estimating pressure and rest. Contractility changes and multiscale wall motion are studied using the apparent flow approach. Every aspect explains an oriented velocity and a cardiac ROI at a specified place [16].

The transformation of digital photos into usable data is known as region-based analysis. The region-based feature provides the classification of the image's different nature and structural properties by analyzing the data using various statistical and mathematical procedures [17]. The heart chambers' more advanced and intricate properties are quantified using region-based analysis which may be seen directly (Table 2). Region-based analysis, like clinical imaging indices, requires the definition of cardiac structures before features can be retrieved, as shown in Fig. 3.

The region-based model, introduced in 2012, was mostly used in oncology for a long time. Several recent studies have demonstrated the potential of region-based analysis coupled by ML for image-aided diagnosis of CVD. About ten region-based variables integrated into an ML model are sufficient to distinguish several major CVDs. More recently, Harvard University researchers developed an ML model that uses six radiomic characteristics estimated as T1 mapping sequences toward distinguishing between HHD and HCM. Several studies have used LRs for their specific purposes in the literature. For example, utilizing formed characteristics collected from cine MRI each segment, researchers used a succession of four LRs to classify patients as per heart disease. As a result, they created a basic and easy-to-understand model with just three information highlighted for every classifier. Another study employed SPECT images to detect obstructive CAD using a mix of

Table 2 Region-based features' overview

Type	Description	Example
Feature extraction	Cardiac analysis of geometric feature analysis	Angle, shape, flatness, and rectangular box modeling
Resolution estimation	Statistical analysis of resolution in ROI at a pixel density	Entropy, intensity, and skewness assumptions in cardiac intensity
Texture estimation with second-order modeling	The ROI with relationship modeling and pixels is estimated through the CNN technique	Preprocessing with aspect ratio and resolution
Higher-order modeling	Quantify the medical image geometric parameters and intensity-level adjustment	Long- and short-run image enhancement with entropy adjustment
Texture analysis	Color and gray-level intensity adjustment using ROI	Brightness and ROI analysis
Factorial analysis	Ratio and scale of intensity adjustment	Feature level ML application
Texture-based image analysis	An exact image scale defense model with DL analysis	Deep learning-based image enhancement

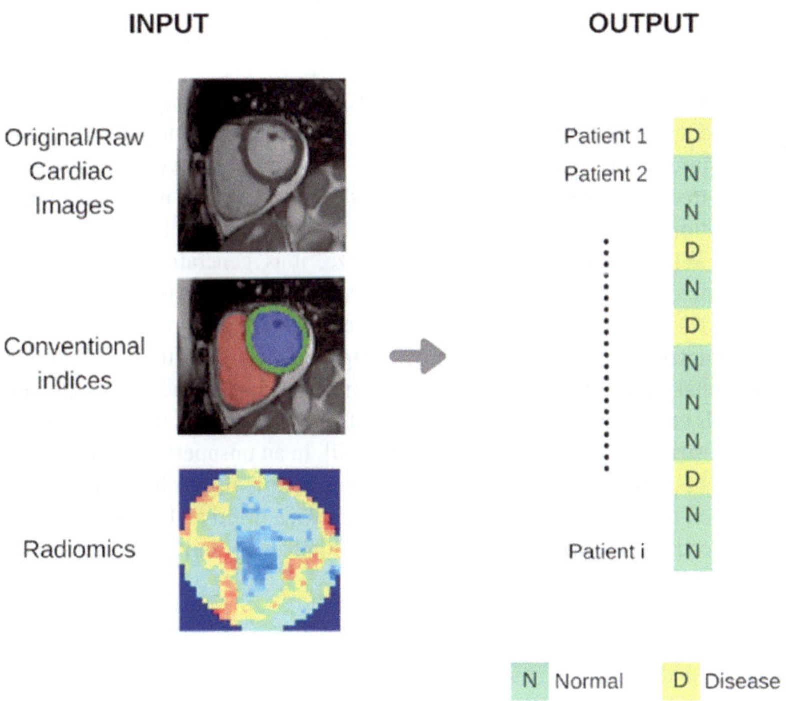

Fig. 3 Detection of coronary artery disease

classifiers improved with an LR. Finally, an LR was used to diagnose myocarditis-like acute or chronic heart failure. ACNNs: Implementations of cardiovascular disease image segmentation and classification and ACNNs' algorithms enhanced SCI diagnosis classification rate and overall performance. Uk's country health center provided a Heart CT scan dataset that has been imported for ML training. RFO classification, advanced model, and adaptive Gaussian filter [18].

Computed tomography (CT) and Magnetic resonance imaging (MRI) scanned heart samples are used to diagnose heart illness through various methodologies, such as Stratified Decision Forests for Accurate Anatomical, Landmark Localization in Cardiac Images Advanced Model, MLMachine learning (ML) Techniques. The k-Nearest Neighbor Algorithm Advanced Model: A Machine-to-Machine (M2M) Telemedicine Systems for Rural areas Cardiovascular diseases Patients using Auto-Diagnosis, Decreasing Over Noise and Classifying Hcaa Using Ml Technique, Machine to Machine (M2M), (Heart Coronary Injury). Logistic regression is a binary classification-based extension of linear regression. It does not involve empirical parameter adjustment or input feature normalization, and it is simple and easy to understand. Advanced model, which is ineffective for nonlinear issues, is prone to overfitting; thus, a support vector machine is used to find the best class border. It can handle a variety of nonlinear set segmentation and doesn't need a big number of training data. Advanced Model, hyperparameter adjustment, and nonlinear kernel selection are required but are not appropriately designed for extremely large information [19].

RF (random forest) builds a set of hierarchical decision inquiries based on the input and output data. Features are automatically prioritized; no feature normalization is required. Advanced model, which is susceptible to overfitting, depth, and number of trees, must be defined. Input data is propagated via a network of nonlinear transformations in an artificial neural network, which models difficult categorization problems. When trained on large sample size, it is generalized well. Advanced model, which is complex to understand, needs the previous assortment of system structural design (e.g., network depth) and requires a big amount of training data. ANNs adapted for image data processing and classification are known as convolutional neural networks (CNNs). Flexible design that adapts to the application's needs can learn the best characteristics from photographs directly. ANNs have the same restrictions as the advanced model [20]. In an unsupervised way, clustering identifies subdivisions of input feature extent, which is useful for discovering subgroups when the labels of the groups are not known a priori and is simple and quick. For advanced model that is susceptible to initialization and scale, estimating the number of subgroups is difficult [21, 22].

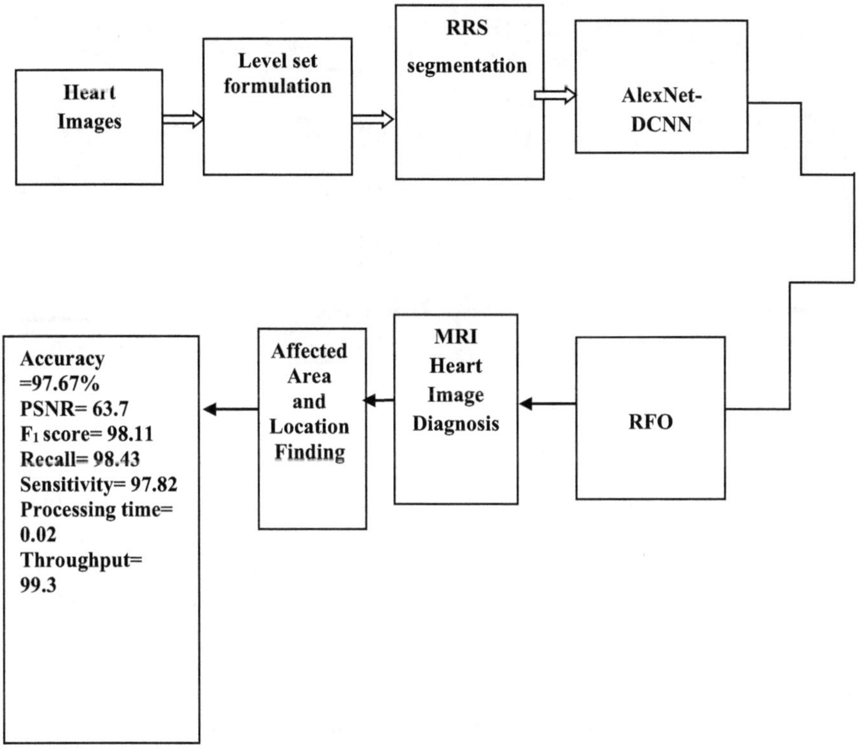

Fig. 4 Block diagram of proposed work

3 Methodology

The proposed model has a color constancy index (CCI) = $1 - a/b$, where a is the actual space in the shading space among the test images under the first and second illuminants and b is the distance in the shading space amid the onlooker's match to the match that would be made if shading consistency were awesome. CCI = 1 if shading steadiness is incredible ($a = 0$), and CCI = 0 if color constancy isn't present ($a = b$). CCI normalizes color space distances, which may differ for various samples, as a ratio. The abnormal and normal diseases-affected heart samples have been trained through the GHLB approach.

Figure 4 clearly shows the block diagram of the proposed model; in the first stage, local images are applied for training. The level set formulation mechanism uses like preprocessor. The RRS segmentation provides information on the object of heart disease-affected area. The RFO and AlexNet DCNN models train and test the model and then classify the abnormality and performance measures to be calculated.

BCI = $-\log(c/d)$, in which c is the outright contrast in luminance among the spectator's match to the match that would be made if splendor consistency were

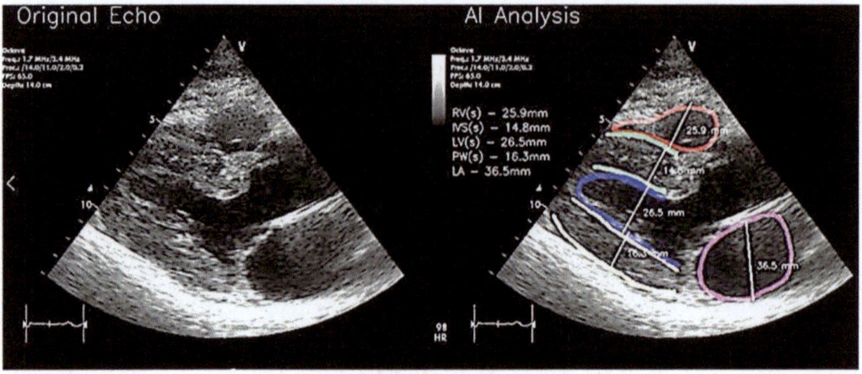

Fig. 5 Sample images of segmented artery

magnificent, and then $d > 0$ is the outright worth of the real distinction in luminance among the focal patches beneath the first and second illuminants as shown in Fig. 5.

This list doesn't separate among brilliance and intricacy (Fig. 6), which are intently relative in multi-chromatic Mondrian's pattern where nearby surface differences will result in general average out; overlooks the reliance of splendor on immersion, as immersion will influence c and d comparably in the wake of coordinating; and does exclude reaction pressure, which just applies to higher powers. Even though easing up and obscuring impacts might contrast as a general rule, the outright qualities respect over- and under-assessments of the matches similarly, as these are commonly modest. The log change of (irrefutably the) c/d proportions is utilized to decide the degree to which we saw brilliance as corresponding to improvement log27 instead of boost force. (The log exists as long as $d > 0$ and $c > 0$, which this information did.) The negative sign before the log characterizes BCI as a file of consistency instead of incorrectness irregularity; it has no impact on the connections or inclinations other than transforming their signs. The skew in the c/d ratios was also minimized using the log transform.

We used the mean simulated illuminant coordinates ($u'0 = 0.188$, $v'0 = 0.440$) as the origin, accepting that the subjects were similarly fit to the two presentations. S0.40 is 29.30. Each example had four arrangements of organized HSB: one for the main illuminant, one for the subsequent illuminant, one for the subject's surface appearance, and one for amazing steadiness, which was utilized to decide CCI and BCI. Member matches uncovered huge differences and were read independently for every person for both synchronous and successive sessions [28]. Two key issues may restrict the accuracy of quality score prediction. The first is accurate foreground segmentation. Incorrect image attributes such as the mean of the test image and the mean of the edge map can be computed due to inaccurate segmentation. The blur quality index will not correspond with the perceptual quality index if the foreground region is understated or exaggerated. The algorithm's sensitivity to the size of the filter is the second problem as shown in Fig. 7. Gaussian channel approach for a component image with numerous photo locales $L(x, y, \sigma)$ is made with the aid of

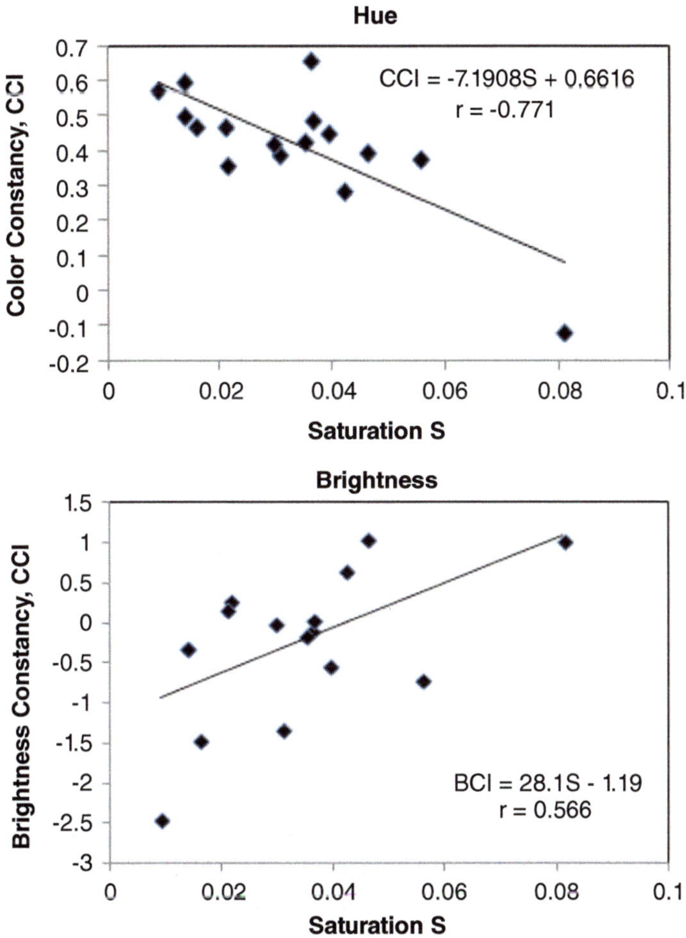

Fig. 6 Coefficient adjustment to saturation in H and B planes

convolving the image I (x, y) with Gaussian component G (x, y, σ) throughout circumstance (Fig. 4):

$$L(x, y, \sigma) = G(x, y, \sigma)\Theta I(x, y)$$

where ⊗ implies the Convol overseer. In Eq. 1, σ addresses the size with the fundamental evaluation of 1.6 repeated logically using K at exceptional stages of the octaves. Scale version factors dependent on the above situations are as follows:

$$SC_{ol} = \sigma.2^{\left(0-1+\frac{l}{LN}\right)} = \sigma.K^{LN(0-1+l)} = 1, 2 \ldots, ; l = 1, 2, \ldots., LN; k = 2\ 1/LN \quad (1)$$

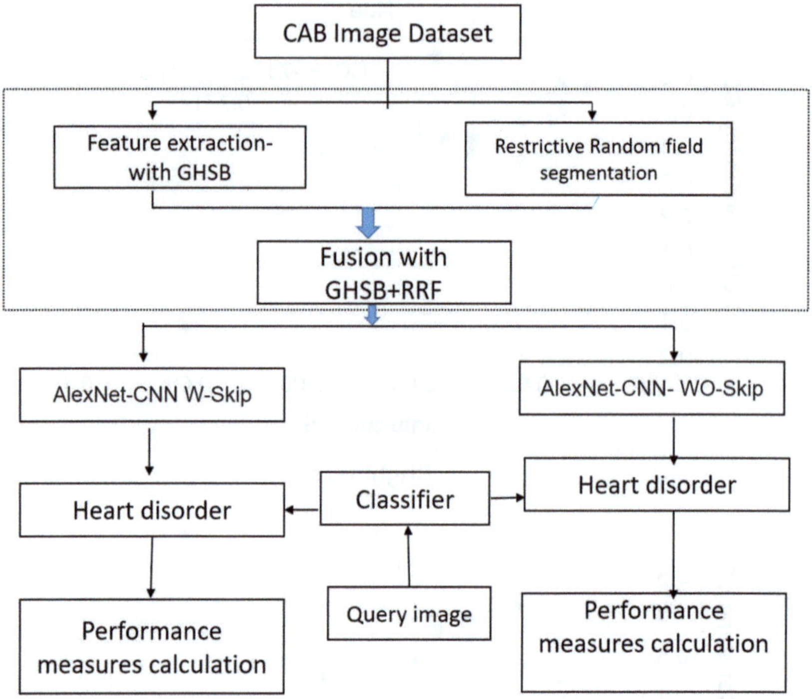

Fig. 7 Block diagram for proposing a scheme

SC_{ol} is the attained angle for stage l of the octave in Fig. 5. The Euclidean distance metric is applied on two-component images. The Euclidean distance-based analysis provides a Region where the coronary artery has been blocked moreover abnormality was classified as a rectangular or circular shape.

Figure 8 clearly shows image extraction analysis based on Gaussian filtering; the risk of heart failure is extracted easily. Various curves are used to make the system critical and define impulse outcomes to model.

AlexNet was proposed by Krizhevsky and was the winning model in the 2012 ImageNet competition, more than doubling ImageNet's recognition accuracy. In Fig. 7, an eight-layer architecture was shown based on this 17-layer architecture implemented in our proposed model shown in Fig. 9a. To present nonlinearity, the ReLU initiation work is used rather than Tanh. It speeds up by multiple times while keeping up with similar accuracy. To manage the overfit, use dropout instead of regularization. With a dropout pace of 0.5, in any case, the preparation time is multiplied as shown in Fig. 9b. Cross-over pooling is a strategy for diminishing the size of an organization. The top one and top five blunder rates are decreased individually by 0.4 percent and 0.3 percent, respectively

AlexNet is comprised of five Convolal layers and three completely associated layers. After an exceptionally Convolal and completely connected layer, ReLU is applied. Before the first and second associated years, dropout is utilized. The

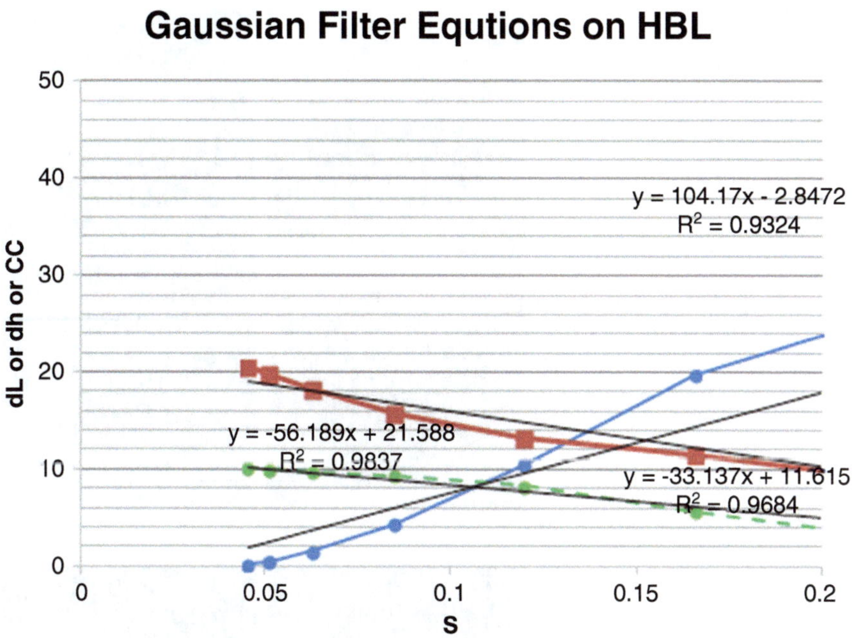

Fig. 8 H and B plane correction using Gaussian filtration

organization contains 62.3 million boundaries in a forward pass and requires 1.1 billion computation units. Convol layers, which represent 6% of all boundaries yet cost 95% of the work, may likewise be seen in Fig. 10 and Table 3.

4 Results and Discussion

In this section, a brief study on future random forest advance mechanical coronary artery segmentation and DCNN centerline origin process in CTA cardiac volume has been measured [27]. In this model, the preprocessing is done with prior usage of segmentation [29]. After that decision, a random forest algorithm is used for classification as shown in Fig. 11.

Figure 12 clearly shows ML- and DL-based heart disease classification outcomes. This RRS (restrictive random field segmentation) has been attained at the primary stage [24, 25]. Finally, for feature extraction and classification purposes, RFO and DCNN models are imported (Table 4).

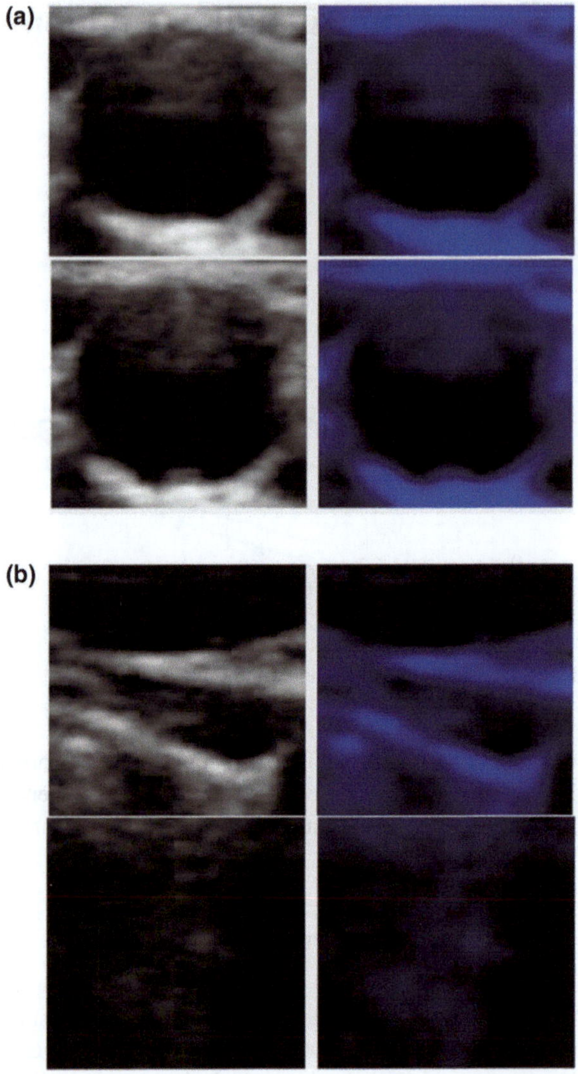

Fig. 9 (**a**) Results for positive *sample* artery using GHBL. (**b**) Results for negative *sample* artery using GHBL

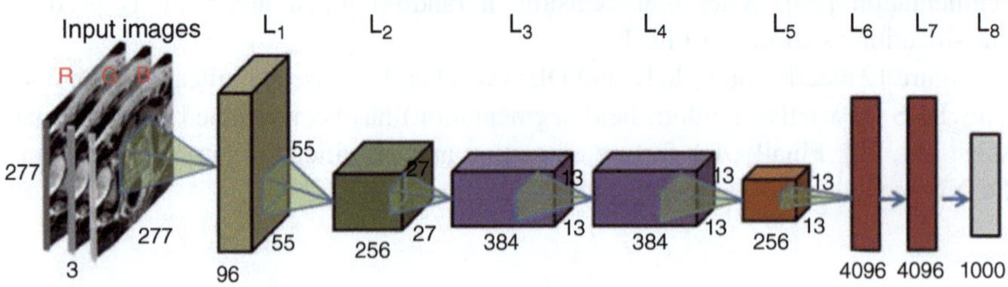

Fig. 10 DCNN architecture

Table 3 AlexNet architecture

1	'data'	Image information	227×227×3 normalization
2	'Convol1'	Convol	96 11×11×3 convols through step [4 4] and packing [0000]
3	'ReLu1'	RecLU	RecLU
4	'Norm1'	Balancing and normalization using metrics	5 channels are adjusted to cross the normalization
5	'pool1'	MAX pool layer analysis	3×3 layers with max pooling with [2 2] array as well as pad [0 0 0 0]
6	'Convol2'	Convol	512 6×6×56 convolution with stride model of [2 2] and pad [3 3 3 3]
7	RecLU2	Rectified linear unit (RecLU)	RecLU
8	Normalization 2	Channel modeling based on normalization	5-channel basic function through balancing elements
9	'MAX_POOL_2'	Pooling layer analysis	Pooling of 3×3 max with stride [2 2] and padding [0000]
10	'Convol3'	Convol	384 3×3×256 convolvs with stride [1 1] and padding [1111]
11	RecLU3	RecLU	RecLU
12	'Convol4'	Convol	384 3×3×192 convolvs with stride [1 1] and padding [1111]
13	'relu4'	RecLU	RecLU
14	'Convol5'	Convol	256 3×3×192 convolvs with stride [1 1] and padding [1111]
15	'ReLu 5'	RecLU	RecLU
16	'Pool5'	Max pooling	3×3 max pooling with stride [2 2] and padding [3333]
17	'fc 6'	Fully connected	4096 fully connected layers
18	'ReLu 6'	RecLU	RecLU
19	'drop6'	Dropout	60% normalization
20	FCNN &	FCNN	5013 FCNN
21	'ReLu 7'	RecLU	RecLU
22	'droop7'	Dropout	80% FCNN
23	'fc 8'	Fully connected	5000 FCNN layers
24	'Prob'	Softmax layers	RecLU
25	o/p	Output analysis	Cross-validation layer with 3×3 mechanism

5 Conclusion

In this research work, advanced heart disease detection is performed through machine learning feature extraction and deep convolutional neural networks classification. The segmentation can be performed through restrictive random field segmentation. A segmentation and multi-level regression-based probabilistic random

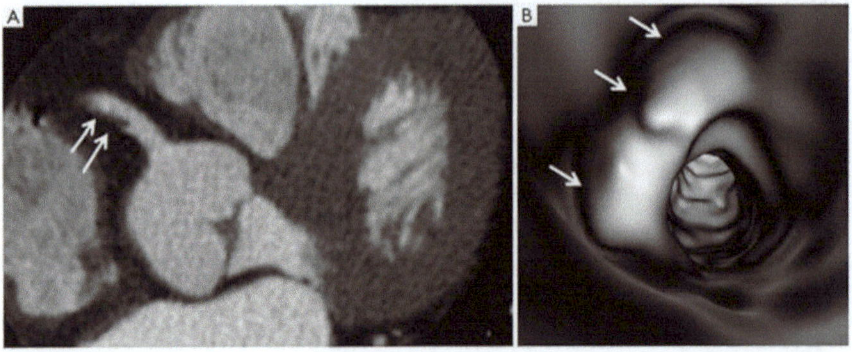

Fig. 11 Segmentation and classification

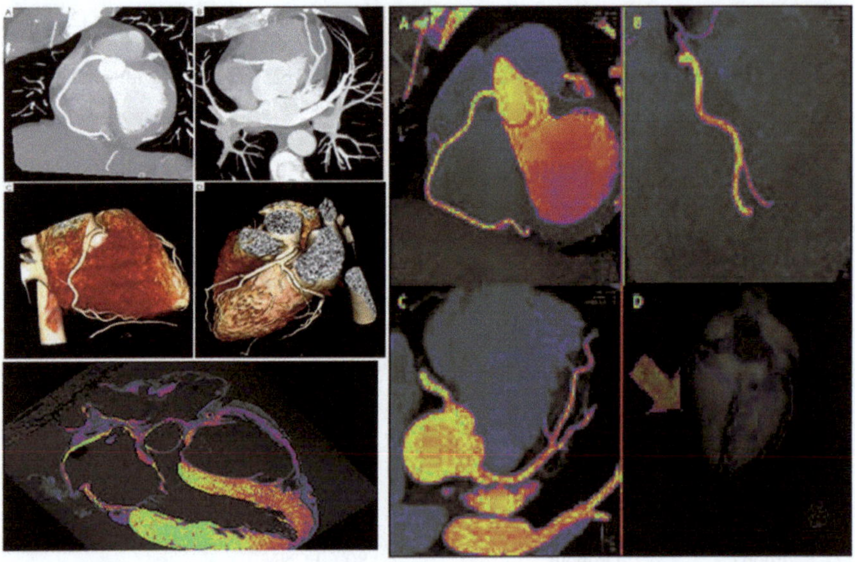

Fig. 12 Heart disease classification

forest (RFO) classification model was used to forecast the diverse problems in the coronary artery. A DCNN (deep convolutional neural network)-based feature selection and image net classification model for coronary artery model is required for healthcare applications. GHSB and RFO models are used on heart/MRI ultrasound images in this study. This model detects the CAB in the applied image and extracts the anomaly from the scanned data accurately. The AlexNet-DCNN classifier is then used to determine the breadth and length of the obstruction. Finally, 99.74 percent accuracy, 98.81 percent precision, 98.14 percent recall, 94.87 percent F1 score, 59.26 percent PSNR, 0.0989 percent CC (correlation coefficient), 99.45 percent sensitivity, and other metrics were achieved. Furthermore, the outcomes of this

Table 4 Comparison of outcomes

Model	LEA-CNN with RRF and GHSB	Meta-analysis [26]	Automatic synthesis [22]	Iterative image deblurring [23]
Measure of dice	74.21	89.12	71.8	70.15
Accurateness	99.74	91.0	91.23	89.78
Precision	98.81	77.91	87.45	91.48
Recall	98.14	81.74	84.78	86.15
F measure	94.87	76	76.28	81.23
PSNR	59.26	41.45	40.56	44.97
Correlation coefficient	0.0989	0.0897	0.091	0.0923
Sensitivity	99.45	92.0	96.12	97.18

technological simulation outperform and challenge current methodologies. This work is most suitable for future level heart diagnosis applications. Moreover, this application with android and iOS modeling can be likely helpful for future generations with easy access.

References

1. Saikumar, K., Rajesh, V. "A Telemedicine Technology for Cardiovascular Patients Diagnosis Feature Using KNN-MPM Algorithm" Journal of International Pharmaceutical Research, 90 (7), 72–77 (2019).
2. Saikumar, K., Rajesh, V. "A deep learning process for spine and heart segmentation using pixel-based Convolal networks" Journal of International Pharmaceutical Research, 90 (7), 72–77 (2019).
3. Saikumar, K., Rajesh, V. "Medical diagnosis for hybrid image fusion using advanced wavelet and contourlet" IEEE, conference 10 (12), 301–319 (2020).
4. K saikumar, V Rajesh "Coronary blockage of artery for Heart diagnosis with DT Artificial Intelligence Algorithm" International Journal of Research in Pharmaceutical Sciences, Volume 11, Issue 1, January (2020).
5. K Saikumar, V Rajesh "Diagnosis of coronary blockage of artery using MRI/cta images through adaptive random forest optimization" JCR, 5, Volume: 7 (2020).
6. Enriko, I. K. A., Suryanegara, M., & Gunawan, D. (2017). Comparative Study of Heart Disease Diagnosis Using Top Ten Data Mining Classification Algorithms. Accepted in Journal of Telecommunication, Electronic and Computer Engineering, (2018).
7. M. S. Sapna and D. A. Tamilarasi, "Fuzzy Relational Equation in Preventing Neuropathy Diabetic," International Journal of Recent Trends in Engineering, Vol. 2, No. 4, p. 126 (2009).
8. L. Carnimeo and A. Giaquinto, "An Intelligent System for Improving Detection of Diabetic Symptoms in Retinal Images," IEEE International Conference on Information Technology in Biomedicine, Ioannina, 26–28, (2006).
9. R. Radha and S. P. Rajagopalan, "Fuzzy Logic Approach for Diagnosis of Diabetes," Information Technology Journal, Vol. 6, No. 1, pp. 96–102 (2007).

10. Waheed, H.J., Abduljalil, M., Alkuraishy, H. Estimation of apolipoprotein A, apo B, apo E and some biochemical markers in type 2 diabetic patients in Iraq. International Journal of Pharmaceutical Research, 10 (3), pp. 493–498 (2018).
11. K. Gopalakrishnan R. Lakshmanan V. Naveen S. TamilKumaran and S. Venkatesh. "Digital Signature Manager." International Journal of Communication and Computer Technologies 5, 53–57 (2017).
12. Bahmani, Kavita, and yashpaul singla. "Enhanced Solubility Of Antihypertensive Drug Using Hydrophilic Carrier- Based Potent Solid Dispersion Systems." International Journal of Pharmacy Research & Technology 9, 24–37 (2019).
13. F. Ensan, M. H. Yaghmaee and E. Bagheri, "Fact: A New Fuzzy Adaptive Clustering Technique," The 11th IEEE Symposium on Computers and Communications, Sardinia, 26–29, pp. 442–447 (2006).
14. UCI Machine Learning Repository. http://www.ics.uci.edu/mlearn/MLRepository.html
15. S. W. Purnami, A. Embong, J. M. Zain and S. P. Rahayu, "A New Smooth Support Vector Machine and Its Applications in Diabetes Disease Diagnosis," Journal of Computer Science, Vol. 5, No. 12, pp. 1006–1011 (2009).
16. The Mathworks-Fuzzy Logic Toolbox, 2006. http://www.mathworks.ch/access/helpdeskr13/help/toolbox/fuzzy/fuzzy.html. Mavrides N, Nemeroff C. Treatment of depression in cardiovascular disease. Depression and Anxiety. (2013).
17. Celano CM, Huffman JC. Depression and cardiac disease: a review. Cardiology in Review, 19(3):130–142 (2011).
18. Carney RM, Freedland KE. Depression in patients with coronary heart disease. The American Journal of Medicine, 121, 11, supplement 1: S20–S27 (2008).
19. Lespérance F, Frasure-Smith N, Juneau M, Théroux P. Depression and 1-year prognosis in unstable angina. Archives of Internal Medicine;160(9):1354–1360 (2000).
20. Sk. Hasane Ahammad, V.Rajesh, "Image Processing based segmentation for spinal cord in MRI", Indian Journal of Public Health Research and Development 9 (6), pp. 317–323 (2018).
21. Schleifer SJ, Macari-Hinson MM, Coyle DA, et al. The nature and course of depression following myocardial infarction. Archives of Internal Medicine, 149 (8):1785–1789 (1989).
22. Haase R, Schlattmann P, Gueret P, Andreini D, Pontone G, Alkadhi H, Hausleiter J, Garcia MJ, Leschka S, Meijboom WB, Zimmermann E, Gerber B, Schoepf UJ, Shabestari AA, Nørgaard BL, Meijs MFL, Sato A, Ovrehus KA, Diederichsen ACP, Jenkins SMM, Knuuti J, Hamdan A, Halvorsen BA, Mendoza-Rodriguez V, Rochitte CE, Rixe J, Wan YL, Langer C, Bettencourt N, Martuscelli E, Ghostine S, Buechel RR, Nikolaou K, Mickley H, Yang L, Zhang Z, Chen MY, Halon DA, Rief M, Sun K, Hirt-Moch B, Niinuma H, Marcus RP, Muraglia S, Jakamy R, Chow BJ, Kaufmann PA, Tardif JC, Nomura C, Kofoed KF, Laissy JP, Arbab-Zadeh A, Kitagawa K, Laham R, Jinzaki M, Hoe J, Rybicki FJ, Scholte A, Paul N, Tan SY, Yoshioka K, Röhle R, Schuetz GM, Schueler S, Coenen MH, Wieske V, Achenbach S, Budoff MJ, Laule M, Newby DE, Dewey M; COME-CCT Consortium. Diagnosis of obstructive coronary artery disease using computed tomography angiography in patients with stable chest pain depending on clinical probability and in clinically important subgroups: meta-analysis of individual patient data. BMJ. Jun 12;365: l1945 (2019). https://doi.org/10.1136/bmj.l1945. PMID: 31189617; PMCID: PMC6561308.
23. Renuka J Bathi, Sameena Parveen, Krishna Burde, The Role of Gutka Chewing in Oral Submucous Fibrosis: A Case-Control Study, Quintessence International, Volume 40, Issue 6, pages e19–e25. 7p. 5 (2009).
24. Sameena Parveen, Neeraj Taneja, Renuka J Bathi, AC Deka, Evaluation Of Circulating Immune Complexes And Serum Immunoglobulins In Oral Cancer Patients – A Follow Up Study, Indian Journal of Dental Research, Volume 21, Issue 1, Pages 14–19, (2010).
25. Renuka J Bathi, Sameena Parveen, Neeraj Taneja, Oral Tuberculous Ulcer – A Report of Two Cases, Journal of Indian Academy of Oral Medicine and Radiology, Volume 15, Issue 2, Pages 62–65 (2003).

26. Parveen S. Bathi R, Taneja N, Dermoid Cyst in The Floor of The Mouth-A Case Report, Karnataka State Dental Journal, Vol. 25, no. 2, pp. 52–54 (2006).
27. Sameena Parveen, Impact of Calorie Restriction and Intermittent Fasting on Periodontal Health, Periodontology 2000, Vol. 87, no. 1, pp. 315–324 (2021).
28. T. Radhika K Mohideen, C Krithika, N Jeddy, S Parveen, A Meta-Analysis in Assessing Oxidative Stress Using Malondialdehyde in Oral Submucous Fibrosis, European Journal of Dentistry, (2021).
29. Parveen S Taneja N, R Bathi, Serum Glycoproteins as Prognosticator in Head and Neck Cancer Patients – A Follow Up Study, Oral Oncology Head and Neck Oncology, Vol. 47 (2011).

A Dynamic Perceptual Detector Module-Related Telemonitoring for the Intertubes of Health Services

Vaibhav Rupapara, S. Suman Rajest, Regin Rajan, R. Steffi, T. Shynu, and G. Jerusha Angelene Christabel

1 Introduction

Scientists and doctors are becoming more interested in the future generation of healthcare systems. Medical gadgets, ubiquitous tracking, and applications connected to health information systems through structures can be quite utilized in the medical field. These technologies would improve the efficiency of health outcome trials or keep track of patients in real time. On the one hand, hospital-based therapy and procedures may be much more efficient. As an alternative, home care can be made available, which saves money for the government while also improving the patient's quality of life. The market is anticipated to be worth $136 billion by

V. Rupapara
School of Computing and Information Sciences, Florida International University, Miami, FL, USA
e-mail: vupap001@fiu.edu

S. S. Rajest
Present Address: Department of Research, Bharath Institute of Higher Education and Research, Chennai, Tamil Nadu, India

R. Rajan (✉)
Department of Computer Science and Engineering, SRM Institute of Science and Technology, Chennai, Tamil Nadu, India

R. Steffi
Department of Electronics and Communication, Vins Christian College of Engineering, Nagercoil, Tamil Nadu, India

T. Shynu
Department of Biomedical Engineering, Agni College of Technology, Chennai, Tamil Nadu, India

G. J. A. Christabel
Sathyabama Institute of Science and Technology, Chennai, Tamil Nadu, India

P. Agarwal et al. (eds.), *Artificial Intelligence for Smart Healthcare*, EAI/Springer Innovations in Communication and Computing,
https://doi.org/10.1007/978-3-031-23602-0_15

2021 [1]. For example, the Internet of things (IoT) paradigm allows for seamless data collection from a wide range of sources, which could then be explored to extract useful data about a patient's state. New sensor technology also makes it possible to gather precise, inexpensive, and accessible samples of vital parameters and bio-signals. However, advancements in scalability, reactivity, security, and privacy are required to make IoMT pervasive and effective. The majority of efforts in this area aim to establish a strategy for edge computing. Using a proper portable/wearable processing platform, digital data obtained using detectors can be analyzed, at minimum in portion, at the periphery until being transferred cloud-based. This has a lot of advantages. To begin with, it reduces the amount of bandwidth required. Near-sensor system allowed more compact information to be extracted from raw data.

As a result, the centralized server requires less communication bandwidth, and the energy consumption associated with wireless data transfer is dramatically decreased. It can also improve grid stability by using near-sensor computing. Monitoring doesn't rely on network availability, and network delays can if rapid notification toward the user and/or local activation is necessary; this should be avoided. Data must be protected from the internet to protect personal confidentiality and compassionate data. Heart disease and stroke treatment, a serious health issue that kills millions of people each year and costs the government a lot of money, is an important application field for IoMT. For example, in 2016, 17.6 million fatalities (95 percent confidence interval: 17.3–18.1 million) were due to CVD worldwide. Since 2006, there has been a 14.5 percent growth (95 percent confidence interval: 12.1 percent–17.1 percent) [2]. The economic effects of CVD in Europe [3], and expected that the total cost of the project will be roughly C210 billion. In most cases, electrocardiogram (ECG) signals are analyzed during CVD treatment using remote monitoring. Edge-processing presents additional complications in this situation.

Because of the large bandwidth generated by ECG sensors, sending raw data wirelessly necessitates a significant amount of energy, which might be neglected in an accessible, transportable, and low-power gadget. The operation module features where the obtained data is conveyed outside the node are important to balance the operation mode in which the raw data is processed directly in the node. It is possible to monitor your health with low-cost devices that are reliable and accurate. They can assist in compensating for a shortage of medical competence and surgical supplies, such as in nations where medical costs are too expensive. When balanced to standard rule for detecting unknown on the ECG trace, cutting-edge deep learning techniques can save time and energy while providing excellent accuracy. Deep learning is used in a variety of ways to detect irregularities in the ECG trace. Nonetheless, as illustrated in Sect. 2, they typically overlook energy consumption or use platforms that aren't designed for handheld equipment with low-power consumption. There are also no studies on precision after deployment. This work examines how to execute self-development and self-data handling in CVD, extending hardware/software optimization adaptivity. A quantized neural network is used in the system, particularly scaled and configured to run on a small controller. After the system has been installed, we continue to evaluate it, focusing on accuracy losses caused by complications while dealing with real-world scenarios. As a result, this document concentrates on two main activities:

As a reference microcontroller platform, we chose SensorTile from STMicroelectronics. IoMT node's system will be described in detail first, in terms of hardware and software. In addition to the activities that implement the sensor, the system contains an ADAM component for monitoring and onboard processing that may dynamically adjust the device's hardware/software settings to optimize power usage and staging. ADAM establishes and maintains a meshwork of FIFO-based processes for data sharing. The architecture of the activity network changes depending on the mode of operation during accomplishment. ADAM can be stirred by external environment re-layout signals or certain strain-related characteristics in explored streams. When ADAM is turned on, it modifies the task network's morphology by turning on and off processes and reordering under-task FIFOs. Furthermore, the new arrangement alters the CPU system's physical layout, modifying power-related factors including clock frequency, supply voltage, and auxiliary gating.

Another example of a linked set of sensing devices is shown using a SensorTile-based microcontroller node. The detector thread built the hardware required to receive and digitize ECG data, contact pressure, temperature, and breathing activities. To ensure a smooth integration, a suitable acquired front-end has been designed that connects to SensorTile on-board. The ensuing is the rest of the article: A description of the composition can be found in Sect. 2, followed by a description of the comprehensive SoS picture in Sect. 3, a description of the suggested template for nodes and reference target systems in Sect. 4, the type of application chosen in Sect. 5, the ADAM process in Sect. 6, the use-case chosen as either an illustration in Sect. 7, the peak detection method in Sect. 8, and the co-authoring of the paper in Sect. 9. A summary of our findings is presented in Sect. 11. The chapter structure is as follows: Related work is explained in detail. Then data transmission layout adaptation is discussed. Node structure of the IoMT, which involves planning, is studied in detail. Outlining the approaching model that we used to construct and assess the app is also discussed. Adaptive environment scheduler is taken as assistance for flexibility. Peek detection and activation of neural networks are also taken into considerations.

2 Related Work

Multiple solutions have been proposed in the literature, including the use of detectors in clinics and at home, as well as the Internet of things [4–6]. Most such investigations employ Internet research, which involves encoding data in common compositions and transmitting it to remote servers for analysis. Most research considers adaptable and transportable as the main aims for creating data detecting methods that rely on IoMT. As a result, gadgets on the market can provide days or weeks of autonomy [7, 8]. If cognitive computing at the periphery is effective, it must use more powerful and precise algorithms powered by AI or deep learning. On elevated software systems, their use has been convincingly demonstrated [9], which has a 3.60 ttHz Intel Core i7-4790 CPU; an NVIDIA GeForce GTX 1080 Ti (11 GB), [10], a 32 GB RAM, and a GPU NVIDIA Titan X (Pascal, 12 GB); and [11] a 3.5 ttHz Intel Core i7-7800X CPU, a 32 GB RAM, and a GPU NVIDIA Titan X (Pascal; on the other hand, the topic of how to integrate cutting-edge cognitive computing onto resource-constrained platforms remains unanswered). The variety of machine learning models is growing all the time.

To recognize particular events in seen data, artificial intelligence and machine learning are applied. Artificial neural networks (ANNs) are used by the authors of [12] and [13] to recognize specific circumstances in the provided information. In [13], an ANN is used to determine the patient's inner states. On the other hand, network structures are still relatively fundamental and must be fine-tuned and suited toward the objective device. For example, [14] enhances power efficiency by utilizing manufacturing in the vicinity of the detector to reduce information communication and dynamically altering entreaty configuration and periodicity of the structure to an external user's operating mode and data-dependent workload. For example, to detect irregularities in ECG data, a CNN is utilized. Several studies have shown that using ECG monitoring on tailored chips allows for real-time classification of cardiac abnormalities with low-energy consumption, even when using AI techniques [15–18]. Further research focuses on creating effective commercial neighborhood technologies that are off-the-shelf acceptance of these tactics. The literature has used a variety of target technologies, like FPGAs or systems with microcontrollers. Much research has been done on Internet devices in healthcare, namely, invigilation of ECG and anomaly detection [2]. Local processing is frequently used to perform rudimentary actual data verification and/or dispatching duties to wrap the detected information contained within traditional network methods. The advantage concept is only partially utilized [15–17]. If cognitive computing at the edge is genuinely effective, more advanced and precise technologies powered by AI and supervised learning, for example, must be handled.

When differentiated to other normal methodologies put together or not to artificial reasoning calculations, the intellectual technique, including utilizing convolutional neural organizations, guarantees high precision in perceiving ECG signal arrhythmias [14–16]. Often, CNNs can group an ECG signal regardless of whether it hasn't been pre-prepared. Moving deduction activities to the edge, picking a low-power gadget, and using quantized ways to accelerate the web execution of the surmising stage are the most pervasive procedures highlighted in various cutting-edge works that permit upgrading the exhibition of these IoT hubs [15]. announced one more intriguing review in which latent semantic analytical procedures were used to work on the organization's unwavering quality and look at other ECG follow appraisal techniques. Both preparing and deduction are made in the cloud; as it may, we wish to migrate translation to the outskirts of a limited zone gadget to decrease inactivity and energy use brought about by remote networks [7]. announced exceptional outcomes for the order of ventricular and supraventricular arrhythmias, with exactness upsides of 99.6% and 99.3%, affectability upsides of 98.4% and 90.1 percent, and positive prescient upsides of 99.2% and 94.7 percent, individually [7]. uses a double CNN, one of which receives the ECG signal's frequency domain information as input. Despite the excellent accuracy results, this methodology was not considered in our circumstance because running on a microcontroller is highly expensive. As shown in [36–38], when evaluated to methods like K-nearest neighbors (KNN) and unpredictable forest (RF), neural nets produce good results (according to the MIT-BIH Atrioventricular Arrhythmia Database, 95.98 percent). The IoT node makes this determination directly, but the power consumption remains high because they're employed in quasi gadgets like televisions (the Raspberry Pi 4) [6]. explored the architecture of the deep CNN that has been better suited for inferences on ECG signals, and the network we utilized has a shape that is quite close to that established in [6]. Although the reasoning is done on the cloud, [8] achieves incredible precision (96 percent using the MIT Arrhythmia dataset). Even with low latency, the node must still transmit a large amount of raw data, and this increased power consumption in our sample refers to edge-side interpretation [39].

- An embedded device capable of making an immediate node interpretation was chosen like [9]. Chen et al. [9] conducted a swotting on the fluctuation of precision as a function of incompatible quantization levels; they chose a precision of 12-bits with 97 percent accuracy. However, accuracy levels exceed 90 percent already from 6 bits upward. During computation, the node consumes roughly 200 mW of power, based on FPGA technology.
- We will likewise use the quantization methodology in our study, but with 8-bit precision, which will greatly increase the speed of prediction processes. The CMSIS libraries are particularly utilized to take advantage of the microcontroller's SIMD capabilities [40].
- Baloglu et al. [4] are some of the other works with which we are confronted. The key articles referenced in the article from the classics are summarised in Table 1.
- We extend [14] in this paper, considering that technologies, infrastructure components, and the organization knows might be significantly a supplemental complex in today's state-of-the-art scenario [41]. On one side, the group has developed novel ultralow-power processor systems that provide hitherto unmatched computational capabilities for popular computing and data analytic workloads.
- The creation of a structural template for hardware, software, and firmware for deployment in an IoT scenario of an autonomous unmanned perceptual module that can process located close intellectual data.
- As an illustration of computation complexity, a legislature statistical analysis employing a CNN was used to validate it [42–45].
- Another real-life example, including the platforms of ECG data, was used to evaluate and to minimize the node's power consumption by using in-place computation and dynamic operating model optimization on an ARM microcontroller architecture consumption [46].

Table 1 The architecture of certain proposed technologies in the literature

Credential	Technology of node	Operation placement	Energy consumption	Validity	Categorization method
[11]	–	–	–	MIT-BIH categorizes sinus and involves direct interaction arrhythmias: reliability values of 99.6% and 99.3%, respectively, and classification values of 90.1 and 98.4% percent	CNN
[10]	–	Cloud-based education and interpretation	–	99.2 percent for responsiveness and 94.7 percent for accuracy, respectively On an observation system, the being was 94% and the accuracy was 99.3%	CNN + LSA method
[8]	–	–	–	Ventricular ectopic rhythms had a 93.63 percent exactness, and supraventricular ectopic beats had a 95.57 percent accuracy rate	RBM and DBN
[7]	–	–	–	NSVFQ classifications for correctness, sensitivities, and specificity for the MIT-BIH sample are 99.09 percent, 98.55 percent, and 99.52 percent, respectively	DNN
[3]	The Intel I7-4700MQ has eight CPUs and 16GB of memory, although it's meant to work on less efficient platforms	Assumption on the cliff	–	Thoracic ectopic beats have a 99 percent accuracy rate, while supraventricular aberrant beats have a 97.6% accuracy rate	MIT's flexible development of 1-D CNNs
[16]	Framework with a succession	Interpretation on the perimeter, retraining in the cloud	–	On the MIT Arrhythmia sample, the prediction accuracy was 96 percent	Arrhythmia dataset CNN
[15]	FPGA	An assumption on the cliff	**200** mW[I]	97% on custom dataset	Numeral CNN

[10]	Raspberry Pi 4 (Quad-core CortexA72 @ 1.5GHz), Raspberry Pi 3 (Quad-core CortexA57 @ 1.43GHz)	An assumption on the cliff	–	On the MIT-BIH Atrioventricular Heart rhythm Database, the precision for NSVF classes is 95.27 percent	CNN
[12]	3 (Quad-core Cortex-A53 @ 1.4GHz) Raspberry Pi 3	Reasoning on the periphery, retraining in the cloud	–	96 percent of the time, the regular heartbeat, the LBB, the RBB, the Ventricular Flutter We used the ventricular escape beat (VEB) and wave (VFW) beats on the MIT Arrhythmia collection to diagnose arrhythmia diseases	CNN
Our work	SensorTile ST	Assumption on the cliff	**9** mW[II]	NLRAV and NSVFQ classes in the MIT-BIH dataset: 98.37 percent and 97.76 percent, respectively	Numeral CNN

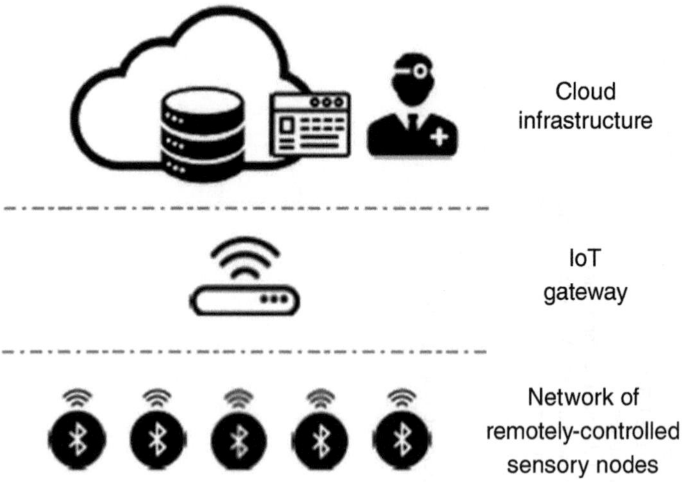

Fig. 1 A description of the planned process in particular

3 Data Transmission Layout Adaptation

Figure 1 shows how the system architecture is implemented as described in this article. The network has three strengths. The bottom strength comprises sensor nodes that collect data from the environment [47–49]. To connect to the top level, they employ Bluetooth technology. The nodes can respond to directives provided from higher levels or workload changes noticed near-sensor by altering their operating model, thanks to an internal core known as ADAptive dynamic coordinator, which will be explained later. Several gateways at the intermediate level gather information from a set of nodes and deliver it to the upper level. To test the methodologies presented in this paper, a Raspberry Pi 3 with a Linux operating system was used to build the gateway [50]. Google App Engine was leveraged on top of the stack to build cloud-based infrastructure for the same purpose. Data is securely stored in the cloud, where a healthcare professional may examine or view it. The user may also transmit downstream commands to the nodes through the web interface, such as modifying the needed detail of patient parameter acquisition to indicate the required change in operating mode [51].

The detector will be the sole center of attention in this paper.

4 Node Structure for IoMT

The structure of the member nodes could be seen as a composite material, as shown in Fig. 2. Every stage is explained in detail in the accompanying areas. The computer system is at the end of the list.

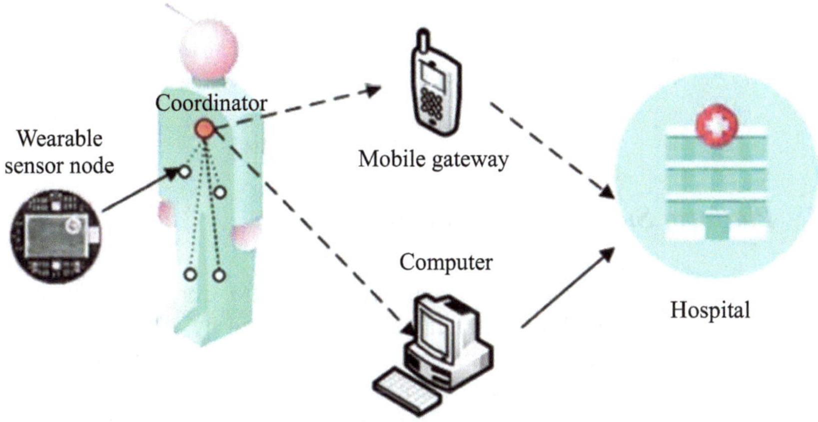

Fig. 2 Description of the IoMT involving planning

For a modified microcontroller with gadgets for information gathering, at least one processor parts for a sufficient arrangement of availability peripherals for contribution to the passage, just as sterilization and pre-preparing [52]. The A sensor level deals with the information base motor at execution, containing some working framework (OS) backing to work with the organization and booking of programming strings. This level should likewise uncover a couple of diminished neanderthals to set up the significance subtleties (e.g., interface with connectors, routineness, authority method of activity, proficiency counting, and so forth) and a bunch of estimating technology platform to control the glory of the list of capabilities reliably (e.g., electrical limit status, keeping the rest administration life, and so on) and to change the condition of the figuring stage [53]. At the top of the planning process, the software product level performs activities in an appropriate integrative framework of traditional process nodes that can be developed and changed in real time. The program receives an employee named ADAM (ADAptive deployment Manager) to respond to users' wants. ADAM monitors all events that could lead to running mode changes (workflow fluctuations, battery status, remote orders) and then reshapes the activity networking to save power and energy. Task activation, deactivation, and restructuring inter-task linkages are reconfiguration actions. As discussed earlier, we used a single-core microcomputer, especially the process SensorTile off-the-shelf system, to evaluate the practicality of our strategy based on the dynamic redesign. SensorTile was chosen to represent a market category of low-power single-core IoT nodes that commonly include several sensors and peripherals to boost usability. Mid-to-limited computation units capable of performing essential near-sensor data processing on small budget optimized collections for capacity recovery and ultralight software products are common components of such systems that allow several software processes to coexist. The primary aspects of the platforms employed in this study will be discussed in the following sections.

Table 2 Present usage of SensorTile in various operational situations

RUN (Range I) at 80 MHz	120 μA/MHz
RUN (Range 2) at 26 MHz	100 μA/MHz
LPRUN at 2 MHz	112 μA/MHz
SLEEP at 26 MHz	35 μA/MHz
LPSLEEP at 2 MHz	48 μA/MHz

4.1 Platform Surface of Hardware

The SensorTile has a width of 13.5 mm. A 32-bit ARM Cortex-M4 low-power microprocessor drives it. The gadget can also be powered by a battery due to its small size and low-energy consumption, resulting in good autonomy without sacrificing portability. To customize the technology to various situations, several architectural knobs can be used. SensorTile offers two main modes of operation: run and sleep, which utilize different subsets of the hardware. Furthermore, the chip can be tuned to a separate system periodicity in each mode. The technology uses several power supplies to power the chip and information about system frequency and operational conditions. In Table 2, we've put together a list of options that can be selected when using framework retailer's modulation APIs.

- We used two ways to dynamically reduce power consumption in our experiments: changing system frequency over time in response to workload.
- Whenever feasible, we are using the microcontroller's switch. When no computational operations are scheduled to complete, the operating system puts the computer into sleep mode. If necessary, a countdown awaken will be employed to continue marathon mode.

4.2 OS/Layer of the Load Balancer

Several backend pieces were used to handle different computing processes at a time and to achieve satisfactory accuracy for CNN-based near-sensor analytics, in addition to the manufacturer's API.

4.2.1 FreeRTOS

As a ROTS, SensorTile is powered by FreeRTOS. This software component is intended for developers who want to use an actual-time operating system without worrying about their applications' memory footprint. The software is between 4 and 9 kB in size. It has the capability of specifying processing activities using thread-level abstract. On the stage and managing their scheduling at runtime was one of the most important elements in our decision to use FreeRTOS. Actual sequencing synchronized, and data set includes real-world scheduling examples provided by the operating system. FreeRTOS creates an idle system task using the greatest completion priority feasible, the subsystem tick counter is stopped, and the Arduino is put to rest once this phase is done. The idle job will only run if no other jobs are waiting to be called because of the priority setting. The speed variation of the system isn't size by FreeRTOS. All timing functions would be entirely desynchronized once the frequency was altered. Permitting frequency control has alterations without disturbing the rest of the OS operation and used to have to alter part of both the OS support.

4.2.2 Cortex Microcontroller

We used the Cortex Microcontroller (CMSIS), a component that has been modified especially targeting Cortex-M processor cores, to do in-place processing of the detected data. It consists of multiple modules with numerous optimized dependents on the structure used in arithmetic operations. The CMSIS-NN module is particularly intriguing because it has various optimized characteristics that enable executive function computation implementations. While CMSIS offers a lot of support for artificial serotonin in the brain, we had to make changes to enable single convolution layers on one-dimensional sensor data streams for the use-case described below.

5 Approach Model

We outline the approach model that we used to construct and assess the app in this part. Tasks are represented as separate processes that communicate using delayed speak and read interaction neanderthals and FIFO structures to prevent data loss during busy pipeline phases. In the case of available processing resources, processes could be run in parallel, potentially enhancing performance utilizing a software pipeline.

In particular, we create a chain of activities that function on the edge devices to every reported parameter to be examined in Fig. 3.

For each sensor node, a series of events occur so that the functional and semi-aspects can be dynamically turned on and off, if necessary, by changes in the operating mode.

We envision four types of broad duties for each sensor:

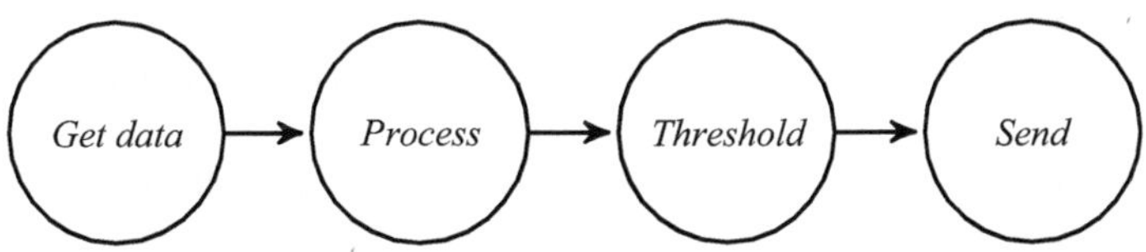

Fig. 3 Sequence of routine things

- Get data task: this job is in charge of collecting data from the node's sensing hardware.
- Process task: this sort of job might have numerous instances, each representing a different stage of an in-place data analysis method. Existing multi-tasking options allow a specific level of analysis to be selected, which affects the required connection bandwidth, data retrieval detail, and power/energy usage. Its goal is to reduce information being moved from one node to another in a minimum.
- Threshold task: you could use this activity to filter data based on in-place analysis results. A threshold job, for example, could only be used to transfer information to the server when necessary particular events or alert circumstances are recognized.
- Send task: this task is in charge of communicating with the gateway outwardly. Provocation/deactivation of tasks or complete chains related to sensors can be implemented using the process network model chosen:
- Enabling/disabling the associated task's periodic execution.
- Reshaping the process chain by redesigning the FIFOs.

These above ponits allow for selecting multiple application configurations matching operation modes with varying Throughout processing effort, network needs, and monitoring precision are all factors to consider.

6 Assistance for Flexibility: The ADAptive Environment Scheduler

A specialized task system was created throughout the procedure to administer solely the platform's rearchitecting of operating systems on the fly. We performed such a change in ADAptive Runtime Manager, a software agent (ADAM). An inbuilt timer allows ADAM to be activated regularly, and it assesses the system's health by tracking:

- Gateway reconfiguration orders.
- Workload changes, such as the rate at which events must be handled. For example, a task may need to be performed regularly, at an outlay determined by the number of particular subsets in sensor data. This creates actual time limits, which may change over time as data changes.
- Additional factors have to be taken.
- ADAM can react to such input by changing platform parameters and conducting several operations:
- Enable or disable specific sequence of detector tasks or the complete sensor task chain.
- Select whether or not to put the microcontroller into sleep mode.

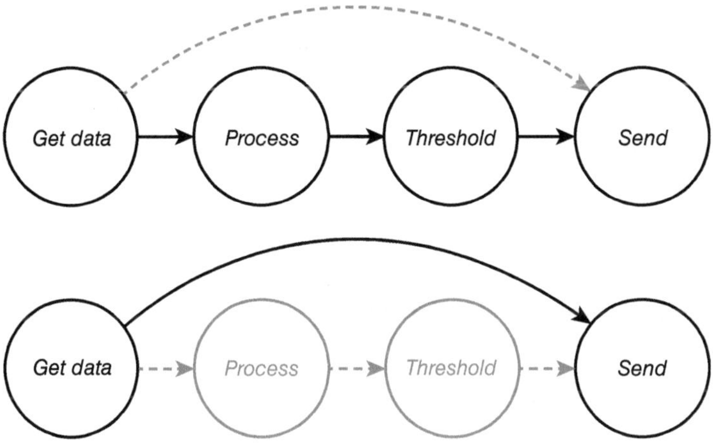

Fig. 4 A modular controller is programmed in two ways

- Change the microcontroller's operating frequency to improve or decrease performance.
- Reroute the FIFO-managed data flow following the active tasks.

An example of how ADAM could terminate a process is shown in Fig. 4. The challenge was to switch one functioning model to another, one that sends the information to the server and another that gives raw information to the server.

7 Use-Case Evaluation

A case that is already containing a node that measures a patient's ECG was used to validate our technique. We created a prototype utilizing an Analog Devices AD8232 sensor module, which was coupled to the reference platform's ADC converter. First, we tested our technique on the SensorTile, allowing the user to choose between three different operating modes by sending appropriate orders from the cloud. Figure 5 depicts the various operating modes.

7.1 Information Collected Is the First Intraoperative Phase

The first working model envisions forwarding the sensor node's whole data stream to the gateway. As a result, there will be no near-sensor statistical software, and it is possible and the bandwidth requirements are quite large.

- A variety of instances is aggregated and placed the contents of a package 20 bytes in this operating mode (8 ECG data 16 bits, 1 timestamp 32 bit).

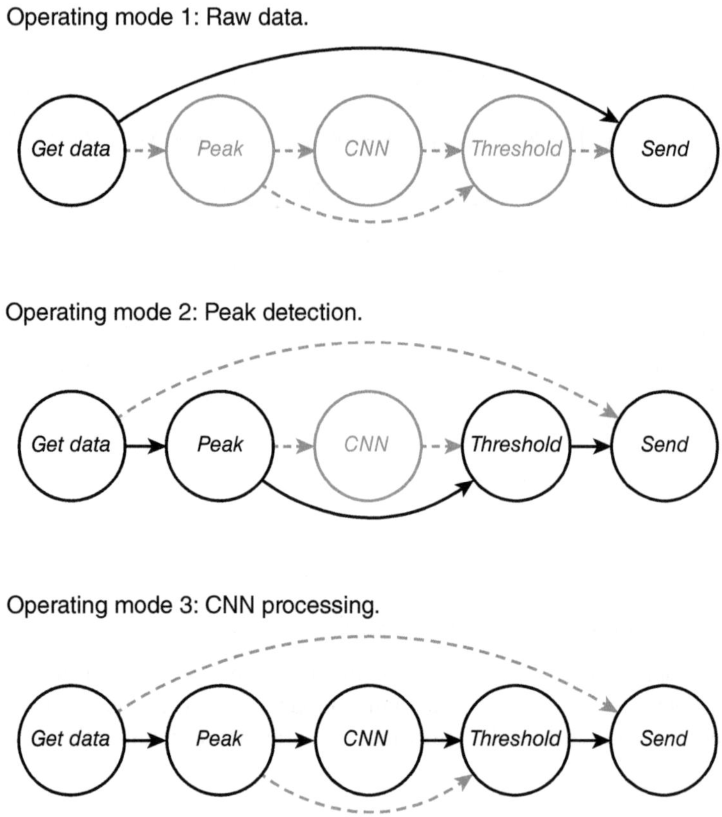

Fig. 5 Schema of EEG use

- The ADC frequency of collection is set to 330 Hz because numerous samples are sent at once and that each second, a wireless transmission is being sent at 24 ms.

7.2 Saturation Identification Is the Client Operating Mode

This module does not allow you to see the entire ECG waveform. When viewing the data, a healthcare practitioner can choose to monitor merely cardiac rate, needing a reduced degree of facts in great detail provided by the Internet. It might also set limits and only allow certain things to enter; thus, a notification will be shown when those thresholds were reached. Four tasks are active in this operating mode:

- Gather data.
- Analyze data.
- Boundary challenge.
- Assign a task.

This way of operation examines data for electrical maxima and quantifies the cardiac rate as an indicator. The first operation receives signal (as in raw data form of electrical energy), the second processes the signal and estimates the cardiac output, and the third permits system operation. If data should be transmitted to the cloud, the threshold assignment decides if it should be done. If the pulse rate is changed among two elevated/low warning settings, for illustration, no data is delivered. The gradient is utilized in the algorithm for detecting a potential in terms. In addition to increased power consumption, it isn't critical. The size of the delivered item was 5 bytes. The data rate is plotted due to the number of peaks found; under the worst assumption, a packet is sent for each maximum found.

7.3 Analysis of CNN o.m. in the Mode of Operation 3

Through the latter working style, a further degree of evaluation is introduced. This challenge uses a neural network to identify and differentiate different tissue circumstances from the ECG waveform. This categorization method permits users to keep track of the signal's shape sans requiring them to transmit the complete data stream to the cloud, conserving the drive system's energy. The deployed neural network detects strange events in the ECG trace; in this scenario, contacts with the gateway are only initiated when an abnormality is detected. The following tasks are available:

- Get information goal.
- Protocol data 1 task.
- Task 2: integrate information (CNN).
- Criterion complexity.
- Assign a goal.

Transmission is required. Canny edge detection o.m. has more accessible capacity than actual data o.m.; nevertheless, peak detection o.m. requires more processing work. A 1D deep neural network is implemented in this node, similar to that described in [15]. The artificial network has two CNN architectures, two flip levels, and a second connection layer, as illustrated in Fig. 6, and has an input size of 198. The network's outputs are divided into two categories, each of which has five NLRAV classes. In addition to NSVFQ (see Fig. 6), the data delivered to the cloud is 6 bytes in size [18–21].

8 Peak Detection

You can pick either ghastly investigation or CNN o.m. The R tops in the sign should be identified in both working modes [22]. Therefore, during information assortment from the sensor, an improved form of the Pan-Tompkins approach was utilized to decide the situation of the R tops. Figure 7 shows the interaction control block graph

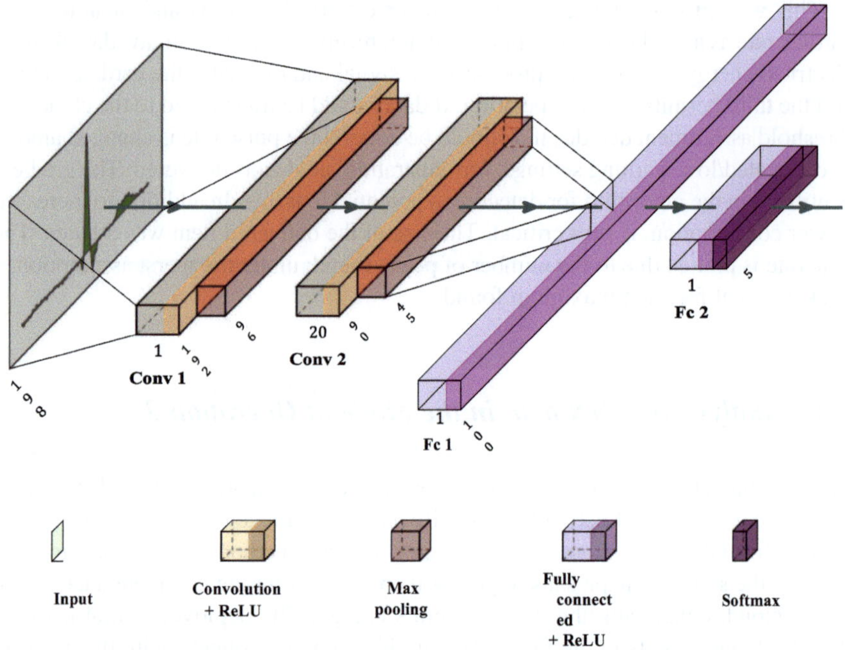

(N) Normal beats	(N) Normal beats
(L) Left bundle branch block	(S) Superventricular ectopic beats
(R) Right bundle branch block	(V) Ventricular premature contraction
(A) Atrial premature contraction	(F) Fusion beats
(V) Ventricular premature contraction	(Q) Unclassificable beat

Fig. 6 The construction of a CNN and the two kinds of identifiers that can be used

from [6], a benchmark study for fostering the R top got consent. Figure 8 shows the crude (blue) and sifted (red) signals from two unique accounts [7]. At the point when a sifted signal surpasses a predefined limit and afterward bounce back to a nearby least point while representing the said channel's postponements, a pinnacle is distinguished; the edges' esteem changes for each recording [23–26].

A maximum detected by the system is regarded as a genuine positive in this circumstance if its location is within a 20-sample interval of the real peak [27]. Equations 1 and 2 show the peaked detection method's responsiveness (positive predictive value) and accuracy using the MIT-BIH atrial database:

$$\mathrm{TPR} = \frac{\mathrm{TP}}{\mathrm{TP} + \mathrm{FN}} = 0.98883, \tag{1}$$

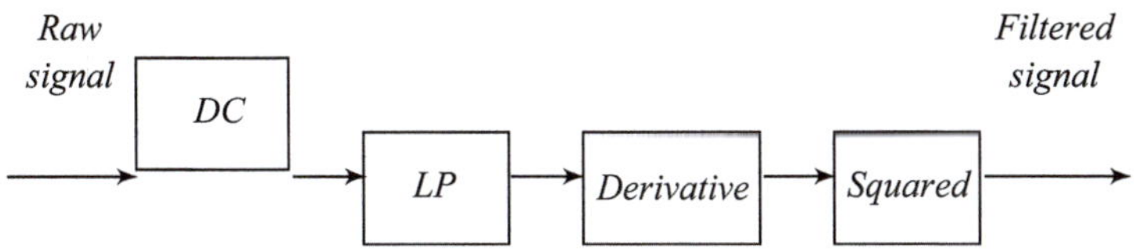

Fig. 7 Schematic representation for screening

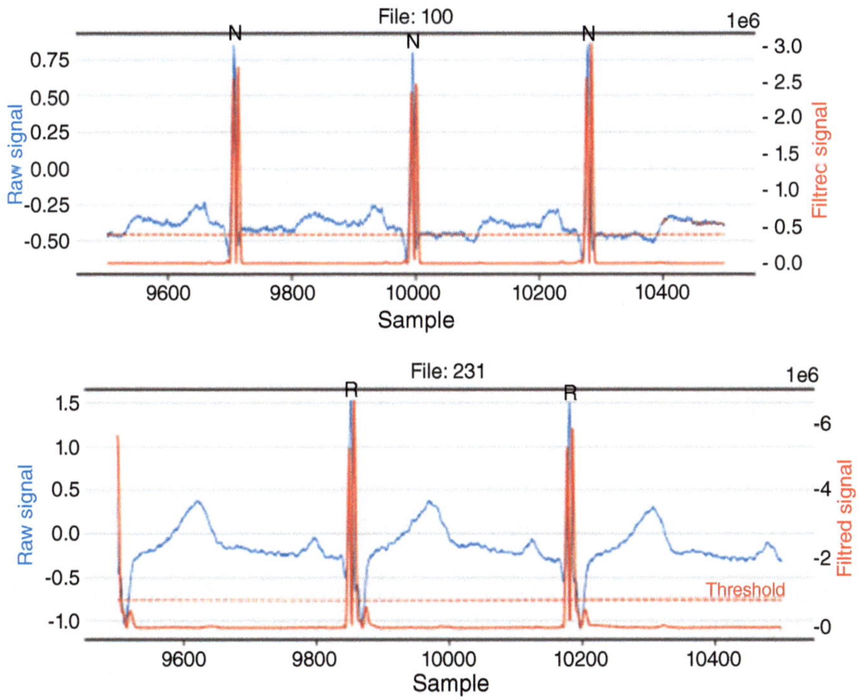

Fig. 8 Two separate signals, one uncooked and one adjusted recordings

$$\text{PPV} = \frac{\text{TP}}{\text{TP} + \text{FP}} = 0.98629. \tag{2}$$

Figure 9a shows the peak detection algorithm's true-positive, false-positive, and false-negative results with a 20-sample tolerance. The human brain was taught to detect an ECG frame with a peak within 50 samples of the center. Calculations 3 and 4 specify relevant reliability data if the proposed tolerance obtains 50 samples:

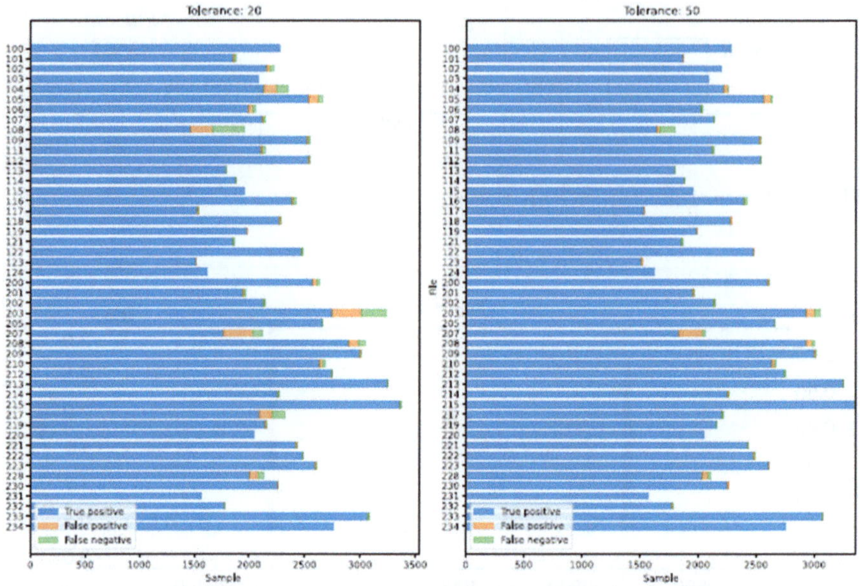

(a) 20 acceptability specimens.

(b) 50 acceptability specimens.

Fig. 9 The peak detection algorithms. There are three types of false positives: true positives, false positives, and false negatives, each with a distinct confidence interval. (**a**) Twenty acceptability specimens. (**b**) Fifty acceptability specimens

$$\text{TPR} = 0.99674, \tag{3}$$

$$\text{PPV} = 0.99421. \tag{4}$$

Figure 9b shows the canny edge detection algorithms with a 50-sample threshold; massively positive, optimistic, and false-negative outcomes are possible.

9 Activation for Neural Networks

The neural network is trained using the PyTorch framework. A static quantization step converts the loads and activations from float to int precision once training is completed1. CMSIS-NN optimized procedures that take input with an accuracy of 8 bits are simple to use in this manner [28].

9.1 *Quantization*

An inspector module is placed in numerous network locations that understand how the extracted features of each tier are distributed, and measurements on a level and at zero points are determined based on this distribution, which allows data conversion [29]. A simple transformation is not required for this technique. A MinMax observer2 is used to update the parameters, with the bias values set to zero. The CMSIS convolutional and densely integrated layered functions [30] allow you to alter the outputs by moving them on a scale of -128 to 127. On the other hand, quantization in the PyTorch application requires a scale that is not always a multiple of a power of 2 [31]. As a result, CMSIS functions have been changed to scale outputs using a scale value comparable to the PyTorch framework. This improvement lowers execution times by 2.87 percent and 10.52 percent for the 20_20_100 and 4_4_100 networks, respectively [32]. fc1_ Conv1OutputFeatures_ Conv2OutputFeatures_ Conv1OutputFeatures_ Conv2OutputFeatures_ Conv1OutputFeatures_ Conv The model identifiers are the outputs [33].

9.2 *Investigation of Archetypes*

The findings for the NLRAV and NSVFQ classes are shown in Fig. 10 to help us figure out which neural network model is best for our situation [34]. As demonstrated in Eqs. 5 and 6, the NLRAV 20 20 100 and NSVFQ 20 20 100 acquire the best detection value; they attain about 100 percent accuracy during training using 70 percent of the data as shown in the training set (Fig. 11):

$$\mathrm{TS}_{\mathrm{NLRAV\_20\_20\_100}} = \frac{\mathrm{TP}}{\mathrm{TP}+\mathrm{FP}+\mathrm{FN}} = 0.99224, \quad (5)$$

$$\mathrm{TS}_{\mathrm{NSVFQ\_20\_20\_100}} = \frac{\mathrm{TP}}{\mathrm{TP}+\mathrm{FP}+\mathrm{FN}} = 0.98885. \quad (6)$$

Models within 0.5 percent of the most accurate estimate of that school organization have been chosen for testing within each class group [35]. Figure 12 shows the concepts used only for NLRAV and NSVFQ tags; the gray line indicates the 0.5 percent limit compared to the more accurate models. The energy required for a single CNN task call is depicted in Fig. 12. The models NLRAV 4 4 100 and NSVFQ 4 4 100 were chosen that lie within the region and use less power.

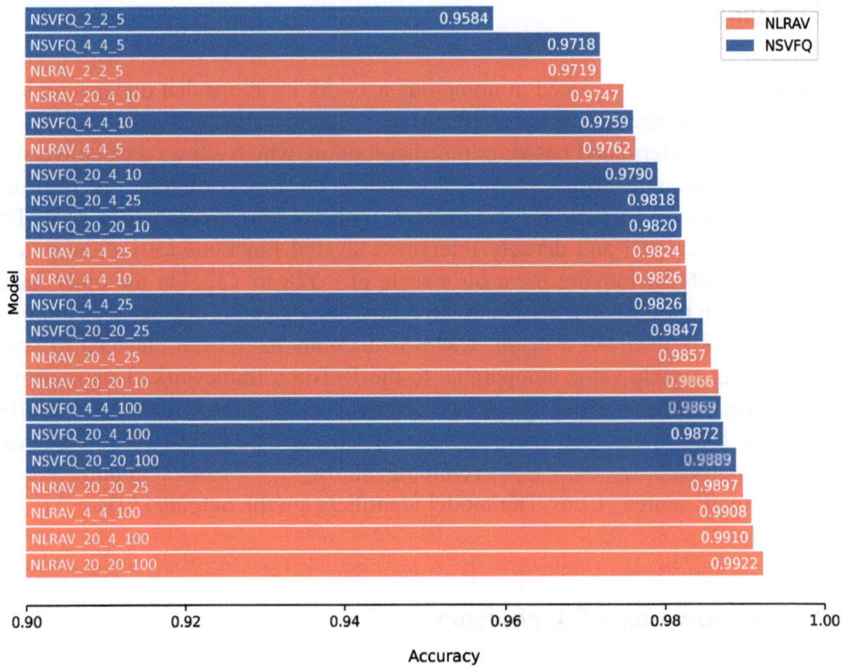

Fig. 10 Categories conv1OutputFeatures_ conv2OutputFeatures_ fc1Outputs are used to investigate the specified machine learning algorithm

9.3 *Amplification*

Clusters in the output are centered like input areas to train the system, and the position from both the peak's center and the predetermined point in the collection is set by the record label. The network detects the selected classes as long as the peak is in the signal frame's center. Peak detection algorithms doing the maximum are sometimes not detected at the same spot, resulting in errors as stated in the dataset. As a result, the selected system has undergone retraining. To train it is to recognize non-centered peaks. As a result, the network was trained with frames featuring centered peaks and frames containing decentralized peaks, as illustrated in Fig. 13. The chosen augmentation design entails using 33 pictures per centered apex in it and 3 samples apart.

The exactness of the series of checks is diminished by expansion, with 98.37 percent and 97.76 percent for classes NLRAV and NSVFQ, respectively. ECG records with deviant pinnacles that are hard to focus on utilizing the pinnacle recognizable proof strategy, then again, are distinguished undeniably more precisely. Table 3 shows the number of bogus cautions instigated by the pinnacle identification approach. The extra cases, yet obvious upsides, were arranged to utilize the neural organization picked for the NLRAV and NSVFQ classes. The crate plot related to the calculation's derivation of genuine positive pinnacles is displayed in Fig. 14.

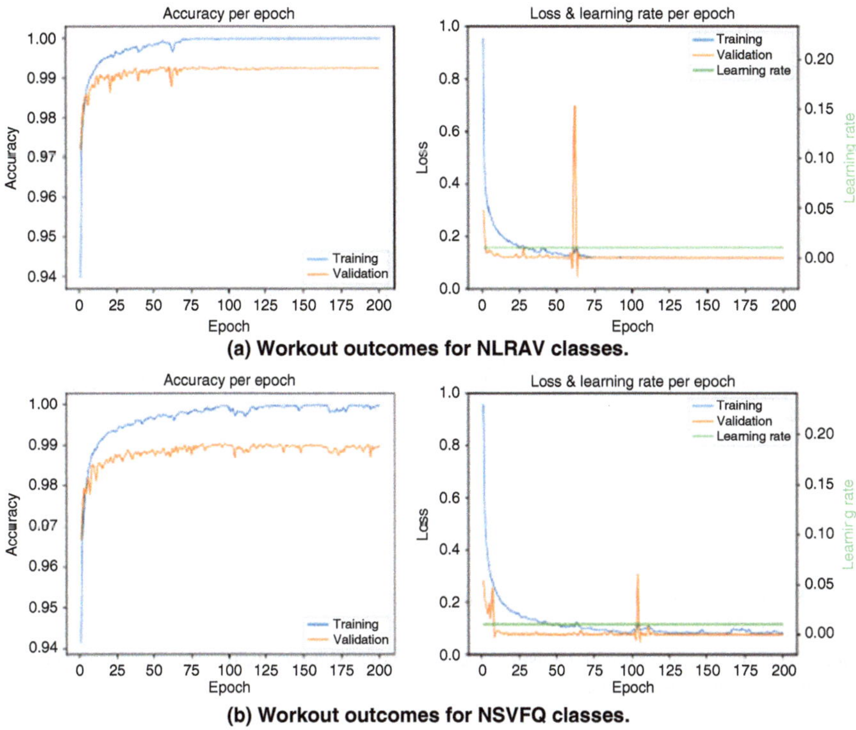

Fig. 11 The system was built with 20 extracted Conv1, 20 output values for Conv2, and 100 output elements for Fc1. (**a**) Workout outcomes for NLRAV classes. (**b**) Workout outcomes for NSVFQ classes

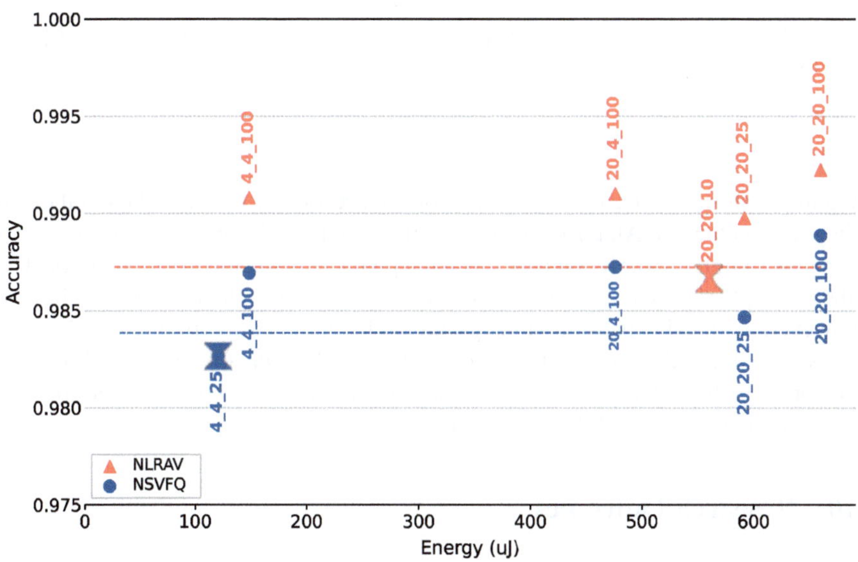

Fig. 12 After selecting the best useful prediction, the energy usage for a single CNN task call is displayed. The model-based entry requirements are represented by the dotted lines and the dashed lines for each class equal that class's highest accuracy minus 0.5 percent

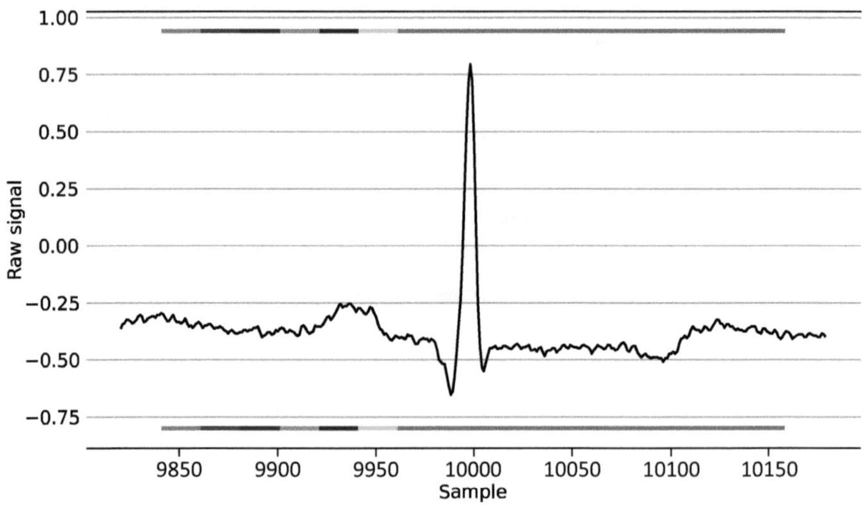

Fig. 13 An illustration of enhancement in its descriptive way

Table 3 Completely bogus and falsified cases coming from the peak detection technique and segmentation with true positives for NLRAV and NSVFQ classes

Predicted \ True	N	L	R	A	V	FP
N	22,166	13	7	65	46	635
L	49	2424	1	1	21	
R	54	0	2092	26	4	
A	132	2	13	626	7	
V	60	6	2	1	2087	
FN	356					

Predicted \ True	N	S	V	F	Q	FP
N	26,885	68	44	4	91	635
S	331	476	2	0	29	
V	117	25	1986	5	7	
F	74	0	41	127	1	
Q	23	0	1	0	2439	
FN	356					

Figure 14 shows the exactness esteems for each recording for each class in the two diagrams on the left. All through the deduction, the precision esteem with each chart depends straightforwardly on how much the pinnacle is suitably focused or not. The above graph shows how improvement prompts a little fall in middle rightness; however, a critical expansion in the group model in the most "troublesome" conditions, essentially diminishing the number of anomalies. Finally, Table 4 shows the outcomes of the inference on edge works reported in Sect. 2 in terms of artificial neural efficiency on the MIT-BIH database.

10 Research Outcomes

The critical aspects of implementing real-time analytics are estimated to take and create the optimizer architecture, select the correct software system, and resolve equipment and software challenges. However, because of a few technological

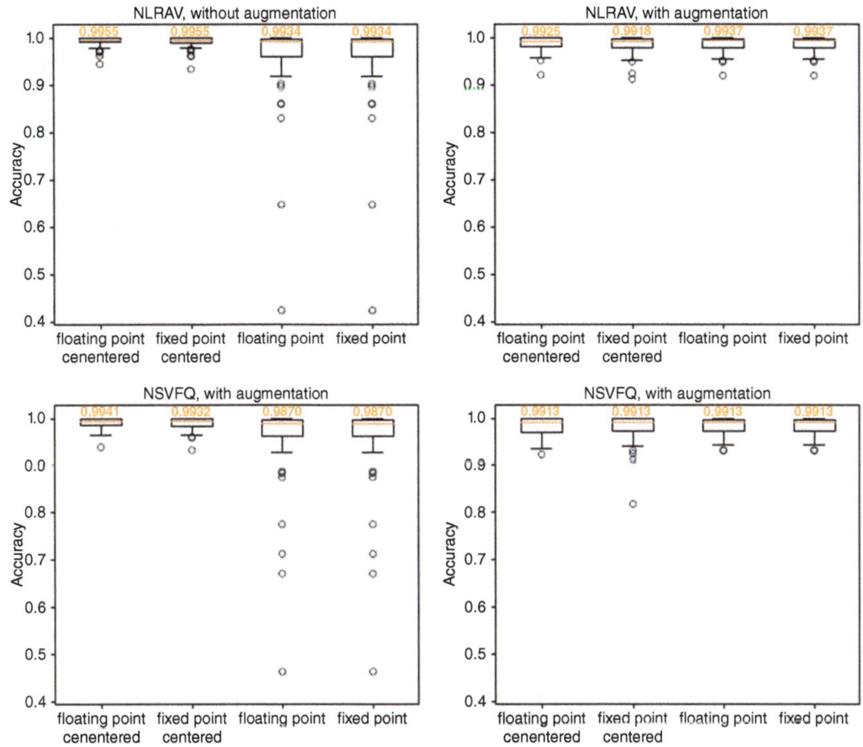

Fig. 14 The empirical dispersion of the correctness value calculated out from identification on the classification model for each ECG recorded is displayed using correct positive peaks produced with a tolerance of 50 samples. Inference using centered and non-centered peaks in the frame and fixed-point models is examined and suspended. The resulting data is shown in orange

Table 4 On the MIT-BIH sample, the efficiency of human brains was tested (see class names in Fig. 6)

Work	Responsive to correction precision			Diseases
[11]	95.98%	–	95.9%	NSVF
[17]	96%	–	–	NSVFQ
[13]	96%	–	–	[1]
Our	97.76%	90.9%	95.85%	NSVFQ
Our	98.37%	96.45%	97.06%	NLRAV

responsibilities, businesses frequently overlook the issue of what to do with their core operations. In this part, the overall system's power consumption and the energy expenditures of each activity are presented.

10.1 *Assessment of Energy Utilization*

The findings were utilized to develop a model that highlighted the impact of each task on the node's electricity usage.

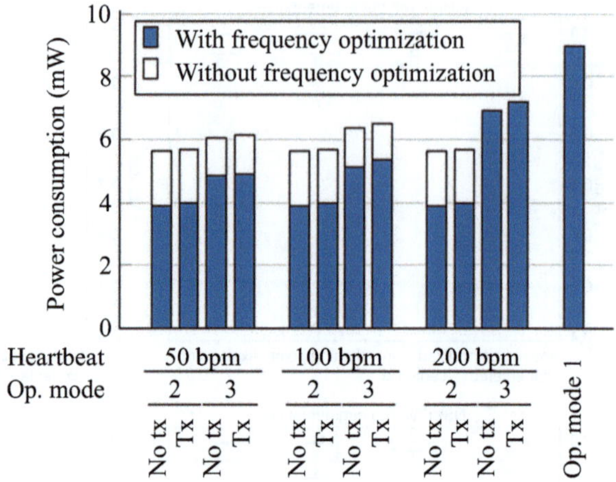

Fig. 15 This data shows the energy consumption for the various senses to add whenever the barrier task allows data transmission (Tx) or does not allow data transmission (No Tx). Raw o.m. is unaffected by pulse or criterion settings

The phrases left benefits. It can help nerve block, right bundle branch block, inhabitants' beat, premature ventricular retraction, atrial neonatal problem contraction, cardiac flutter wave, and left ventricle escape Beat to the same event.

10.2 Indicators of Electricity Consumption

We used an analyzer and shunt resistors to test the device's power usage to display the current absorption. Figure 15 shows statistics on power usage resulting from experimental findings, with particular examples being examined and addressed.

10.2.1 Instance: 50 bpm

Even without adjusting the system frequency to the task, low heart rates result in significant energy savings. Much more energy is saved by adjusting system frequency according to workload; in this case, the adaptive filtering o.m. is 2 MHz, and the CNN processing o.m. is 4 MHz. In any case, the worst scenario, raw data o.m., works at 8 MHz. As originally said, the threshold job makes the final decision. The graph also depicts what they would be or how much they would consume if data were not transmitted to the cloud (Tx, No tx).

10.2.2 Instance: 100 bpm

Basic data o.m. and compressive sensing o.m. remain at the same frequency as before, while CNN processing o.m. jumps to 8 MHz. In terms of power consumption, there is no change in raw data o.m., but there is a minor increase for the remainder modes.

10.2.3 Instance: 200 bpm

The importance of the barrier task is highlighted in this situation. The raw data o.m. and peak detection o.m. have not changed since the previous example. The variations in energy usage of the CNN processing o.m. compared to the preceding scenario are barely discernible due to the extremely high workload.

10.3 Estimation of Energy Usage Related to Power Model and Operation Mode

A series is conducted in studies in which we measured energy usage under various setup settings. The findings were utilized to develop a model highlighting each task's contribution to the node's energy usage. By approximating the observational evidence on resource usage in different use cases and knowing the start and finish dates, a model for effective estimating the app's energy consumption under every feasible scenario is constructed. Table 5 shows the energy levels for each task in the process network. Table 6 shows the product's idle energy consumed and the power consumption of the ECG sensor.

At around this level, estimating the power usage for each operation is simple; the calculations that determine the energy consumption for each mode of operation are as follows:

- *P*raw data o.m.
- *P*peak detection o.m.
- *P*cnn processing o.m.

Table 5 For every operation, an overview of utilization and performance evaluation is provided

Target type	Numeral of cycle	Implementation time (8 MHz)	Power contribution
Obtain data	841	105 μs	$E_g = 2.96$ μJ
Obtain data + peak	1550 + 841	300 μs	$E_{gp} = 3.76$ μJ
CNN 4_4_100	361,360	45 ms	$E_c = 148.781$ μJ
CNN 20_20_100	1,719,582	215 ms	$E_c = 660.37$ μJ
Threshold	910	114 μs	$E_t = 2.73$ μJ
Send data	~25,000	~3 ms	$E_s = 83.96$ μJ

Table 6 Expenditure of accessories in a nutshell

Device	Power consumption 2 MHz	4 MHz	8 MHz
Platform in idle state	2.609 mW	3.101 mW	4.546 mW
ECG sensor	237 uW	237 uW	237 uW

$$\left(E_g + aE_s\right) \cdot f_s + P_{\text{idle}} + P_{\text{sensor}}$$
$$E_{gp} \cdot f_s + (E_t + E_s) \cdot f_p + P_{\text{idle}} + P_{\text{sensor}}$$
$$\left(E_g + E_p\right) \cdot f_s + E_t \cdot f_p + (E_c + E_s) \cdot f_{hr} + P_{\text{idle}} + P_{\text{sensor}}$$

Here:

- f_s is the number of collecting.
- f_{hr} is the pace of cardiac.
- f_p is the periodicity of optimum information scrubbing.
- α^{-1} is the total number of variables in a BLE container.
- P_{idle} is the network's inactive energy usage determined by the switching frequency.
- P_{sensor} is ECG laser's power usage.

Figure 16 illustrates the device's estimated power consumption and the outputs of each task when the heart muscle is around 60 beats per minute.

11 Conclusion

Medical alert sensors are placed on humans to continually gather and communicate biomedical parameters to a nearby gateway, sending the data to a cloud-based healthcare platform. This strategy, on the other hand, frequently fails to meet the stringent criteria of healthcare systems. The battery life of portable sensor sensors is limited, and the system's reliance on the cloud makes it subject to bandwidth and latency difficulties. The compressive sensing (CS) principle has been widely used in electrocardiogram (ECG) monitoring applications to reduce the power consumption of wearable sensors. The suggested method addresses these restrictions by enabling an entry point connected health system that performs the most power-intensive operations locally on a core processor. A hardware and system foundation for establishing a controlled IoMT node that can analyze physiological data in real time is developed in this publication. The workload consisted of CNN-based computation identifying anomalies on ECG traces, and the program was validated on two low-power devices. The device may restructure itself according to the appropriate operation modes. The ADAM element, which manages the device's reconstruction, has a big impact on energy efficiency. For NLRAV and NSVFQ diseases, a quantized neural network trained on the MIT-BIH Arrhythmia dataset yields above 98 percent classification accuracy. This could save up to 50% on energy by starting in-place analysis and adjusting the vehicle's system components. This study highlights the need for data-dependent runtime architectural control while demonstrating how near-sensor processing might enhance battery life.

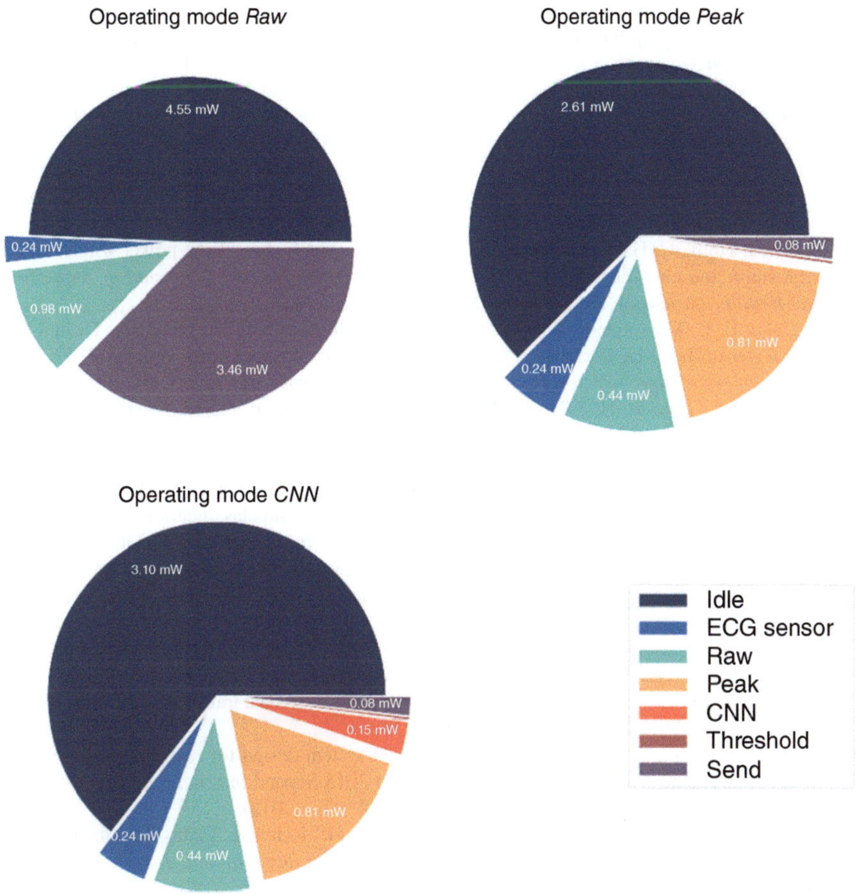

Fig. 16 At 60 beats per minute, estimate power consumption for each task in each operational state

References

1. Silvia Macis, Daniela Loi, Danilo Pani, Luigi Raffo, Serena La Manna, Vincenzo Cestone, and Davide Guerri.: Home telemonitoring of vital signs through a tv-based application for elderly patients. In 2015 IEEE International Symposium on Medical Measurements and Applications (MeMeA) *Proceedings* pages 169–174, (2015).
2. Kanitthika Kaewkannate and Soochan Kim.: The Comparison of Wearable Fitness Devices. 10 (2018).
3. Reetu Kumari and D. K. Sharma.: Generalized 'Useful non-symmetric divergence measures and Inequalities.' *Journal of Mathematical Inequalities*, 13(2), pages 451–466, (2019).
4. Ulas Baran Baloglu, Muhammed Talo, Ozal Yildirim, Ru San Tan, and U Rajendra Acharya.: Classification of myocardial infarction with multi-lead ECG signals and deep CNN. *Pattern Recognition Letters*, 122:23 – 30, (2019).

5. M. Magno, M. Pritz, P. Mayer, and L. Benini.: Deepemote: Towards multi-layer neural networks in a low power wearable multi-sensors bracelet. In 2017 7th IEEE *International Workshop on Advances in Sensors and Interfaces*, pages 32–37, June (2017).
6. Matteo Antonio Scrugli, Daniela Loi, Luigi Raffo, and Paolo Meloni.: A runtime-adaptive cognitive IoT node for healthcare monitoring. *CF '19: Proceedings of the 16th ACM International Conference on Computing Frontiers*. Pages 350–357, 04, (2019).
7. A. Amirshahi and M. Hashemi.: ECG classification algorithm based on stdp and r-stdp neural networks for real-time monitoring on ultra-low-power personal wearable devices. *IEEE Transactions on Biomedical Circuits and Systems*, 13(6):1483–1493, (2019).
8. S. Lee, J. Hong, C. Hsieh, M. Liang, S. Chang Chien, and K. Lin.: Low-power wireless ECG acquisition and classification system for body sensor networks. *IEEE Journal of Biomedical and Health Informatics*, 19(1):236– 246, (2015).
9. T. Chen, E. B. Mazomenos, K. Maharatna, S. Dasmahapatra, and M. Niranjan.: Design of a low-power on-body ECG classifier for remote cardiovascular monitoring systems. *IEEE Journal on Emerging and Selected Topics in Circuits and Systems*, 3(1):75–85, (2013).
10. N. Bayasi, T. Tekeste, H. Saleh, B. Mohammad, A. Khandoker, and M. Ismail.: Low-power ECG-based processor for predicting ventricular arrhythmia. *IEEE Transactions on Very Large Scale Integration (VLSI) Systems*, 24(5):1962–1974, (2016).
11. Shuenn-Yuh Lee, Jia-Hua Hong, Cheng-Han Hsieh, Ming-Chun Liang, Shih-Yu Chang Chien, and Kuang-Hao Lin.: Low-power wireless ECG acquisition and classification system for body sensor networks. *IEEE Journal of Biomedical and Health Informatics*, 19(1):236–246, (2014).
12. U. Satija, B. Ramkumar, and M. Sabarimalai Manikandan.: Real-time signal quality-aware ECG telemetry system for IoT-based health care monitoring. *IEEE Internet of Things Journal*, 4(3):815–823, (2017).
13. E. Spanò, S. Di Pascoli, and G. Iannaccone.: Low-power wearable ECG monitoring system for multiple-patient remote monitoring. *IEEE Sensors Journal*, 16(13):5452–5462, (2016).
14. G. Xu.: IoT-assisted ECG monitoring framework with secure data transmission for health care applications. *IEEE Access*, 8:74586–74594, (2020).
15. G. R. Deshmukh and U. M. Chaskar.: IoT enabled system design for real-time monitoring of ECG signals using tiva c-series microcontroller. In 2018 Second *International Conference on Intelligent Computing and Control Systems* page 976–979, (2018).
16. Aakanksha Singhal, D.K. Sharma.: Generalized 'Useful' Rényi & Tsallis Information Measures, Some Discussions with Application to Rainfall Data. *International Journal of Grid and Distributed Computing*, 13(2), pages 681–688, (2020).
17. G. Sannino and G. De Pietro.: A deep learning approach for ECG-based heartbeat classification for arrhythmia detection. *Future Generation Computer Systems*, 86:446–455, (2018).
18. Serkan Kiranyaz, Turker Ince, and Moncef Gabbouj.: Real-time patient-specific ECG classification by 1-d convolutional neural networks. *IEEE Transactions on Biomedical Engineering*, 63(3):664–675, (2016).
19. N.T. El-dabel; A.Refaie Ali; A. El-shekhipy, A.; and A. Shalaby, G.: "Non-Linear Heat and Mass Transfer of Second Grade Fluid Flow with Hall Currents and Thermophoresis Effects," *Applied Mathematics & Information Sciences*: Vol. 11: Iss. 1, Article 73 (2017).
20. G. S and S. R. Raja.T.: "A Comprehensive Survey on Alternating Fluids Used For The Enhancement of Power Transformers," 2021 IEEE International Conference on the Properties and Applications of Dielectric Materials, pp. 57–60 (2021).
21. F. J. John Joseph, R. T, and J. J. C.: "Classification of correlated subspaces using HoVer representation of Census Data," in 2011 International Conference on Emerging Trends in Electrical and Computer Technology, Mar. 2011, pp. 906–911 (2011).
22. S. Bhoumik, S. Chatterjee, A. Sarkar, A. Kumar, and F. J. John Joseph.: "Covid 19 Prediction from X-Ray Images Using Fully Connected Convolutional Neural Network," in CSBio '20: Proceedings of the Eleventh International Conference on Computational Systems-Biology and Bioinformatics, pp. 106–107 (2020).

23. F. J. J. Joseph.: "Effect of supervised learning methodologies in offline handwritten Thai character recognition," *International Journal of Information Technology*, vol. 12, no. 1, pp. 57–64, Mar. (2020).
24. S. Sudhakar and S. Chenthur Pandian.: "Authorized Node Detection and Accuracy in Position-Based Information for MANET", *European Journal of Scientific Research*, Vol. 70, No. 2, pp. 253–265 (2012).
25. K. Ganesh Kumar and S. Sudhakar.: Improved Network Traffic by Attacking Denial of Service to Protect Resource Using Z-Test Based 4-Tier Geomark Traceback (Z4TGT), *Wireless Personal Communications*, Vol. 114, No. 4, pp. 3541–3575, (2020).
26. M. Govindaraj, R. Rathinam, C. Sukumar, M. Uthayasankar and S. Pattabhi.: Electrochemical oxidation of bisphenol-A from aqueous solution using graphite electrodes, "*Environmental Technology*", 34: 4, 503–511 (2013).
27. R. Rathinam, M. Govindaraj, K. Vijayakumar and S. Pattabhi.: Removal of Colour from Aqueous Rhodamine B Dye Solution by Photo electrocoagulation Treatment Techniques, *Journal of Engineering, Scientific Research and Application*, 1: 2, 80–89 (2015).
28. K. Jayanthi, R. Rathinam and S. Pattabhi.: Electrocoagulation treatment for removal of Reactive Blue 19 from aqueous solution using Iron electrode, "*Research Journal of Life Sciences, Bioinformatics, Pharmaceutical and Chemical Sciences*", 4: 2, 101–113 (2018).
29. M. Nomani & R Parveen.: COVID-19 pandemic and disaster preparedness in the context of public health laws and policies. *Bangladesh Journal of Medical Science*, Volume 20, issue 5, pages 41–48 (2021).
30. B. Prabhu Kavin, S. Ganapathy, P. Suthanthiramani, and A. Kannan, "*A modified digital signature algorithm to improve the biomedical image integrity in cloud environment*," in Advances in Computational Techniques for Biomedical Image Analysis, Elsevier, pp. 253–271 (2020)
31. B. Panjwani, V. Singh, A. Rani, and V. Mohan.: Optimum multi-drug regime for compartment model of tumour: cell-cycle-specific dynamics in the presence of resistance, *Journal of Pharmacokinetics and Pharmacodynamics*, vol. 48, no. 4, pp. 543–562, (2021).
32. V. Mohan, H. Chhabra, A. Rani, and V. Singh.: Robust self-tuning fractional order PID controller dedicated to non-linear dynamic system, *Journal of Intelligent & Fuzzy Systems*, vol. 34, no. 3, pp. 1467–1478, (2018).
33. G. A. Ogunmola, B. Singh, D. K. Sharma, R. Regin, S. S. Rajest and N. Singh.: "Involvement of Distance Measure in Assessing and Resolving Efficiency Environmental Obstacles," 2021 International Conference on Computational Intelligence and Knowledge Economy, pp. 13–18, (2021).
34. H. Chhabra, V. Mohan, A. Rani, and V. Singh.: Multi-objective PSO tuned fractional order PID control of robotic manipulator, in The international symposium on intelligent systems technologies and applications, pp. 567–572: Springer (2016).
35. A. Rawat, S. Jha, B. Kumar, and V. Mohan.: Nonlinear fractional order PID controller for tracking maximum power in photo-voltaic system, *Journal of Intelligent & Fuzzy Systems*, vol. 38, no. 5, pp. 6703–6713, (2020).
36. J. Kubiczek and B. Hadasik.: Challenges in Reporting the COVID-19 Spread and its Presentation to the Society, *J. Data and Information Quality*, vol. 13, no. 4, pp. 1–7, (2021).
37. Reetu Kumari and D. K. Sharma.: "Generalized 'Useful' AG and 'Useful' JS-Divergence Measures and their Bounds", *International Journal of Engineering, Science and Mathematics*, Vol. 7 (1), pp. 441–450, (2018).
38. D.S. Hooda, Reetu Kumari and D. K. Sharma.: Intuitionistic Fuzzy Soft Set Theory and Its Application in Medical Diagnosis, International Journal of Statistics in Medical Research, Vol. 7, pp. 70–76, (2018).
39. D.K. Sharma and Sonali Saxena.: Generalized Coding Theorem with Different Source Coding Schemes, *International Journal on Recent and Innovation Trends in Computing and Communication*, Vol. 5(6), pp. 253 – 257, (2017).

40. H. Pallathadka, M. Mustafa, D. T. Sanchez, G. Sekhar Sajja, S. Gour, and M. Naved.: Impact of machine learning on management, healthcare and agriculture, *Materials Today: Proceedings*, (2021).
41. Guna Sekhar Sajja, Malik Mustafa, R. Ponnusamy, Shokhjakhon Abdufattokhov, Murugesan G., P. Prabhu.: Machine Learning Algorithms in Intrusion Detection and Classification, *Annals of RSCB*, vol. 25, no. 6, pp. 12211–12219, (2021).
42. D. S. Q. Al-Yasiri and A. J. Obaid.: A New Approach for Object Detection, Recognition and Retrieving in Painting Images, *Journal of Advance Research in Dynamic and Control System*, vol. 10, no. 2, pp. 2345–2359, (2018).
43. Surinder Singh and Hardeep Singh Saini.: Detection Techniques for Selective Forwarding Attack in Wireless Sensor Networks, *International Journal of Recent Technology and Engineering*, Vol. 7, Issue-6S, 380–383 (2019).
44. Sharma, S. K., Jain, A., Gupta, K., Prasad, D., & Singh, V.: An internal schematic view and simulation of major diagonal mesh network-on-chip. *Journal of Computational and Theoretical Nanoscience*, 16(10), 4412–4417 (2019).
45. D. K. Sharma, B. Singh, E. Herman, R. Regine, S. S. Rajest and V. P. Mishra.: Maximum Information Measure Policies in Reinforcement Learning with Deep Energy-Based Model, 2021 International Conference on Computational Intelligence and Knowledge Economy, pp. 19–24 (2021).
46. Ghai, D., Gianey, H. K., Jain, A., & Uppal, R. S.: Quantum and dual-tree complex wavelet transform-based image watermarking. *International Journal of Modern Physics* B, 34(04), 2050009 (2020).
47. T. A. Al-asadi and A. J. Obaid.: Object detection and recognition by using enhanced speeded up robust feature, *International Journal of Computer Science and Network Security*, vol. 16, no. 4, pp. 66–71, (2016).
48. Jain, A., & Kumar, A.: Desmogging of still smoggy images using a novel channel prior. *Journal of Ambient Intelligence and Humanized Computing*, 12(1), 1161–1177 (2021).
49. Kumar, S., Jain, A., Shukla, A. P., Singh, S., Raja, R., Rani, S., . . . & Masud, M. A Comparative Analysis of Machine Learning Algorithms for Detection of Organic and Nonorganic Cotton Diseases. *Mathematical Problems in Engineering*, (2021).
50. Misra, N. R., Kumar, S., & Jain, A.: A Review on E-waste: Fostering the Need for Green Electronics. In 2021 International Conference on Computing, Communication, and Intelligent Systems (ICCCIS) (pp. 1032–1036). IEEE (2021).
51. D. S. Gupta and G. P. Biswas.: A novel and efficient lattice-based authenticated key exchange protocol in C-K model, *International Journal of Communication Systems*, vol. 31, no. 3, Art. no. e3473 (2018).
52. T. A. Al-asadi, A. J. Obaid, R. Hidayat and A. A. Ramli.: "A survey on web mining techniques and applications," *International Journal on Advanced Science Engineering and Information Technology*, vol. 7, no. 4, pp. 1178–1184, (2017).
53. D. K. Sharma, B. Singh, M. Raja, R. Regin and S. S. Rajest.: An Efficient Python Approach for Simulation of Poisson Distribution, 2021, 7th International Conference on Advanced Computing and Communication Systems, 2021, pp. 2011–2014.

ConvNet-Based Deep Brain Stimulation for Attack Patterns

Angel Sajani Joseph, Arokia Jesu Prabhu Lazar, Dilip Kumar Sharma, Anto Bennet Maria, Nivedhitha Ganesan, and Sudhakar Sengan

1 Introduction

Deep brain stimulation (DBS) is a neurosurgical procedure that allows reducing the symptoms of tremor, sluggishness of movement, soreness, and issues of advancement opportunities by motion disorders. DBS could be a standard therapy for Parkinson's disease, dystonia, and essential tremor that are not controlled well with medications [1]. Successful DBS enables individuals to manage their symptoms, decrease consumption of prescription drugs, and improve their standard of

A. S. Joseph (✉)
Department of Computer Science and Engineering, Anna University, Chennai, Tamil Nadu, India

A. J. P. Lazar
Department of Computer Science and Engineering, CMR Institute of Technology, Hyderabad, India

D. K. Sharma
Department of Mathematics, Jaypee University of Engineering and Technology, Guna, Madhya Pradesh, India

A. B. Maria
Department of Electronics and Communication Engineering, Vel Tech Rangarajan Dr Sagunthala R & D Institute of Science and Technology, Chennai, Tamil Nadu, India
e-mail: drmantobenet@veltech.edu.in

N. Ganesan
Department of Information Technology, Muthayammal Engineering College, Rasipuram, Tamil Nadu, India
e-mail: nivedhitha.g.it@mec.edu.in

S. Sengan
Department of Computer Science and Engineering, PSN College of Engineering and Technology, Tirunelveli, Tamil Nadu, India

P. Agarwal et al. (eds.), *Artificial Intelligence for Smart Healthcare*, EAI/Springer Innovations in Communication and Computing,
https://doi.org/10.1007/978-3-031-23602-0_16

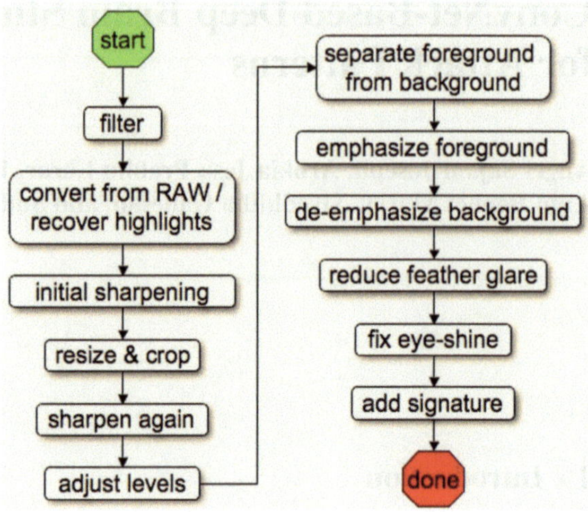

Fig. 1 Clinical workflow of DBS

living. In DBS, a pacemaker-like device is transplanted in the nervous system to transmit electrical pulses to the brain areas responsible for corporal movement. Conditional on the preserved indications, electrodes are positioned in a particular brain area. The sensors are placed in a battery-operated enhancer under the chest, in which an extension wire is insulated and passed under the skin of the head, neck, and shoulder. The patient is prepared to use a handheld regulator to activate and disable the DBS. The surgeon takes a Zigbee device to configure the stimulator settings. Once activated, it sends electric pulses to block faulty nerve signals that cause tremors, soreness, and other health conditions [2]. The activation configuration can be adapted as the condition adjustment for a healthcare provider [3].

In contrast to other operations, DBS does not harm the brain tissue. It is a reversible procedure, ensuring that the method could be altered if better medical conditions are established in the future. DBS can help in classifying many of the side effects of the mentioned motion illnesses (Fig. 1) [4]:

- *Parkinson's Disease:* Shock, inflexibility, and leisureliness of measure triggered by the death of neurotransmitter-producing nerve cells answerable for communicating messages that rheostat body measure [5].
- *Essential Tremor:* Unavoidable rhythmic shocks of hands and arms currently happening in a 'no-no' mobility throughout rest and severe movement and head tremors.
- *Dystonia:* Unintentional actions and continuous blood clotting leading to spinning/wriggling motions of the digestive system, tremor, and abnormal posture can necessitate an entire body or just alienate the area. Deep brain stimulation is used to treat diverse diseases and disorders related to the brain. It involves implanting electrodes within specific areas of the brain that generate electrical pulses and regulate irregular pulses. A pacemaker-like device that is implanted under the skin in the upper chest controls the quantity of activation. Deep brain

stimulation can treat various conditions such as dystonia, epilepsy, Parkinson's disease, and seizures [6].

1.1 Planning and Positioning of DBS

DBS is a surgical procedure performed by implanting a device that sends electrical signals directly to areas of the brain. Electrodes are implanted in the human brain and linked to a neurostimulation smartphone. Like a heart pacemaker, a spinal cord stimulator helps control activities in the brain with electrical impulses [7]. DBS is now mainly practised under general anaesthesia. The omission is a unique occurrence in which an unresolvable measure of illness prevents sustainable positioning, which could be used for general anaesthesia. STN, GPi, and Vim of the thalamus are the most frequent victims. STN and GPi are being used for Alzheimer's disease, including three main aspects. GPi is preferred to STN if the patient's feeling is questioned due to the noticeable prospective significant depression effect of STN stimulation. GPi motivation is presently used for dystonia surgery. Vim stimulus is used to treat Parkinson's disease tremors and considerable muscle spasms in a diagnosable way [8]. A few other forms of digital atlas for strategy development are used worldwide. It is pointless to memorise each aim of the goal's anterior commissure, posterior commissure, and stereotactic responsive neurochirurgical mid-coordinates. The brand Schalten and the atlas Bailey could retrieve coordinates when necessary. All dimensions vary with body frame, age, degree of brain atrophy, and the anatomical brain's potential asymmetry. Suppose a detailed prediction of the edge user's scientific code is deemed the traditional system for measurement. Treatment is performed in two steps:

- The position of one or more DBS sensors, and the second is to place a DBS generator and integrate it into the sensors.
- THE placement on one side of one DBS electrode is bilateral, attempting to place the electrode; on the other edge, the same processes are performed.

1.1.1 The Objective of Machine Learning (ML) Model

- Similarly, classic statistics measure how much a set of explanatory variables is correlated to a target variable. In this case, the interest of ML is its ability to take advantage of large databases and its higher ability to model nonlinear relations between variables compared to classic statistics. The ability of the ML model to predict unknown samples successfully by comparing its predictions to the ground truths represents the degree of correlation between inputs and outputs.
- The most common purpose is towards using the model prospectively. The model will not be restricted to a retrospective analysis of a database but instead execute

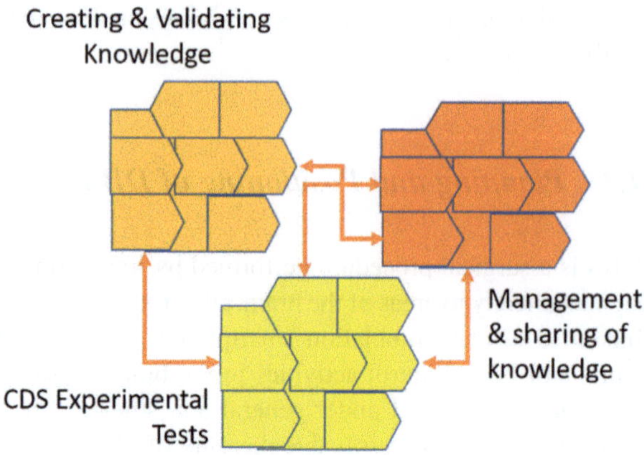

Fig. 2 Analysis of knowledge-based CDSS vs non-knowledge-based CDSS

the prediction task prospectively, providing that the test performance of the model is satisfying enough, allowing for the automation of the process.

Each step of DBS presents many challenges to both the domain brain and ML due to the procedure's powerfully complex and multi-modal nature. The success of this methodology demands a high level of knowledge and experience and technical requirements. Clinical decision support systems (CDSSs) have been required to empower neurosurgery healthcare professionals since the 1980s. Knowledge-based and non-knowledge-based CDSSs are the two different types of CDSSs most frequently selected. All the machine's intelligence comes from the human in a knowledge-based CDSS. The CDSS's primary intention is to extract data, analyse training, and show the output with a graphical interface. According to medical training, evaluation criteria are directly regulated; however, the CDSS's primary intention is to extract data, evaluate practice, and display the result with a user interface (UI). In non-knowledge-based CDSSs, machine learning (ML) takes advantage of experienced professional expert treatment to address the new issues and achieve higher levels of success. Figure 2 shows the comparison of the two approaches. In knowledge-based CDSSs, we can see that the CDSS's intelligence is encoded as a set of rules explicitly created by the clinician experts, thanks to their interaction with the domain knowledge. The intelligence in non-knowledge-based CDSSs is developed artificially by ML from a dataset using ML advanced tools by data analysts, without the need for artificial expertise and knowledge.

2 Literature Survey

DBS is among the most effective tactics of anaerobic glycolysis treatment. Researchers have formed a simulator to create different electrical impulses to enhance DBS's effect. Non-periodic and frequent signals can be obtained and set to four channels in both. Studies were performed to confirm whether the rat's nervous system characterised the device's stimulation system. Electrical impulses were stated to be well transmissible and impacted the actions of neurons. By modifying electrical signals following the illnesses and signs of patients, DBS should stimulate correct brain areas. Therefore, the opportunity to define the acceptable variable and parameters for a stimulator is essential [9]. People with diabetes use injectable medical equipment and insulin pump psychiatric treatment to control blood glucose levels. For this purpose, this work using the on-chip neural network systems for diabetes treatment. This paper has developed an artificial neural multilayer perceptron (MLP) model to clean medical devices connected to the network. This method produces 98.1% accuracy in fake vs actual glucose measurements. The prediction methodology was moderately assessed with a 90.17% linear support vector machine (SVM) [10]. ChMS is a comparatively recent brain stimulation method that offers both the benefits of VMS and CMS. A compact crossover load-mode stimulator is described in this article, where a new technique is built for load balancing injected into the tissue [11].

Brain jacking is defined as the unauthorised control of the computerised brain implant of the other. In innovative and actual environments, hacking a BCI has already been demonstrated. There's a real reason to assume that the software configurations of IPGs that play an essential role in DBS processes will be fast affected [12]. The potential outcome of brandjacking DBS tends to raise notably deep concerns about personal liberty. The opportunity of equitation such phones raises third parties' possibility of influencing the neural circuits underlying the subject's reasoning, expressive, and motivational conditions. Nevertheless, researchers recommend that the implications of brain jacking for personal liberty are complex and challenging since technologies focused on brain jacks often continue improving certain aspects of consumer independence. In the neuro-ethical and philosophical literature, the problems of identifying brain consequences for patient autonomous individuals are amplified by the varied awareness of autonomy. Wireless Body Area (WBAN) is a communication device of sensors [13]. WBANs' primary concern is the sustainability of client security and privacy. This article presents a new ESDS based on ECG, which protects the rights of IMD data from harmful treatments and other attack methods. The scheme establishes a secure communication link in which a discrete ECG bit string is encrypted for the secret. An IMD programmer can only verify this hidden message to evaluate the ECG signals sequentially with the IMD in real time. Because no keys are pre-deployed, physicians can access the IMD without specific approval [14].

2.1 Findings of Machine Learning in DBS

For a long time, there has been a great deal of interest in using machine learning, artificial intelligence, and deep learning to concern humans in healthcare. Several recommendations have been made on the area of study. To aid in decision-making in neurosurgery, researchers have conducted a review and meta-analysis of ML.

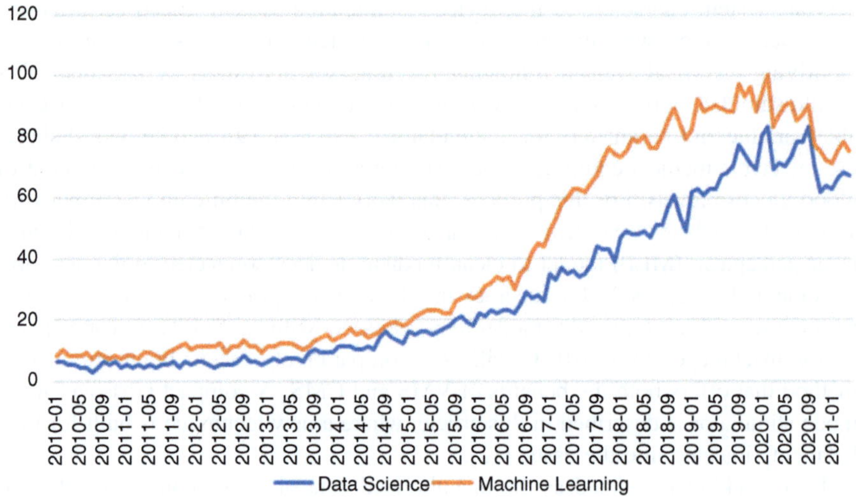

Fig. 3 Google trends of the term 'artificial intelligence' worldwide [16]

Senders also conducted a literature review of ML in neurosurgery and recommended comparing ML results to domain analysts in neurosurgery diagnosis, surgery decision-making, and outcome prediction activities. These testimonials discussed some unique ML applications, but none addressed DBS. Because there are so many techniques, data modalities, and essential functions to use ML in DBS, it's a wide-ranging subject of investigation. We performed a comprehensive review emphasis on ML in DBS (Fig. 3) [15] in the hopes of creating a synthetic landscape of this field of research, capturing recent developments, recognising significant recurrent shortcomings, and thus improving tracking performance described in this study.

3 Proposed Work

3.1 Objectives of Machine Learning

In 1959, the phrase 'machine learning' was formulated for perhaps the first time. It's a type of artificial intelligence (AI) that enables an automated system to understand better to perform the task using a database of views rather than the user's human input. Supervised classification correctly predicted an optimal solution from a combination of functionalities in its most primitive form. The algorithm is implemented with a set of inputs and outputs that are recognised to be in sets (Fig. 4). If the treatment goes well, the qualified and experienced model should estimate the unidentified result of a test sample given the input inputs [17].

The designed practice is DBS, a Wi-Fi health device injectable that treats psychological disorders by stimulating the patient's central nervous system

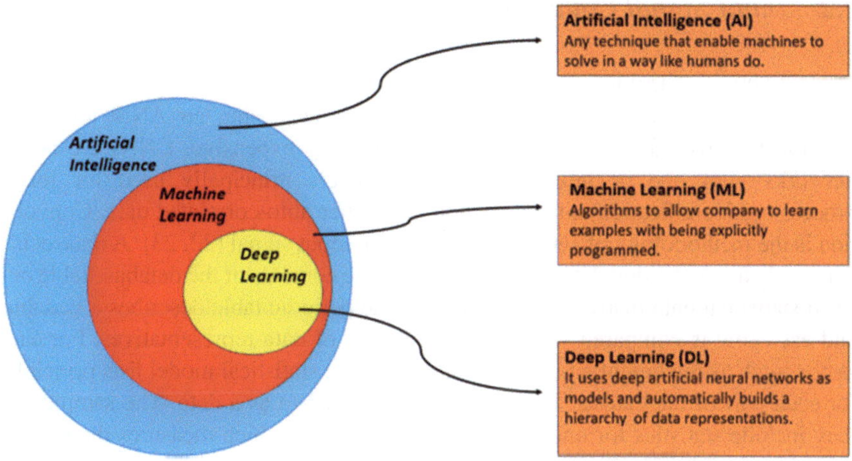

Fig. 4 The flow of artificial intelligence with ML and DL

(Fig. 6). The DBS has progressively benefited patients but has safety awareness implications in parallel. The security of these devices is paramount because they can directly influence patients' physical and mental orientation. This project uses LSTM, a CNN, to predict DBS's pattern. The frequency of neurological disorders is analysed in rest tremor velocity (RTV). Researchers studied RTV values in developing and motivating CNN [18]. A few attack behaviours have been introduced to emulate and classify various attack strategies in the DBS system. The results demonstrate that the method can identify numerous vulnerabilities with slighter impairment principles and minimal exercise time in the DBS. In short, the planned basis will be enforced with precise RTV measurement techniques in a natural deep brain stimulating environment. To evaluate the model's effectiveness concerning correctness and consistency, accurate and incorrect measurements are classified and expected on time [19]. The first phase distributes the information in which all new control signal varieties have been accumulated [20]. The second step is to separate the classes with the LSTM, a classifier method in the CNN. The third phase is RTV, the tremor's speed when the individual rests. Authors have to set RTV for legitimate and false messages at this point. The next step sets received frequency variables such as activity in the brain rate, pulse width, mode, electron beam selection, code, etc. The next step is to prepare CNN through the AlexNet training device. Databases are created after the CNN training [21]. The first step is to analyse a specific person's digital signals; the next stage is training and testing, where the frequency distribution will consider removing radio interference and signals. The third stage is to set the surviving tremor velocity of the person. The next step is to forecast an attack with the trained datasets.

3.2 Input Signal Collection

The extraction of features from an image is used to look for patterns in a dataset. Because the trainable parameters become enormous, using an ANN for image classification would be highly computationally very expensive. CNNs are neural networks with one or more convolutional layers principally used for image processing, identification, edge detection, and other auto-correlated data. Convolution is the methodology of sliding a filter over an input signal [22, 23]. A dataset is a data analysis. A training dataset coincides with the contents of the database table or a fixed statistical data matrix. Each column of the periodic table describes a variable, and each row is compared with the reference set of data representatives. For each factor, such as the height and mass of an object, the statistical model lists principles for each part of the dataset. Each concept is referred to as a date. The sample size may include statistics for one or more representatives, which measures the proportion of rows [24–31].

3.3 Class Separation

The class identification was carried out by the CNN classification model LSTM (Fig. 5). The author designed and trained an LSTM classification for all patients to identify successive brain stimulation patterns [32–39]. And we emulate and predict various kinds of attack patterns for individual patients in deep brain implants, which enables us to determine what type of offensive attack the attacker can use. More specifically, a classification tool is proposed through different combinations of attacks that the intruder can use to change cognitive-behavioural variables for deeper biometric sensors [40–44].

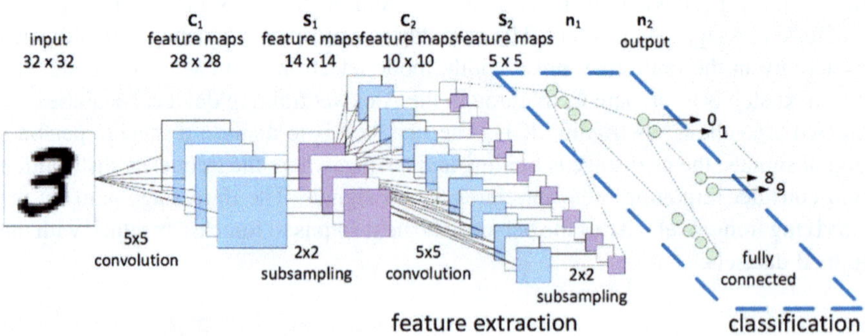

Fig. 5 CNN classification of LSTM

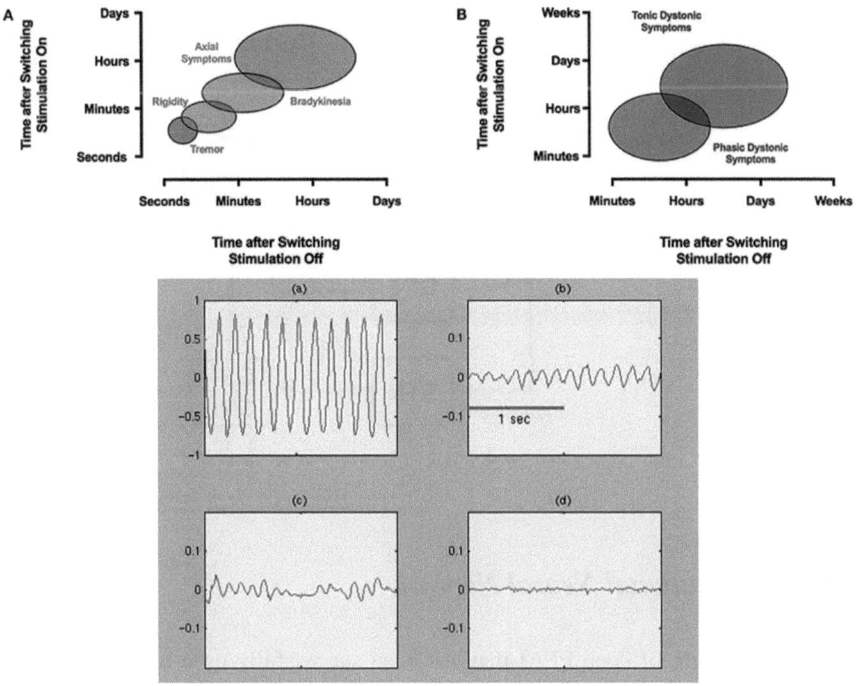

Fig. 6 Rest tremor velocity

3.4 *Rest Tremor Velocity*

The datasets in this computer system are in the index finger with MRTV. RTV is the crucial element to assess the frequency of Parkinson's tremors. It is described as the tremor that ensues if the muscle fibres do not move voluntarily. The very first sign of the nervous illness is deemed [45–49]. The valuation of RTV is insignificant/close to '0' for uncommon patients and people with controlled Alzheimer's disease. It is ascertained that the RTV is generally *null* when legitimate stimuli regulate the DBS [50]. Figure 6 shows the RTV for a patient with Parkinson's disease on different conditions: stimulation on, medications on, stimuli on, drugs off, inspiration off, and medication off [51–53]. The graph represents that the RTV is checked after the DBS's implantation and that the valuation is outstanding characteristics nil, particularly compared to other scenarios [54, 55].

3.5 *Parameter Setting*

As shown in Fig. 7, a standard head stimulator has the following criteria that are used to regulate discrete pain.

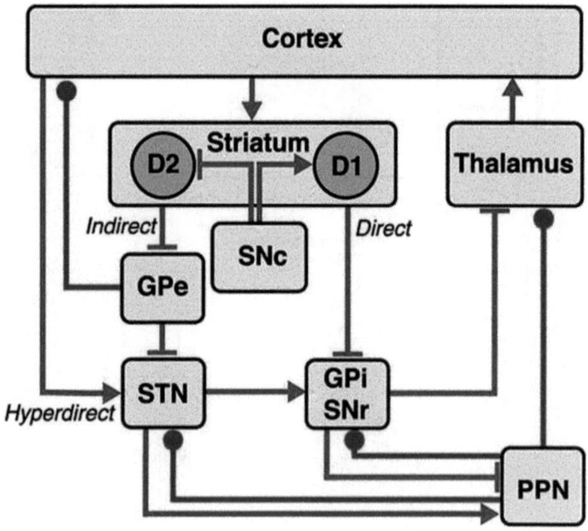

Fig. 7 Parameters of signal

3.6 Convolutional Neural Network

A CNN is a form of deep FFAI that has been successfully used to analyse visual elements in ML. CNNs use a form of multi-layer perceptron that needs very little pre-processing. Their shared-weights structure and translation invariance features are also regarded as SIANN. The connection pattern between neurons in CNN was influenced by biological processes in that it looks like the organisation of the animal visual cortex. A small portion of the visual field is individual cortical neurons that react to stimuli only in the receptive field. Different neurons' receptive fields partly overlap, occupying the whole visible area (Fig. 8).

In comparison to several other image classifications, CNNs require very little pre-processing. This means the organisation learns that the filters are hand-made in traditional algorithms. Designing features without relying on prior information or human effort is a huge benefit. A CNN contains a layer of input and output and several hidden layers. Convolutional, pooling, fully connected, and normalisation layers are common hidden layers in CNNs. By convention, the process is described as a CNN. It's a cross-correlation, not a convolution, in terms of mathematics. This only matters for the matrix indices and hence the weights at which index. CNN layers perform a convolution operation on the input and then pass the output to the next layer. The convolution simulates an individual neuron's response to visual stimuli. Respectively, the convolutional nerve cell only processes data for the receptive field in which it is located. Although the wholly integrated FF-NN is used to automatically extract and classify the data, it is not feasible to use these architectural features to perform classification. Because of the prominent feature sizes linked with images, each pixel is an important variable; even in a relatively thin structure, many brain areas would be considered necessary.

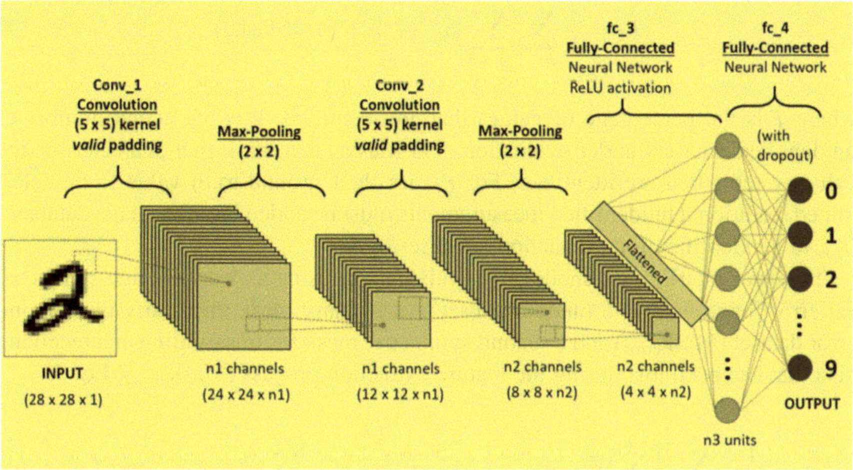

Fig. 8 Process of CNN

- Pooling: Current networks can include global pooling layers incorporating neuron clusters' outputs on one layer in the next layer into one neuron. For instance, max-pooling utilises the maximum value of each neuron cluster in the last layer. Average pooling, which further employs each set of brain regions' optimum rate in the previous layer, is another example.
- Fully Connected: In fully connected layers, every neurotransmitter with one network is connected to every brain cell in another layer. In concept, it works on the same principle as a traditional multi-layer feed-forward neural network.
- Weights: Using the same filter for each CNN layer while communicating their weights decreases memory space and ensures that improvements are being made in real time.

3.7 Performance Measures for Precision, Error Rate, and Fully Connected Layers

Each error checking method has been assessed for diagnosis and staging, and two precision support in measuring based on the data, i, and values for transformation, $\bar{i}$, were cast-off, Eqs. 1 and 2:

$$P_1 = \frac{1}{T}\sum_{a=1}^{n}\sum_{b=1}^{m}\{\bar{i}_b^a - i_b^a\}^2 \times \text{Mask}_a^b \tag{1}$$

$$P_2 = \frac{1}{V}\sum_{a=1}^{n}\sum_{b=1}^{m}\left\{\overline{i_b^a} - i_b^a\right\}^2 \times \left(1 - \text{Mask}_a^b\right) \quad (2)$$

where T is the percentage of values that are identified, V is the actual number of unidentified datasets under evaluation, and $\text{Mask}_{i,j}$ is a mask that characterises the value systems that are identified. For P_2, for their ground-truth value to be determined, additional unidentified measurements must be added into the image database, (i_b^a), to be identified for calculation purposes.

The error metric was functionally equivalent to using a mean average symmetrical error function with a random subset and a binary mask to classify the training error dataset ($\text{Mask}_{\text{error}}$) and a second symmetric mask for transmitting and receiving data that has been lost during the feature extraction process ($\text{Mask}_{\text{error}}$), Eq. 3:

$$P_3 = \frac{1}{T+V}\sum_{a=1}^{n}\left(\sum_{a=b}^{n}\overline{i_b^a} - i_b^a\right)^{2*}\left(1 - \text{Mask}_{\text{error},b}^a\right) + \sum_{a=b}^{\text{Mask}}\left(\overline{i_b^a} - i_b^a\right)^{2*}\text{Mask}_{\text{error},b}^a\Big) \quad (3)$$

The index is equivalent to putting a high value on reconstructing the error data value, which predominantly enhances the CNN's P_2 precision. The most significant findings emerged from a scale factor.

4 Experimental Results

The broadly applied or regional onset of brain activity spills in preterm and term babies and children can occur after focal or simplified brain perturbations. Multiple acute intensity pulses exploited at the patient can allow these patterns. When the EEG is predicted or mild to reasonably abnormal, diagnostic seizure activity is much more ubiquitous than when the history is severely irregular. The method by which an intelligent organism can identify a sensory input pattern as completely undiscovered is known as novelty diagnosis. During the Cold War, once unusual aircraft-reflection variations could imply a threat by a new type of plane, the philosophy became necessary for infrared investigative techniques. The hypothesis is now widely used in machine learning and data mining, with the corresponding primary references as feature extraction and anomaly analysis. On the other hand, a medical problem is an illness that develops over time, such as hypertension or asthma. It's important to note that osteoporosis, a chronic disease, can contribute to a fractured wrist, an acute situation. Tobacco, excessive drinking, poor diet, sedentary lifestyle, and inadequate relief of prolonged inflammation are significant contributors to the growth and progression of completely avoidable illnesses such as overweightness, blood pressure, etc. A severe defence strategy bears a striking resemblance to an incremental offensive attack, with a narrative format of increases or decreases in the RTV sequence. The portion of noise sufficient to break these disabilities varies. We uncovered that loud noise (100 dBA) creates ultrastructural changes in the rat cardiomyocytes preceded by DNA damage. A reduction of DNA integrity was evaluated in the adrenal glands of noisy noise-exposed rats. Injury to these distant tissues is most likely affected by differences in sympathetic nerve fibres, impacted by brain circuitry improvements. Loud noise is estimated to influence internal organs through its genetic gateway, the ear, altering brain areas that control neuroendocrine activities. RTV levels can discover unexpectedly high variations to noise defects triggered by attacker equipment failures.

4.1 Software Environment

The PCA (Fig. 9) and classifier versions from scikit-learn were implemented, and the Python script used to perform the multiple tests is accessible. IBM SPSS *Ver.* 22.0 had been used to execute the quantitative models. The Statistical Package for the Social Sciences (SPSS) is a statistical data programme used by many researchers. The SPSS application software was developed to address and subject to statistical social science statistics. Scientific researchers use SPSS, a genuinely innovative software package, to store large amounts of data in a matter of minutes. Working with data is a complex and confusing and time-consuming activity, but with the additional assistance of specific techniques, this software can easily actually control and operate data. SPSS is Logo icon, v27 is the latest version of the software, and it is working under Windows (x86-64), macOS (x86-64), and Linux (x86-64, ppc64le, IBM Z) with JAVA platform. A highly regarded but more nuanced process of the information estimation method fits a linear statistical model. By trying to eliminate the PCA eigenvector components corresponding to sampling error when predicting PCA findings but using the full eigenvector when helping to transform the scores back into the data matrix, principal component analysis (PCA) can equally be applied to complete present and future imputation. Numerous methods can decide

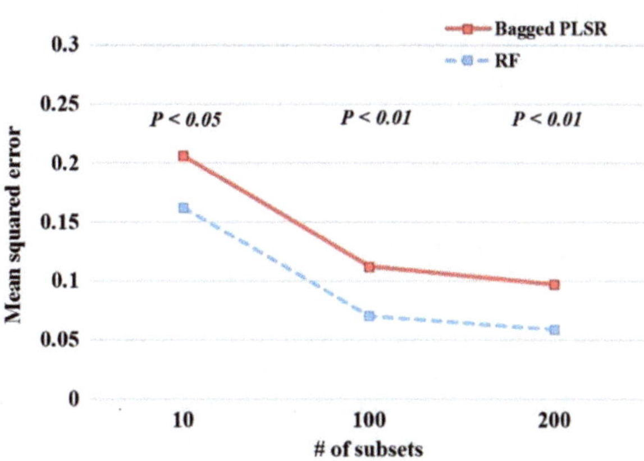

Fig. 9 Caudate nucleus (left), putamen (right), MSE of PCA test

the PCA decomposition if the training dataset also contains standard errors. PCA is also a commonly used feature extraction technique, producing it even more appropriate for the patient pre-processing phase. On the other hand, their time-dependent nature can be problematic when challenges are applied in combination in a primarily non-linear measured way.

Step 1. There is an optimal internal representation (IR) size for minimising error. The network's A2 efficiency is negatively affected by a great deal of flexibility in its results. This is expected for PCA, where factors allow the IR to 'remember' measure error as the mean predicts the behaviour rather than attributes them after a certain point.

Step 2. When data vectors are more complete, the CNN reconstructs them more precisely, but as data becomes unavailable, effectiveness endures.

Step 3. There is an advantage to learning from sparse data points. Even though reliable data vectors are significantly better, using case extraction to reduce the training examples to only those sample points increases accuracy.

5 Conclusion

DBS is a generation of artificial intelligence heart health devices that enhance the patient's nervous system to treat neurological diseases. Even though DBS has improved patients quality of life, it has also promoted safety issues in the long run. Security is essential because such interfaces can significantly affect a patient's physical and mental orientation. This work evaluates LSTM, a sort of CNN, to forecast and predict DBS's pattern. The intensity of neurological disorders is researched using RTV. We looked at RTV values required to formulate and train the CNN. The DBS framework introduced various attack patterns to rival and classified different bout policies. The research outcomes demonstrate that the prototypical example was able to identify distinct known vulnerabilities in the DBS with lower loss attributes and less skill exercise. The conceptual methodology will soon be screened with accurate RTV measurements in a genuinely emotional brain stimulator ecosystem. Legitimate and false information readings were classed and assumed at run time to analyse the new framework's performance, accuracy, and robustness.

5.1 Future Work

Because the physical displacements of specific structures are more significant in some problems than in many others, we predicted that specific brain features would cause deformation in an inhomogeneous approach over time. We attempted to find a pattern in the diffusion of relevant clusters of locations over the class of the human disease emergence, but we couldn't find anything consistent. More investigation would be required in this field. In addition, a clear interpretation of the most relevant structures of each problem could not be found. Longitudinal patient monitoring would be an appropriate follow-up for this study in this regard. Since the interpopulation bias is removed by following a patient over time, it is possible to draw more reliable conclusions about striatal shape alteration patterns.

References

1. Aleesa B, Zaidan A, Zaidan and Sahar NM: Review of Intrusion Detection Systems Based on Deep Learning Techniques: Coherent Taxonomy, Challenges, Motivations, Recommendations, *Substantial Analysis and Future Directions, Neural Computing and Applications,* Springer, Berlin, Germany, (2019).
2. Ferrag M.A, Maglaras L, Moschoyiannis S and Janicke H.: Deep learning for cybersecurity intrusion detection: approaches, datasets, and comparative study, *Journal of Information Security and Applications*, 50, 102419, (2020).
3. Gophika T, Aarthi R, Akash R and Anish V.: Different Attack Patterns for Deep Brain Implants by Using CNN, *International journal of scientific & Technology research,* 9 (6), (2020).
4. Henna Rathore, Abdulla Khalid Al-Ali, Amr Mohamed, Xiaojiang Du2 and Mohsen Guizani.: A Novel Deep Learning Strategy for Classifying Different Attack Patterns for Deep Brain Implants, *in Proc. IEEE*, 7, (2019).
5. S. Sudhakar and S. Chenthur Pandian "Secure packet encryption and key exchange system in mobile ad hoc network", *Journal of Computer Science*, vol. 8, no. 6, pp. 908–912, (2012).
6. S. Sudhakar and S. Chenthur Pandian, "Hybrid cluster-based geographical routing protocol to mitigate malicious nodes in mobile ad hoc network", *International Journal of Ad Hoc and Ubiquitous Computing*, vol. 21 no. 4, pp. 224–236, (2016).
7. A. U. Priyadarshni and S. Sudhakar, "Cluster-based certificate revocation by cluster head in mobile ad-hoc network", *International Journal of Applied Engineering Research*, vol. 10, no. 20, pp. 16014–16018, (2015).
8. S. Sudhakar and S. Chenthur Pandian, "Investigation of attribute aided data aggregation over dynamic routing in wireless sensor," *Journal of Engineering Science and Technology*, vol. 10, no. 11, pp. 1465–1476, (2015).
9. S. Sudhakar and S. Chenthur Pandian, "A Trust and co-operative nodes with effects of malicious attacks and measure the performance degradation on geographic aided routing in mobile ad hoc network", *Life Science Journal*, vol. 10, no. 4s, pp. 158–163, (2013).
10. S. Sudhakar and S. Chenthur Pandian, "An efficient agent-based intrusion detection system for detecting malicious nodes in MANET routing", *International Review on Computers and Software*, vol. 7, no. 6, pp. 3037–304, (2012).
11. Jokstad A and Ganeles J.: Systematic review of clinical and patient-reported outcomes following oral rehabilitation on dental implants with a tapered compared to a non-tapered implant design, *Clin Oral Implants Res,* 29 (16), 41–54, (2018)
12. Junyu Lin, Lei Xu, Yingqi Liu and Xiangyu Zhang.: Composite Backdoor Attack for Deep Neural Network by Mixing Existing Benign Features. In Proceedings of the 2020 ACM SIGSAC Conference on Computer and Communications Security (CCS '20). *Association for Computing Machinery*, New York, NY, USA, 113–131, (2020).
13. Moctezuma L.A, Torres-García A.A, Villaseñor-Pineda L and Carrillo M.: Subjects identification using EEG-recorded imagined speech, *Expert Systems with Applications,* 118, 201–208, (2019).
14. Ramanauskaite A, Borges T and Almeida B.L.: Dental implant outcomes in grafted sockets: a systematic review and meta-analysis, *J Oral Maxillofac Res*, 10 (8), 1–13, (2019).

15. Rathore H, Badarla V and Shit S.: Consensus-aware sociopsychological trust model for wireless sensor networks, *ACM Trans. Sensor Netw.*, 2 (3), 21, (2016).
16. Wang Z, Chen K and Shang Wu H.: Label-removed generative adversarial networks incorporating k-means, *Neurocomputing*, 361, 126–136, (2019).
17. https://trends.google.com/trends, Accessed by April 25, (2021).
18. Wilaiprasitporn T, Ditthapron A, Matchaparn K, Tongbuasirilai T, Banluesombatkul N and Chuangsuwanich E.: Affective EEG-based person identification using the deep learning approach, *IEEE Transactions on Cognitive and Developmental System*, 1 (1), (2019).
19. Yao L, Sheng X, Mrachacz-Kersting N, Zhu X, Farina D and Jiang N.: Sensory stimulation training for BCI system based on somatosensory attentional orientation, *IEEE Trans. Biomed.* Eng., 66 (3), 640–646, (2019).
20. Yingdong Wang, Qingfeng Wu, Chen Wang and Qunsheng Ruan.: DE-CNN: An Improved Identity Recognition Algorithm Based on the Emotional Electroencephalography, *Computational and Mathematical Methods in Medicine,* Article ID 7574531, 12, (2020).
21. Zhang X, Yao L, Kanhere S.S., Liu Y., Gu T and Chen K.: Mind ID: person identification from brain waves through attention-based recurrent neural network, *Proceedings of the ACM on Interactive, Mobile, Wearable and Ubiquitous Technologies,* 2 (3), 1–23, (2018).
22. Zheng W, Liu W, Lu Y, Lu B and Cichocki A.: Emotion-meter: a multi-modal framework for recognising human emotions, *IEEE Transactions on Systems, Man, and Cybernetics,* 49 (3), 1110–1122, (2018).
23. Rosak-Szyrocka, J.; Żywiolek, J.; Kulinska, E.; Matulewski, M. Analysis of Enterprises' Readiness in for Industry 4.0 Implementation: The Case of Poland. *ERSJ*, XXIV, 615–628 (2021).
24. Żywiolek, J.; Molenda, M.; Rosak-Szyrocka, J. Satisfaction with the Implementation of Industry 4.0 Among Manufacturing Companies in Poland. *ERSJ,* XXIV, 469–479 (2021).
25. Sharma, S. K., Jain, A., Gupta, K., Prasad, D., & Singh, V. (2019). An internal schematic view and simulation of major diagonal mesh network-on-chip. Journal of Computational and Theoretical Nanoscience, 16 (10), 4412–4417 (2019).
26. Ghai, D., Gianey, H. K., Jain, A., & Uppal, R. S. (2020). Quantum and dual-tree complex wavelet transform-based image watermarking. International Journal of Modern Physics B, 34 (04), 2050009 (2020).
27. Jain, A., & Kumar, A. (2021). Desmogging of still smoggy images using a novel channel prior. *Journal of Ambient Intelligence and Humanized Computing*, 12 (1), 1161–1177 (2021).
28. B. Panjwani, V. Singh, A. Rani, and V. Mohan, "Optimum multi-drug regime for compartment model of tumour: cell-cycle-specific dynamics in the presence of resistance," *Journal of Pharmacokinetics and Pharmacodynamics*, vol. 48, no. 4, pp. 543–562, 2021/08/01 (2021).
29. Kumar, S., Jain, A., Shukla, A. P., Singh, S., Raja, R., Rani, S., ... & Masud, M. (2021). A Comparative Analysis of Machine Learning Algorithms for Detection of Organic and Nonorganic Cotton Diseases. *Mathematical Problems in Engineering*, (2021).
30. Misra, N. R., Kumar, S., & Jain, A. A Review on E-waste: Fostering the Need for Green Electronics. In 2021 International Conference on Computing, *Communication, and Intelligent Systems*, (pp. 1032–1036). IEEE (2021).
31. Jain, A., Kumar, A., & Sharma, S. Comparative Design and Analysis of Mesh, Torus and Ring NoC. *Procedia Computer Science*, 48, 330–337 (2015).
32. B. Panjwani, V. Singh, A. Rani, and V. Mohan, "Optimizing Drug Schedule for Cell-Cycle Specific Cancer Chemotherapy," Singapore, pp. 71–81: Springer Singapore (2021).
33. Jain, A., Dwivedi, R., Kumar, A., & Sharma, S.: Scalable design and synthesis of 3D mesh network on chip. In Proceeding of International Conference on Intelligent Communication, Control and Devices (pp. 661–666). Springer, Singapore (2017).
34. B. Panjwani, V. Mohan, A. Rani, and V. Singh, "Optimal drug scheduling for cancer chemotherapy using two degree of freedom fractional order PID scheme," *Journal of Intelligent & Fuzzy Systems,* vol. 36, no. 3, pp. 2273–2284, (2019).

35. V. Mohan, H. Chhabra, A. Rani, and V. Singh, "An expert 2DOF fractional order fuzzy PID controller for nonlinear systems," *Neural Computing and Applications*, vol. 31, no. 8, pp. 4253–4270, (2019).
36. V. Mohan, A. Rani, and V. Singh, "Robust adaptive fuzzy controller applied to double inverted pendulum," *Journal of Intelligent & Fuzzy Systems*, vol. 32, no. 5, pp. 3669–3687, (2017).
37. V. Mohan, H. Chhabra, A. Rani, and V. Singh, "Robust self-tuning fractional order PID controller dedicated to non-linear dynamic system," *Journal of Intelligent & Fuzzy Systems,* vol. 34, no. 3, pp. 1467–1478, (2018).
38. H. Chhabra, V. Mohan, A. Rani, and V. Singh, "Multi objective PSO tuned fractional order PID control of robotic manipulator," in the *international symposium on intelligent systems technologies and applications,* 2016, pp. 567–572: Springer (2016).
39. H. Chhabra, V. Mohan, A. Rani, and V. Singh, "Robust nonlinear fractional order fuzzy PD plus fuzzy I controller applied to robotic manipulator," *Neural Computing and Applications,* vol. 32, no. 7, pp. 2055–2079, 2020/04/01 (2020).
40. H. Chhabra, V. Mohan, A. Rani, and V. Singh, "Trajectory tracking of Maryland manipulator using linguistic Lyapunov fuzzy controller," *Journal of Intelligent & Fuzzy Systems,* vol. 36, no. 3, pp. 2195–2205, (2019).
41. Jain, A., Gahlot, A. K., Dwivedi, R., Kumar, A., & Sharma, S. K. Fat Tree NoC Design and Synthesis. In Intelligent Communication, Control and Devices (pp. 1749–1756). Springer, Singapore (2018).
42. A. Rawat, S. Jha, B. Kumar, and V. Mohan, "Nonlinear fractional order PID controller for tracking maximum power in photo-voltaic system," *Journal of Intelligent & Fuzzy Systems,* vol. 38, no. 5, pp. 6703–6713, (2020).
43. Jain, A., AlokGahlot, A. K., & RakeshDwivedi, S. K. S. Design and FPGA Performance Analysis of 2D and 3D Router in Mesh NoC. *International Journal of Control Theory and Applications,* ISSN, 0974–5572 (2017).
44. Agrawal, N., Jain, A., & Agarwal, A. Simulation of Network on Chip for 3D Router Architecture. *International Journal of Recent Technology and Engineering*, 8, 58–62 (2019).
45. Renuka J Bathi, Sameena Parveen, Neeraj Taneja, Oral Tuberculous Ulcer – A Report of Two Cases, *Journal of Indian Academy of Oral Medicine and Radiology*, 2003, Volume 15, Issue 2, Pages 62–65 (2003).
46. A.K. Gupta, Y. K. Chauhan, and T Maity, "Experimental investigations and comparison of various MPPT techniques for photovoltaic system," *Sādhanā,* Vol. 43, no. 8, pp. 1–15, (2018).
47. J. Kubiczek and B. Hadasik, "Challenges in Reporting the COVID-19 Spread and its Presentation to the Society," *J. Data and Information Quality,* vol. 13, no. 4, pp. 1–7, (2021).
48. Sameena Parveen, Impact of Calorie Restriction and Intermittent Fasting on Periodontal Health, *Periodontology 2000*, Vol. 87, Issue 1, Pages 315–324 (2021).
49. A.K. Gupta, "Sun Irradiance Trappers for Solar PV Module to Operate on Maximum Power: An Experimental Study," *Turkish Journal of Computer and Mathematics Education*, Vol. 12, no. 5, pp. 1112–1121, (2021).
50. T. Radhika K Mohideen, C Krithika, N Jeddy, S Parveen, A Meta-Analysis in Assessing Oxidative Stress Using Malondialdehyde in Oral Submucous Fibrosis, *European Journal of Dentistry*, (2021).
51. A.K. Gupta, Y.K Chauhan, and T Maity and R Nanda, "Study of Solar PV Panel Under Partial Vacuum Conditions: A Step Towards Performance Improvement," *IETE Journal of Research*, pp. 1–8, (2020).
52. Parveen S Taneja N, R Bathi, Serum Glycoproteins as Prognosticator in Head and Neck Cancer Patients – A Follow Up Study, *Oral Oncology Head and Neck Oncology*, Volume 47 (2011).
53. A.K. Gupta, Y.K Chauhan, and T Maity, "A new gamma scaling maximum power point tracking method for solar photovoltaic panel Feeding energy storage system," *IETE Journal of Research*, vol. 67, no. 1, pp. 1–21, (2018).
54. Parveen S. Bathi R, Taneja N, Dermoid Cyst in The Floor of The Mouth-A Case Report, *Karnataka State Dental Journal*, Vol. 25, Issue 2, pages 52–54 (2006).

55. A. K. Gupta et al., "Effect of Various Incremental Conductance MPPT Methods on the Charging of Battery Load Feed by Solar Panel," in *IEEE Access*, vol. 9, pp. 90977–90988, (2021).

Web-Based Augmented Reality of Smart Healthcare Education for Machine Learning-Based Object Detection in the Night Sky

Sriram Veeraiya Perumal, Sudhakar Sengan, Dilip Kumar Sharma, Amarendra Kothalanka, Rajesh Iruluappan, and Arjun Subburaj

1 Introduction

The psychological investigation of celestial bodies is called meteorology, and it attempts to explain the known formation and development of the universe. A planetarium is a critical approach to analysing planetary systems and atmospheric theories. Reflected light assessment in glittering sky stars and planets is not simple because it could be blocked by climatic conditions, geographic locations, and time intervals. It is not easy for the students to identify unreachable celestial objects of the glittery night sky associated with the Sun/Moon to have access. AR is a powerful

S. Veeraiya Perumal (✉)
Acharya Bangalore B School (ABBS), Bengaluru, Karnataka, India

S. Sengan
Department of Computer Science and Engineering, PSN College of Engineering and Technology, Tirunelveli, Tamil Nadu, India

D. K. Sharma
Department of Mathematics, Jaypee University of Engineering and Technology, Guna, Madhya Pradesh, India

A. Kothalanka
Department of Computer Science and Engineering, Koneru Lakshmaiah Education Foundation, Vijayawada, Andhra Pradesh, India
e-mail: amarendra@kluniversity.in

R. Iruluappan
Department of Computer Science and Engineering, Knowledge Institute of Technology, Salem, Tamil Nadu, India

A. Subburaj
Tranxit Technology Solutions Private Limited, Chennai, Tamil Nadu, India
e-mail: aj@sentientlabs.io

P. Agarwal et al. (eds.), *Artificial Intelligence for Smart Healthcare*,
EAI/Springer Innovations in Communication and Computing,
https://doi.org/10.1007/978-3-031-23602-0_17

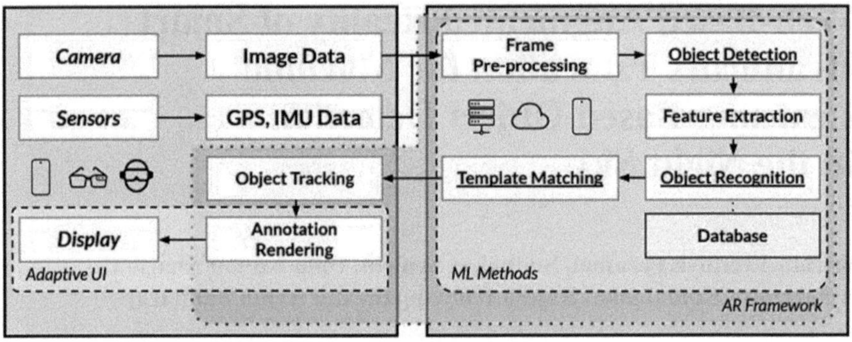

Fig. 1 ML-based AR functions

tool that can be used for astronomical purposes [1]. The information and communications technology can assist and support in avoiding accidents and help mitigate the public, physical, and emotional issues that the ageing persons commonly face. Numerous primary healthcare systems and old-age supporting activities are being advanced by combining many sensors and recent network trends. Home automation systems for older adults and the technological advances, devices, and development and validation with active assisted living are two examples. Vital signals, behavioural data, and other contextual data can be collected in these homes using gestures, locators, gravity, and vision sensors [2]. The data composed can be evaluated to track the behaviour and health of the ageing persons. Vision and audio-visual sensors, in particular, are ubiquitously used in aged people. An entire house is fitted with vision cameras that monitor the residents' movements and behaviours. Researchers have used RGB-depth cameras to conduct many research investigations on fall prevention and detection and physiotherapy practices after a fall accident.

Overview of augmented reality (AR): Figure 1 presents the typical pipeline of an AR system. The components in AR systems can be approximately grouped into AR device and tasks, where the tasks may be executed on a device or an external server. Generally, hardware sensors on the AR device first capture images and sensor data, which are then fed into the AR tasks. The first is frame pre-processing, where data is cleaned and prepared to be inputted into the analysis tasks to retrieve information on which objects are in the environment, e.g. object detection and reorganisation, feature extraction, and template matching tasks. These tasks can be classed as ML tasks, where ML techniques are used to complete the tasks more efficiently due to their complexity [3]. After data analysis, successful results and associated annotations are returned to the AR device for object tracking and annotation rendering on the client. This can form an AR framework with ML methods where developers can use pre-built frameworks to create their AR applications. The AR device's annotation rendering and display components can be grouped as part of adaptive UI; the contents and interaction with the rendered augmentations are essential for users as this allows them to experience AR [4].

AR provides a composite view by imposing computer-generated images' statements. These requests identify planetary figures, such as gatherings using GPS. Many AR stargazing apps for detecting stars can be utilised in global environments [5]. In recent times, various investigations have been directed to education and the advancement of informative material in astronomy. The astronomical apps present in the market fulfil the primary objective of observing the night sky but don't create a learning environment to reach the educational goal required. Space 360 is a desktop application that will provide a virtual planetarium experience to the user [6]. This paper presents a CNN model for quick and accurate star image detection based on the YOLO model. The need for hard-coding specific features such as particular star shapes, colours, and other attributes was eliminated using those DL techniques. Several convolutions and pooling layers have been twisted and transformed from the basic prototype to create this network. The modifications improve the ML model's accuracy in detecting objects of the same class nearby. Although the model was trained with training data images, it is highly accurate with other stars and Mars with similar attributes [7]. The paper's outline is described as object detection in the night sky and astronomical philosophies. Section 2 is represented as related works. Section 3 is Space 360-based object findings. Section 4 is the result and discussion. Section 5 concluded the paper.

2 Related Works

Skymap is a project that tries to replicate the environment of a planetarium virtually. Skymap is not an extensive language work because pictorial data creates a virtual experience. The intended audience who will benefit from this work is enthusiasts interested in astronomy [8]. The work can also be extended for educational purposes, which is helpful for students. After extensive research about the topic, we got valuable insights and answers to pondering questions. The Sky Map explorer provided insights about the coordinates. These coordinates were not calculated and were assumed to be when the map was wholly zoomed out; an oval was observed instead of a sphere. AstroViewer gave us an idea about how the stars and constellations were plotted in the night sky with insights about coordinates' mathematical calculations on their position using attributes like declination, distance, etc. [9]. The problem with the above product is that it was static [10]. Sky Live had the feature of zooming in and out. Still, when those operations have been performed, the map was motionless, and there was no rendering in the position of the constellations, which wasn't that informational but became irrelevant. Sky.org planetarium website suggested adding an interactive option with the static map by rendering the place accordingly when zooming in and zoom out options were bought under action. The original display parameters are stored in memory and can be recovered using zoom-out operations. The automatic grid spacing is defined, so the programme's optimum spacing is taken care of, which provides a legit way to display the contents. In addition to the sky map, an encyclopaedia [11] is also incorporated into the website, and it is purely for educational purposes, giving some basic information about astronomical objects.

The future scope can be extended by making the map more interactive and developing it to a bigger picture of the entire universe [12]. The sky map can also be interactive by hovering options to pop up information about the particular celestial body. Printable sky maps can be used for educational purposes like atlas to make the product more interactive. To conclude, if the above methods are incorporated, the production efficiency will increase, making the product more user reliable and efficient. An important subfield of ML, DL, is the study and application. However, while both fall under the artificial intelligence (AI) umbrella, deep learning (DL) controls the most human-like AI-based real-time applications. This model is designed to continuously analyse data with a logical design comparable to how a human would make conclusions. As a result, DL employs an artificial neural network (ANN), a layered structure of algorithms [13]. The biological ANN of the human brain inspired the design of an ANN. For example, supervised training with DL allows for automatic learning of the valuable training feature sets from the images and efficient exploitation of them in order to construct an accurate detector. As a general rule, the local visual characteristics of an image are extracted by a convolutional neural network (CNN), and the next classifier is a fully connected network (FCN) [14]. By learning internal feature representations with little input data cubes, CNNs preserve the spatial relationship between pixels. Objects in the image can be transitioned or converted in this professional way while still being observable by the CNN. The purpose of using a faster R-CNN model was to implement a precise, rapid, and efficient system designed to detect stars and Mars. In cognitive training, the prototype detected functionalities with 0.838 precision and recall. They also aggregated RGB and NIR image data using a multi-modal segmentation technique. The model used in an accurate simulation model requires at least 8 Gb internal storage [15].

3 Materials and Methods

This work was performed to study the different celestial objects in the Milky Way galaxy. Space 360 is a web application that aims to provide a virtual planetarium experience (Fig. 2). It serves as an encyclopaedia for planets and constellations visible from the earth. Using Space 360, different celestial objects visible in other geographical locations and times can be examined. Space 360 aims to provide an interactive user experience [16].

Regarding the tools and technology used, the webpages are structured in HTML (HyperText Markup Language) and made attractive in CSS (Cascading Style Sheet). JavaScript facilitates interactive features on the website [17]. All the data regarding the celestial objects are stored in JSON (JavaScript Object Notation) format and extracted when necessary, using jQuery when the website is loading. The sky map is made using a JavaScript library, three.js, creating 3D computer graphics. The result

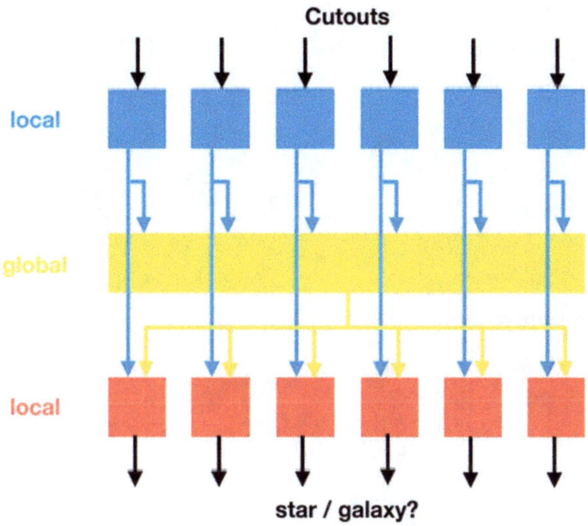

Fig. 2 A high-level overview of the Context Net architecture

is rendered using WebGL (Web Graphics Library). The website runs in the local host of the computer provided by XAMPP Apache. Space 360 can be divided into two modules, and this section explains them extensively [18].

3.1 Sky Map

The sky map feature of Space 360 visualises the night sky and exhibits the different planets and constellations visible from the earth. The objective is to provide the stargazers with a virtual planetarium. A celestial sphere is constructed to simulate the night sky in this study. The celestial sphere is a fictitious sphere whose centre is the earth around which all celestial bodies are projected. Figure 3 illustrates the celestial sphere with the earth as the centre. The planets and stars of the constellations are plotted as celestial spheres [19].

An HYG database schema was implied from the original star training dataset for this investigation. The HYG repository was preferred as the performance measure, observing various sources' comprehensive comparative analysis with the star dataset. An implementation of phenomenal data from a series of books and magazines is the HYG database [20]. The HYG database is the type of data as catalogues: the Hipparcos Catalogue, the Yale Bright Star Catalogue, and the Nearby Stars Gliese Catalogue. The dataset includes many domains from which the visual magnitude (Mag) of the Henry Draper ID (HD), the right ascension (RA), the declining (Dec), and the location were retrieved. There have been over 100,000 stars in the training dataset. A database schema with all the above domains allowed a comparison of only 88 stars (around 650). The stars' digital camera (P, Q, R) was determined to correlate the stars as a celestial sphere. The appropriate ascent and decline

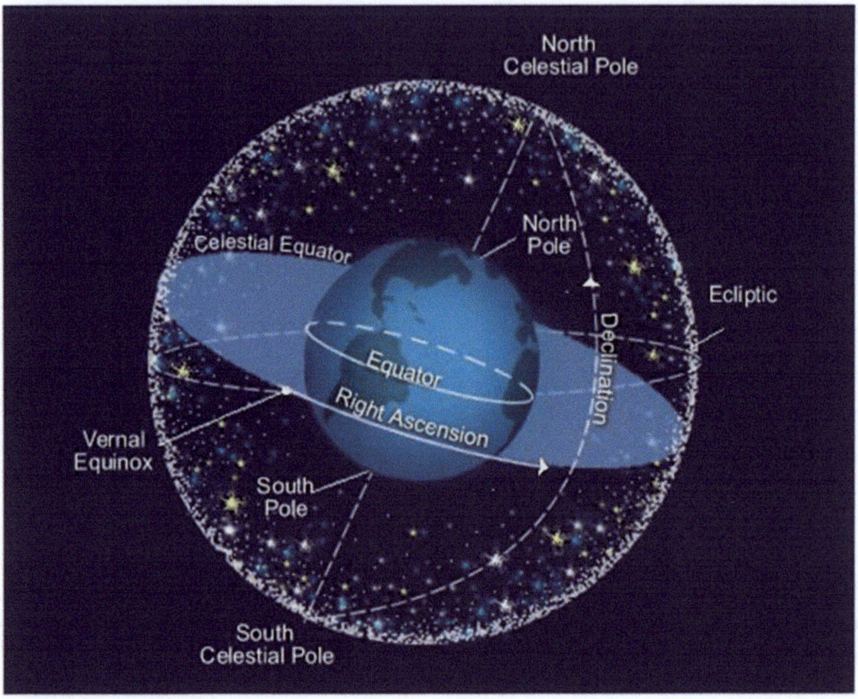

Fig. 3 Celestial sphere

coordinates were computed for precise configuration instead of the HYG database Cartesian coordinates. The distance from the sky's earth and latitude is exposed in Fig. 2 [21], RA (suitable ascent) and Dec (decline). RA aims to measure the object's geometric distance from the autumnal equinox to the hour circle, passing the image to the east of the celestial equator [22–26]. Decline actions the pointed remoteness of an entity diagonal to the northern beneficial, south-destroying equatorial plane (Wikipedia 2021 Equatorial Coordinate System) [27]. And here's the equation for the measurement of the latitude and longitude Eqs. 1, 2, and 3.

$$P=[C\times\varphi(B)]\times\varphi(A)] \tag{1}$$

$$Q=[C\times\varphi(B)]\times\theta(A)] \tag{2}$$

$$Z=[C\times\theta(B)] \tag{3}$$

The database was inferred from Satellitium's constellation ship database (Fig. 4). *A* represents the RA in degrees, *B* represents the Dec in degrees, and *C* represents the distance in light-years or parsecs. The coordinates calculated were plotted in three.js as a particle system [28–32]. The size of each star is unique according to its magnitude extracted from the HYG database. After plotting the stars, the stars

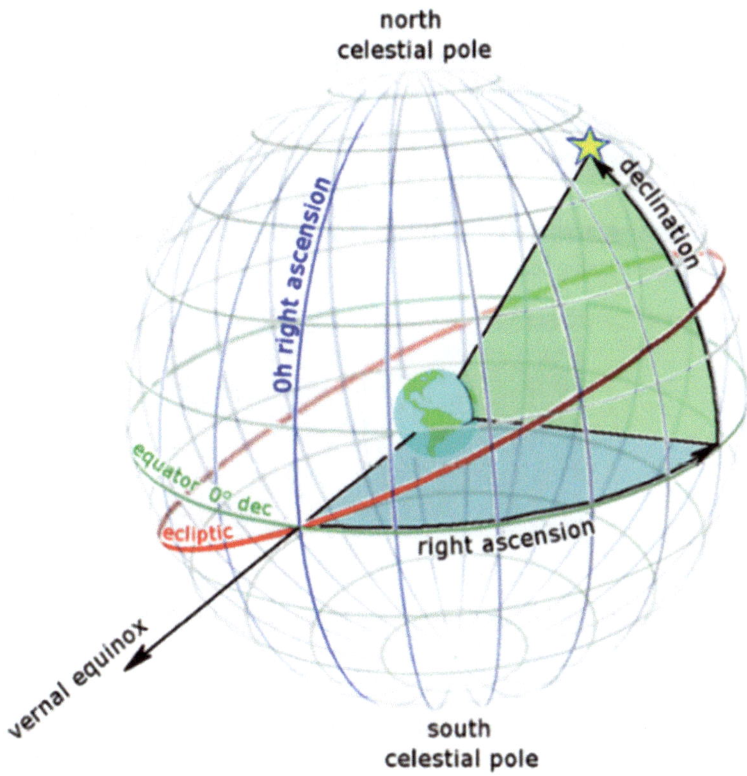

Fig. 4 RA (blue) and Dec (green) of a celestial sphere. (Image Courtesy: Wikipedia)

were joined by line according to the constellations' patterns. The stars which should be joined were stored as pairs in the database [33–37].

3.2 Space Catalogue

Space 360 also provides a Space Catalogue feature, an encyclopaedia for the celestial bodies presented in the galaxy's Milky Way. The objective is to create a reserve for the 88 constellations and eight planets [38–42]. The web page displays these celestial bodies' basic information with a slideshow of pictures that symbolise the celestial object. A database was created currently containing information about the 88 constellations and eight planets for this study [43–47]. The definitions of the night sky, semantics, areas in degrees, meridian crossings, visibility between latitudes, and declinations in degrees of stars and planets. For planets, the subheadings were Description, Diameter, Mean Distance from the Sun, Rotational Period, Orbital Period, Surface Temperature, and Main Atmospheric Component [48–52].

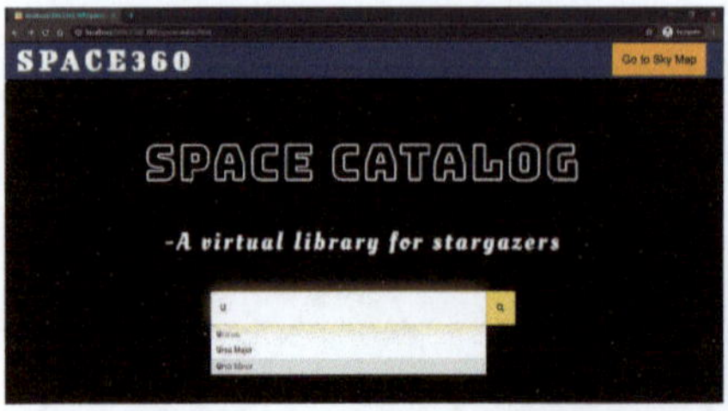

(a) Space Catalog search bar

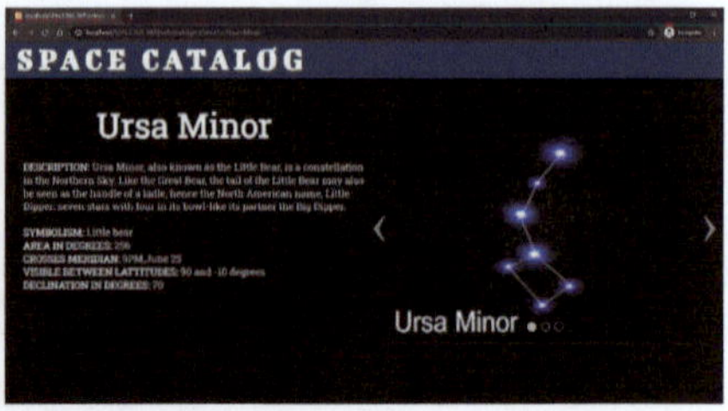

(b) Space Catalog search result

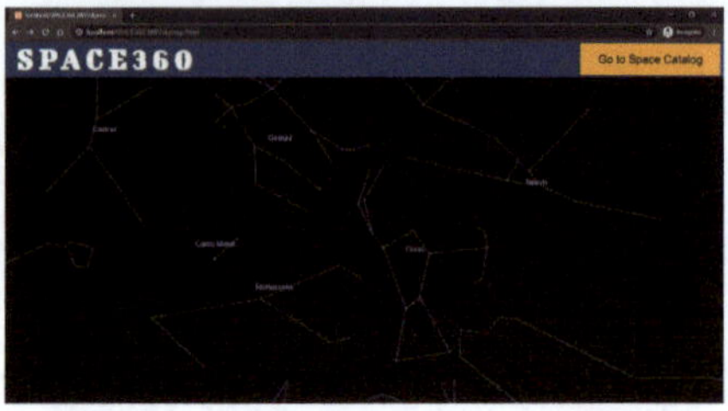

(c). Sky Map

Fig. 5 Screenshots of implementation. (**a**) Space Catalogue search bar. (**b**) Space Catalogue search result. (**c**) Sky Map

Space 360 serves two primary goals. The first is that it provides a platform for the user to observe the night sky's celestial bodies [53–55]. This map is created using three.js and is user interactive and responsive (Fig. 5a, b, and c). The map can be dragged, zoomed in, and zoomed out to view other constellations and planets [56–59]. Space 360, in addition to the above feature, provides insights into the celestial body. The Space Catalogue feature was developed using HTML, CSS, and JS, and all the data regarding the celestial bodies are stored in a JSON file [60–62]. When a planet or constellation is searched, information about the same is presented.

This paper was inspired by the thought of bringing an experience of the virtual planetarium to their place. The sky map projects referred to were not user interactive and were static. These projects didn't give the user the experience of gazing at the stars. It was more like seeing a piece of information wherein Space 360 provides a virtual platform for stargazing. Most of the sky maps give the user only the option of observing the night sky, and there is no learning happening. In this pandemic situation, where going to the planetarium is impossible, Space 360 helps bridge this gap and provides the user with hands-on experience about gazing at the night sky and giving information about those celestial bodies. Space 360 has an additional feature to facilitate the above process and provide information about the celestial bodies. Space 360 is a platform that can be used for stargazing and acquiring knowledge. Currently, this project is limited only to our solar system, and it can be further extended, but it's beyond the scope of this project. The constellations and planets' database should be updated regularly, which is an extensive admin work and will consume much time.

Table 1 Specification of AR

Parameter	Specification
CPU	Dual Core 2 GHz
RAM	4 GB
GPU	PowerVR SGX540
Camera	8 MP
OS	Android
Display	1024×800
Board	T1OMAP 4430

Table 2 Testing of learning applications

Test property	Metrics
Correctness	Accuracy-precision-recall-F-score
Group discrimination	Disparate impact
Discrete discrimination	Flip-rate
Error sensitivity	
Procedural sensitivity	
Minor linear change	Big linear transformation
Un-ordered information	
Big linear transformation	

3.3 Experimental Setup

This learning application was created using the following tools, materials, and software: As shown in Table 1, the mobile phone hardware used to develop the application is described. The minimum operating system requirement for a mobile phone is using OpenCV.

3.4 Validation

Learning applications must be tested to ensure that they meet all of their needs at this stage. All functions that are tested in the real-time application can be fixed (Table 2). Black-box testing will be used to test this application. Several factors, such as digital camera distance, light intensity, and the pointer itself, were responsible for identification not being detected during black-box testing.

3.5 ML and OpenCV to Detect Objects

We need (1) to detect the webcam stream efficiently and (2) to identify the object detection to each frame to construct our ML-based real-time image detection with

OpenCV (Fig. 6). If you want to study and detect objects, you need to train your models on labelled images. Each image in the training dataset must be accompanied by a dataset containing the edge detection and classes. OpenCV includes many before classifiers that can be used to classify images such as trees, license plate numbers, continues to face, eyes, and so on. To detect the object, researchers can do any of those classifiers. OpenCV (Open-Source Computer Vision Library) is CV's and ML's software framework. More than 2500 optimal process techniques are shown in the library, which provides a complete sequence of classic and cutting-edge CV and ML algorithms. These object classification methods can be pre-trained or designed from the initial concept. We use pre-trained weights from pre-trained modelling techniques in most cases and then fine-tune them to satisfy our needs, and the diagram can identify the difference. OpenCV is a small open library for CV, ML, and image processing, and it now plays an essential role in real-time operation, which is essential in today's modern systems. Pictures and videos can recognise objects, faces, and even human hand geometry. CNN (R-CNN, region-based CNN), fast R-CNN, and YOLO (You Only Look Once) are three of the most popular object detection algorithms. The R-CNNs are necessarily applied to the R-CNN group, whereas the single-shot detection systems belong to the single-shot detector group.

- High Specificity: YOLO is a correlation method that yields accurate and consistent performance with a minimum noisy environment.
- Cognitive Functioning: The method has efficient and effective learning abilities, allowing it to learn object expressions and implement them into object classification.

4 Dataset

Many different angles of the same tree have been used, as well as various tree species and cultivars and other times of the year and weather conditions (Table 3). As a result, over 5000 test images are required to train the ML models. There were 100 images of stars and 50 images of Mars. The images were considered before the stars began to turn red, so they were all still green when captured. Pears have a lower number than stars, but in this case, we wanted to observe some transfer AR learning methods from stars, so this number was sufficient to carry out this research.

4.1 Data Preparation

Before building an ML algorithm, preparing the data and performing pre-analysis is crucial. Following the collection of images together, we started the exploratory data analysis. In order to capture the entire tree, each image was taken from a different angle. Only 1/5 of the top and bottom images do not have any stars. When the model

```
# import the necessary packages
from imutils.video import VideoStream
from imutils.video import FPS
import numpy as np
import argparse
import imutils
import time
import cv2
# construct the argument parse and parse the arguments
ap = argparse.ArgumentParser()
ap.add_argument("-p", "--prototxt", required=True,
    help="path to Caffe 'deploy' prototxt file")
ap.add_argument("-m", "--model", required=True,
    help="path to Caffe pre-trained model")
ap.add_argument("-c", "--confidence", type=float, default=0.2,
    help="minimum probability to filter weak detections")
args = vars(ap.parse_args())
# initialize the list of class labels MobileNet SSD was trained to
# detect, then generate a set of bounding box colors for each class
CLASSES = ["background", "aeroplane", "bicycle", "bird", "boat",
    "bottle", "bus", "car", "cat", "chair", "cow", "diningtable",
    "dog", "horse", "motorbike", "person", "pottedplant", "sheep",
    "sofa", "train", "tvmonitor"]
COLORS = np.random.uniform(0, 255, size=(len(CLASSES), 3))

    # loop over the detections
    for i in np.arange(0, detections.shape[2]):
        # extract the confidence (i.e., probability) associated with
        # the prediction
        confidence = detections[0, 0, i, 2]

        # filter out weak detections by ensuring the `confidence` is
        # greater than the minimum confidence
        if confidence > args["confidence"]:
            # extract the index of the class label from the
            # `detections`, then compute the (x, y)-coordinates of
            # the bounding box for the object
            idx = int(detections[0, 0, i, 1])
            box = detections[0, 0, i, 3:7] * np.array([w, h, w, h])
            (startX, startY, endX, endY) = box.astype("int")

            # draw the prediction on the frame
            label = "{}: {:.2f}%".format(CLASSES[idx],
                confidence * 100)
            cv2.rectangle(frame, (startX, startY), (endX, endY),
                COLORS[idx], 2)
            y = startY - 15 if startY - 15 > 15 else startY + 15
            cv2.putText(frame, label, (startX, y),
                cv2.FONT_HERSHEY_SIMPLEX, 0.5, COLORS[idx], 2)
```

Fig. 6 Using ML and OpenCV in real-time object recognition

Table 3 The source of the image and the augmentation of stars and mars

Digital camera	Count	Image size	Image resize	AR	Synthetic
Web camera	21	1290×780	610×610	90	1
Smartphone IR camera	110+25	2460×4618	1230×1230	250	110
DSLR Canon camera	40	5671×8791	1217×1217	150	0

Table 4 Correctness of detection

Ground truth		Predicted value	
		True	False
	T	TP	FN
	F	FP	TN

detects falling stars, it is measured as an FP, F1-score. In some cases, the bottom part even had fallen stars. We scaled and cropped a set of images to the desired size and shape using a Python script. The captured images had to be trimmed and cropped to fit the ML model. All of the images were cropped to avoid this and better provide the image into a square dimension. For M1 and M2, the image size was cropped to 608608 pixels, and for M3, to 612168 pixels. Training and testing sets of images are created. Only images from a smartphone camera were used for testing, and those images were subjected to all of the same methodologies as other image data before validating the algorithm. Training does not see these images because it is important to test the accuracy of the models on images that have never been seen before. This allows us to determine whether the model is over-fitting on the training images or whether it can still generalise and detect stars and Mars.

4.2 Metrics

The assessment of ground truth and projected information was used to calculate pixel-level accuracy. Confusion matrix, precision, recall, F1-score (Table 4), and intersection over union are used as accuracy metrics. For example, precision measures the portion of true positives (TP) sensed bounding boxes in a pool of all TP calculations. In contrast, recall measures the fraction of TP detected threshold boundaries in the pool of all TP and false-positive (FP) predictions, Eqs. 4, 5, and 6.

$$\text{Precision} = \frac{\text{TP}}{\text{TP} + \text{FP}} \tag{4}$$

$$\text{Recall} = \frac{\text{TP}}{\text{TP} + \text{FN}} \tag{5}$$

We can only use the F1-score to calculate the score and how well the estimate matches the ground truth because precision and recall are closely related.

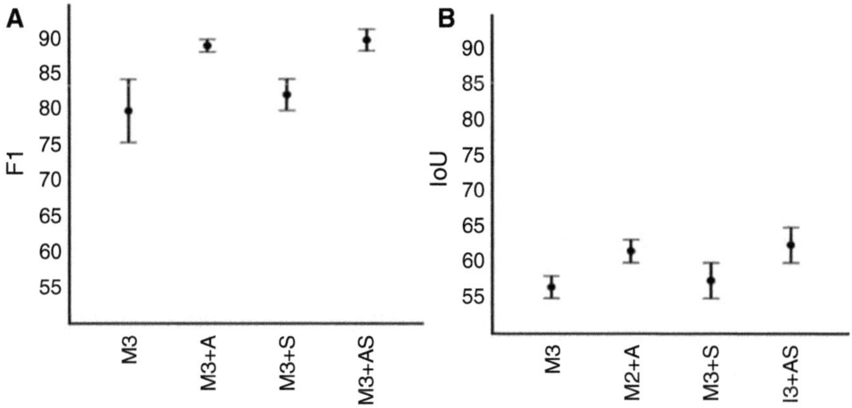

Fig. 7 Intuition-based accuracy of images with ML

$$\text{F1-score} = \frac{2 \times \text{Precision} \times \text{Recall}}{\text{Precision} + \text{Recall}} \tag{6}$$

As a result, we use IoU to determine whether or not detection is correct. To calculate IoU, one must calculate the overlap between prediction and ground truth. The prediction bounding box image size is P_w and P_h, respectively, and the ground truth bounding box image size is G_w and G_h. It is considered positive if the threshold exceeds 0.5 IoU, but less than that, it is deemed poor detection. A second metric we used to gauge speed was framed per second. NVIDIA Jetson TX2 with 300 cores (CUDA) and GeForce GTX960M (96 cores) were used to test the model. It was considered by dividing a second by the time it took to process a single image in ms (Fig. 7), Eq. 7.

$$\text{AOC} = \frac{(P_w \times P_h) \cap (G_w \times G_h)}{(P_w \times P_h) \cup (G_w \times G_h)} \tag{7}$$

5 Conclusion

The learning environment is limited to virtually observing the constellations, and a significant difference can be observed between reality and the user's imagination. Using Space 360, the user can get hands-on experience gazing at the night sky and getting information about celestial objects without being physically present in a planetarium. Space 360 is a non-profit project and was developed purely for educational purposes. The above project is intended for an audience interested in astrophysics and people fascinated by the scientific phenomenon.

References

1. Chen H.Y., Yang C.Y, Liu X.Y and Chou C.F.: On Deep Learning-Based Feedback and Precoding for Multi-user Millimeter-Wave Enabled VR/AR, IEEE International Conference on Consumer Electronics – Taiwan (ICCE-Taiwan), 1–2, (2020).
2. Cheng Q, Zhang S, Bo S, Chen D and Zhang H.: "Augmented Reality Dynamic Image Recognition Technology Based on Deep Learning Algorithm," IEEE Access, 8, 137370–137384, (2020).
3. Jifeng, Dai., Yi, Li., Kaiming, He., Jian, Sun, Object detection via region-based fully convolutional networks. In Advances in neural information processing sysems, 379–387, (2016).
4. Le H, Nguyen M, Nguyen Q, Nguyen H and Yan W.Q.: "Automatic Data Generation for Deep Learning Model Training of Image Classification used for Augmented Reality on Pre-school Books," International Conference on Multimedia Analysis and Pattern Recognition (MAPR), 1–5, (2020).
5. Lera, F.J.; Rodríguez, V.; Rodríguez, C.; Matellán, V.: Augmented reality in robotic assistance for the elderly. In International Technology Robotics Applications; Springer, 3–11, (2014).
6. Luyang, Liu., Hongyu. Li., Marco, Gruteser.: Edge Assisted Real-time Object Detection for Mobile Augmented Reality. ACM, (2019).
7. Maleke, B., Paseru, D., Padang, R.: Learning Application of Astronomy Based Augmented Reality using Android Platform, IOP Conf. Series: Materials Science and Engineering vol 306, (2018).
8. S. Sudhakar and S. Chenthur Pandian "Secure packet encryption and key exchange system in mobile ad hoc network", Journal of Computer Science, vol. 8, no. 6, pp. 908–912, (2012).
9. S. Sudhakar and S. Chenthur Pandian, "Hybrid cluster-based geographical routing protocol to mitigate malicious nodes in mobile ad hoc network", International Journal of Ad Hoc and Ubiquitous Computing, vol. 21 no. 4, pp. 224–236, (2016).
10. A. U. Priyadarshni and S. Sudhakar, "Cluster-based certificate revocation by cluster head in mobile ad-hoc network", International Journal of Applied Engineering Research, vol. 10, no. 20, pp. 16014–16018, (2015).
11. S. Sudhakar and S. Chenthur Pandian, "Investigation of attribute aided data aggregation over dynamic routing in wireless sensor," Journal of Engineering Science and Technology, vol. 10, no. 11, pp. 1465–1476, (2015).
12. S. Sudhakar and S. Chenthur Pandian, "Trustworthy position-based routing to mitigate against the malicious attacks to signifies secured data packet using geographic routing protocol in MANET", WSEAS Transactions on Communications, vol. 12, no. 11, pp. 584–603, (2013),
13. Sakib Ashra, Zargar., Fuh-Gwo, Yuan.: Augmented reality for enhanced visual inspection through knowledge-based deep learning, 20 (1), 426–442, (2010).
14. Tasneem, Khan., Kevin, Johnston., Jacques, Ophoff.: The Impact of an Augmented Reality Application on Learning Motivation of Students. Advances in Human-Computer Interaction, (2019).
15. Upadhyay G.K, Aggarwal D., Bansal A and Bhola B.: Augmented Reality and Machine Learning based Product Identification in Retail using Vuforia and MobileNets, International Conference on Inventive Computation Technologies (ICICT), 479–485, (2020).
16. Wenxiao, Zhang., Bo, Han., Pan, Hui.: On the networking challenges of mobile augmented reality. In Proceedings of the Workshop on Virtual Reality and Augmented Reality Network, ACM, 24–29, (2017).
17. Wolf, D.; Besserer, D.; Sejunaite, K.; Riepe, M.; Rukzio, E. cARe, An Augmented Reality Support System for Dementia Patients. In Proceedings of the 31st Annual ACM Symposium on User Interface Software and Technology Adjunct Proceedings, Berlin, Germany, 14(17), 42–44, (2018).
18. Yoon Jung, Park.: Deep-cARe: Projection-Based Home Care Augmented Reality System with Deep Learning for Elderly. Applied Sciences. Sci., 9 (18), (2019).

19. A. Jain, A. Kumar, and S. Sharma, "Comparative Design and Analysis of Mesh, Torus and Ring NoC," Procedia Comput. Sci., vol. 48, pp. 330–337, (2015).
20. A. Jain, R. Dwivedi, A. Kumar, and S. Sharma, "Scalable design and synthesis of 3D mesh network on chip," in Proceeding of International Conference on Intelligent Communication, Control and Devices, pp. 661–666 (2017).
21. A. Jain, A. K. Gahlot, R. Dwivedi, A. Kumar, and S. K. Sharma, "Fat Tree NoC Design and Synthesis," in Intelligent Communication, Control and Devices, Springer, 2018, pp. 1749–1756 (2018).
22. S. K. Sharma, A. Jain, K. Gupta, D. Prasad, and V. Singh, "An internal schematic view and simulation of major diagonal mesh network-on-chip," J. Comput. Theor. Nanosci., vol. 16, no. 10, pp. 4412–4417, (2019).
23. P. Manta, S. Chandra Singh, A. Deep, and D. N. Kapoor, "Temperature-regulated gold nanoparticle sensors for immune chromatographic rapid test kits with reproducible sensitivity: a study," IET Nanobiotechnol., no. nbt2.12024, (2021).
24. D. Ghai, H. K. Gianey, A. Jain, and R. S. Uppal, "Quantum and dual-tree complex wavelet transform-based image watermarking," Int. J. Mod. Phys. B, vol. 34, no. 04, p. 2050009, (2020).
25. P. Manta, R. Chauhan, H. Gandhi, S. Mahant, and D. N. Kapoor, "Formulation rationale for the development of SARS-COV-2 immunochromatography rapid test kits in India," J. Appl. Pharm. Sci. https://doi.org/10.7324/JAPS.2021.1101017 (2021).
26. A. Jain and A. Kumar, "Desmogging of still smoggy images using a novel channel prior," J. Ambient Intell. Humaniz. Comput., vol. 12, no. 1, pp. 1161–1177, (2021).
27. P. Manta et al., "Optical density optimization of malaria pan rapid diagnostic test strips for improved test zone band intensity," Diagnostics (Basel), vol. 10, no. 11, p. 880, (2020).
28. S. Kumar et al., "A Comparative Analysis of Machine Learning Algorithms for Detection of Organic and Nonorganic Cotton Diseases," Math. Probl. Eng., vol. 2021, (2021).
29. N. R. Misra, S. Kumar, and A. Jain, "A Review on E-waste: Fostering the Need for Green Electronics," in 2021 International Conference on Computing, Communication, and Intelligent Systems, pp. 1032–1036 (2021).
30. P. Manta, N. Wahi, A. Bharadwaj, G. Kour, and D. N. Kapoor, "A statistical quality control (SQC) methodology for gold nanoparticles based immune-chromatographic rapid test kits validation," Nanosci. Nanotechnol.-Asia, vol. 11, no. 6, pp. 1–5, (2021).
31. A. Jain, A. K. AlokGahlot, and S. K. S. RakeshDwivedi, "Design and FPGA Performance Analysis of 2D and 3D Router in Mesh NoC," Int. J. Control Theory Appl., pp. 0974–5572, (2017).
32. N. Gupta and A. K. Agarwal, "Object Identification using Super Sonic Sensor: Arduino Object Radar," 2018 International Conference on System Modeling & Advancement in Research Trends, pp. 92–96 (2018).
33. P. Manta et al., "Analytical approach for the optimization of desiccant weight in rapid test kit packaging: Accelerated predictive stability (APS)," Systematic Reviews in Pharmacy, vol. 11, no. 8, pp. 102–113, (2020).
34. P. Manta, D. N. Kapoor, G. Kour, M. Kour, and A. K. Sharma, "critical quality attributes of rapid test kits – a practical overview," Journal of Critical Reviews, vol. 7, no. 19, pp. 377–384, (2020).
35. S. Shukla, A. Lakhmani and A. K. Agarwal, "A review on integrating ICT based education system in rural areas in India," 2016 International Conference System Modeling & Advancement in Research Trends, pp. 256–259 (2016).
36. Agarwal, A.K., Jain, A., Synthesis of 2D and 3D NoC Mesh Router Architecture in HDL Environment, Jour of Adv Research in Dynamical & Control Systems, 11(04) (2019).
37. Ishaq, A., Sadiq, S., Umer, M., Ullah, S., Mirjalili, S., Rupapara, V., & Nappi, M. (2021). Improving the Prediction of Heart Failure Patients' Survival Using SMOTE and Effective Data Mining Techniques. IEEE Access, 9, 39707–39716 (2021).

38. Rustam, F., Khalid, M., Aslam, W., Rupapara, V., Mehmood, A., & Choi, G. S. A performance comparison of supervised machine learning models for Covid-19 tweets sentiment analysis. PLOS ONE, 16(2), e0245909 (2021).
39. Yousaf, A., Umer, M., Sadiq, S., Ullah, S., Mirjalili, S., Rupapara, V., & Nappi, M. (2021b). Emotion Recognition by Textual Tweets Classification Using Voting Classifier (LR-SGD). IEEE Access, 9, 6286–6295. 1
40. Sadiq, S., Umer, M., Ullah, S., Mirjalili, S., Rupapara, V., & NAPPI, M. Discrepancy detection between actual user reviews and numeric ratings of Google App store using deep learning. Expert Systems with Applications, 115111. https://doi.org/10.1016/j.eswa.2021.115111 (2021).
41. B. Panjwani, V. Mohan, A. Rani, and V. Singh, "Optimal drug scheduling for cancer chemotherapy using two degree of freedom fractional order PID scheme," Journal of Intelligent & Fuzzy Systems, vol. 36, no. 3, pp. 2273–2284, (2019).
42. B. Panjwani, V. Singh, A. Rani, and V. Mohan, "Optimizing Drug Schedule for Cell-Cycle Specific Cancer Chemotherapy," Singapore, pp. 71–81: Springer Singapore (2021).
43. B. Panjwani, V. Singh, A. Rani, and V. Mohan, "Optimum multi-drug regime for compartment model of tumour: cell-cycle-specific dynamics in the presence of resistance," Journal of Pharmacokinetics and Pharmacodynamics, vol. 48, no. 4, pp. 543–562, 2021/08/01 (2021).
44. V. Mohan, H. Chhabra, A. Rani, and V. Singh, "An expert 2DOF fractional order fuzzy PID controller for nonlinear systems," Neural Computing and Applications, vol. 31, no. 8, pp. 4253–4270, (2019).
45. G. S and S. R. Raja.T, "A Comprehensive Survey on Alternating Fluids Used For The Enhancement of Power Transformers," 2021 IEEE International Conference on the Properties and Applications of Dielectric Materials, pp. 57–60 (2021).
46. V. Mohan, A. Rani, and V. Singh, "Robust adaptive fuzzy controller applied to double inverted pendulum," Journal of Intelligent & Fuzzy Systems, vol. 32, no. 5, pp. 3669–3687, (2017).
47. V. Mohan, H. Chhabra, A. Rani, and V. Singh, "Robust self-tuning fractional order PID controller dedicated to non-linear dynamic system," Journal of Intelligent & Fuzzy Systems, vol. 34, no. 3, pp. 1467–1478, (2018).
48. Żywiołek, J.; Rosak-Szyrocka, J.; Mrowiec, M., Knowledge Management in Households about Energy Saving as Part of the Awareness of Sustainable Development. In: Energies, 14 (24), S. 8207 (2021).
49. H. Chhabra, V. Mohan, A. Rani, and V. Singh, "Multi objective PSO tuned fractional order PID control of robotic manipulator," in the international symposium on intelligent systems technologies and applications, 2016, pp. 567–572: Springer (2016).
50. H. Chhabra, V. Mohan, A. Rani, and V. Singh, "Robust nonlinear fractional order fuzzy PD plus fuzzy I controller applied to robotic manipulator," Neural Computing and Applications, vol. 32, no. 7, pp. 2055–2079, 2020/04/01 (2020).
51. Nora Omran Alkaam, Ahmed J. Obaid, Mohammed Q. Mohammed. A Hybrid Technique for Object Detection and Recognition Using Local Features Algorithms, Journal of Advanced Research in Dynamical and Control Systems, Vol. 10, No. 2: 2330–2344 (2018).
52. Rosak-Szyrocka, J., Żywiolek, J., Kulinska, E., Matulewski, M. Analysis of Enterprises' Readiness in for Industry 4.0 Implementation: The Case of Poland. ERSJ, XXIV, 615–628 (2021).
53. K. Balachander, S. Ramesh, Ahmed J. Obaid. Simulation Of 1KW Multi-Level Switch Mode Power Amplifier, International Journal of Innovations in Scientific and Engineering Research, Vol. 5, No. 9: 85–92 (2018).
54. Saba Alyasiri, Ahmed J. Obaid. A New Approach for Object Detection, Recognition and Retrieving in Painting Images, Journal of Advanced Research in Dynamical and Control Systems, Vol. 10, No. 2: 2345–2359 (2018).
55. H. Chhabra, V. Mohan, A. Rani, and V. Singh, "Trajectory tracking of Maryland manipulator using linguistic Lyapunov fuzzy controller," Journal of Intelligent & Fuzzy Systems, vol. 36, no. 3, pp. 2195–2205, (2019).

56. A. Rawat, S. Jha, B. Kumar, and V. Mohan, "Nonlinear fractional order PID controller for tracking maximum power in photo-voltaic system," Journal of Intelligent & Fuzzy Systems, vol. 38, no. 5, pp. 6703–6713, (2020).
57. O. M. Abo-Seida, N. T. M. El-dabe, A. Refaie Ali and G. A. Shalaby, "Cherenkov FEL Reaction with Plasma-Filled Cylindrical Waveguide in Fractional D-Dimensional Space," in IEEE Transactions on Plasma Science, vol. 49, no. 7, pp. 2070–2079, July (2021).
58. Osama M. Abo-Seida, N.T.M.Eldabe, Ahmed Refaie Ali, & Gamil.Ali Shalaby. Far-Field, Radiation Resistance and temperature of Hertzian Dipole Antenna in Lossless Medium with Momentum and Energy Flow in the Far- Zone. Journal of Advances in Physics, 18, 20–28 (2020).
59. Żywiołek, J.; Rosak-Szyrocka, J.; Jereb, B. Barriers to Knowledge Sharing in the Field of Information Security. Management Systems in Production Engineering, 29, 114–119 (2021).
60. N.T.M. El-Dabe, A.Refaie Ali, A.A. El-shekhipy, Influence of Thermophoresis on Unsteady MHD Flow of Radiation Absorbing Kuvshinski Fluid with Non-Linear Heat and Mass Transfer, American Journal of Heat and Mass Transfer (2017).
61. Osama M. Abo-Seida, N.T.M.Eldabe, M. Abu-Shady, A.Refaie Ali, " Electromagnetic non-Darcy Forchheimer flow and heat transfer over a nonlinearly stretching sheet of non-Newtonian fluid in the presence of a non-uniform heat source", Solid State Technology, Vol. 63 No. 6 (2020).
62. N.T. El-dabel; A.Refaie Ali; A. El-shekhipy, A.; and A. Shalaby, G. "Non-Linear Heat and Mass Transfer of Second Grade Fluid Flow with Hall Currents and Thermophoresis Effects," Applied Mathematics & Information Sciences: Vol. 11: Iss. 1, Article 73 (2017).

The Role of Augmented Reality and Virtual Reality in Smart Health Education: State of the Art and Perspectives

M. Raja and G. G. Lakshmi Priya

1 Introduction

Over the last twenty years, the corporate world has been changing drastically. The use of the web and social applications and systems, including smartphones, tablets, and PCs, is closely attributed to the majority of such changes. Such technologies are constantly improving and gaining greater significance in our everyday lives. Artificial intelligence (AI), the Internet of things (IoT), robotics, augmented reality (AR), and virtual reality (VR) are the most recent technological advancements. Specific industries have delayed understanding how to safeguard or divert their present operational paradigms from disruptive technologies since more enterprises adjust to such emerging technologies. The system of education, notably higher education, has battled to embrace this digital revolution fully. Two main issues are causing this resilience. The first issue is comprehensive. It relates to institutions' incapacity to support the digital investments required to develop innovative hardware and software tools while perhaps abandoning current infrastructure. The second issue is teachers' incompetence or unwillingness to adjust and use the most up-to-date innovations to satisfy students' changing needs. Yet, the employment of digital technologies in educational sectors has progressed dramatically in current years at every degree of education, from primary schools to postgraduate universities. As a result, administrators now have greater possibilities to adopt new tools and enhance the academic knowledge for the digital inhabitants. While using digital technology could enable learners to become more motivated to learn and improve their abilities, administrators confront the issue of finding, assessing, and choosing the appropriate

M. Raja · G. G. L. Priya (✉)
Department of Multimedia, VIT School of Design, Vellore Institute of Technology, Vellore, Tamil Nadu, India
e-mail: raja.m@vit.ac.in; lakshmipriya.gg@vit.ac.in

P. Agarwal et al. (eds.), *Artificial Intelligence for Smart Healthcare*,
EAI/Springer Innovations in Communication and Computing,
https://doi.org/10.1007/978-3-031-23602-0_18

technology to meet these objectives. Administrators need to stay current on subjects relating to their field to identify acceptable technology that could improve their students' education [1].

AR and VR are promising methodologies with a wide range of benefits and applicability in various fields. They offer sophisticated platforms for communication, navigating, and participation in the education system. A variety of benefits and applications of these technologies can assist both students and teachers. Yet, specific considerations should be addressed when integrating AR and VR into the educational process. First and foremost, they should assist pupils in their academic endeavors. Secondly, their health, protection, and data security should not be jeopardized. In terms of virtual reality, it could be employed to achieve a variety of goals, including providing students with new general understanding (e.g., technical information, illustrations, and explanations), specialized techniques and abilities (e.g., technological records, processes, and prototypes), and enhancing developed technical skills (e.g., measurements, maneuvers, and technical expertise). AR, primarily a learning environment, shall utilize magic books, learning items, or unique locations. Physical books with virtual material have been incorporated into genuine manuals, students' instructions and tutorials, activities, and exam sheets for magic books. Students can use particular and intriguing materials and study using AR for artifacts (e.g., an electrical circuit and a fossil). They offer intriguing information about the locations, institutions, and objects in ancient, geological, and fossil areas for AR applications depending on locales. Several instructional goals could be met by incorporating AR and VR into the educational process. They could be utilized to teach and learn much about a difficult idea and supplement a course and conduct an experiment. To avoid overloading pupils with data and causing health problems, they must be used for limited periods and just a few times per day. Furthermore, the use of AR over VR must be emphasized for children and elementary school pupils. Whether adults and children, pupils are more aware and can perform secure AR and VR educational experiences [2].

VR can be used to achieve various goals, including providing students with new general understanding (i.e., analytical information, descriptions, and explanations), specialized technologies, and talents (i.e., analytical documentation, processes, and prototypes). It also enhances sophisticated practical knowledge (e.g., measurements, maneuvers, and technical expertise) [3]. AR, primarily a teaching approach, can use magic books, educational items, or unique locations [4]. In teaching, augmented reality has proven to be highly beneficial. The young students now visualize complex spatial linkages and abstract ideas. This platform allows pupils to participate in events that are impossible to replicate in the actual world. Furthermore, AR can easily visualize invisible phenomena such as magnetic fields [5].

Several computer-based solutions were developed to create novel experiences in teaching and learning because it is such an important concept. Various investigators have focused on incorporating AR and VR into educational settings during the last two decades. Students and academics, for example, can utilize virtual legacy as a medium in their investigations of historical incidents, according to [6]. AR has been proved in studies to improve educating and studying practices in the educational field [7]. Educating, learning, and instructional strategies have all benefited from the use of AR and VR. Nevertheless, there is presently no study that investigates the academic impacts of AR and VR technology empirically. AR is a methodology that integrates digitalized content with data from real-world settings, allowing students to communicate with virtual things while concurrently viewing the real world (typically with the assistance of a digital camera on a smartphone or tablet). VR, on the other hand, uses digital images to create real-time immersive simulations. Consequently, AR incorporates virtual things into a physical location, while VR isolates information from the physical world and sends people to a completely virtual world. To put it another way, VR gives users the sensation of being mentally engaged in a virtual world, while AR lets them communicate with both virtual and real-world objects. As a result, the benefits of AR and VR are vastly different [8].

We gathered papers published between 2010 and 2020 from Google Scholar using the keywords augmented reality, virtual reality, and education to acquire a complete overview of the topic for our study. A total of 250 publications appropriate for this research were chosen and assessed utilizing inclusion criteria. The research must provide experimental outcomes, one of the inclusion requirements (the user study). We excluded articles that used augmented reality and virtual reality in domains apart from education, bringing the total number of publications to 39. The collected journals and conference articles were briefly inspected, and only those significant to this study's topic were chosen for a more thorough examination. A sum of 39 papers was chosen for final reading based on this survey's requirements. This paper is structured as follows: A detailed discussion on the role of augmented reality and virtual reality is available in Sects. 2 and 3, respectively. Intending to address the current trends and issues in adopting AR and VR in education, Sect. 4 discussed the recent advancements of AR/VR in education, followed by challenges of adopting AR/VR in education in Sect. 5. Finally, the future scope of AR/VR in education is discussed in Sect 6, followed by the conclusion as the final chapter.

2 Augmented Reality (AR) in Education

The adoption of AR in the educational sector is similar to that of mobile learning (mLearning). While learning hailed as a game-changer in the classroom, it evolved into a valuable supplement rather than an essential element of instruction. Many concerns, particularly screen size limitations, difficulties developing and creating educational content, and excessive pricing, have contributed to mLearning's inability to reach original academic predictions. These same concerns are affecting the widespread utilization of AR in the educational sector. Furthermore, many AR applications rely on mobile technology and mobile devices like tablets and smartphones. The impact of current AR innovations, like smart glasses, has yet to be assessed, although early indications are promising [9]. The "reality–virtuality continuum" displayed in Fig. 1 can be used to describe the AR paradigm. The real world is depicted on the left, while the virtual environment is depicted on the right.

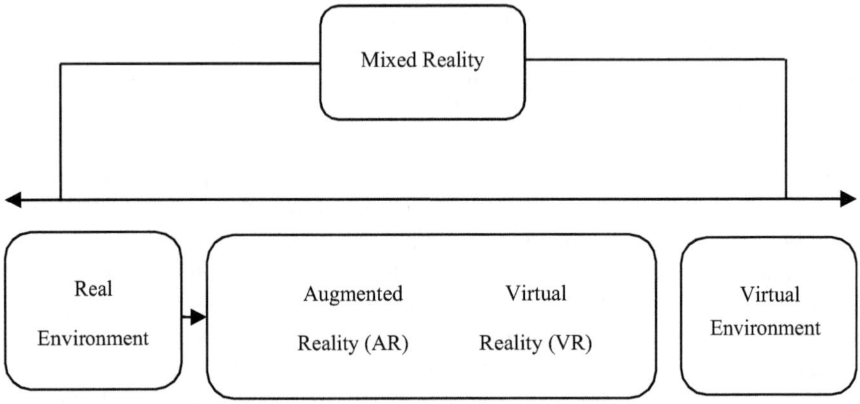

Fig. 1 Reality–virtuality continuum

As a result, AR is closer to the actual surroundings, VR is more relative to the virtual surroundings, and MR is somewhere in between because it combines both AR and VR.

The use of augmented reality on a mobile device can help students learn more effectively. Mayer's spatial and continuity theories from the multimodal learning hypothesis describe these findings. As per the authors, offering appropriate data (e.g., images, documents, videos) that are well-integrated and arranged may assist in decreasing inadvertent cognitive burdens—the students' learning efficiency increases as a result of this [10]. Most research found that using AR technology in education led to "improved educational performance" in classrooms. AR has been shown in various studies to improve educational outcomes [11, 12]. According to [13], the learners had a favorable attitude toward the AR-improved educational process in their analysis. They seemed to be having a good time as they "learned through play." They concluded that AR improved students' academic achievement. In a further investigation, the researchers determined that using a portable AR device could boost learners' educational outcomes [14]. AR that may be used in a variety of settings is indeed accessible in an education setting. AR could be applied in various school environments, including physics, chemistry, biology, mathematics, geometry, and foreign language teaching. The application of augmented reality in educational contexts can give information in three dimensions, generate concurrent and cooperative learning possibilities, render the hidden visible, and connect formal and informal education. On the other side, this innovation piques students' curiosity, boosts their desire, allows them to pass on events that aren't possible in the actual world, and improves collaboration and engagement between instructors and students. It also enhances students' creativeness, guarantees that they choose their preferred learning style and finish the learning experience at their own pace, and allows for the creation of distinct academic settings suited to different ways of education. In the educational process, AR additionally offers the opportunity to solve various challenges. Certain students, for instance, have trouble visualizing the micro and macro environments in their brains. AR may educate very small microstructures like atoms and molecules and model extremely vast macro systems like planets and galaxies [15]. AR has several educational benefits. These advantages for pupils can be outlined as follows: enjoyable courses, reduce cognitive load, boost interest and enthusiasm in the course, provide more possibilities for students to ask questions, enhance student engagement, provide new opportunities for individual learning, concretize complex ideas, and increase achievement. For teachers, these advantages include promoting innovation in students, assuring good student involvement in the course, and allowing students to complete the course at their own pace [16].

3 Virtual Reality (VR) in Education

It is widely known that the usage of communication and information technology improves students' learning and academics. It is a fast-expanding field of study that is constantly evolving and seeking new technical remedies. In recent years, VR that creates an interacting computer-developed world has progressed from entertainment to professional development areas like defense, psychology, healthcare, and education [17]. Virtual reality has several features that can help student participation. It is a fresh approach to studying for pupils, giving compelling, unique experiences they might not have experienced previously, as it is a hands-on, engaging, interactive experience. For instance, Google Expeditions enables teachers to take students on virtual field trips to Mars, the lower part of the oceans, and a variety of other locations that can pique students' curiosity, create mutual experiences for greater classroom debate, and boost overall participation. Novel and innovative educational opportunities like this entice kids and stimulate their interest, proactively investigating and exercising their interest. This enhanced involvement may present a chance to discuss subjects that are generally dull or unappealing. VR has sparked a renewed enthusiasm in archaeology, particularly in areas where attention had previously waned. Virtual reality's uniqueness and enjoyment factor could be carefully exploited to attract the attention of distracted and disengaged pupils, even in areas that are generally uninteresting or unimportant to them. Compared to conventional learning environments, VR increases students' engagement by giving a powerful sensation of existence and engagement. Everyone has varying degrees of existence, reading books in a classroom, casually watching movies, seeing performance theatre, and the most engaged, literally embodied characters and things in VR. VR brings a topic matter to life by immersing students in immersive, multisensory experiences. In The Body VR, learners can, for example, explore within the human body's bloodstream like a red blood cell. One of the most crucial prospects for VR to develop more engaging learning opportunities is its capacity to imitate an environment and increase a child's sense of existence [18]. VR is utilized in different ways to support the teaching–learning process; a few examples are mentioned in Fig. 2.

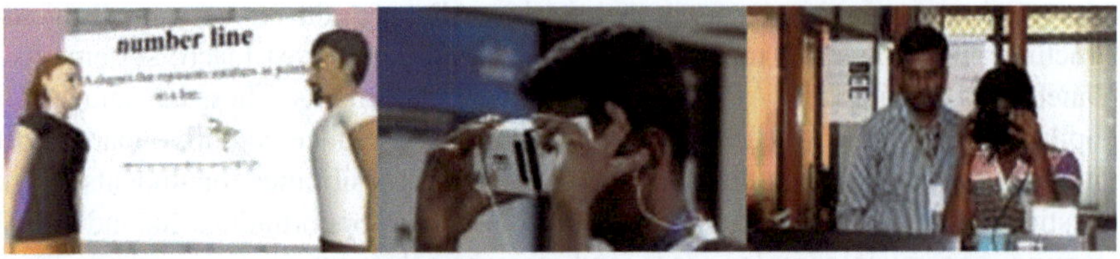

(a) (b) (c)

Fig. 2 Various kinds of VR utilized for education. (**a**) PC VR without the need of HMD, (**b**) a student experiencing cardboard VR, (**c**) a student experiencing Oculus Rift

"Immersive environments" are the constantly changing types of digital and computer-dependent education [19]. Students can be completely engaged in a self-contained simulated or virtual surrounding while perceiving it as if it were realistic. Virtual settings can provide students with comprehensive and complicated content-based educational experiences while enhancing their technological, imaginative, and problem-solving abilities. Users tend to be very interested in virtual reality since they are so rich and appealing. Virtual reality, web-based game consoles, hugely multiplayer digital games, multiuser virtual worlds, simulations, and augmented reality are all examples of immersive environments [20]. Some may claim that VR isn't essential for teaching because movies and presentations are sufficient for teaching topics. VR, on the other hand, creates a degree of engagement that conventional media cannot match. Clients feel more engaged with information in VR since they can communicate with it and distribute it individually. Unlike televisions, where the experience is from a third-person viewpoint, VR provides a realistic first-person viewpoint. This essential feature provides VR with a lot of instructional possibilities. A novel, creative education systems, technological developments, and programs geared to render technology available to as many schools as possible are reshaping education for students and teachers alike. Education has changed in several aspects in the last five years, so it's hard to predict the destination of this turbulence. In a wide context, AR and VR reforms head in the same direction to expand the educational experience for all children. Instructors are delivering material to students in whole-class education, which is transforming class methods. More lectures are now offered online or in a hybrid format, which combines online and face-to-face instruction. Educators are also flipping courses, in which children receive a video lecture as an assignment and use classroom time to collaborate and use what they've learned to diverse issues [21].

Furthermore, virtual reality makes the learning process essential because it can bring practical experience into the classrooms without abandoning it. Through simulations and virtual encounters, VR may supplement traditional teaching. Several advantages of using VR in the educational sector and training have previously been established [22]. Several educational organizations and universities are already using virtual reality technology for commercial reasons. The great majority of elite universities use it to recruit potential children in many methods. VR is an ideal technique for student recruiting because it allows institutions to approach, interact, and connect to prospective students via virtual campus visits.

4 Recent Advancements of AR/VR in Education

AR can enhance biological teaching and could be a useful teaching tool in situations where visualizing 3D objects is knowledge acquisition. Given the increasing problems encountered in higher education in the post-COVID-19 environment, where immersive contents bolster distant education, efficient development of the learning environment is critical. Consequently, it's conceivable that augmented reality is becoming a more common method of delivering digital material. Significantly, the appropriateness of AR-based tasks in connection to the essential topics being represented and the educational targets specified must be carefully considered. While more research is needed to evaluate if AR improves overall student achievement, there are still chances to broaden the classrooms in several topic areas beyond structural biology [23].

According to studies, AR/VR systems are extremely advantageous to education and can assist students in improving their experience and competencies very effectively. AR/VR technologies can display instructional materials in engaging ways, increasing student motivation and engagement. Students not only love AR/VR education, but they also pursue learning strategies, allowing AR/VR technologies to assist them in gaining correct knowledge. Academic challenges, which have been discussed in the educational literature, can be better understood with AR/VR technology. Some kids, for example, are unable to see 3D representations or envision unseen events like the earth spinning. Students can see 3D models, control things digitally, deduce immeasurable occurrences, and encounter complex ideas via AR/VR (e.g., travel in wormholes). Such virtual insights shall help students think more critically and address mistakes. Recent AR/VR technology advancements enable cooperation and communication between many perceptions and a world using multisensory gadgets. Sensory integration provides learners to construct meaning from experiences [24]. Virtual reality technology can deliver real-time communication and allow children to participate in a virtual classroom simultaneously. Children can use sensory integration to create meaning from their experiences [25]. They shall talk about it, get rapid feedback from others, and feel like they're in the same room as their colleagues [26]. Virtual reality also promotes healthy lifestyle by enabling the students to stay active while they learn. Healthcare workers and graduate students of medical schools can both learn practical skills in a hazard-free environment with the aid of VR software. A hard, risky, or unaffordable scenario in real life can be simulated using this form of healthcare VR.

In reality, the connection between AR/VR and education improves education and learning efficiency and stimulation. Despite this, there is no infrastructure designed exclusively to create AR/VR information, even by nonprogrammers rapidly. So, new technologies must be established to facilitate users to become providers of these encounters quickly. As a result, a novel framework known as ScoolAR was designed to facilitate teachers to design tailored pedagogical initiatives involving students in the instructional activity. This resulted in increased engagement and information recognition, handled in the development of AR and VR technologies, and declined within disciplinary subject matters [27]. Many consumer-oriented activities are now possible because of the latest innovations in virtual reality (VR) technologies and the increasing accessibility of VR-equipped gadgets. Nevertheless, for inexperienced designers, building engaging sceneries for virtual environments is a time-consuming and challenging operation requiring a high level of technical understanding that is frequently lacking. This limits the ability of amateurs to build, alter, and implement their own interactive virtual reality situations. Though current authoring tools for immersive VR scenes seem intriguing, most of them focus on skilled professionals and ignore amateurs with less programming experience. They created VREUD, an open-source web-based end-user development (EUD) platform that facilitates the quick creation and implementation of immersive VR environments to decrease the entrance hurdle. VREUD allows for the characterization of the VR scenario, comprising relationships and activities in terms of architecture. VREUD also facilitates the implementation and engaging storyline of generated immersive VR scenarios on VR head-mounted displays [28].

Instructional technologies have recently demonstrated significant gains in learners' visual short-term memory, problem-solving, situational awareness, and multitasking abilities compared to conventional educational media. Educators are increasingly interested in experiencing instructional information in immersive environments and have developed "digital reality" to incorporate AR, VR, MR, immersive experience, and artificial intelligence. Students are allowed to explore or create instructional content utilizing games in this class. As academics investigated its characteristics, benefits, and restrictions, there has been a gradual growth in the usage of virtual reality in education. Because these virtual environments can affect how people think and behave, they can be used in educational settings. The way students use technology in education has evolved. With the current generation of children preferring visual learning, innovative advancements in technology such as MR, AR, VR, and computer games are gaining momentum. The majority of today's students are primarily reliant on various ways of education and instructing. Only a small percentage of them are willing to devote effort to reading and studying material. Instead, they prefer to watch movies and learn new things, which they feel more comfortable doing. In addition, students in the class express a desire for a different teaching style than the conventional ones. Teachers convey their worries about the test-based teaching methods, that is, educating to the exam [29].

Table 1 Comparative framework of the familiar designs of head-mounted displays (HMD) for AR/VR utilized for educational sectors

Technologies	AR/ V R	Benefits	Drawbacks
HTC Vive Pro	VR	DS: 1440 × 1600 per eye Field of view ~110 Exterior virtual regulators Area of tracing: 10 m × 10 m	Load: 550 g Cost ~1099 $ Longer deployment duration
Oculus Quest	VR	DS: 1440 × 1600 per eye Field of view ~90 Exterior virtual regulators Movable	Load: 571 g Cost ~500 $
Samsung Gear VR	VR	DS: 1480 × 1440 per eye (smartphone-based) Load: 345 g + smartphones Cost: 130 € Movable	Field of view ≈101 Less battery span Computational abilities (smartphone-based) Absence of positional tracing
Google Cardboard	VR	Load ~ smartphones Cost: 7 € Movable	DS: smartphone-based Field of view ~90 Less battery span Computational abilities (smartphone-based) Absence of positional tracing
Microsoft HoloLens	AR	Easy to use Gesture recognition Resolution Clicker	Cost ~3000 $ Vision is limited Bulky and too complicated
Vuzix Blade	AR	Voice control, touchpad Clear camera Easy-to-use features	Cost ~1000 $ Battery requires more work It has a fragile nature
Epson Moverio BT-300	AR	GPS, geomagnetic, accelerometer, gyroscopic, lighting sensors Operated by remotes	Price ~700 $

5 Challenges of Adopting AR/VR in Education

Students can use AR/VR goods to overcome learning obstacles and increase their knowledge, abilities, reasoning, and comprehension. Nevertheless, there are problems and limitations to using AR/VR in most classroom settings as a teaching tool. The first issue is the cost of deploying AR/VR equipment in place. HMDs, as we've seen, are pretty costly. A comparative framework of the familiar designs of head-mounted displays (HMD) for AR/VR utilized for educational sectors is juxtaposed in Table 1. Simulator illnesses are another adverse effect that isn't confined to HMDs and appears predominantly in VR experiences. Simulator illness is caused by a discrepancy between visual perception and motion perception. Nausea, dizziness, and pain are some of the indications of simulator illness [31]. In some circumstances, computers and display equipment must demonstrate the VR/AR items, which may be difficult for many organizations. The inadequacy of realism in VR or AR simulations is the second issue. The quality of a user's graphics display can enhance visual perception and give a more rich experience [32–35]. The third issue is health and its physical consequences for children. HMDs are pretty hefty, and wearing them for an extended amount of time may cause weariness [36]. Although current HMDs have lenses that are close to the eye, they may impair vision. The fourth difficulty stems from hardware restrictions. While recent technological advancements have improved AR and VR presentations, constraints may prevent users from experiencing a higher degree of user experience [37–41]. Inadequacy of efficiency, GPS inaccuracies, maritime issues, the lag between sensor information, and visual system consequences are prevalent issues that can frustrate pupils and disrupt their learning.

In the use of AR and VR in education, three major technological hurdles have been recognized: (1) using an ad hoc interface to regulate the camera, (2) positioning the camera so that it does not interfere with students while still providing the teacher with an ideal angle of view, and (3) layering the media files into a video content that also currently requires proprietary code and thus provides a black box for video editing. Addressing these issues could improve higher education's technical integration into a 360-degree video production process [30].

6 Future Scope of AR/VR in Education

Owing to the utilization of virtual educational facilities, which encourage adaptable, transparent, and cooperative education beyond time, character, and location restrictions within virtual classrooms of academic organizations across the globe, provocative advances in technology like VR/AR shall gain critical significance in the coming days [31]. Furthermore, virtual surroundings offer actual and engaging role-playing scenarios in which children congregate and communicate efficiently, having a distributed sense of being connected in a virtual area where education is an action that is not dependent on an environmental area [40, 48–50]. Moreover, virtual surroundings have been observed to possess distinctive educational benefits, such as producing virtual educational settings and facilitating a more extensive range of classes to be educated. They also communally link people and institutions from all over the nation and the globe "who you would likely never meet in real life" [41].

AR/VR can assist distance learners in education by allowing students to employ AR/VR interfaces to understand topics and concepts more quickly [42]. Students could use AR/VR 3D creations to gain a better understanding of an idea. It's also employed to develop animations and virtual experiences of concepts before they're implemented in the actual world [43]. Aside from schooling, augmented and virtual reality could be utilized to market products. Exhibits and event activations, for instance, employ augmented reality to display content in a more participatory

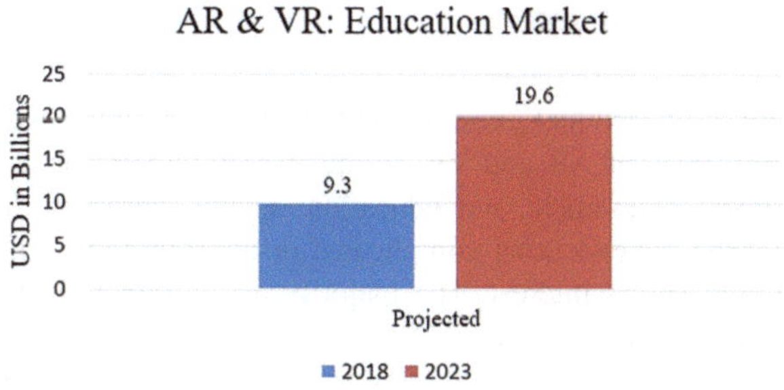

Fig. 3 Opportunities in the AR and VR market concerning education

manner. The AR/VR concept can be developed in various ways and for various areas, including real estate, tourism, education, coaching and training, and the medical world [44–47]. VR could be used in tourism to promote hotel tours and activities, vacation destinations, and tourist packages and deals. For medical purposes, VR could help to reduce anxiety and fear associated with vaccines, injections, and blood draws in children, adolescents, and adults [21]. Though there are many obstacles to the employment of VR environments, including academic property authorities and digitalized media administration architectures, there is proof of their possibility for cooperation, innovation, and learning in private and public education.

Educators can employ augmented reality to help students build higher-level thinking abilities by fostering learning by designs, which requires skills including assessment, analysis, and creativity, all of which contribute to students' overall progress. A future approach would be to reconstruct the virtual environment for VR applications to simplify the development and design procedure and make it a multidisciplinary research field. The market for AR and VR is drastically expanding; especially the educational sector has started embracing these technologies. The project market size during the year 2023 is more than double the size compared to that of the year 2018 (Fig. 3). The "realistic settings" and "basic interaction" design aspects appear across all types of VR systems in our study, according to our findings. As a result, these might be considered the fundamental design criteria for instructional virtual reality applications. VR programs that aim to improve factual knowledge can be suggested to get students interested in VR in the classroom. From our linkage of design features and academic results, we can observe that most declarative knowledge applications use only those two design features. As a result, these aspects can serve as a soft launchpad for VR development. They are simple to utilize by teachers and students and do not necessitate any curricular revisions.

7 Conclusion

We offer a concise, comprehensive, and non-exhaustive literature evaluation of the influences of AR and VR on the educational sector in this article. Students' intellectual assessment and education, which increases the high-level understanding needed for executing complicated or nonroutine activities, has piqued the research community's interest. The majority of the papers in this study were found in the ScienceDirect (Elsevier), Springer Link, and Scopus database journals. Despite a count of limitations and threats to implementing AR/VR environments in the academic areas, the findings revealed that AR/VR apps could be a valuable tool for improving learning and memory because they provide engaged multisensory settings with numerous sensory elements. Users engage with virtual and augmented surroundings in multimodal ways, using the haptic auditory and visual abilities to fulfill the requirements. It's also shown that much proof shows pupils' academic, social, and thinking ideas improve drastically. Such innovations, when used correctly, can improve the modern education system and provide students with more opportunities to learn. In any event, AR/VR shall alter the manner we communicate with the actual environment in the coming years and will be widely accepted across all domains. Future studies may want to look at the survey's upcoming research points on both the sound and adverse effects of VR/AR technologies on learning. While AR and VR are undeniably beneficial to use current technology in the classroom, they are not without hazards or disadvantages. One of the most serious problems is a lack of flexibility. Students can ask questions, receive a response, and participate in discussions in regular courses. Students use a virtual reality headset with specific software to obey the rules and cannot do anything other than what they are instructed to do. Some instructors are naturally averse to change, and thus active involvement and participation are critical for the successful integration of technology into the classroom. Others may over-rely on technology advancements, resulting in a lack of teacher–student interaction.

References

1. McGovern, E., Moreira, G. and Luna-Nevarez, C.: An application of virtual reality in education: Can this technology enhance the quality of students' learning experience? *Journal of education for business*, 95(7), pp. 490–496 (2020).
2. Elkoubaiti, H. and Mrabet, R.: October. How are augmented and virtual reality used in smart classrooms?. In Proceedings of the 2nd International Conference on Smart Digital Environment, pp. 189–196, (2018).
3. Górski, F., Buń, P., Wichniarek, R., Zawadzki, P. and Hamrol, A.: Effective design of educational virtual reality applications for medicine using knowledge-engineering techniques. *EURASIA Journal of Mathematics, Science and Technology Education*, 13(2), pp. 395–416 (2016).

4. Santos, M.E.C., Chen, A., Taketomi, T., Yamamoto, G., Miyazaki, J. and Kato, H.: Augmented reality learning experiences: Survey of prototype design and evaluation. *IEEE Transactions on learning technologies*, 7(1), pp. 38–56 (2013).
5. Aggarwal, R. and Singhal, A.: January. Augmented reality and its effect on our life. In 2019 9th International Conference on Cloud Computing, Data Science & Engineering, pp. 510–515, IEEE (2019).
6. Noh, Z., M.S. Sunar and Z. Pan.: A review on augmented reality for virtual heritage system. Proceedings of the International Conference on Technologies for E-Learning and Digital Entertainment, (EDE'09), Springer, Berlin, Heidelberg, pp: 50–61 (2009).
7. Dalim, C.S.C., Kolivand, H., Kadhim, H., Sunar, M.S. and Billinghurst, M.: Factors influencing the acceptance of augmented reality in education: A review of the literature. *Journal of computer science*, 13(11), pp. 581–589 (2017).
8. Huang, K.T., Ball, C., Francis, J., Ratan, R., Boumis, J. and Fordham, J.: Augmented versus virtual reality in education: an exploratory study examining science knowledge retention when using augmented reality/virtual reality mobile applications. *Cyberpsychology, Behavior, and Social Networking*, 22(2), pp. 105–110 (2019).
9. Wang, M., Callaghan, V., Bernhardt, J., White, K. and Peña-Rios, A.: Augmented reality in education and training: pedagogical approaches and illustrative case studies. *Journal of ambient intelligence and humanized computing*, 9(5), pp. 1391–1402 (2018).
10. Akçayır, M. and Akçayır, G.: Advantages and challenges associated with augmented reality for education: A systematic review of the literature. *Educational Research Review*, 20, pp. 1–11 (2017).
11. Chang, Y.-L., Hou, H.-T., Pan, C.-Y., Sung, Y.-T., & Chang, K.-E.: Apply an augmented reality in a mobile guidance to increase the sense of place for heritage places. *Journal of Educational Technology & Society*, 18(2), 166–178 (2015).
12. Ferrer-Torregrosa, J., Torralba, J., Jimenez, M., García, S., & Barcia, J.: ARBOOK: Development and Assessment of a Tool Based on Augmented Reality for Anatomy. *Journal of Science Education and Technology*, 24(1), 119–124 (2015).
13. Lu, S.-J., & Liu, Y.-C.: Integrating augmented reality technology to enhance children's learning in marine education. *Environmental Education Research*, 21(4), 525–541 (2015).
14. Chiang, T. H., Yang, S. J., & Hwang, G.-J.: An Augmented Reality-based Mobile Learning System to Improve Students' Learning Achievements and Motivations in Natural Science Inquiry Activities. *Journal of Educational Technology & Society*, 17(4), 352–365, (2014a).
15. Altinpulluk, H.: Determining the trends of using augmented reality in education between 2006–2016. *Education and Information Technologies*, 24(2), pp. 1089–1114 (2019).
16. Kurubacak, G. and Altinpulluk, H. eds. Mobile technologies and augmented reality in open education. Igi Global (2017).
17. Kamińska, D., Sapiński, T., Wiak, S., Tikk, T., Haamer, R.E., Avots, E., Helmi, A., Ozcinar, C. and Anbarjafari, G.: Virtual reality and its applications in education: Survey. *Information,* 10(10), p. 318 (2019).
18. Hu-Au, E. and Lee, J.J.: Virtual reality in education: a tool for learning in the experience age. *International Journal of Innovation in Education*, 4(4), pp. 215–226 (2017).
19. M. Burns.: Immersive Learning for Teacher Professional Development, eCampus News, January (2016).
20. Velev, D. and Zlateva, P.: Virtual reality challenges in education and training. International Journal of Learning and Teaching, 3(1), pp. 33–37 (2017).
21. Al-Gindy, A., Felix, C., Ahmed, A., Matoug, A. and Alkhidir, M.: Virtual reality: Development of an integrated learning environment for education. *International Journal of Information and Education Technology*, 10(3), pp. 171–175 (2020).
22. M. Jenner.: 99p Virtual Reality and the implications for video in HE, November (2015).
23. Reeves, L.E., Bolton, E., Bulpitt, M., Scott, A., Tomey, I., Gates, M. and Baldock, R.A.: Use of augmented reality (AR) to aid bioscience education and enrich student experience. *Research in Learning Technology*, 29, p. 2572 (2021).

24. Ardiny, H. and Khanmirza, E.: The role of AR and VR technologies in education developments: opportunities and challenges. In 2018 6th RSI International Conference on Robotics and Mechatronics (IcRoM), pp. 482–487, IEEE (2018).
25. C. Christou.: "Virtual reality in education," in Affective, interactive and cognitive methods for e-learning design: creating an optimal education experience. IGI Global, pp. 228–243 (2010).
26. T. Monahan, G. McArdle, and M. Bertolotto.: "Virtual reality for collaborative e-learning," *Computers & Education*, vol. 50, no. 4, pp. 1339–1353, (2008).
27. Puggioni, M.P., Frontoni, E., Paolanti, M., Pierdicca, R., Malinverni, E.S. and Sasso, M.: A content creation tool for AR/VR applications in education: The ScoolAR framework. In International conference on augmented reality, virtual reality and computer graphics, pp. 205–219. Springer, Cham (2020).
28. Yigitbas, E., Klauke, J., Gottschalk, S. and Engels, G.: VREUD--An End-User Development Tool to Simplify the Creation of Interactive VR Scenes (2021). arXiv preprint arXiv:2107.00377.
29. Vemula, S.: Leveraging VR/AR/MR and AI as Innovative Educational Practices for "iGeneration" Students. In Handbook of Research on Equity in Computer Science in P-16 Education, pp. 265–277. IGI Global (2021).
30. Feurstein, M.S.: Towards an integration of 360-degree video in higher education. Workflow, challenges and scenarios (2018).
31. Lytras MD, Mathkour HI, Abdalla H, Al-Halabi W, Yanez-Marquez C, Siqueira SWM.: An emerging–Social and emerging computing enabled philosophical paradigm for collaborative learning systems: toward high effective next-generation learning systems for the knowledge society. *Comput Hum Behav* 51:557–561 (2015).
32. Furió D, GonzáLez-Gancedo S, Juan MC, Seguí I, Costa M.: The effects of the size and weight of a mobile device on an educational game. *Comput Educ* 64:24–41 (2013).
33. F. J. J. Joseph.: Effect of supervised learning methodologies in offline handwritten Thai character recognition, *Int. J. Inf. Technol.*, vol. 12, no. 1, pp. 57–64, Mar. (2020).
34. Wisetsri, W., & Maaz, U. D.: The Influence of Leadership, Work Motivation and Organizational Culture on Job Performance. *International Journal of Psychosocial Rehabilitation*, 24(5): 7336–7350 (2020).
35. V. Pattana-anake, P. Danphitsanuparn, and F. J. J. John Joseph.: "BettaNet : A Deep Learning Architecture for Classification of Wild Siamese Betta Species," IOP Conf. Ser. *Mater. Sci. Eng.*, vol. 1055, (2021). https://doi.org/10.1088/1757-899X/1055/1/012104.
36. Sadiq, S., Umer, M., Ullah, S., Mirjalili, S., Rupapara, V., & NAPPI, M.: Discrepancy detection between actual user reviews and numeric ratings of Google App store using deep learning. Expert Systems with Applications, 115111 (2021). https://doi.org/10.1016/j.eswa.2021.115111.
37. Listiningrum, H. D., Wisetsri, W., & Boussanlegue, T.: Principal's Entrepreneurship Competence in Improving Teacher's Entrepreneurial Skill in High Schools. *Journal of Social Work and Science Education*, 1(1), 87–95 (2021).
38. F. J. John Joseph, S. Nonsiri, and A. Monsakul.: Keras and Tensorflow – A Hands on Experience, in Advanced Deep Learning for Engineers And Scientists: A Practical Approach, Switzerland: Springer Nature Switzerland AG, (2020).
39. Obaid A.J., Alghurabi K.A., Albermany S.A.K., Sharma S.: Improving Extreme Learning Machine Accuracy Utilizing Genetic Algorithm for Intrusion Detection Purposes. Research in Intelligent and Computing in Engineering. Advances in Intelligent Systems and Computing, vol 1254. Springer, Singapore (2021). https://doi.org/10.1007/978-981-15-7527-3_17
40. Rustam, F., Khalid, M., Aslam, W., Rupapara, V., Mehmood, A., & Choi, G. S.: A performance comparison of supervised machine learning models for Covid-19 tweets sentiment analysis. *Plos One*, 16(2), e0245909 (2021). https://doi.org/10.1371/journal.pone.0245909
41. H. Pallathadka, M. Mustafa, D. T. Sanchez, G. Sekhar Sajja, S. Gour, and M. Naved.: "Impact of machine learning on management, healthcare and agriculture," Materials Today: Proceedings, (2021).

42. Ebrahimi M., Obaid A.J., Yeganegi K.: Protecting Cloud Data Privacy Against Attacks. In: Favorskaya M.N., Peng SL., Simic M., Alhadidi B., Pal S. (eds) Intelligent Computing Paradigm and Cutting-edge Technologies. ICICCT 2020. Learning and Analytics in Intelligent Systems, vol. 21. Springer, Cham (2021). https://doi.org/10.1007/978-3-030-65407-8_37
43. Kumar, S., Kumar, P., Wisetsri, W., Raza, M. & Norabuena-Figueroa, R.P.: Social entrepreneurship education: Insights from the Indian higher educational courses. Academy of Strategic Management Journal, 20(S1), 1–14 (2021).
44. S S Rajest, P. Suresh.: "Impact of 21st century's different heads of learning skills for students and teachers" in International Journal of Multidisciplinary Research and Development, Volume: V, Issue IV, Page No.: 170–178 (2018).
45. J. F. Joe.: "Enhanced sensitivity of motion detection in satellite videos using instant learning algorithms," IET Chennai 3rd International on Sustainable Energy and Intelligent Systems, pp. 1–6, (2012). https://doi.org/10.1049/cp.2012.2250.
46. D. K. Sharma, N. A. Jalil, R. Regin, S. S. Rajest, R. K. Tummala and T. N,.: "Predicting Network Congestion with Machine Learning," 2021 2nd International Conference on Smart Electronics and Communication, 2021, pp. 1574–1579 (2021). https://doi.org/10.1109/ICOSEC51865.2021.9591897
47. Guna Sekhar Sajja, Malik Mustafa, R. Ponnusamy, Shokhjakhon Abdufattokhov, Murugesan G., P. Prabhu, "Machine Learning Algorithms in Intrusion Detection and Classification", *Annals of RSCB*, vol. 25, no. 6, pp. 12211–12219, Jun. (2021).
48. Surinder Singh and Hardeep Singh Saini.: Learning-Based Security Technique for Selective Forwarding Attack in Clustered WSN, *Wireless Pers Commun* 118, 789–814 (2021). https://doi.org/10.1007/s11277-020-08044-0
49. P. Suresh, S S Rajest.: An Analysis of Psychological Aspects in Student-Centered Learning Activities and Different Methods, in *Journal of International Pharmaceutical Research*, Volume: 46, Special Issue 01, Page No.: 165–172 (2019).
50. Amiya Kumar Sahu, Suraj Sharma, M. Tanveer, Rohit Raja.: Internet of Things attack detection using hybrid Deep Learning Model, *Computer Communications*, Volume 176, Pages 146–154, (2021). https://doi.org/10.1016/j.comcom.2021.05.024

Estimation of Thyroid by Means of Machine Learning and Feature Selection Methods

S. Dhamodaran, B. B. Shankar, Bhuvaneswari Balachander, D. Saravanan, and Dinesh Sheshrao Kharate

1 Introduction

A gland in the neck called the thyroid (TH) produces thyroid hormones. These hormones might be too high or too low. An underactive thyroid gland causes hypothyroidism. The body's metabolism and energy utilisation are both influenced by these hormones. When the body doesn't have the right quantity of thyroid hormones, regular bodily processes begin to slow down, and the body is constantly confronted with new challenges. Data mining's uses in human services and clinical research are beneficial and substantial. Thyroid disease research may be a painful ordeal. Data mining is crucial to the medical field's search for new treatments. According to the accuracy of the disease prediction, information mining provides various options for arranging data. As a result of various infections, inactive perception recordings obtained from many medical associations are valuable. The patient's medical history and physical examinations are utilised to diagnose. These tests generate much data, and machine learning may identify the most important

S. Dhamodaran (✉)
Sathyabama Institute of Science and Technology, Chennai, Tamil Nadu, India

B. B. Shankar
N.M.A.M. Institute of Technology, Nitte, Karkala, Karnataka, India

B. Balachander
Department of E.C.E., Saveetha School of Engineering, Saveetha Institute of Medical and Technical Sciences, Chennai, Tamil Nadu, India

D. Saravanan
Department of C.S.E., I.F.E.T. College of Engineering, Villupuram, Tamil Nadu, India

D. S. Kharate
Animal Research Laboratory, P.G. Department of Zoology, Sant Ramdas Arts, Commerce & Science College, Ghansawangi, Maharashtra, India

P. Agarwal et al. (eds.), *Artificial Intelligence for Smart Healthcare*,
EAI/Springer Innovations in Communication and Computing,
https://doi.org/10.1007/978-3-031-23602-0_19

elements. Because of this ML expertise, ML can be used in conjunction with medical research to accurately diagnose hypothyroidism conditions. ML approaches have progressed, and ensembles are often utilised to attain the greatest model accuracy. This work uses three formulas to predict thyroid disease by highlighting several factors at the start of the study period. When everything is said and done, we look forward to knowing exactly what the outcome will be.

Hypothyroidism, or an underactive thyroid, is when the thyroid organ fails to produce enough thyroid hormones to reach the body's tissues. The thyroid organ is a minuscule butterfly formed at the front of the neck. Thyroid chemicals manage how your body utilises energy, which implies they affect every organ in your body, including how your heart beats. A significant number of your body's capacities are delayed on the off chance that you need more thyroid hormones. The thyroid gland may produce an excessive amount of one or more of these hormones. There is a disease known as hyperthyroidism in which the thyroid hormone levels are abnormally high, causing many of the body's functions to accelerate. This condition is known as "hyperthyroidism". Find out more about hyperthyroidism and pregnancy hyperthyroidism. When your thyroid hormone levels are too low, many of your body's functions are affected. This is known as hypothyroidism. The expression "hypo" alludes to an underactive thyroid. Become familiar with pregnancy-related hypothyroidism. If you have thyroid difficulties, you can still have a safe pregnancy and preserve the health of your baby by getting regular thyroid function testing and following any medications prescribed by your doctor. Thyroid chemicals are vital for your child's cerebrum and sensory system to grow regularly. In the first 3 months of pregnancy, your baby relies on your supply of thyroid chemicals, which pass via the placenta. At 12 weeks old, your child's thyroid begins to regulate itself independently. Pregnancy hormones are not delivered until the foetus is between 18 and 20 weeks old. Pregnancy-related hormones such as hCG and oestrogen enhance your blood levels of thyroid hormones. During pregnancy, the thyroid grows to some degree in healthy ladies; however, it is insufficient for a medical services provider to distinguish during an actual test.

Because of the more prominent degrees of thyroid chemicals and different indications in pregnancy and thyroid illnesses, thyroid issues can be hard to analyse during pregnancy. Some manifestations of hyperthyroidism and hypothyroidism are more self-evident, prompting your primary care physician to test you for these thyroid issues. Post-pregnancy thyroiditis is a thyroid ailment that can develop after your child is conceived. During pregnancy, Graves' disease is the most well-known reason for hyperthyroidism, influencing 1–4 out of every 1000 pregnancies in the United States. First, Graves' disease is an immune system illness that influences the body's susceptibility framework. Your invulnerable framework produces antibodies that cause the thyroid to create a lot of thyroid chemicals because of this condition. Thyroid-animating immunoglobulin, or TSI, is the name of the neutraliser. Graves' disease may show itself in the first trimester of pregnancy. In the second and third trimesters, nonetheless, if you, as of now, have Graves' disease, your side effects may improve. Later in pregnancy, a few segments of your invulnerable framework become less dynamic. Hence your insusceptible framework delivers less TSI. This could clarify why your manifestations have improved. As TSI levels rise, Graves' ailment habitually deteriorates initially, not many months after your child is conceived. On the off chance that you have Graves' infection, your primary care physician will, in all probability, test your thyroid capacity month to month during the time of pregnancy, along with possibly endorsing medicine for your hyperthyroidism treatment. Initially, a very high thyroid chemical level may destroy both your and your child's well-being. Hyperthyroidism in pregnancy is frequently associated with hyperemesis gravidarum national institutes of health (NIH), which is characterised by severe sickness and retching and can cause weight loss and parchedness. Specialists accept that raised levels of hCG in pregnancy are blamed for outrageous sickness and regurgitating. Thyroid chemical creation might be excessive because of high hCG levels. During the second half of pregnancy, hyperthyroidism regularly dies down. In rare cases, at least one knob or tumour in your thyroid may produce an excess of thyroid chemicals.

1.1 A General Overview of Thyroid Disease

Figure 1 shows the thyroid as an endocrine gland. Thyroid gland hormones must be withdrawn from the body to achieve this capacity. Through the circulatory system, it mimics and controls the digestion or improvement of every single nasty component. The thyroid's functions include breathing, blood circulation, digestion, temperature management, muscular movement, assimilation, and the brain's functioning. The

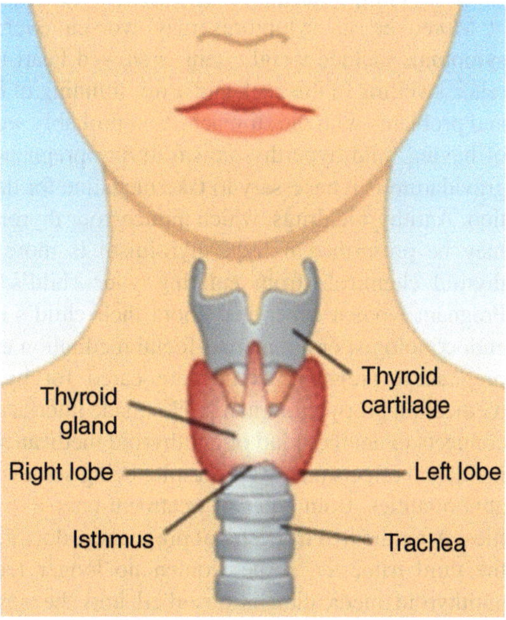

Fig. 1 Thyroid organ

normal functioning of the ethnic body may be affected by any colouring in the thyroid area. Thyroid hormone impacts growth and improvement by claiming immunity as a justification.

Thyroid gland hormone production is now significantly reduced, a condition known as hypothyroidism. Figure 1 depicts the prevalence of hyperthyroidism due to thyroid hormone intoxication, which is now at a high level.

1.1.1 The Role of the Thyroid in the Body's Health

Thyroid difficulty is a common primary endocrine infection around the world. In an Indian study, 42 million people reported experiencing these disorders. Thyroid disorders are distinct in their similarity to others, as well as their relative deception, utterance ease, and scientific treatment mode accessibility. The incorrect advent of thyroid hormone influences health conditions.

1.1.2 Hyperthyroidism

It is hyperthyroidism that results from an increase in the production of thyroid hormones. As a result of Graves' condition, hyperthyroidism is caused by immune system difficulties. Preventive measures include glacial skin, an increase in the body's sensitivity to heat and cloud decrease, a rise in the pulse, hypertension, excessive perspiration, neck extension, and worry, among other symptoms. Hypo is a medical term that refers to a lack or deficiency. A decrease in thyroid hormones causes hypothyroidism.

Moreover, its symptoms may worsen over time if it isn't recognised. The symptoms include weight gain, a slowed heart rate, an increase in the capacity to relax, swelling of the neck and arms, thinning of the hair, irregular menstrual cycles, and problems with the stomach. You probably won't need therapy on the off chance of having mild hyperthyroidism during pregnancy. Only if you have hyperemesis gravidarum is it necessary to take medicine for the vomiting sensation and dehydration. Antithyroid drugs, which induce your thyroid to produce less thyroid hormone, may be prescribed if hyperthyroidism is more severe. This therapy keeps your thyroid chemicals from entering your child's dissemination in overabundance. Pregnant women concerned about their child's health should seek advice from an endocrinologist or a maternal-foetal meditation expert. During the first 3 months of pregnancy, pregnant women are cared for by specialists using the antithyroid medication propylthiouracil NIH outside interface (PTU). Methimazole NIH outside connects to another kind of antithyroid medication, is simpler to take, and has fewer incidental effects than PTU, despite being somewhat bound to cause significant birth abnormalities. Both types of treatment have a low risk of inducing birth abnormalities. After the first trimester of pregnancy, doctors may transition to methimazole. In the third trimester, some women no longer require antithyroid medication. The antithyroid medication is absorbed into the newborn's circulation and decreases the amount of thyroid hormone generated. If you take antithyroid medication, your primary care physician will prescribe the lowest dose possible to prevent hypothyroidism in your child while also addressing increased thyroid chemical levels, which might again injure your child.

1.1.3 Thyroid Hormones

The thyroid hormones produced by the body (T3) are thyroxin (T4) and triiodothyronine (T3). For example, thyroid hormones control the ageing of carbohydrates, protein, and fat. The pituitary gland is in charge of the arrival of L-thyroxin and triiodothyronine, as well as the utilisation of iodothyronine hormones. Now that thyroid hormone is required, the "thyrotrophic-stimulating hormone" from the pituitary gland is released and then circles via habit control according to the entrance at the thyroid organ. The thyroid hormone is essential. As a result of the introduction of T4 and T3 endocrine hormones, TSH animates the thyroid organs. The pituitary glands' input configuration restricts thyroid hormone onset. There is a larger spread of TSH when T3 and T4 are higher and a higher onset of TSH when they are lower.

The thyroid chemical is responsible for directing digestion, growth, and other body exercises. The hypothalamus has three organs: the thyroid, the front pituitary, and the nerve. This is an automated circuit. The thyroid gland's main function is to generate two essential hormones: thyroxin (T4) and triiodothyronine (T3). Thyrotropin releasing hormone (TRH), a molecule that delivers thyroid-stimulating hormone (TSH) from the brain's nerve centre, as well as T4 from the body's main pituitary organ, all work together to maintain the body in balance. Bradycardia, cold sensitivity, blockage, fatigue, and weight gain are all symptoms of hypothyroidism caused by an underactive thyroid gland. Weight reduction, heat intolerance, looseness of the bowels, quake, and muscle shortcomings are, for the most part, manifestations of hyperthyroidism, which is brought about by expanded thyroid organ work. Iodine is an important trace element because it's found in our food in such small amounts. It's still important for T3 and T4. Iodine may be found in various foods, including iodised table salt, seafood, seaweed, and veggies. A decline in iodine intake may lead to an iron deficit and a reduction in thyroid hormone production. Iodine deficiency causes cretinism, goiter, myxedema coma, and hyperthyroidism. Recent technologies have focused more on the proposed thyroid disease diagnosis, but the level or stage of effecting rate is impossible to predict. The latest technologies like ML (machine learning), feature selection, SVM, KNN, Naive Bayes(NB), and decision trees (DT) are imported, but proper functionality is not attained.

2 Literature Survey

When treating thyroid disease [1]. the author examines the item and then recommends it. Malady's determination takes on an essential role as a top doctor. The augur is the most difficult task in the fight against thyroid disease. Thyroid disorders (hyperthyroidism and hypothyroidism) are nearly universal in the population, according to Irina Ioniă and Liviu Ioniă [2, 3]. [4, 5] N.B., D.T., multilayer perception, and "Radial Basis Function Network" were all explored by the inventors [4, 5]. Ali Keeps and colleagues developed one of the most often used frameworks for estimating thyroid [6]. For this ESTD, neuron fuzzy rules achieved a 95.33% success rate. Heart disease patients may now be diagnosed utilising classification mining techniques developed by a researcher named S.B. Patel [7]. Data mining techniques have evaluated classification function strategies for predicting heart disease.

Author	Technique	Key point	Advanced model
Ha et al. [14]	Thyroid estimation using machine learning	This model cannot overcome future, prior-stage thyroid issues	SVM
Razia et al. [15]	Thyroid estimation using deep learning	This work cannot overcome prior-stage thyroid issues	RFO
Dharamkar et al. [3]	Thyroid estimation using ML technology	This methodology cannot overcome future, prior-stage thyroid issues	CNN

2.1 Problem Declaration

2.1.1 Existing System

Diagnosing thyroid disease entails a long list of time-consuming but crucial steps. Several blood tests are traditionally used to diagnose thyroid disease. However, one of the most difficult tasks will be determining the disease's early stages with high accuracy [16–19]. Data mining is an essential part of disease diagnosis in the medical field. Data mining provides a variety of methods for determining the accuracy of a disease diagnosis [20]. An examination of multiple diseases' risk factors requires data from a variety of healthcare organisations. Doctors have traditionally relied on their instincts when making clinical decisions. It is possible that this could have disastrous consequences. Many clinical findings and outcomes are incorrect, resulting in astronomical medical costs [21–25].

Limitations of Current Material

- No action was taken as a result of the ML approaches used in health information during current excursions.
- No attempt was made to test the preceding data.

2.1.2 Proposed System

In healthcare services, the data mining method will be significantly utilised for identifying the disease, making a decision, and providing the best medical care to every affected person in a moderately inexpensive way [26–30]. The classification of thyroid gland disorders will be a significant task in disease prediction. Several blood tests may be conducted in the future, the thyroid may be reduced, and the time taken to diagnose illness may be reduced due to the dimensionality reduction effort. It is planned to use data from the "UCI data repository site" for the thyroid study. Thyroid patient information is included in the databases [31–35]. The patient's history has diverse attributes depicted in the dataset description, and various data mining methods have been applied to obtain a thyroid prediction [36]. For the survey, data mining methods such as NB, KNN, and SVM were considered [37].

2.2 System Overview

System overview as a conceptual method describes behaviour, structure, and many views of the framework [38–42]. An architecture depiction will be a formal explanation and demonstration of the system, organised in a way that helps to reason about behaviours and framework structures. First, we collect information from various individuals [43]. We narrowed the list of qualities to 15 using feature selection. NB, SVM, and KNN are used to categorise features once they have been extracted. Admin will train the data and, depending on the accuracy of the results, could suggest a superior categorisation technique [44–47].

2.3 Machine Learning Implementation

The implementation of machine learning (ML) employs three special types of key algorithms, which are discussed below:

2.3.1 SVM Algorithm (Support Vector Machine)

SVM is a type of lesson fabric tab used by function characterisation among outstanding precisely and utilising two-class classifiers, referred to as having more "choice power" than the choice surface. The quadratic enchantment problem is described as a set of points arranged straightforwardly by the graphs [48–51]. The atypical plane identifies acceptable preparation by looking at the lack of preparation in an arrangement [52].

2.3.2 KNN Algorithm (K-Nearest Neighbor)

KNN is one of the finest regular AI computations used for the order; it provides a structured information point about whether or not its neighbours are described. KNN keeps track of the densities of all the litigants and organisations that can be reached by themselves. The k-nearest neighbours tab (or KNN for short) may be accessed in a way that's easy to understand but difficult to implement. However, even though the Iris flower categorisation difficulty remains, the use option remains clear due to association difficulties. A KNN model incorporates the whole preparation dataset. As a result of the hidden facts, for example, we need a foretell; the KNN calculation appears through the coaching dataset due to the k-most comparative examples. As a result of this inconspicuous event, the augury faith that accumulated over similar but not identical situations is summarised above and then lower back [53–57]. The kind of information influences the resemblance measure. Using the Euclidean severance makes it possible to get reliable, trustworthy information. The hammering split may be used for several types of information, such as entire and twofold knowledge. Because of the possibility of relapse, the anticipated stress level may revert to its normal course.

2.3.3 NB (Naïve Bayes)

Naïve Bayes [8] classifiers are a kind of classifier that uses Bayes's hypothesis and some autonomous presumptions to make simple probabilistic classifiers. In terms of complexity, they are among the simplest Bayesian models. As the closeness to a specific object in the category follows the immediacy of the partial mean element, it shares representative governance.

2.3.4 The Dataset Description

The UCI AI data vault has been used to store this dataset [9]. There are thyroid entries in the database that are troubling for thyroid patients. A thyroid patient's file comprises 15 subfiles describing their unique features [10, 11]. Boolean (genuine or

	A	B	C	D	E	F	G	H	I	J	K	L	M	N
1	age	sex	cp	trestbps	chol	fbs	restecg	thalach	exang	oldpeak	slope	ca	thal	target
2	52	1	0	125	212	0	1	168	0	1	2	2	3	0
3	53	1	0	140	203	1	0	155	1	3.1	0	0	3	0
4	70	1	0	145	174	0	1	125	1	2.6	0	0	3	0
5	61	1	0	148	203	0	1	161	0	0	2	1	3	0
6	62	0	0	138	294	1	1	106	0	1.9	1	3	2	0
7	58	0	0	100	248	0	0	122	0	1	1	0	2	1
8	58	1	0	114	318	0	2	140	0	4.4	0	3	1	0
9	55	1	0	160	289	0	0	145	1	0.8	1	1	3	0
10	46	1	0	120	249	0	0	144	0	0.8	2	0	3	0
11	54	1	0	122	286	0	0	116	1	3.2	1	2	2	0
12	71	0	0	112	149	0	1	125	0	1.6	1	0	2	1
13	43	0	0	132	341	1	0	136	1	3	1	0	3	0
14	34	0	1	118	210	0	1	192	0	0.7	2	0	2	1
15	51	1	0	140	298	0	1	122	1	4.2	1	3	3	0
16	52	1	0	128	204	1	1	156	1	1	1	0	0	0
17	34	0	1	118	210	0	1	192	0	0.7	2	0	2	1
18	51	0	2	140	308	0	0	142	0	1.5	2	1	2	1
19	54	1	0	124	266	0	0	109	1	2.2	1	1	3	0
20	50	0	1	120	244	0	1	162	0	1.1	2	0	2	1
21	58	1	2	140	211	1	0	165	0	0	2	0	2	1

Fig. 2 Dataset

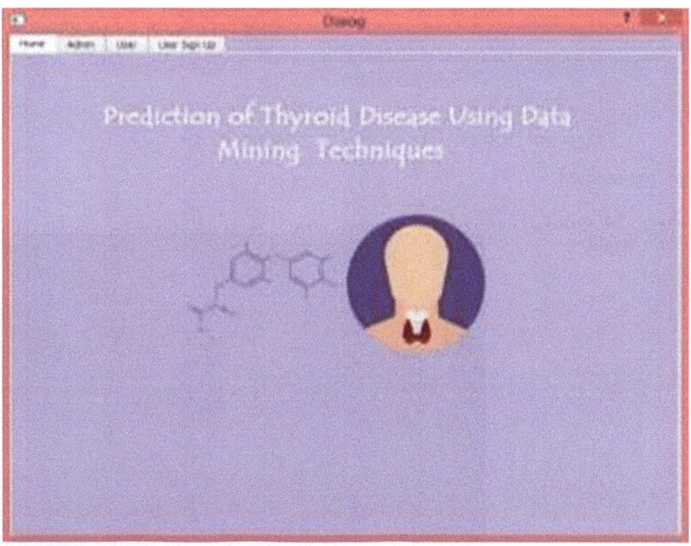

Fig. 3 Dialogue flow

bogus) characteristics persist, and those consistently seen as such stay so. Figure 2 presents the Hypothyroid.csv dataset. User registration is shown in Fig. 4, while the discussion flow is shown in Fig. 3.

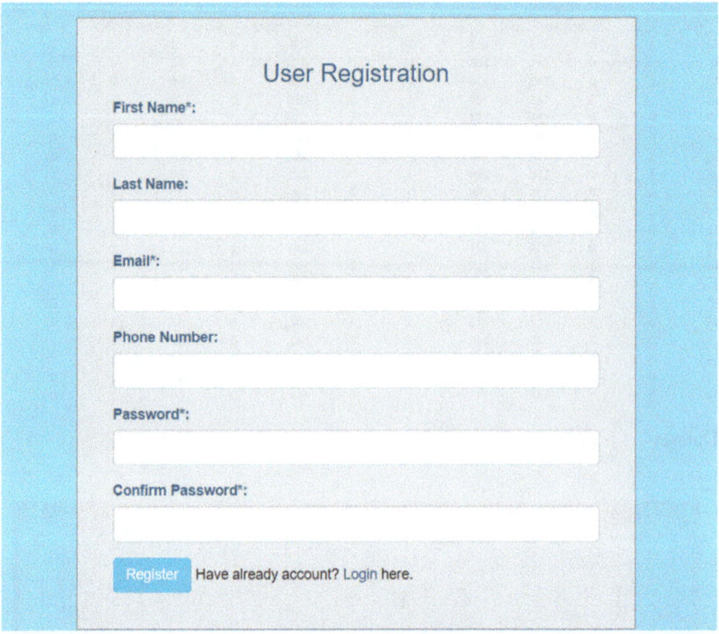

Fig. 4 User registration

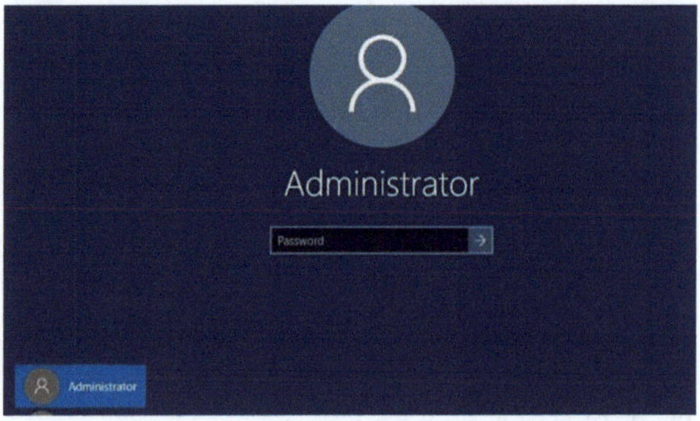

Fig. 5 Admin window

2.4 *Modules*

2.4.1 Admin

Users are assigned classification algorithms by the system administrator [12]. After logging in, use the appropriate computations to train the dataset [13]. SVM, KNN, and naive bayes (NB). The administrative team may handle the categorisation. The administrator performs the following tasks (Fig. 5):

- Following the training, the administrator divides 30% of the training devices to evaluate reliability.
- The administrator would then use the Naïve Bayes categorisation algorithm to determine the optimum classification method.
- Admins may also view the reliability graphs for the three methods and the attribute selection rating graph.

2.4.2 User

The user is the program's final consumer, and our application intends to assist the customer by directing the previous patient dataset and classification algorithms to imitate the consumer by utilising thyroid contamination. To determine whether the user has a thyroid illness, he or she must provide medical information. The user's responsibilities are outlined below:

- After logging in, consumers may create an account with their information and upload a single patient record in a CSV file.
- After that, users can notice the results through the forecast of the calculation.

Figures 4 and 5 clearly explain the registration and administrative modelling of the thyroid estimation process. ML and DL work can concentrate on medical data to get access.

3 Result and Analysis

Figures 6 and 7 illustrate the classification window and feature selection graph, respectively. Figure 8 depicts the accuracy of the forecast for several machine learning algorithms. Figure 9 depicts the accuracy analysis graph utilising SVM, the Naïve Bayes method, and KNN. Figure 10 indicates whether or not a person has

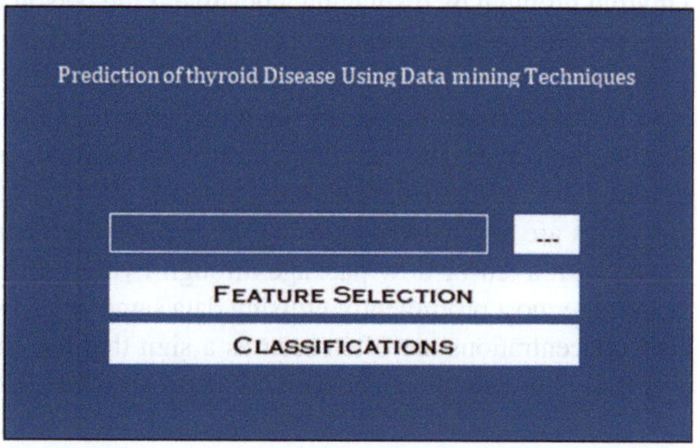

Fig. 6 Classification window

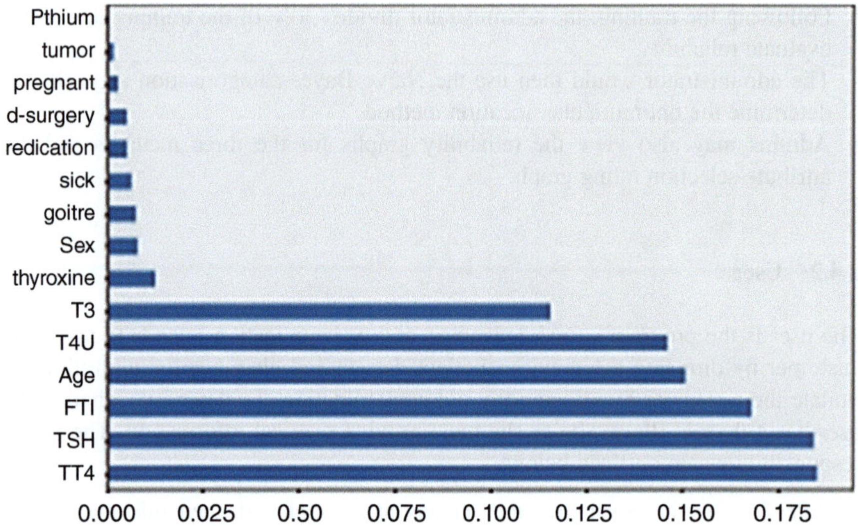

Fig. 7 Graph of feature selection

Fig. 8 Accuracy prediction

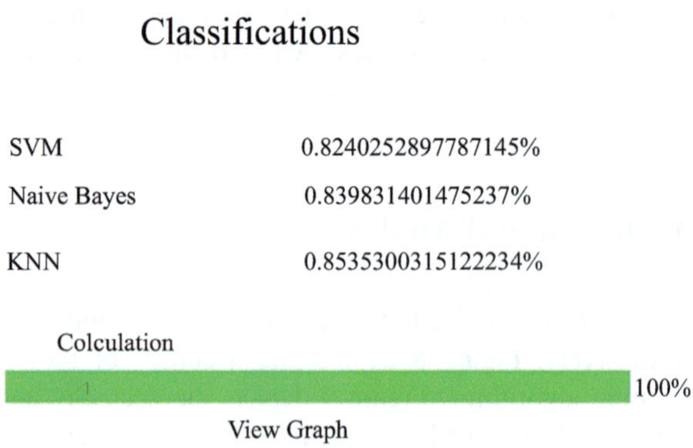

a thyroid problem by displaying a positive if the person has a thyroid problem and a negative if the person does not have a thyroid problem.

Figure 6 clearly explains thyroid disease estimation using data mining technology. The prediction of thyroid stage recognition is the most important function in data mining; here, the feature selection and classification buttons perform their commands with mathematical computations. The classification and feature extraction terms are continually focusing on updated Excel data. The dataset CSV file is loaded with a tensor flow package through Python software. The machine learning models are most prominently utilising data samples in a systematic manner. Medical TSH concentrations are often seen as a sign that the entire network is functioning properly, although this is, at most, an approximation. Healthy T3 levels range from

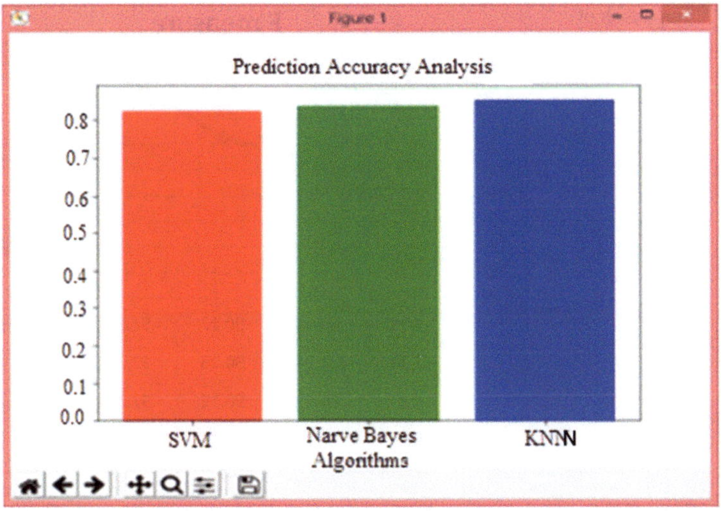

Fig. 9 Graph of accuracy analysis

Fig. 10 Showing results (positive or negative)

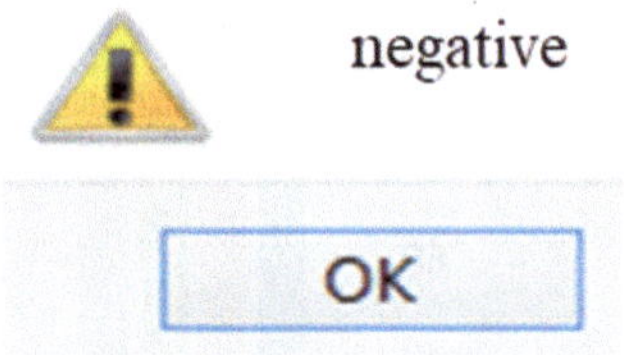

Table 1 Comparison of results

S. no.	Accuracy	Sensitivity	Recall	*F* measure
[5]	87.23	82.34	84.35	89.23
[6]	89.23	88.94	89.23	91.28
[7]	90.12	90.23	90.12	92.29
Proposed	97.36	93.23	97.23	94.56

100.00 to 200.00 nanometres per millilitre (ng/dL), whereas typical T4 levels range from 5.00 to 12.00 milligrammes per millilitre (g/dL).

Figure 7 clearly explains different hormone-balancing graphical analyses; this model calculates D-surgery, medication, and TT4 gland hormones.

Figure 8 explains the accuracy analysis of SVM, KNN, and Naïve Bayes technologies. Here, KNN attains more improvement compared to earlier models.

Figures 9 and 10 clearly explain various graphs' mathematical analysis and numerical methodology. Here, bar graphs represent the comparison of three models where KNN attains more improvement.

Table 1 and Fig. 11 clearly explain the *F* measure and comparison of results. Here, the proposed model improves at all stages: accuracy, recall, *F*, and sensitivity measures.

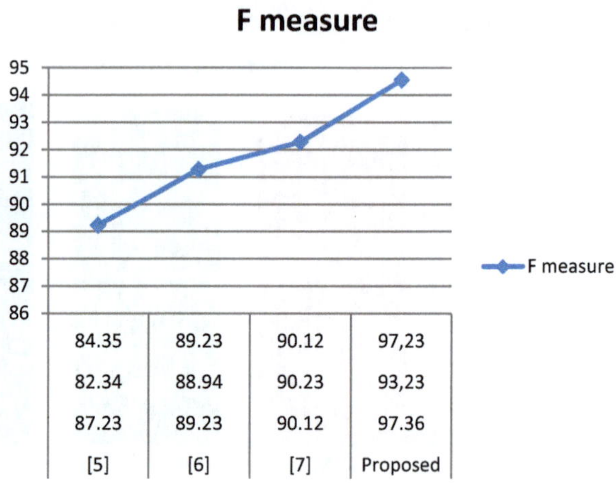

Fig. 11 Comparison of results

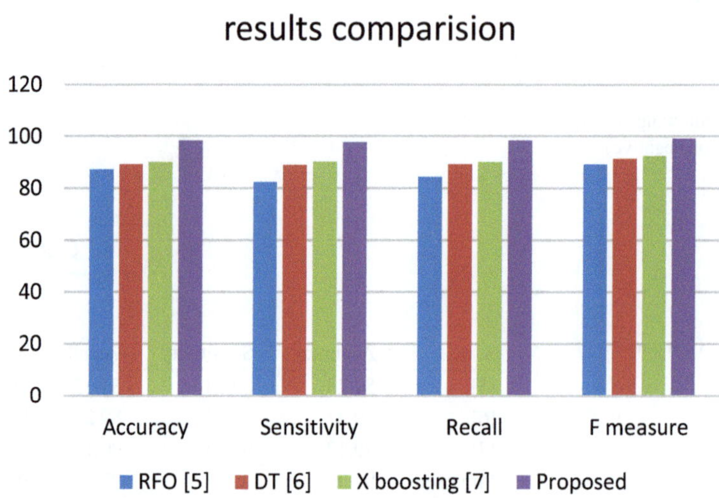

Fig. 12 Comparisons of results

Table 1 and Fig. 12 clearly explain the comparison of measures compared to earlier models like RFO and DT. The X-boosting proposed model is attaining more improvement in all metrics. The accuracy of 98%, the recall of 97%, and the sensitivity of 99% had been attained. This outperforms the methodology and competes with the present models.

4 Conclusion

At the outset of this research project, data mining methods will be used to identify thyroid gland disorders. Data mining classification methods have been utilised to diagnose thyroid issues. Thyroid disease detection is a more complex mechanism that must be detected earlier. The suggested model aids in the reduction of a patient's noisy data. Data mining algorithms such as NB, KNN, and SVM are being considered for research. The accuracy and transparency of the procedure have been crucial to the results of various categorisation systems. With this data classification, it will be simpler to locate medicines for thyroid patients that are less expensive and easier to sustain. The accuracy of SVM, Naïve Bayes, and KNN for the given dataset is 0.82%, 0.83%, and 0.85%, respectively. The proposed model outperforms the methodology and competes with current technology. The performance measures with ESTTD giving accuracy 98.53%, recall 97.23%, throughput 98.34%, and sensitivity 99.23% were achieved and competed with current trending technologies.

References

1. Ioniţă, I., & Ioniţă, L.: Prediction of thyroid disease using data mining techniques. BRAIN. Broad Research in Artificial Intelligence and Neuroscience, 7(3), 115–124 (2016).
2. Roshan Banu D, then K. C. Sharmili. "A Study of Data Mining Techniques after Detect Thyroid Disease" International Journal concerning Innovative Research into Science, Engineering and Technology, Vol. 6, SI. 11 (2017).
3. Khushboo Taneja, Parveen Sehgal, Prerana.: "Predictive Data Mining because of Diagnosis over Thyroid Disease the use of Neural Network" International Journal regarding Research of Management, Science & Technology. Vol. 3, No. 2 (2016).
4. Hanung Adi Nugroho, Noor Akhmad Setiawan, Md. Dendi Maysanjaya, "A Comparison regarding Classification Methods about Diagnosis of Thyroid Diseases" IEEE International Seminar of Intelligent Technology and Its Applications (2017).
5. K. Rajam and R. Jemina Priya darsini "A Survey on Diagnosis of Thyroid Disease Using Data Mining Techniques", I.J.C.S.M.C., Vol. 5, no. 5, pg.354–358 (2016).
6. Keleş, A., & Keleş, A. E.S.T.D.D.: Expert system for thyroid diseases diagnosis. Expert Systems with Applications, 34(1), 242–246 (2008).
7. Udhan, S., & Patil, B. A systematic review of Machine learning techniques for Heart disease prediction. International Journal of Next-Generation Computing, 12(2) (2021).
8. Lewis, D. D. Naive (Bayes) at forty: The independence assumption in information retrieval. In European conference on machine learning (pp. 4–15). Springer, Berlin, Heidelberg (1998).
9. U.C.I. Machine learning repository (patient's data) (online). Available: http://archive.ics.uci.edu/ml/machine- learning- databases/thyroid-disease/hypothyroid, Accessed by 21, Sep., 2021.
10. Dr. k. Raju, A. Sampath Dakshina Murthy, Dr B. Chinna Rao, Sindhura Bhargavi, G. Jagga Rao, K. Madhu, K. Saikumar.: A Robust and Accurate Video Watermarking System Based On S.V.D. Hybridation For Performance Assessment International Journal of Engineering Trends and Technology, 68(7), 19–24 (2020).
11. Saba, S. S., Sreelakshmi, D., Kumar, P. S., Kumar, K. S., & Saba, S. R. Logistic regression machine learning algorithm on M.R.I. brain image for fast and accurate diagnosis. International Journal of Scientific and Technology Research, 9(3), 7076–7081 (2020).

12. Saikumar, K., & Rajesh, V. Coronary blockage of artery for Heart diagnosis with D.T. Artificial Intelligence Algorithm. International Journal of Research in Pharmaceutical Sciences, 11(1), 471–479 (2020).
13. Saikumar, K., Rajesh, V. A novel implementation heart diagnosis system based on random forest machine learning technique International Journal of Pharmaceutical Research 12, pp. 3904–3916 (2020).
14. Ha, E. J., & Baek, J. H. Applications of machine learning and deep learning to thyroid imaging: where do we stand?. Ultrasonography, 40(1), 23 (2021).
15. Razia, S., Kumar, P. S., & Rao, A. S. Machine learning techniques for Thyroid disease diagnosis: A systematic review. Modern Approaches in Machine Learning and Cognitive Science: A Walkthrough, 203–212 (2020).
16. Dharamkar, B., Saurabh, P., Prasad, R., & Mewada, P. An Ensemble Approach for Classification of Thyroid Using Machine Learning. Progress in Computing, Analytics and Networking, 13–22 (2020).
17. C. Saravana Murthi, C. R. Rathish, J. Indirapriyadharshini, Deepak V, A. Sagai Francis Britto, A Novel and Effective Method for Automatic Paper Trimming and Cutting process in Paper Industries, International Journal of Advanced Science and Technology, Vol. 29, no. 6, pp. 4136–4143 (2020).
18. A. Sagai Francis Britto C. R. Rathish, C. Saravana Murthi, J. Indirapriyadharshini, Deepak V, A Novel and Effective Method for Automatic Paper Trimming and Cutting process in Paper Industries, International Journal of Advanced Science and Technology, Vol. 29, no. 6, Pp. 4136–4143 (2020).
19. Rathish Radhakrishnan & Karpagavadivu Karuppusamy, Cost Effective Energy Efficient Scheme for Mobile Adhoc Network, International Journal of Computing, Vol. 19, no.1, Pages 137–146 (2020).
20. CR Rathish & A Rajaram, Hierarchical Load Balanced Routing Protocol for Wireless Sensor Networks, International Journal of Applied Engineering Research, Vol. 10, no. 7, pp. 16521–16534 (2015).
21. P. Manta, S. Chandra Singh, A. Deep, and D. N. Kapoor, "Temperature-regulated gold nanoparticle sensors for immune chromatographic rapid test kits with reproducible sensitivity: a study," I.E.T. Nanobiotechnol., no. nbt2.12024, (2021).
22. Siva Agora Sakthivel Murugan, K. Karthikayan, Natraj N.A, Rathish C.R, Speckle Noise Removal Using Dual Tree Complex Wavelet Transform, International Journal of Scientific & Technology Research, Vol.2, no. 8, Pp. 4 (2013).
23. Renuka J Bathi, Sameena Parveen, Krishna Burde, The Role of Gutka Chewing in Oral Submucous Fibrosis: A Case-Control Study, Quintessence International, Vol. 40, no.6, pages e19–e25. 7p. 5 Charts (2009).
24. Sameena Parveen, Neeraj Taneja, Renuka J Bathi, AC Deka, Evaluation of Circulating Immune Complexes and Serum Immunoglobulins in Oral Cancer Patients – A Follow Up Study, Indian Journal of Dental Research, Vol. 21, no.1, pp. 14–19 (2010).
25. T. Radhika K Mohideen, C Krithika, N Jeddy, S Parveen, A Meta-Analysis in Assessing Oxidative Stress Using Malondialdehyde in Oral Submucous Fibrosis, European Journal of Dentistry, (2021).
26. Parveen S Taneja N, R Bathi, Serum Glycoproteins as Prognosticator in Head and Neck Cancer Patients – A Follow Up Study, Oral Oncology Head and Neck Oncology, Vol. 47 (2011).
27. P. Manta, N. Wahi, A. Bharadwaj, G. Kour, and D. N. Kapoor, "A statistical quality control (S.Q.C.) methodology for gold nanoparticles based immune-chromatographic rapid test kits validation," Nanosci. Nanotechnol.-Asia, vol. 11, no. 6, pp. 1–5, (2021).
28. N. Srinivasan and D. Sathyanarayanan, "Pharmacognostical investigation of Indigofera barberi Gamble (Fabaceae)–A Threatened medicinal herb," Hygeia: journal for drugs and medicines, vol. 6, no. 2, pp. 45–56, (2014).

29. K. Kavitha, N. Srinivasan and Y. Haribabu, "A review on quinazolinone and its derivatives with diverse biological activities," World Journal of Pharmacy and Pharmaceutical Sciences, vol. 7, no. 4, pp. 628–649, (2018).
30. N. Babu, S. Kodithala, R. Murali and N. Srinivasan, "Anthelmintic activity of methanolic bark extract of Buchanania axillaris (Desr.)," Research Journal of Pharmacy and Technology, vol. 11, no. 4, p. 1298, (2018).
31. K. Kavitha, N. Srinivasan and Y. Haribabu, "Review of quinazolinone scaffold as anticancer agents," World Journal Pharmaceutical Research, vol. 7, no. 9, pp. 434–454, (2018).
32. G. Kamala, N. Srinivasan, K. Shankar and R. Suresh, "Synthesis, Characterization and Antimicrobial Evaluation of N-Mannich Bases of (2-Substituted Phenyl) Benzimidazole Derivatives," Asian Journal of Pharmaceutical Research, vol. 8, no. 2, p. 87, (2018).
33. K. Govindarao, N. Srinivasan and R. Suresh, "Synthesis, Characterization and Antimicrobial Evaluation of Novel Schiff Bases of Aryl Amines Based 2-Azetidinones and 4-Thiazolidinones," Research Journal of Pharmacy and Technology, vol. 13, no. 1, p. 168, (2020).
34. N.T.M. El-Dabe, A. Refaie Ali, A.A. El-shekhipy, Influence of Thermophoresis on Unsteady MHD Flow of Radiation Absorbing Kuvshinski Fluid with Non-Linear Heat and Mass Transfer, American Journal of Heat and Mass Transfer (2017).
35. Osama M. Abo-Seida, N.T.M. Eldabe, M. Abu-Shady, A. Refaie Ali, "Electromagnetic non-Darcy Forchheimer flow and heat transfer over a nonlinearly stretching sheet of non-Newtonian fluid in the presence of a non-uniform heat source", Solid State Technology, Vol. 63 No. 6 (2020).
36. G. S and S. R. Raja. T, "A Comprehensive Survey on Alternating Fluids Used for The Enhancement of Power Transformers," 2021 IEEE International Conference on the Properties and Applications of Dielectric Materials, pp. 57–60 (2021).
37. F. J. John Joseph, R. T, and J. J. C, "Classification of correlated subspaces using HoVer representation of Census Data," in 2011 International Conference on Emerging Trends in Electrical and Computer Technology, pp. 906–911 (2011).
38. S. Bhoumik, S. Chatterjee, A. Sarkar, A. Kumar, and F. J. John Joseph, "Covid 19 Prediction from X Ray Images Using Fully Connected Convolutional Neural Network," in CSBio '20: Proceedings of the Eleventh International Conference on Computational Systems-Biology and Bioinformatics, pp. 106–107 (2020).
39. S. Sudhakar and S. Chenthur Pandian, "Authorized Node Detection and Accuracy in Position-Based Information for MANET", European Journal of Scientific Research, Vol.70, No.2, pp.253–265, (2012).
40. K. Balachander, S. Ramesh, A. J. Obaid. Simulation Of 1KW Multi-Level Switch Mode Power Amplifier, International Journal of Innovations in Scientific and Engineering Research, Vol. 5, No. 9: 85–92, (2018).
41. Saba Alyasiri, A. J. Obaid. A New Approach for Object Detection, Recognition and Retrieving in Painting Images, Journal of Advanced Research in Dynamical and Control Systems, Vol. 10, No. 2: 2345–2359 (2018).
42. K. Ganesh Kumar and S. Sudhakar, Improved Network Traffic by Attacking Denial of Service to Protect Resource Using Z-Test Based 4-Tier Geomark Traceback (Z4TGT), Wireless Personal Communications, Vol.114, No. 4, pp:3541–3575, (2020).
43. Govindaraj, M., Rathinam, R., Sukumar, C., Uthayasankar, M, Pattabhi, S. Electrochemical oxidation of bisphenol-A from aqueous solution using graphite electrodes: Environmental Technology, 34(4), 503–511 (2013).
44. Surinder Singh and Hardeep Singh Saini, "Learning-Based Security Technique for Selective Forwarding Attack in Clustered W.S.N.", Wireless Pers Commun 118, 789–814 (2021).
45. Rathinam, R., Govindaraj, M., Vijayakumar, K., Pattabhi, S. Decolourization of Rhodamine B from aqueous by electrochemical oxidation using graphite electrodes: Desalination and Water Treatment, 57(36), 16995–17001 (2016).

46. Jayanthi, K., Rathinam, R., Pattabhi, S. Electrocoagulation treatment for removal of Reactive Blue 19 from aqueous solution using Iron electrode: Research Journal of Life Sciences, Bioinformatics, Pharmaceutical and Chemical Sciences, 4(2), 101–113 (2018).
47. ThirumalaiRaj Brindha, Ramasamy Rathinam, Sivakumar Dheenadhayalan. Antibacterial, Antifungal and Anticorrosion Properties of Green Tea Polyphenols Extracted Using Different Solvents: Asian Journal of Biological and Life Sciences, 10(1),62–66 (2021).
48. Umadevi, M., Rathinam, R., S. Poornima, S., Santhi, T., Pattabhi, S. Electrochemical Degradation of Reactive Red 195 from its Aqueous Solution using RuO2/IrO2/TaO2 Coated Titanium Electrodes: Asian Journal of Chemistry, 33(8), 1919–1922 (2021).
49. Nora Omran Alkaam, Ahmed J. Obaid, Mohammed Q. Mohammed. A Hybrid Technique for Object Detection and Recognition Using Local Features Algorithms, Journal of Advanced Research in Dynamical and Control Systems, Vol. 10, No. 2: 2330–2344 (2018).
50. Surinder Singh and Hardeep Singh Saini "Intelligent Ad-Hoc-On Demand Multipath Distance Vector for Wormhole Attack in Clustered W.S.N.", Wireless Pers Commun (2021).
51. Kumar Sandeep, Arpit Jain, Anand Prakash Shukla, Satyendr Singh, Rohit Raja, Shilpa Rani, G. Harshitha, Mohammed A. AlZain, and Mehedi Masud. "A Comparative Analysis of Machine Learning Algorithms for Detection of Organic and Nonorganic Cotton Diseases." Mathematical Problems in Engineering (2021).
52. Amiya Kumar Sahu, Suraj Sharma, M. Tanveer, Rohit Raja, Internet of Things attack detection using hybrid Deep Learning Model, Computer Communications, Vol. 176, Pages 146–154, (2021).
53. Laxmikant Tiwari, Rohit Raja, Vineet Awasthi, Rohit Miri, G.R. Sinha, Monagi H. Alkinani, Kemal Polat, Detection of lung nodule and cancer using novel Mask-3 F.C.M. and T.W.E.D.L. N.N. algorithms, Measurement, Vol. 172, 108882, (2021)
54. Rohit Raja, Hiral Raja, Raj Kumar Patra, Kamal Mehta, Akanksha Gupta, Assessment methods of Cognitive ability of human brains for inborn intelligence potential using Pattern Recognition, IntechOpen – Biometric Systems ISBN 978-1-78984-188-6 (2021).
55. M. Nomani & R Parveen, COVID-19 pandemic and disaster preparedness in the context of public health laws and policies. Bangladesh Journal of Medical Science, Volume 20 issue 5, pages 41–48 (2021).
56. J. Kubiczek and B. Hadasik, "Challenges in Reporting the COVID-19 Spread and its Presentation to the Society," J. Data and Information Quality, vol. 13, no. 4, pp. 1–7, Dec. (2021).
57. B. Prabhu kavin and S. Ganapathy," Data Mining Techniques for Providing Network Security through Intrusion Detection Systems: A Survey," International Journal of Advances in Applied Sciences, vol. 7, no. 1, pp. 7–12, (2018).

A Multiuser-Based Data Replication and Partitioning Strategy for Medical Applications

V. Devi Satya Sri and Srikanth Vemuru

1 Introduction

Cloud computing offers the medical business the possibility of providing different medical care assets and applications for patients, specialists, medical laborers, and managers. By using the cloud infrastructure, the hospitals and healthcare societies can save their investment and used it to develop emergency wings to provide a high-quality hospital environment and reduce patient risks. Using the cloud structure, the patient records are easily stored and secured. But due to security threats, many hospitals are not interested in outsourcing their patient's sensitive data; if any of the patient's sensitive data is misused, then patients' lives will be at risk. Like the financial sector, the healthcare sector should also be significantly protected [1]. The medical field requires high safety security and innovations that are very cost-effective and innovative [2]. The data is generated and maintained wisely from time to time, so data handling is critical in the medical field. The medical field needs technical support, cloud infrastructure, etc. [3]. The medical records and reports have been managed through a cloud computing system according to legal conditions followed by government rules and regulations, staffing, budget, organizational culture, and policies in the assessment of the capabilities to reach the objective in recognizing the approaches developed for shifting system forward [4]. For computing the novel model, the promising technique is cloud computing to necessitate efficient work, minimal cost, and flexible operation in the respective IT field within the end-users [5]. To enhance the adoption of HER, it is providing opportunities in the research field of healthcare services. Many issues and challenges

V. D. S. Sri (✉) · S. Vemuru
Department of Computer Science and Engineering, Koneru Lakshmaiah Education Foundation, Guntur, Andhra Pradesh, India
e-mail: vsrikanth@kluniversity.in

P. Agarwal et al. (eds.), *Artificial Intelligence for Smart Healthcare*,
EAI/Springer Innovations in Communication and Computing,
https://doi.org/10.1007/978-3-031-23602-0_20

are faced toward fostering healthcare in the novel model designed [6]. The leading cloud services providers like Google, Microsoft, and Amazon have been facing security issues, which can be overcome through blockchain mechanisms. The proposed method has been solving the above security limitations with accurate operations. Providentially, the commitments of various providers such as Google, Microsoft, and Amazon need to progress the policies and practices at the best point of securing the privacy and data of customer profiles [7].

Data replication makes duplicates of a current copy. For easy and efficient access, data replication is essential [8]. In data replication, data is stored in replicas. The data has been processed through the hash key through the blockchain mechanism, which has been completed with image Net deep learning modeling [9]. The models are stored in different servers. If any one of the servers breaks down, then there is no issue of data loss. By using replication, we get the replicated data from another server [10, 11]. So, in case of system failure, repetition is beneficial. So, the copy supports backup, high availability, and disaster recovery. There are mainly two types of replication processes: one is dynamic and the other is static [12, 13]. In the static process, the required number of replicas and required bandwidth and host nodes is predefined, while in the dynamic process, since it is an ongoing process, the required number of replicas is changed according to usage patterns. Bandwidth consumption also changes, so dynamic replication has more issues than the static image; all the medical application data is dynamic, so the active copy is needed for this [14]. The user data is stored at different data centers. If the user wants to access the data, then the near data site will be available for access, thereby reducing the bandwidth consumption and improving run time and access time [15, 16].

Figure 1 shows the architecture of data replication. Firstly, the user sends the task to the scheduling manager. Then the scheduling manager guides the correct path to the user to avoid a collision. With the help of the scheduling manager, the user accesses the data in the data center; there may be different data nodes in different data centers [17]. Data partitioning is a mechanism that divides the entire data into small partitions. Applying the data encryption is made easy for small cells rather than massive data, and also, if any threat happens, it only ends to that small partition, so it does not affect the entire data [18]. While uploading the data in the cloud, the data is processed and then partitioned and uploaded in the cloud [19]. Thus, cloud replication and partitioning are offering high availability and performance without any additional software. Data partitioning is done in many ways by using several machine learning techniques. The data is partitioned in different ways based on hash, range, and list and is generally typed by considering the database [20].

Clinical findings could be predicted using biological data such as biomarkers or illness patterns to diagnose patients using medical data analysis. On the other hand, medical data is highly dimensional and sparsely described, making classic statistical methods challenging to utilize [21–23]. Hence, classification and prediction-based machine learning techniques are applied [24]. A feature selection strategy based on correlation was also utilized to decrease illness features to improve the algorithms' accuracy [25–27]. However, no machine learning algorithm consistently outperforms the others, and the dataset's nature appears to impact algorithm performance significantly [28–31]. The strategy for correlation-based feature selection enhanced

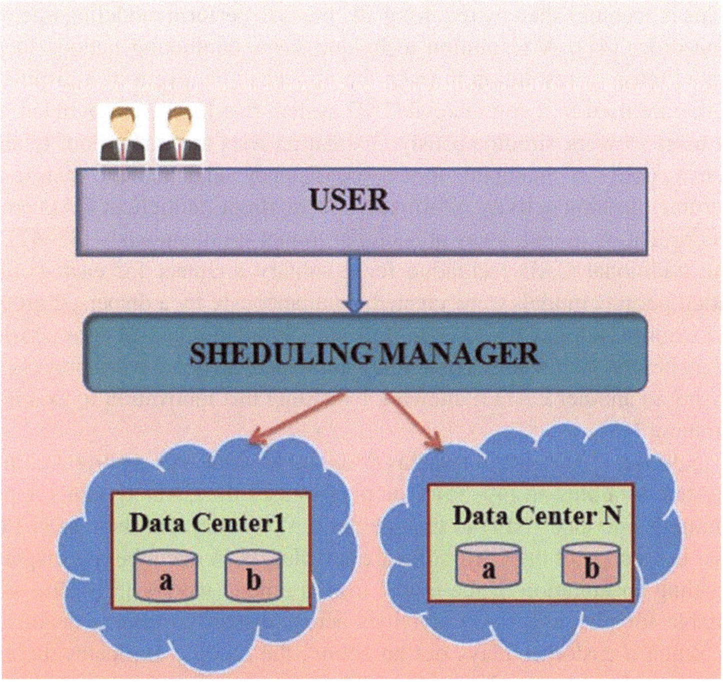

Fig. 1 The architecture of data replication

the prediction accuracy of all models by deleting irrelevant genes [32]. Several thousands to tens of thousands of gene/protein sequences make up medical data [33].

Each piece of medical data is scanned and turned into continuous, normalized data. The large dimensionality and unbalanced nature of medical datasets are the key challenges [34–36]. Traditional machine learning classifiers classify and predict diseases using a subset of characteristics, with a high actual negative rate and error rate. Several thousands to tens of thousands of gene/protein sequences make up a biological dataset [37]. Each distributed medical dataset is scanned and translated into continuous data that is normalized. The large dimensionality and unbalanced nature of remote medical data are the primary challenges [38]. Traditional machine learning classifiers classify and predict disease using a subset of characteristics, with a high actual negative rate and error rate. The well-known measure in information theory, i.e., entropy, is utilized to estimate the impurity of the random samples to manage uncertain data effectively using the information gained correctly. The impurity level in a group of models is measured using entropy [39].

Multiple designers can work on the same model simultaneously using simultaneous multiuser computer-aided design (CAD) [40]. Product development cycles are shortened as a result of the parallel design methodology. Modeling data must be kept consistent among clients in a replicated, simultaneous multiuser CAD system. This paper describes a solution for keeping dispersed CAD clients' versions of models in sync. This is accomplished by requiring all clients to perform modeling operations in the same order [41]. A resolution technique saves conflicting actions locally for subsequent reuse or resolution through the utilizer in the event of a dispute. These techniques are used in a commercial CAD system that has been upgraded to allow several users to work simultaneously. Validation tests are carried out to show the procedures used to maintain model consistency and resolve clashes while safeguarding clashing activity information. Concurrent multiclient CAD empowers various originators to chip away at a similar model simultaneously [42–47]. Rather than the traditional CAD technique for a solitary architect for each model, this innovation permits models to be created simultaneously by a dispersed group. This newly distributed approach allows entirely completing product designs considerably faster than before. Companies can quickly implement an equal work process without progressing to another CAD framework by adding this innovation to existing CAD programming [48].

Our multiuser CAD system remains designed to work with a current commercial CAD system as a plug-in [49–55]. The plug-in uses the CAD system's application programming interface (API) to change the CAD model. On their local PC, each customer has a copy of the CAD software and plug-in. A client begins displaying by downloading an imitation of the model from a unified worker [56]. The worker is accountable for planning CAD activities across distant customers dealing with a model. When a customer plays out an action, the module extricates the essential information and sends it to the worker [57]. Every activity is sent to any remaining customers in a similar model by the worker, who then, at that point, stores it in a focal dataset for long haul stockpiling. The module plays out the tasks in the CAD programming when customers get new far-off activities from the worker.

Asynchronous communications are used in the simultaneous multiuser system to provide concurrent communication between CAD client customers and the worker. Albeit this correspondence method permits various customers to chip away at a similar body simultaneously, it may prompt model irregularities if not painstakingly planned. Business CAD frameworks, like Siemens NX, are ordinarily single-strung, permitting only each activity to be acted in turn. Other clients' activities may finish and begotten while a customer is completing an action. Any remaining clients' tasks should be deferred until the dynamic client's move is finished. Models can veer into conflicting many states because of this deferral, which is compounded by network inertness. The possibility of model disparity increases as more clients are added to the multiclient areas.

2 Related Works

Almetwaly et al. [3] proposed a new model that addresses the issues of primary backup replication. In this model, all the data is stored in one single node called primary node. If it crashes, the entire data will be lost. To overcome this, they recommended a new approach, i.e., the whole data is divided into small subsets and these subsets are stored to separate nodes and treat one primary node as the master node and the remaining replicas as slaves. Hence, if one slave will crashed, the remaining slaves and the master will back up the data. They follow an object creation, that is, the owner has the right to lock or unlock the object whenever necessary [3].

Alexander Stiemer et al. [4] found that data replication and partition decrease the data access latency. In this paper, they examine three methodologies for data in the cloud, specific Read-One-Write-All-Available (ROWAA), Majority Quorum (MQ), and Data Partitioning (DP) – all in a configuration that ensures solid consistency. They present BEOWULF, a meta convention dependent on an exhaustive cost model that incorporates the three methodologies and powerfully chooses the pattern with the most minimal inertness for a given responsibility. In the assessment, they analyze the expectation of the BEOWULF cost model with a gauge assessment. Their outcomes pleasantly show the adequacy of the scientific model and the exactness in choosing the most appropriate convention for a given responsibility.

Krunal [5] found that the client does not directly upload the data into the cloud. Before uploading the data, they need to perform two steps to ensure data security and privacy. In the first step, the data is partitioned. In the second step, the information is encrypted using parallelism [5]. In any application, customer satisfaction is of utmost priority, so the security of customer data is highly maintained.

Xiao et al. [15] extended the KP-ABE method and introduced a unique technique they called HASE. In a cloud context, it provides data security and user revocation capabilities. The authors combined Lazy Re-encryption and Usually Re ideas so that individuals' permissions could be kept private. Users could be held responsible for their private key while also reducing data operating costs [13]. Even though this approach provides perfectly acceptable accessing policy, it also has a disadvantage, i.e., it takes a long time to compute differentiated to conventional approaches. Upcoming projects may be performed to overcome this disadvantage and decrease calculation time. Data protection and perfectly acceptable security systems have subsequently been addressed using a variety of new methods. [6] proposed a methodology called software-defined network in that the load balances in nodes are managed and several machine learning methods like supervised learning and naive Bayes clustering and also host-based monitoring and network-based monitoring are observed. Tao Chan [7] proposed a framework called scalable service-oriented replication (SSOR). It is used for service-level applications. For this, they apply two techniques: multi-fixed sequencer protocol and region-based election protocol. By applying the methodology, the efficiency and integrity are increased and scalability is upheld [8, 9]. The proposed scheme was based on an RDF graph partitioning algorithm for cloud storage.

The cloud security [10] alliance: a nonprofit organization and a group of trusted companies attain the vision of progression into the guidelines of a comprehensive system in both software and hardware technologies to construct the inability of the applications for trustworthy fields [11, 12]. To secure the privacy and data of the cloud users, certain rules and regulations are implemented by the government.

Moreover, issues can be solved in a legal way using evaluations or negotiations contracted in cloud computing [14, 15].

Poster used an advanced feature gene selection methodology with an affinity propagation clustering strategy to build an advanced feature gene selection methodology for adult acute lymphoblastic leukemia (ALL) microarray data. Microarray data analysis has become a more prominent and widely used method for detecting diseases. It has a total of 10,000 genes in the input dimension. It's a severe computing problem in the data analysis process. They used affinity propagation clustering in the case of feature gene selection in adult acute lymphoblastic leukemia microarray data in this study. In the case of affinity propagation clustering, the total number of clusters is solely dependent on identifying feature genes. Affinity propagation clustering is a type of advanced clustering that requires message exchange between different data points. Aside from that, it's also in charge of reducing the size of each sample. It does not necessitate any prior knowledge of the total number of clusters. Specific genes with AP clustering can give adequate learning in categorization and prediction by analyzing the outcomes of the above-presented methodology. For Bayesian categorization of microarray data, Remeseiro suggested partition-conditional ICA.

In the field of medical decision-making, precise and appropriate classification of microarray data is critical. Based on the findings of earlier studies, we may conclude that class-conditional independent component analysis (CC-ICA) effectively improves the performance of the naive Bayes classifier in microarray data processing. The microarray dataset may contain a small number of samples for numerous classes in some circumstances. Some CC-ICA applications appear to be infeasible in the conditions mentioned above. The classic CC-ICA technique is extended in this study article. The partition-conditional independent component analysis is the newly enlarged and improved version of CC-ICA (PC-ICA). PC-ICA delivers a better and more efficient feature extraction procedure than existing techniques.

To put it another way, we can say that the technique mentioned above improves the overall performance of naive Bayes classification of microarray data. ICA-NN used neural action to perform independent component analysis on a multivariate distribution to make it statistically mutually independent. These models must converge to estimate the separate medical data components correctly [16]. ICA uses the imperialistic competition concept to optimize the objective function. As a biomedical node, each member of this population is a vector of random numbers, and the cost of the objective function will determine the biomedical activity in a relationship. The use of ICA with neuronal action in classification, learning, and optimization functions has proven successful.

2.1 Partitioning Strategies

Select a partitioning plan based on the needs of the users:

- Start at the top and work your way down.
- Top-down partitioning is a technique for dividing a database among several processors, servers, or computers, increasing database scalability, reliability, and performance. Create a separate application for each partitioned database to get the most outstanding results from top-down partitioning.
- Start at the bottom and work your way up.
- To control data flow between various connected databases, use bottom-up partitioning, increasing the quality and accessibility of data in databases.
- Divide databases into subsets based on attribute values associated with base dimensions (a standard measurement related to one or more attribute dimensions).
- Use this strategy to extract data based on dimension attributes like flavor or size.

2.2 *Proposed Model*

This section aims to provide a brief explanation of AwS-based virtual machine 1, virtual machine 2, and virtual machine 3 functionalities.

Figure 2 shows the data analyzed statistically to accomplish the task of dynamically partitioning graph data and the prior information questioned by the user profile in monitoring the data to be managed further. The proposed method achieves the data analyzed statistically by the previous questions made for the practical outcome of the graph of dynamic RDF environment in the process of situation raised by the potential user. The AWS-based cloud load balancing can be performed with users on the application, which was decreasing the performance at dynamic operations. Additionally, data for partitioning the graph at locations can be provided relying on the frequency questions and size of the question in related stages of graph partitioning. Based on the concept of the architecture of master-salve, the proposed method is developed to gather the statistics data as shown in Fig. 2. They are storing the RDF partitioning for subgraphs in server distribution and questions processing for the user in collecting the information for computation complexity created at the additional level.

Consequently, edges and vertices have been ordered in every slave utilized in the processing of questions. The edge and vertex information is used to identify the questions and later stored by the individual slave. By gathering the edges and vertices of the entire slave field, the query is performed by the master in producing the updates for the creation of a complete slave.

The database has been processed with a deep learning mechanism for statistical analysis. The patterns helped to detect security violation issues. Nevertheless, the updation for the statistical data has not been modified since the proposed technology has been utilized for collecting the queries of previous information. For instance, queries at the server cloud of the processing system at the User-1D, Virtual Machine1, and Virtual Machine3 are stored in the prior query to identify the count of edges and vertices from the outcome.

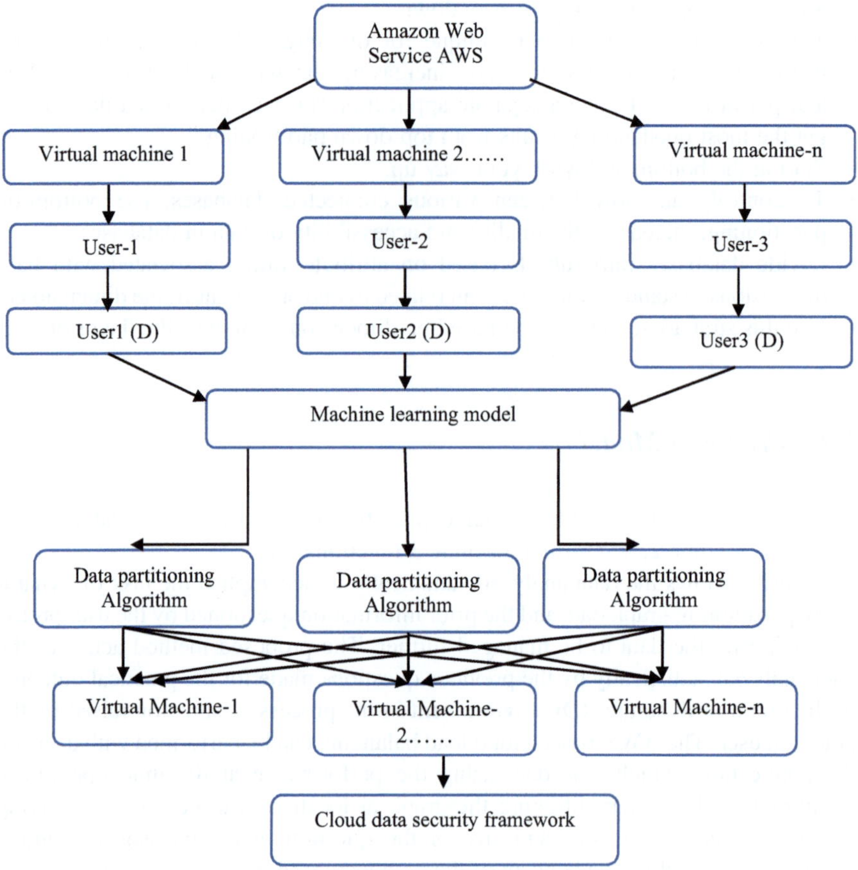

Fig. 2 Proposed multiple data partitioning load balancing parameter selections

The change in the graph of RDF with continuous operation is needed to count for the query for the vertices inclusive for the updated version of the periodic information in the related vertices of the outcomes at the data statistically provided. Consequently, the periodical updation of the resulting query is proposed for the dynamic knowledge required for the system's update for performing the RDF graph environment. The overall performance of the dynamic process in partitioning the data has been shown in Fig. 2. The queries of the high load are maintained in the situation for the data created at the initial level. The proposed method achieves the data analyzed statistically by the prior questions made for the practical outcome of the graph of dynamic RDF environment in the process of situation raised by the potential user. Users need to send acknowledgments continually when facing any security issues, therefore clustering concept has been applied to make application accuracy faster. To finalize the dynamic data for the RDF graph, prior information of the potential users of the monitored data is partitioned. The efficient communication for the queried user for the emotional purpose requested by the frequency sample at the environment issued at the managing queries for sample rate.

The information on the server was taken into account and updated same acknowledgment was to clients in less time. Based on the concept of the architecture of master-slave, the proposed method is developed to gather the data of statistics. They are storing the RDF partitioning for subgraphs in server distribution and question processing for the user in collecting the information for computation complexity created at the additional level. Consequently, edges and vertices have been ordered in every slave utilized in the processing of questions. The edge and vertex information is used to identify the questions and later stored by the individual slave. The individual server can be associated with the subgraphs in plotting the query processing in calculating the different featured characteristics.

Therefore, the listed information is crucial for the query's resulting outcome, such as ID, identification of distributed server, server, query, sampling rate, frequency, query identifier, mean of the identified cross-section, vertices' count, and so on individually. The classification of questions and servers is based on the user's requested queries. To group the frequency, the cluster family is associated with the subcluster family for dynamic change in the partitioning of the balanced loads for the servers. To evaluate the size of the data partition, the storage level of each server distributed results in the count of vertices individually. The subgraphs' size can be mapped separately for the further requirement of the vertices' count in the storage of the queries related to the additional question of edges in the symmetry region of 2019, 11, and 9267 of the division fields of 24 for recognizing the information stored in the IDs of the managed statistical data (Figs. 3 and 4).

Replication algorithm
Output: Replicas of cloud data files
Input: Cloud data files
Procedure

1. Initialize the dynamic and static parameters of the data files D.
2. Distribute the virtual machine with path nodes.
3. Each data node is divided into sub-nodes (SN)
4. And for each sub-node, SN path node is assigned
5. As D (SN) with path node.
6. And for every sub-node, SN replica is generated and stored as SNR.
7. Then, find the path node for each replica SNR and assign a bandwidth.
8. Done.

In this replication algorithm, cloud data files are first taken as inputs and assigned static and dynamic parameters based on the average virtual machine path nodes identified. For every node, the sub-node SNR is replicated and then generate the replicas of the cloud data files, and for each cloud data replica file, the bandwidth is assigned.

Table 1 shows the performance analysis of the data replication model compared with the traditional models in a multiuser environment. Considering the size of the

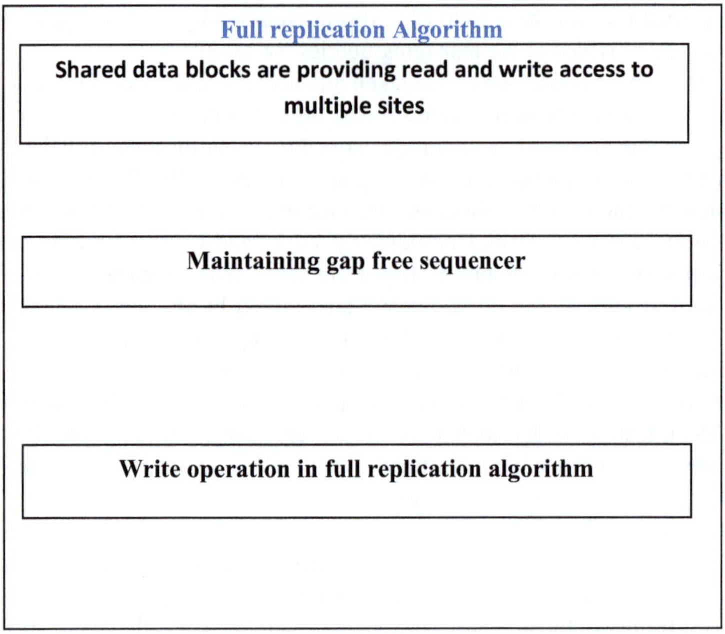

Fig. 3 Replication algorithm

Fig. 4 FSM proposed work

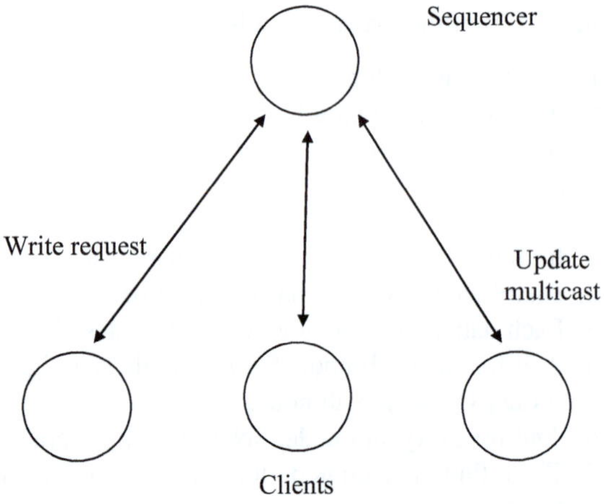

data, different virtual machines' performance values are observed and treated as average virtual machines' performance values.

Figure 5 shows the replication in the cloud. The efficiency of the replication method on the cloud is demonstrated on different test cases and compared with the Tabu Search and practical swarm optimization, ant colony optimization, and HPSOTS.

Table 1 Data replication model performance analysis comparison with traditional models on multiuser environment

Size of the data – 10 KB	3.23	5.26	2.89	4.03
Size of the data – 20 KB	3.22	5.3	2.13	4.68
Size of the data – 30 KB	3.32	5.65	2.65	4.22
Size of the data – 40 KB	3.41	5.84	2.78	4.63
Size of the data – 50 KB	3.62	5.37	2.41	4.12
Size of the data – 60 KB	3.33	5.64	2.02	4.74
Size of the data – 70 KB	3.64	5.26	2.69	4.58
Size of the data – 80 KB	3.73	5.42	2.23	4.91
Size of the data – 90 KB	3.12	5.72	2.59	4.83
Size of the data – 100 KB	3.08	5.18	2.88	4.41

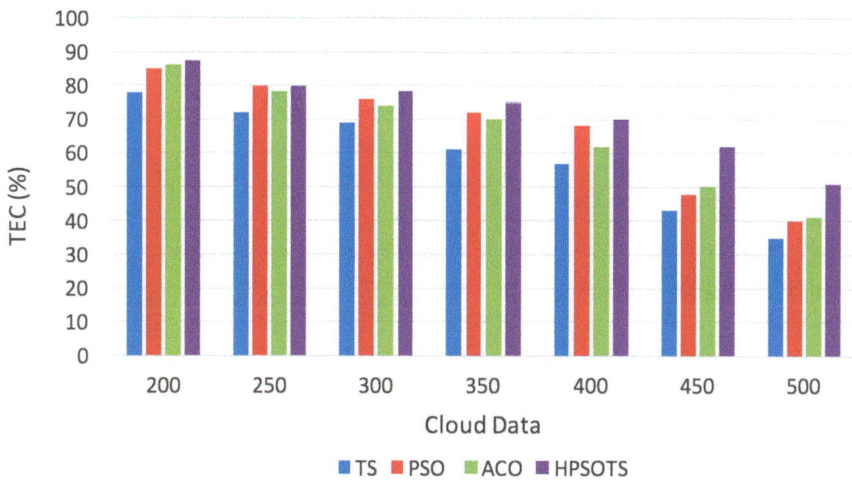

Fig. 5 Data replication in the multiuser environment (cloud)

The efficiency and scalability of the replication are shown and also attain efficient bandwidth usage and avoid bandwidth collisions (Fig. 5).

Figure 6 and Table 2 clearly show the differentiation of results, where accuracy, sensitivity recall, and F measures are identified and concluded that the proposed model is accurate.

3 Conclusion

For potential operators, those who come up with projects related to cloud computing, this study is beneficial in planning actions. To further determine the strategy, direction, and resource allocation, a novel designed model is projected named HC2SP employed by the health organization to transfer with the cloud paradigm. Nevertheless, the four critical stages in the model comprised identification,

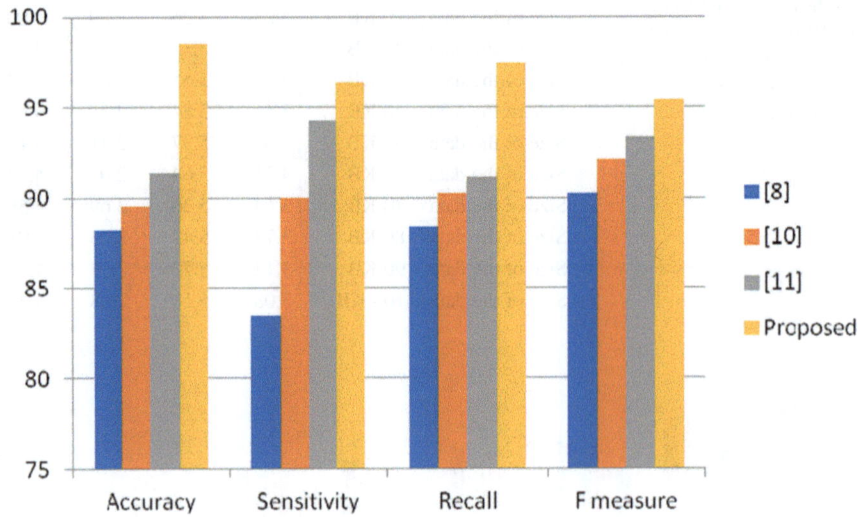

Fig. 6 Differentiation of results

Table 2 Comparison models

S. no	Accuracy	Sensitivity	Recall	F measure
[8]	88.22	83.49	88.39	90.28
[10]	89.51	89.98	90.28	92.08
[11]	91.43	94.29	91.16	93.36
Proposed	98.49	96.32	97.38	95.39

evaluation, action, and follow-up. Firstly, the organizations analyze the present scenario of the provided service in identifying the benefit of the fundamental objective. Secondly, the challenges and openings are approving the cloud computing technology. The organization could estimate the internal and external strength and the weak stage factors for employing the SWOT analysis, including the chances at outer region and factors threatening the system of approving the novel model. Also, the solutions for potential users to grip the cloud issues have been highlighted. Thirdly, a cloud computing plan for employment has been strained. Finally, the suggestions made by the author provide minimal knowledge in defining the service at the cloud stage as well as distribution of model, obtaining assurance in choosing the provider for the cloud system, comparing the various providers, initiating the implementation through the pilot, and reflecting the migrated future data. The measures like accuracy 98.23%, sensitivity 94.53%, and recall 92.29% had been attained. In the end, the cloud computing is deployed for proper infrastructure and plan to quantify the enhancements of healthcare services.

References

1. V.Devisatyasri, Dr V.Srikanth survey on data security issues related to multi-user environment in cloud computing, *Journal of critical reviews*, vol. 7, Issue 4, (2020).
2. V.Devisatyasri, Dr V.Srikanth: A Hybrid Based Outlier Detection Machine Learning Models On Medical Databases, *European Journal of Molecular & Clinical Medicine*, Volume 07, Issue 08, (2020).
3. A. M. Mostafa and A. E. Youssef, "A multi-primary ownership partitioning protocol for highly scalable and available replication services," 2013 Saudi International Electronics, Communications and Photonics Conference, pp. 1–5, (2013).
4. Alexander Stiemer, I. Fetai and H. Schuldt, "Analyzing the performance of data replication and data partitioning in the cloud: The BEOWULF approach," 2016 IEEE International Conference on Big Data (Big Data), pp. 2837–2846, (2016).
5. K. Patel, N. Singh, K. Parikh, K. S. S. Kumar and N. Jaisankar, "Data security and privacy using data partition and centric key management in cloud," International Conference on Information Communication and Embedded Systems (ICICES2014), pp. 1–5, (2014).
6. A.M El-Shamy "Anomaly Detection Bottleneck identification of the distributed application in the cloud data center using software-defined networking" Egyptian informatics journal, Jan. (2021).
7. Tao Chen, and R. Bahsoon, "Scalable Service Oriented Replication in the Cloud," 2011 IEEE 4th International Conference on Cloud Computing, pp. 766–767, (2011).
8. Al-Ghezi, A.I.A.; Wiese, L. Adaptive Workload-Based Partitioning and Replication for RDF Graphs. In Proceedings of the International Conference on Database and Expert Systems Applications, Regensburg, Germany, 3–6 September; pp. 250–258, (2018).
9. Stanton, I.; Kliot, G. Streaming graph partitioning for large distributed graphs. In Proceedings of the International Conference on Knowledge Discovery and Data Mining, Beijing, China; pp. 1222–1230. 37, (2012).
10. Yang, S.; Yan, X.; Zong, B.; Khan, A. Towards effective partition management for large graphs. In Proceedings of the ACM SIGMOD International Conference on Management of Data, Scottsdale, AZ, USA, pp. 517–528, (2012).
11. Hayes, J.; Gutiérrez, C. Bipartite Graphs as Intermediate Model for RDF. In Proceedings of the International Semantic Web Conference, Hiroshima, Japan, pp. 47–61, (2004).
12. Tomaszuk, D.; Skonieczny, L.; Wood, D. RDF Graph Partitions: A Brief Survey. In Proceedings of the International Conference on Beyond Databases, Architectures and Structures, Ustro'n, Poland, pp. 256–264 (2015).
13. Akhter, A.; Ngomo, A.N.; Saleem, M. An Empirical Evaluation of RDF Graph Partitioning Techniques. In Proceedings of the International Conference on Knowledge Engineering and Knowledge Management, Nancy, France; pp. 3–18 (2018).
14. M. Nomani & R. Parveen, Contextualizing Epidemic Diseases (Amendment) Ordinance, 2020 in Epidemic-Pandemic Syndrome of COVID-19 in India. *Systematic Reviews in Pharmacy,* Wolters Kluwer Medknow India, Volume: 11, Issue 8 pages 156–160 (2020).
15. Amiya Kumar Sahu, Suraj Sharma, M. Tanveer, Rohit Raja, Internet of Things attack detection using hybrid Deep Learning Model, *Computer Communications,* Volume 176, Pages 146–154, (2021).
16. M. Nomani & R. Parveen, Covid-19 Pandemic and Application of Disaster Management Act, 2005: Promises and Pitfalls, *International Journal of Pharmaceutical Research, Advanced Scientific Research*, India, volume 12, issue 4, pages 3730–3734, (2020).
17. Saikumar, K., & Rajesh, V. Coronary blockage of artery for Heart diagnosis with DT Artificial Intelligence Algorithm. *International Journal of Research in Pharmaceutical Sciences*, 11(1), 471–479 (2020).
18. Metwaly, A. F., Rashad, M. Z., Omara, F. A., & Megahed, A. A. Architecture of multicast centralized key management scheme using quantum key distribution and classical symmetric encryption. *The European Physical Journal Special Topics*, 223(8), 1711–1728, (2014).

19. Farouk, A., Zakaria, M., Megahed, A., & Omara, F. A. A generalized architecture of quantum secure direct communication for N disjointed users with authentication. *Scientific reports*, 5(1), 1–17, (2015).
20. Naseri, M., Raji, M. A., Hantehzadeh, M. R., Farouk, A., Boochani, A., & Solaymani, S. A scheme for secure quantum communication network with authentication using GHZ-like states and cluster states controlled teleportation. *Quantum Information Processing*, 14(11), 4279–4295 (2015).
21. Wang, M. M., Wang, W., Chen, J. G., & Farouk, A. Secret sharing of a known arbitrary quantum state with noisy environment. *Quantum Information Processing*, 14(11), 4211–4224 (2015).
22. Zhou, N. R., Liang, X. R., Zhou, Z. H., & Farouk, A. Relay selection scheme for amplify-and-forward cooperative communication system with artificial noise. *Security and Communication Networks*, 9(11), 1398–1404, (2016).
23. Zhou, N. R., Li, J. F., Yu, Z. B., Gong, L. H., & Farouk, A. New quantum dialogue protocol based on continuous-variable two-mode squeezed vacuum states. *Quantum Information Processing*, 16(1), 1–16, (2017).
24. Abdolmaleky, M., Naseri, M., Batle, J., Farouk, A., & Gong, L. H. Red-Green-Blue multi-channel quantum representation of digital images. *Optik,* 128, 121–132 (2017).
25. Naseri, M., Heidari, S., Baghfalaki, M., Gheibi, R., Batle, J., Farouk, A., & Habibi, A. A new secure quantum watermarking scheme. *Optik*, 139, 77–86 (2017).
26. Heidari, S., Naseri, M., Gheibi, R., Baghfalaki, M., Pourarian, M. R., & Farouk, A. A new quantum watermarking based on quantum wavelet transforms. *Communications in theoretical Physics*, 67(6), 732 (2017).
27. Nagata, K., Nakamura, T., & Farouk, A. Quantum cryptography based on the Deutsch-Jozsa algorithm. *International Journal of Theoretical Physics*, 56(9), 2887–2897 (2017).
28. Nagata, K., Nakamura, T., Geurdes, H., Batle, J., Abdalla, S., & Farouk, A. Creating Very True Quantum Algorithms for Quantum Energy Based Computing. *International Journal of Theoretical Physics*, 57(4), 973–980 (2018).
29. Abulkasim, H., Farouk, A., Hamad, S., Mashatan, A., & Ghose, S. Secure dynamic multiparty quantum private comparison. *Scientific reports*, 9(1), 1–16, (2019).
30. Abulkasim, H., Alsuqaih, H. N., Hamdan, W. F., Hamad, S., Farouk, A., Mashatan, A., & Ghose, S. Improved dynamic multi-party quantum private comparison for next-generation mobile network. *IEEE Access*, 7, 17917–17926, (2019).
31. A. J. Obaid, "Critical Research on the Novel Progressive, JOKER an Opportunistic Routing Protocol Technology for Enhancing the Network Performance for Multimedia Communications," in Research in Intelligent and Computing in Engineering. *Advances in Intelligent Systems and Computing*, vol 1254. Springer, Singapore., Springer, Singapore, pp. 369–378, (2021).
32. A. J. Obaid, K. A. Alghurabi, S. A. K. Albermany and S. Sharma, "Improving Extreme Learning Machine Accuracy Utilizing Genetic Algorithm for Intrusion Detection Purposes," in *Advances in Intelligent Systems and Computing*, Springer, Singapore, pp. 171–177 (2021).
33. Agarwal, A. K., & Jain, A. (2019). Synthesis of 2D and 3D NoC mesh router architecture in HDL environment. Journal of Advanced Research in Dynamical and Control Systems, 11(4), 2573–2581.
34. Agrawal, N., Jain, A., & Agarwal, A. (2019). Simulation of Network on Chip for 3D Router Architecture. International Journal of Recent Technology and Engineering, 8, 58–62.
35. C. Meshram, R. W. Ibrahim, A. J. Obaid, S. G. Meshram, A. Meshram and A. M. Abd El-Latif, "Fractional chaotic maps based short signature scheme under human-centered IoT environments," *Journal of Advanced Research*, (2020).
36. D. K. Sharma, B. Singh, E. Herman, R. Regine, S. S. Rajest and V. P. Mishra, "Maximum Information Measure Policies in Reinforcement Learning with Deep Energy-Based Model," 2021 International Conference on Computational Intelligence and Knowledge Economy, pp. 19–24, (2021).

37. D. K. Sharma, B. Singh, M. Raja, R. Regin and S. S. Rajest, "An Efficient Python Approach for Simulation of Poisson Distribution," 2021 7th International Conference on Advanced Computing and Communication Systems, pp. 2011–2014 (2021).
38. D. K. Sharma, B. Singh, R. Regin, R. Steffi and M. K. Chakravarthi, "Efficient Classification for Neural Machines Interpretations based on Mathematical models," 2021 7th International Conference on Advanced Computing and Communication Systems, pp. 2015–2020, (2021).
39. F. Arslan, B. Singh, D. K. Sharma, R. Regin, R. Steffi and S. Suman Rajest, "Optimization Technique Approach to Resolve Food Sustainability Problems," 2021 International Conference on Computational Intelligence and Knowledge Economy, pp. 25–30, (2021).
40. Farouk, A., Alahmadi, A., Ghose, S., & Mashatan, A. Blockchain platform for industrial healthcare: Vision and future opportunities. *Computer Communications,* 154, 223–235, (2020).
41. G. A. Ogunmola, B. Singh, D. K. Sharma, R. Regin, S. S. Rajest and N. Singh, "Involvement of Distance Measure in Assessing and Resolving Efficiency Environmental Obstacles," 2021 International Conference on Computational Intelligence and Knowledge Economy, pp. 13–18 (2021).
42. Ghai, D., Gianey, H. K., Jain, A., & Uppal, R. S. (2020). Quantum and dual-tree complex wavelet transform-based image watermarking. International Journal of Modern Physics B, 34(01), 2050009.
43. Gupta, N., Jain, A., Vaisla, K. S., Kumar, A., & Kumar, R. (2021). Performance analysis of DSDV and OLSR wireless sensor network routing protocols using FPGA hardware and machine learning. Multimedia Tools and Applications, 80(14), 22301–22319.
44. Gupta, N., Vaisla, K. S., Jain, A., Kumar, A., & Kumar, R. (2021). Performance Analysis of AODV Routing for Wireless Sensor Network in FPGA Hardware. Computer Systems Science and Engineering, 39(2), 1–12.
45. Jain, A., & Kumar, A. (2021). Desmogging of still smoggy images using a novel channel prior. Journal of Ambient Intelligence and Humanized Computing, 12(1), 1161–1177.
46. Jain, A., Dwivedi, R. K., Alshazly, H., Kumar, A., Bourouis, S., & Kaur, M. Design and Simulation of Ring Network-on-Chip for Different Configured Nodes Computers, Materials, & Continua; Henderson Vol. 71, Iss. 2, (2022): 4085–4100.
47. Jain, A., Dwivedi, R., Kumar, A., & Sharma, S. (2017). Scalable design and synthesis of 3D mesh network on chip. In Proceeding of International Conference on Intelligent Communication, Control and Devices (pp. 661–666). Springer, Singapore.
48. Jain, A., Gahlot, A. K., Dwivedi, R., Kumar, A., & Sharma, S. K. (2018). Fat Tree NoC Design and Synthesis. In Intelligent Communication, Control and Devices (pp. 1749–1756). Springer, Singapore.
49. Jain, A., Kumar, A., & Sharma, S. (2015). Comparative Design and Analysis of Mesh, Torus and Ring NoC. Procedia Computer Science, 48, 330–337. 20.
50. Kumar, A., & Jain, A. (2021). Image smog restoration using oblique gradient profile prior and energy minimization. Frontiers of Computer Science, 15(6), 1–7.
51. Kumar, S., Jain, A., Kumar Agarwal, A., Rani, S., & Ghimire, A. (2021). Object-Based Image Retrieval Using the U-Net-Based Neural Network. Computational Intelligence and Neuroscience, 2021.
52. Kumar, S., Jain, A., Shukla, A. P., Singh, S., Raja, R., Rani, S., ... & Masud, M. (2021). A Comparative Analysis of Machine Learning Algorithms for Detection of Organic and Nonorganic Cotton Diseases. Mathematical Problems in Engineering, 2021.
53. Misra, N. R., Kumar, S., & Jain, A. (2021, February). A Review on E-waste: Fostering the Need for Green Electronics. In 2021 International Conference on Computing, Communication, and Intelligent Systems (ICCCIS) (pp. 1032–1036). IEEE.

54. Sharma, S. K., Jain, A., Gupta, K., Prasad, D., & Singh, V. (2019). An internal schematic view and simulation of major diagonal mesh network-on-chip. Journal of Computational and Theoretical Nanoscience, 16(10), 4412–4417.
55. Zhu, F., Zhang, C., Zheng, Z., & Farouk, A. Practical Network Coding Technologies and Softwarization in Wireless Networks. *IEEE Internet of Things Journal,* 8(7), 5211–5218, (2021).
56. Rao AN, Vijayapriya P, Kowsalya M, Rajest SS. Computer Tools for Energy Systems. In International Conference on Communication, Computing and Electronics Systems, pp. 475–484, Springer, Singapore (2020).
57. J. Kubiczek and B. Hadasik, "Challenges in Reporting the COVID-19 Spread and its Presentation to the Society," *J. Data and Information Quality*, vol. 13, no. 4, pp. 1–7, (2021).

A Deep Study on Thermography Methods and Applications in Assessment of Various Disorders

Komali Dammalapati, P. S. N. Murty, Ibrahim Patel, Prabha Shreeraj Nair, and K. Saikumar

1 Introduction

Thermography employs a photo camera that consists of infrared sensors in greater count that can detect and quantify differences in small temperatures. On a portable computer, these obtained insignificant temperature variations can be downloaded and further demonstrated in the colour of the grey-scale diagram. Usually, there exist two different kinds of thermography: passive and active thermography [1]. In the case of passive thermography, the construction of a temperature map is created by a thermal image by pointing the camera at the region of the test piece. In the case of active thermography, the temperature decays concerning time by critically heating the outer part of the object precipitously applying heat source externally [2]. Disproportions of the material will be obtained at the variations in the rate of temperature decay. Because of the medical thermography, the methodology is a non-obtrusive

K. Dammalapati (✉)
Department of CSE, Koneru Lakshmaiah Education Foundation, Guntur, Andhra Pradesh, India

P. S. N. Murty
Department of ECE, Vignan's Institute of Information Technology (A) Duvvada, Visakhapatnam, Andhra Pradesh, India

I. Patel
Department of Electronics and Communication Engineering, B V Raju Institute of Technology, Narsapur, India
e-mail: ibrahim.patel@bvrit.ac.in

P. S. Nair
CSE Department, S B Jain Institute of Technology Management and Research, Nagpur, India

K. Saikumar
Department of ECE, Koneru Lakshmaiah Education Foundation, Guntur, Andhra Pradesh, India
e-mail: saikumarkayam4@ieee.org

P. Agarwal et al. (eds.), *Artificial Intelligence for Smart Healthcare*,
EAI/Springer Innovations in Communication and Computing,
https://doi.org/10.1007/978-3-031-23602-0_21

and nonionizing structure that captures the image in a real-time environment for the skin of the surface to be associated. The dependency of the distribution for the temperature of the skin usually relies on the exchange of the heat transferred between the skin tissues, the regional vascularization, and the activity involved in the metabolism [3].

Moreover, in the survey of the rate of sensitivity, the commonly measured temperature is nearly at the range of 0.04 °C for the limitation value of 30–40 °C and so forth due to the areas in which heat is absorbed for the period of noticeable count in comparison with the areas in which heat is emitted [4]. The heat cast in the area of skin influenced by the infrared rays relatively exchanges further in the process of quantitative and qualitative relationships scientifically reported with various disorders. Such disorders for the survey highlighted are the region of facial structures and the temporomandibular joints (TMJ) [5]. The skin temperature and temporomandibular joint (TMJ) are daily enhancing in human's inclusive joints discomfort. In contrast, the skin's temperature is at the minimum level for the pain in the myofascial area. The particular personalities have the disorder to the temporomandibular (TMD) conditions to demonstrate the disproportionateness at the greater count for the skin's temperature than those irregularities inside the area. Majorly, the places like the surface of the body and the layers of tissues at superficies can be relatively associated with the more profound movement of the range in specific points at 6–10 mm depth for the symbolic concept in utilizing the methodology involved the thermography [6]. The heat balance and the dysfunctions of the biological means can be significantly influenced due to the variations in the temperature of the regional skin. The measuring device can be emitted for the heat due to specific area configuration in which the sensor is allocated for the radiations of the infrared regions in the spectrum of electromagnetic surface for the device of thermostat consisting of an optical mirror and system of lens connected with an analogy transducer specifically for the specific software in the computer [7]. The investigation illustrates applied inflammation in the region of thermography for associating the pain in the form of oral maxillofacial surgery. Recording the variations in the thermal problem on the exterior of the skin and the inflammation minimization supervised the area that has been inspected. Therefore, thermography is a device in which it allows diagnostics to achieve comprehensive knowledge concerning the patient's situation (shown in Fig. 1).

Evaluation in the scientific system is for fever testing utilizing thermography. As per clinical analysis, an investigational setting is rendered to describe the thermal image to tripod utilized for full-face covered to the structure at the body region. Using MATLAB and IRTs, the graphical user interface (GUI) remained established [8]. The measurements at the four observations are noted to limit the effect at the exterior surface temperature and more profound range movement at a certain point at 6–10 mm depth for the symbolic concept in utilizing the methodology involved in the thermography for 15 min. The heat balance and the dysfunctions of the biological means can be focused on the facial regions. The oral thermometry is applied to establish reference temperature in the corresponding readings of temperature in the model, which modulated for two temperatures in monitoring the model at a fast rate

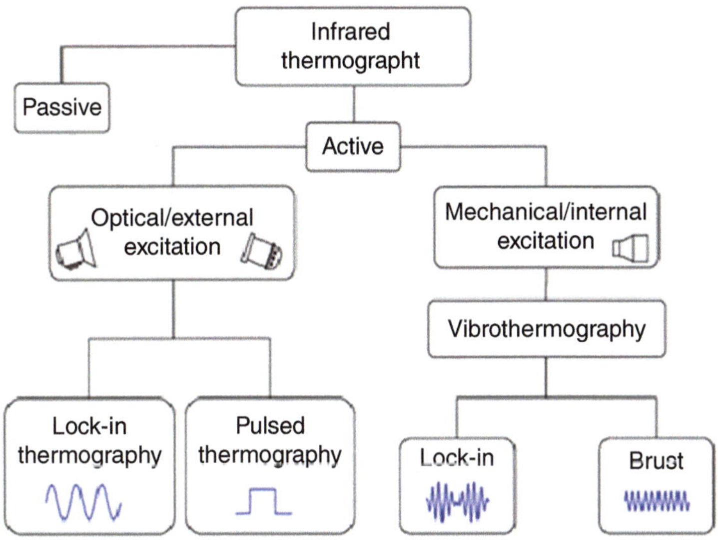

Fig. 1 Approaches of infrared thermography

for monitoring data [9, 10]. The model's accuracy in which the temperature for the oral measurement is around ±1.5 [11]. Concerning temperature, the average throughput value will be assessed. The facial region of the count is depicted in several areas of delineation point in the surface, the procedure for registration in the thermal image for a kind of TMD disorder in the method of relations for prominent facial positions to be recorded in the measurements of the temperature.

The temperature determined for various standards in the regions selected for comparison to the reference for the differences pairwise has been verified [12]. The result was generated at the temperature of different regions in five measurement standards as per the data. The approach monitors the anterior section of the pain to improve image capture in real-time for skin association. The dependency of the distribution for the temperature of the skin usually relies on the exchange of the heat transferred between the skin tissues, the regional vascularization, and the activity involved in the metabolism. Moreover, in the survey of the sensitivity rate, the affected elements are to puzzle for identifying the fluctuation in the clinical investigation (shown in Fig. 2).

An ascent in internal heat level is a typical indication of affliction. For observing internal heat levels, infrared thermography (IRT) gives a fast, aloof, non-contact, and non-intrusive option in dissimilarity to standard clinical thermometers. IRT can likewise plan external body temperature in a good way. The utilization of warm imaging cameras to acquire relationships between warm physiology and skin temperature has consistently expanded during the 50 years. Bosom malignancy, diabetic neuropathy, and fringe vascular sicknesses have all been effectively determined to have IRT. It's additionally been utilized in gynaecology, kidney transplantation, dermatology, cardiology, neonatal physiology, fever screening, and mind imaging.

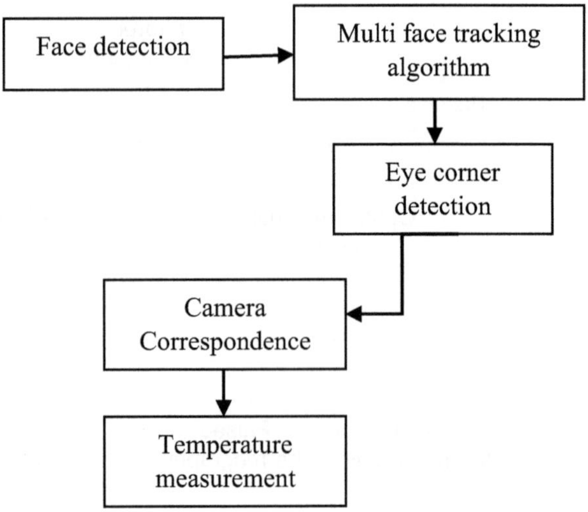

Fig. 2 Procedure for fever-screening at multilevel utilizing thermal and camera

Ongoing high-goal thermographic pictures are currently attainable because of modern infrared cameras, information gathering, and preparing procedures, which will probably prod more exploration in this area. The current spotlight is on the programmed investigation of temperature dispersion in premium locales, just as an objective examination of the information for anomaly distinguishing proof. The accomplishments in the field of clinical IRT are the focal point of this primary appraisal. This outline covers the essentials of IRT, just as the critical hypothetical establishment, conventions for different estimations, and IRT applications in numerous clinical areas. Likewise, foundation material is provided for novices to assist them with grasping the subject better.

The temperature has been demonstrated to be a decent indicator of wellbeing before, and the temperature has been used for clinical conclusions since 400 BC. People, as homeotherms, are fit for keeping a consistent internal heat level, which may contrast with the ambient temperature. The inner core and the outer perimeter of homeotherms' bodies can be separated into two components. The core temperature is kept within a restricted range (about 42–33 degrees Celsius). The management of the inner core temperature is critical for the human body's optimal functioning. A change of a few degrees in core temperature is regarded as a strong indicator of impending sickness. Thermoregulation is a physiological mechanism that regulates the body's temperature.

Thermometers were invented in the seventeenth century. George Martine utilized thermometers to track diurnal temperature fluctuations in healthy people regularly. Carl Wunderlich was the first to rigorously study the temperature of fevered people and compare it to that of healthy subjects in 1868, establishing temperature as a scientific predictor of sickness. He determined that a temperature range of 36.3 to 37.5 °C may remain deemed usual and also that a temperature above this range must be measured as a sign of disease. Liquid-based thermometers were utilized in the beginning. Sir William Herschel's discovery of infrared radiation in 1800 was immediately followed by his son John Herschel's recording of the first thermal image, which unlocked up new sizes in the realm of temperature monitoring. Hardy hypothesized that human skin could be measured by a blackbody radiator when he outlined the physiological position of infrared emission from the human body in 1934. He discovered the diagnostic value of infrared temperature measurement, paving the path for infrared thermography (IRT) in medical disciplines. However, due to a lack of quality equipment and technological know-how, the first use was only documented in 1960.

Thermography is a noninvasive technology for measuring and recording temperatures, allowing for the viewing of heat transfer. Liquid crystal thermography (LeT), infrared thermography (IRT), and microwave thermography are the three forms of thermography (MWT). This paper gives a review of the literature on different sorts of thermography's biomedical uses. The thermographic systems are useful diagnostic and therapeutic tools due to their noninvasive nature and excellent resolution. Blood flow detection, joint inflammation and cancer diagnosis, thermal modeling of diverse body portions, and application in procreative difficulties are common study topics. The survey reveals that thermography has uses in medicine, veterinary medication, pharmacy, and dentistry, among other professions. This can be accomplished by completing an operation to learn more about the situation. This option has numerous disadvantages. The patient suffers a considerable deal of suffering, expense, risk, and time due to exploratory surgery. Alternative procedures that allow a physician to "see" beneath the skin's external deprived of operating are desirable. In many circumstances, it's preferable to see the body in its natural state. A clinician, for example, could want to keep track of a medicine that has been vaccinated into the bloodstream. If required, an operation cannot remain conducted since the body's normal state will be altered. Some techniques allow you to see the confidentiality of the human body from the external. Outside the body, radioactive isotopes can remain injected and followed. Radiology visualizes the interior structure of the body by using the interactions of X-rays and matter. These methods are not without their drawbacks. Any use of radiation for imaging comes with risks, especially when the exposure time is prolonged. As a result of this risk, nonionizing radiation-free testing approaches are being sought. Thermography is a technique for mapping temperature differences in a flattened picture. This strategy distinguishes electromagnetic energy delivered by a body of liquid at a higher temperature than the general climate. The warm radiation produced by a body is relative to the distinction among the fourth force of the body and also the fourth force of its environmental factors, according to Boltzmann's law. As a result, even minor temperature variations can result in significant numbers of released photons, making thermography a potent instrument for detecting even the tiniest temperature variances.

Thermography is a procedure that involves measuring and recording temperatures to visualize heat flow. The three types of thermography are liquid crystal thermography, infrared thermography, and microwave thermography (MWT). LeT makes use of the optical anisotropy of some organic molecules in the liquid phase. A colour change is thus connected to a change in temperature in the case of certain cholesterol molecules. However, IRT and MWT enable the reflection and identification of light produced by heated substances in the infrared and microwave spectrums. In LeT, the study surface is usually painted with a specific paint; in MWT, the receiving antenna is likewise in interaction with the character. As a result, there is the worry that the technique may affect surface thermal circumstances in some instances. IRT, on the other hand, does not necessitate such a touch. The thermography technique does not utilize radiation and may be used repeatedly over extended periods without harming the user's health. Since the 1950s, scientists have studied both people and animals and found a link between their body temperature and health. An area's temperature is determined by the cellular metabolism and local blood flow, and these problems often cause temperature increases. An abnormally high body temperature is an early sign of illness. Here are some of the recent applications of thermography. E Diniz de Lima et al. [19] used artificial intelligence and infrared thermography as supplementary diagnostic techniques for temporomandibular dysfunction. Snekhalatha Umapathy et al. [20] used machine learning and deep learning to identify orofacial discomfort using thermograms. Using infrared thermography to diagnose patients with symptoms of peripheral arterial disease who have infratemporal percutaneous revascularizations is a promising approach authored by Gladiol Zenunaj and colleagues [21]. Ale Procházka et al. [22] study the use infrared thermographs and computational intelligence to analyse facial video recordings.

2 Materials and Methods

Representing the thermography has for paraclinical examination in the irradiation to the functional prognostics in completing the treatment employed. Medical care for the internal aspects is in the department for the study of rheumatology to attain information for the inflammation, pain, and muscular spasm. The differences in the inherent characteristics of the pain that occurred at myofascial introduce various physical attributes in the outbreak regions of the palpation technique in disorder at TMD in the clinical process for associating at the facial criticisms for alterations in TMJ of the surfaced skin [22–26].

The test room's temperature and relative humidity may simply be controlled. The camera is naturally positioned to reduce temperature measuring geometric mistakes. Look at Fig. 3.

Sample 1: A potato was skinned, cleaned, and diced to make the catecholase extract. In a kitchen blender, 30.0 g diced potato and then 150 mL of distilled water were combined and mixed for 2 min. Four layers of cheesecloth were used to filter the resultant solution, and the extract was kept in a sealed, clean container. The following reagents were used in varied proportions (as shown in Fig. 1) to make four individually labelled spectrophotometer tubes: a pH 7 buffer, a 0.1 percent catechol substrate, and distilled water. The Spectronic 20 spectrophotometer's frequency was set to 540 nm. A clear regulator tube made with no catechol substrate and assigned

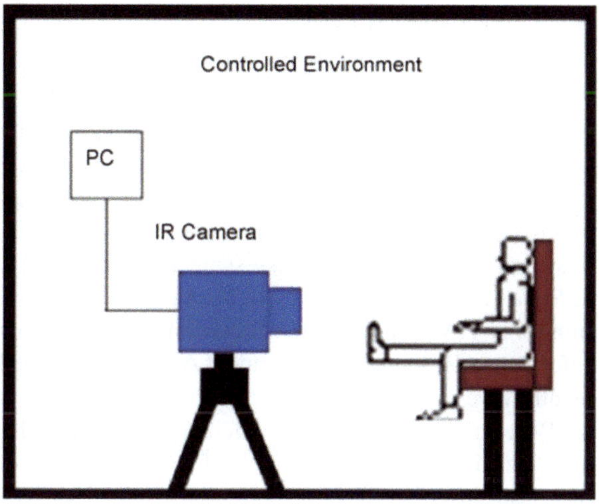

Fig. 3 A diagram of a common health thermography exam

"tube 1" was reversed and acquainted into the spectrophotometer with aligning the spectrophotometer at zero absorbance [26–31].

Significantly, the concentration to be examined was added to each cylinder just before turning on the spectrophotometer. Cylinder 2 got 1.0 mL of catecholase separately pipetted into it. Cylinder 2 was modified and set in the spectrophotometer immediately [32]. For time zero (t0), the 10-min imprint (t10), and then every moment in the middle, the absorbance was perused and recorded. Cylinder 2 was taken out from the spectrophotometer, and estimations were acquired utilizing the indistinguishable technique for tubes 3 and 4.

Sample 2: For this experiment, a potato and a knife were obtained. In addition, eight spectrophotometer tubes, distilled water, a blender, cheesecloth, a clean container by a lid, and then a blender were utilized. For this experiment, a Spectronic 20 spectrophotometer was employed and buffers with pHs of 4, 6, 7, and 8. This experiment also required a catechol substrate, parafilm covers, Kimwipes, a black pen, and a pipette. Finally, a pencil and paper were obtained to keep track of the findings [33–37].

Sample 3: A potato was skinned, cleaned, and diced to make the catecholase extract. To obtain 30.0 g of chopped potato, a balance was utilized. A beaker was filled with 150 mL of distilled water. The diced potato was soaked in water. The lid of a kitchen mixer was taken off. In a blender, combine the potato and water. The fluid had a potato odour to it. The blender's cover was placed on top; then, the power button was pressed. The time remained kept until the second hand circled twice on the clock. To stop the blender, the power button was pressed once again. Four layers of cheesecloth were used to filter the resultant solution. The extract was kept in a sealed, clean container. The above all mechanism concentrates on the tomography-based disease diagnosis process. Here, all types of disorders are discussed through various radiology techniques. Finally, it is identified that the machine intelligence mechanism is suitable for abnormal disorders [38].

3 Literature Survey

A study was undertaken on 46 patients with a flaring or degenerative rheumatic condition and temporomandibular joint difficulties, 24 women and 22 men. With the consent of the Ethics Committee, the investigation took place between November 2016 and March 2018. Patients completed an educated assent structure for clinical, practical, and paraclinical examinations, as well as physiotherapy treatment before the investigation began. The assessment and treatment were tailored to the individual at Stefan cel Mare University in Suceava, Romania's Complex Building of Swimming and Physical Therapy. According to the authors, Brioschi, M. L. [14], The Information Resources Management Association in the United States researched oral health care and technology. Thermography was suggested by A. Dionisio, L. Roseiro, Fonseca, and P. Nicolau to evaluate Facial Temperature Recovery after Elastic Gum. The accuracy of two techniques of infrared image analysis of the masticatory muscles in identifying myelogenous temporomandibular tangle was investigated by D. Rodrigues-Bigaton, A.V. Dibai-Filho, and A.C. Packer [15].

Various thermology effects and facial telethermography were discussed by B.M. Grant and M. Anbar in current and future dent maxillofacial therapeutic applications. "Electronic face thermography: an analysis of asymptomatic adult subjects" was proposed by B.M. Gratt and E.A. Sickles. J Orofac Pain is a journal dedicated to the study of orofacial pain. After orthodontic action, S.B. McBeth and B. M. Gratt investigated the thermographic assessment of temporomandibular messes symptomology [16]. Facial temperature can be calculated in a sitting position, both static and dynamically. Also, images of affected facial regions can be calculated and stored in under 3 min [39–42]. Because of the anatomical imbalance of this location, the ordinary thermograms of the temporary district should be balanced, according to the standard convention proposed thru Schwartz in 2006. Two hours before the assessment, the participants were told not to use any salves or dust on their skin, not to use a hairdryer or hairstyles, and then not to smoke. It's also a good idea to avoid skeletal controls, needle treatment, and physiotherapy during the 12 h before up to the test and for the 24 h following the test [43–44].

Also, avoid drinking espresso, medicine drops, analgesics, sedatives, or anything that could impair your ability to think clearly [45–48]. During the thermographic exam, the patients are instructed not to touch or press on the facial skin. Another suggestive treatment for orofacial suffering is thermovision [17]. K. Wozniak, L. et al. spoke on evaluating thermography's sensitivity, specificity, and correctness in classifying TMD patients. A moral investigation of present procedures in the detection and treatment of temporomandibular messes. The American Academy of Thermology's associated guidelines for neuromusculoskeletal thermography were given by R.G. Schwartz et al.

3.1 Proposed System

In the context of thermography, the variations of the temperatures differentiate for mean and standard deviations for the observed counts in the masseter muscles and temporal in enhanced sensitivity of 1.5% in the clinical investigation [18]. The advancement of the treatment requested in the thermal is essential in the clinical assessment to monitor the muscles. Communal areas are in the study of evaluation in the density of the secondary analyses of the correlated knowledge of the VAS observed scale in the sensitivity. At the limited surface temperature of the skin in the temporomandibular joint, the level of joint severity inbuilt in the infrared sensors for the joints leads to a higher rate of disorders like osteoarthritis, osteoporosis, and arthralgia. For people in healthy conditions, there is a more profound movement of the range at a certain point at 6–10 mm depth for the symbolic concept of utilising the methodology involved in the thermography [49].

The heat balance and the dysfunctions of the biological means can be focused on the facial regions [50, 51]. The oral thermometry is applied to establish reference temperature in the corresponding temperature readings in the model it modulates. The applied knowledge of the thermography is a unique system in TMD that critically evaluates the diagnosis in TMD for data that is insufficiently based on the models of the more significant dynamic effects to utilize the outcomes in the oral facial measurements in the correlation of the variated temperature for TMJ and TMD in different modifications in the prognostics (Shown in Fig. 4).

4 Result Analysis

Based on the diagnostics made, the study has been created that the weight of the different genders was obtained at the rate of approximately 51.3% for the female candidate and 48.7% for the male candidate. Moreover, in the survey of the rate of

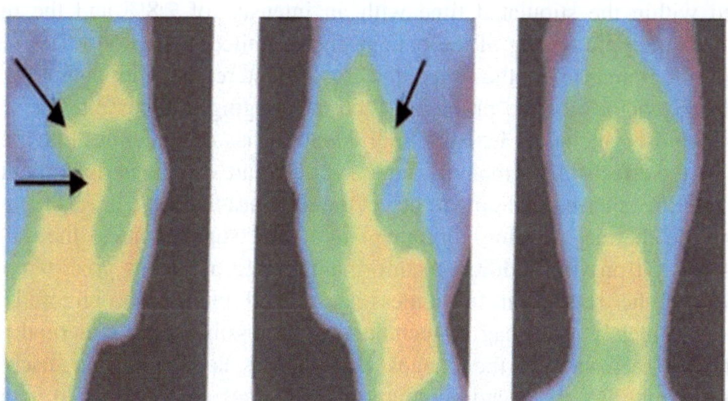

Fig. 4 Thermographic images with maxillary upper hyperthermia, hyperthermia, TMJ asymmetry, osteoarthritis cervical spine

sensitivity, the commonly measured temperature is nearly at the range of 0.04 °C for the limitation value of 30–40 °C and so forth due to the areas in which heat is absorbed for the period of the noticeable count. The patient's age group will be varied from 24 to 75 years, in which the batch-wise average count is at the deviation of 55 ± 13.88 years. The frequency at a higher rate in patients is of various kinds of disorders such osteoarthritis investigated at the average rate of 75.83% inclusive with the abnormalities studied for the years of deviation as shown in the graph around 13 ± 8.39 years until the difference of 5 to 45 age group. The intensity of the pain obtained from the VAS (Visual Analog Scale) in the rate survey for the average count of 2 months decreased in scores for all disciplines.

Overall, the muscle masseter has the rate in the average temperature of 34 °C at the level of muscle in the temporal. The group of the study evaluated for the pain on the scale of VAS is depicted in Fig. 5. The TMJ Algo-Efficient indices indicate a minimum rate onset obtained value of 18 ± 3.65, 12 ± 4 for 5 months, and 9.26 ± 2.96 for 7 months. The TMD dysfunction has an abnormality rate of 25% for women compared with 23% for men. Nevertheless, dangerous dysfunction has been detected rarely in the surveyed group in mutual women (10%) and men (8%).

5 Conclusion

This paper reviews the various materials and methods of thermography at the stage of clinical investigation and in the environment of laboratory thermography emphasized the mutilation of the muscle at the adjacent of the groups in the specific effect of temporomandibular joint over the existence of spasm and muscle at confined disproportions, pain, and swelling. Out of particular findings, it is recommended to utilize a device known as thermography to detect the problem and for proper assessment of temporomandibular disorders, which serves as an overall diagnosis. Furthermore, the analysis gives additional knowledge regarding regional cardiovascular practice and nerve variations. The performance over some time has been recorded within the stipulated time with an intensity of 2.8% and the reach of 86.3 s with multiple testing of the patient under limited restrictions. The visibility of the thermogram is under the area of the conditioned region, with pathology linked easier to the vicinity of the problem. Thermal imaging systems may be used for various purposes, including isolating individuals at risk of epidemics like the flu. In this study, the effects of thermal imaging on children are examined. In particular, it is critical to utilize thermal imaging to detect the illnesses that have been suggested. In addition, the thermal imaging equipment is a great supplement to the diagnostic process since it provides additional information. Because of its great temperature sensitivity, higher resolution, frictionless nature, and ability to do remote imaging, IRT is a completely safe imaging technique. It is possible to save thermal pictures digitally and then analyse the images with various applications to discover the existing thermal pattern. Pseudo-coloured thermographs are simpler to understand

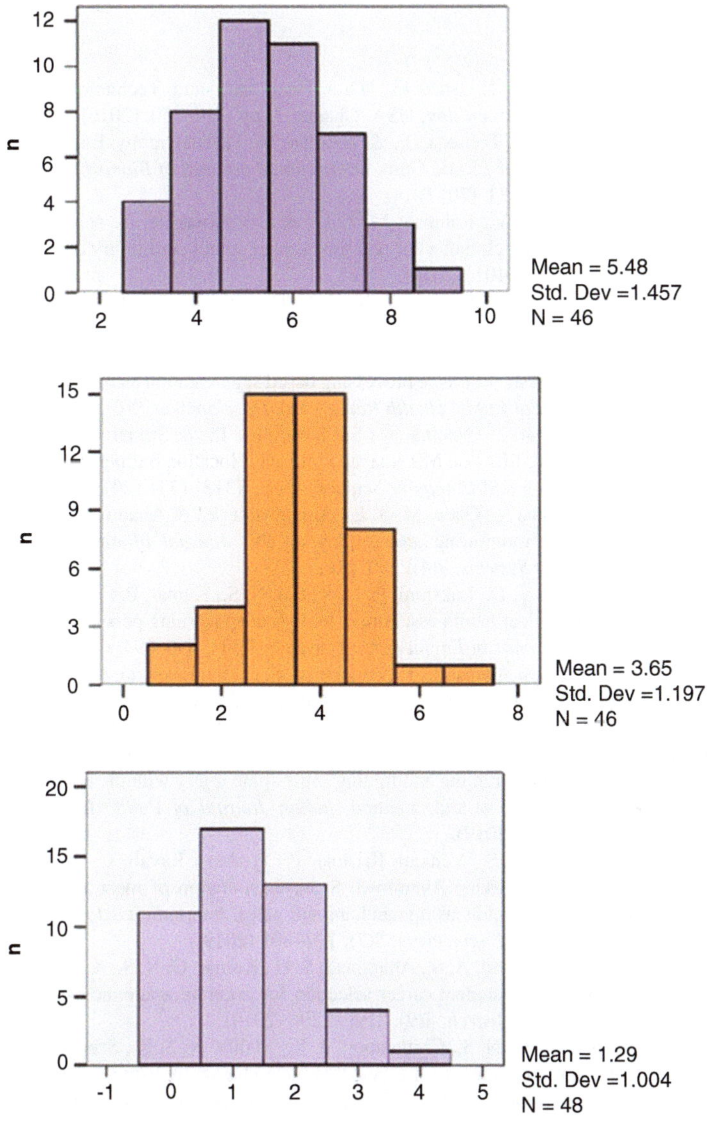

Fig. 5 Group of the study evaluated for the pain on the scale of VAS

and take less time. The results of studies have indicated that IRT is effective in diagnosing many illnesses, including breast cancer and diabetes. This work provided an accuracy of 98.67% and a sensitivity of 94.45%, and a recall of 92.34% had been attained.

References

1. D. Sabbagh Haddad, M. L. Brioschi, "Oral Healt care and Technologies" *Information Resources Management Association*, USA, Chapter 3, pp. 329–350, (2016).
2. Dionisio, A., Roseiro, L., Fonseca, J., & Nicolau, P. Thermography Evaluation on Facial Temperature Recovery after Elastic Gum. *International Journal of Biomedical and Biological Engineering*, 11(5), 269–273, (2017).
3. Ahammad, S. H., Rajesh, V., Rahman, M. Z. U., & Lay-Ekuakille, A. A hybrid CNN-based segmentation and boosting classifier for real time sensor spinal cord injury data. *IEEE Sensors Journal*, 20(17), 10092–10101, (2020).
4. Ahammad, S. H., Rajesh, V., & Rahman, M. Z. U. Fast and accurate feature extraction-based segmentation framework for spinal cord injury severity classification. *IEEE Access*, 7, 46092–46103 (2019).
5. Ahammad, S. K., & Rajesh, V. Image processing based segmentation techniques for spinal cord in MRI. *Indian Journal of Public Health Research & Development*, 9(6), (2018).
6. Ahammad, S. H., Rajesh, V., Neetha, A., Sai Jeesmitha, B., & Srikanth, A. Automatic segmentation of spinal cord diffusion MR images for disease location finding. *Indonesian Journal of Electrical Engineering and Computer Science*, 15(3), 1313–1321 (2019).
7. Vijaykumar, G., Gantala, A., Gade, M. S. L., Anjaneyulu, P., & Ahammad, S. H. Microcontroller based heartbeat monitoring and display on PC. *Journal of Advanced Research in Dynamical and Control Systems*, 9(4), 250–260, (2017).
8. Inthiyaz, S., Prasad, M. V. D., Lakshmi, R. U. S., Sai, N. S., Kumar, P. P., & Ahammad, S. H. Agriculture based plant leaf health assessment tool: A deep learning perspective. *International Journal of Emerging Trends in Engineering Research*, 7(11), 690–694, (2019).
9. Kumar, M. S., Inthiyaz, S., Vamsi, C. K., Ahammad, S. H., Sai Lakshmi, K., Venu Gopal, P., & Bala Raghavendra, A. Power optimization using dual SRAM circuit. *International Journal of Innovative Technology and Exploring Engineering*, 8(8), 1032–1036, (2019).
10. Ahammad, S. H., Rajesh, V., Hanumatsai, N., Venumadhav, A., Sasank, N. S. S., Gupta, K. B., & Inithiyaz, S. MRI image training and finding acute spine injury with the help of hemorrhagic and non-hemorrhagic rope wounds method. *Indian Journal of Public Health Research & Development*, 10(7), 404, (2019).
11. Siva Kumar, M., Inthiyaz, S., Venkata Krishna, P., Jyothsna Ravali, C., Veenamadhuri, J., Hanuman Reddy, Y., & Hasane Ahammad, S. Implementation of most appropriate leakage power techniques in vlsi circuits using nand and nor gates. *International Journal of Innovative Technology and Exploring Engineering*, 8(7), 797–801 (2019).
12. Myla, S., Marella, S. T., Goud, A. S., Ahammad, S. H., Kumar, G. N. S., & Inthiyaz, S. Design decision taking system for student career selection for accurate academic system. *Journal of Scientific & Technology Research*, 8(9), 2199–2206 (2019).
13. Raj Kumar, A., Kumar, G. N. S., Chithanoori, J. K., Mallik, K. S. K., Srinivas, P., & Hasane Ahammad, S. Design and analysis of a heavy vehicle chassis by using E-glass epoxy & S-2 glass materials. *International Journal of Recent Technology and Engineering*, 7(6), 903–905 (2019).
14. Madhav, B. T. P., & Anilkumar, T. Design and study of multiband planar wheel-like fractal antenna for vehicular communication applications. *Microwave and Optical Technology Letters*, 60(8), 1985–1993 (2018).
15. Deepak, B. S., Madhav, B. T., Prabhakar, V. S. V., Lakshman, P., Anilkumar, T., & Rao, M. V. Design and analysis of hetero triangle linked hybrid web fractal antenna for wide band applications. *Progress in Electromagnetics Research* C, 83, 147–159 (2018).
16. Madhav, B. T. P., Rao, T. V., & Anilkumar, T. Design of 4-element printed array antenna for ultra-wideband applications. International *Journal of Microwave and Optical Technology*, 13(1), 8–17 (2018).

17. Gattim, N. K., Pallerla, S. R., Bojja, P., Reddy, T. P. K., Chowdary, V. N., Dhiraj, V., & Ahammad, S. H. Plant leaf disease detection using SVM technique. *International Journal of Emerging Trends in Engineering Research*, 7(11), 634–637 (2019).
18. Ahammad, S. H., Rajesh, V., Venkatesh, K. N., Nagaraju, P., Rao, P. R., & Inthiyaz, S. Liver segmentation using abdominal CT scanning to detect liver disease area. *International Journal of Emerging Trends in Engineering Research*, 7(11), 664–669 (2019).
19. Diniz de Lima E, Souza Paulino JA, Lira de Farias Freitas AP, Viana Ferreira JE, Barbosa JDS, Bezerra Silva DF, Bento PM, Araújo Maia Amorim AM, Melo DP. Artificial intelligence and infrared thermography as auxiliary tools in the diagnosis of temporomandibular disorder. *Dentomaxillofac Radiol.* 2021 Oct 6:20210318 (2021).
20. Snekhalatha Umapathy, Palani Thanaraj Krishnan, "Automated detection of orofacial pain from thermograms using machine learning and deep learning approaches" *Expert Systems*, Volume 38, Issue 7 (2021).
21. Tsolaki, E., Gladiol Zenunaj, Edo Gresta, Stefano Di Mase, and Francesco Mascoli. "Contrast-Enhanced Ultrasound versus Computed Tomography Angiography in the Follow-Up of the Treatment of Abdominal Aortic Aneurysm with Endovascular Techniques." *Journal for Vascular Ultrasound* 36, no. 4: 263–66 (2012).
22. B. Panjwani, V. Singh, A. Rani, and V. Mohan, "Optimum multi-drug regime for compartment model of tumour: cell-cycle-specific dynamics in the presence of resistance," *Journal of Pharmacokinetics and Pharmacodynamics*, vol. 48, no. 4, pp. 543–562, (2021).
23. D. K. Sharma, B. Singh, E. Herman, R. Regine, S. S. Rajest and V. P. Mishra, "Maximum Information Measure Policies in Reinforcement Learning with Deep Energy-Based Model," 2021 International Conference on Computational Intelligence and Knowledge Economy, pp. 19–24 (2021).
24. D. K. Sharma, B. Singh, M. Raja, R. Regin and S. S. Rajest, "An Efficient Python Approach for Simulation of Poisson Distribution," 2021 7th International Conference on Advanced Computing and Communication Systems, pp. 2011–2014 (2021).
25. D. S. Q. Al-Yasiri and A. J. Obaid, "A New Approach for Object Detection, Recognition and Retrieving in Painting Images," *Journal of Advance Research in Dynamic and Control System*, vol. 10, no. 2, pp. 2345–2359, (2018).
26. T. A. Al-asadi and A. J. Obaid, "Object detection and recognition by using enhanced speeded up robust feature," *International Journal of Computer Science and Network Security*, vol. 16, no. 4, pp. 66–71, (2016).
27. F. Arslan, B. Singh, D. K. Sharma, R. Regin, R. Steffi and S. Suman Rajest, "Optimization Technique Approach to Resolve Food Sustainability Problems," 2021 International Conference on Computational Intelligence and Knowledge Economy, pp. 25–30, (2021).
28. F. J. J. Joseph, "Effect of supervised learning methodologies in offline handwritten Thai character recognition," *Int. J. Inf. Technol.*, vol. 12, no. 1, pp. 57–64, Mar. (2020),
29. F. J. John Joseph, R. T, and J. J. C, "Classification of correlated subspaces using HoVer representation of Census Data," in 2011 International Conference on Emerging Trends in Electrical and Computer Technology, pp. 906–911 (2011).
30. G. A. Ogunmola, B. Singh, D. K. Sharma, R. Regin, S. S. Rajest and N. Singh, "Involvement of Distance Measure in Assessing and Resolving Efficiency Environmental Obstacles," 2021 International Conference on Computational Intelligence and Knowledge Economy, pp. 13–18 (2021).
31. Ghai, D., Gianey, H. K., Jain, A., & Uppal, R. S. Quantum and dual-tree complex wavelet transform-based image watermarking. *International Journal of Modern Physics* B, 34(04), 2050009 (2020).
32. Ishaq, A., Sadiq, S., Umer, M., Ullah, S., Mirjalili, S., Rupapara, V., & Nappi, M. Improving the Prediction of Heart Failure Patients' Survival Using SMOTE and Effective Data Mining Techniques. IEEE Access, 9, 39707–39716 (2021).

33. J. Kubiczek and B. Hadasik, "Challenges in Reporting the COVID-19 Spread and its Presentation to the Society," *J. Data and Information Quality*, vol. 13, no. 4, pp. 1–7, (2021).
34. Jain, A., & Kumar, A. Desmogging of still smoggy images using a novel channel prior. *Journal of Ambient Intelligence and Humanized Computing*, 12(1), 1161–1177 (2021).
35. K. Ganesh Kumar and S. Sudhakar, Improved Network Traffic by Attacking Denial of Service to Protect Resource Using Z-Test Based 4-Tier Geomark Traceback (Z4TGT), *Wireless Personal Communications*, Vol. 114, No. 4, pp:3541–3575, (2020).
36. K. Jayanthi, R. Rathinam and S. Pattabhi, "Electrocoagulation treatment for removal of Reactive Blue 19 from aqueous solution using Iron electrode", *Research Journal of Life Sciences, Bioinformatics, Pharmaceutical and Chemical Sciences*, 4:2, 101–113 (2018).
37. Kumar, S., Jain, A., Shukla, A. P., Singh, S., Raja, R., Rani, S., . . . & Masud, M. A Comparative Analysis of Machine Learning Algorithms for Detection of Organic and Nonorganic Cotton Diseases. *Mathematical Problems in Engineering,* (2021).
38. M. Govindaraj, R. Rathinam, C. Sukumar, M. Uthayasankar and S. Pattabhi, "Electrochemical oxidation of bisphenol-A from aqueous solution using graphite electrodes," *Environmental Technology* 34:4, 503–511 (2013).
39. N. O. alkaam, D. M. Q. Mohammed and A. J. Obaid, "A Hybrid Technique for Object Detection and Recognition Using Local Features Algorithms," *Journal of Advance Research in Dynamical and Control Systems*, vol. 10, no. 2, pp. 2330–2343, (2018).
40. Nomani, M. & Parveen, R. Legal Connotations of Biological Resources and its Ripple effect on Conservation Research in India and abroad, *International Journal of Conservation Science.* Vol. 12 Issue 2, 571–576 (2021).
41. Prabhu Kavin, B., Ganapathy, S., Suthanthiramani, P., & Kannan, A. A modified digital signature algorithm to improve the biomedical image integrity in cloud environment. *Advances in Computational Techniques for Biomedical Image Analysis*, 253–271 (2020).
42. Procházka A, Charvátová H, Vyšata O, Kopal J, Chambers J. Breathing Analysis Using Thermal and Depth Imaging Camera Video Records. *Sensors (Basel).* 2017 Jun 16;17(6): 1408 (2017).
43. R. Rathinam, M. Govindaraj, K. Vijayakumar and S. Pattabhi "Removal of Colour from Aqueous Rhodamine B Dye Solution by Photo electrocoagulation Treatment Techniques", "*Journal of Engineering, Scientific Research and Application*", 1: 2, 80–89 (2015).
44. Rehana Parveen. Impact of anti-money laundering legislation in the United Kingdom and European Union. *International Journal of Economics and Management Systems*, 5, 118–122, (2020).
45. Rustam, F., Khalid, M., Aslam, W., Rupapara, V., Mehmood, A., & Choi, G. S. A performance comparison of supervised machine learning models for Covid-19 tweets sentiment analysis. PLOS ONE, 16(2) (2021), e0245909.
46. S. Bhoumik, S. Chatterjee, A. Sarkar, A. Kumar, and F. J. John Joseph, "Covid 19 Prediction from X Ray Images Using Fully Connected Convolutional Neural Network," in CSBio '20: Proceedings of the Eleventh International Conference on Computational Systems-Biology and Bioinformatics, pp. 106–107 (2020).
47. S. Sudhakar and S. Chenthur Pandian "Authorized Node Detection and Accuracy in Position-Based Information for MANET", *European Journal of Scientific Research*, Vol. 70, No. 2, pp. 253–265, (2012).

48. Sadiq, S., Umer, M., Ullah, S., Mirjalili, S., Rupapara, V., & NAPPI, M. Discrepancy detection between actual user reviews and numeric ratings of Google App store using deep learning. *Expert Systems with Applications*, 115111 (2021).
49. Sharma, S. K., Jain, A., Gupta, K., Prasad, D., & Singh, V. An internal schematic view and simulation of major diagonal mesh network-on-chip. *Journal of Computational and Theoretical Nanoscience*, 16(10), 4412–4417 (2019).
50. V. Mohan, H. Chhabra, A. Rani, and V. Singh, "An expert 2DOF fractional order fuzzy PID controller for nonlinear systems," *Neural Computing and Applications*, vol. 31, no. 8, pp. 4253–4270, (2019).
51. Yousaf, A., Umer, M., Sadiq, S., Ullah, S., Mirjalili, S., Rupapara, V., & Nappi, M. Emotion Recognition by Textual Tweets Classification Using Voting Classifier (LR-SGD). *IEEE Access*, 9, 6286–6295 (2021).

A Smart Healthcare Cognitive Radio System for Future Wireless Commutation Applications with Test Methodology

K. R. Swetha, G. Drakshaveni, M. Sathya, Chilukuri Bala Venkata Subbarayudu, and G. Pavithra

1 Introduction

It was first developed at the turn of the century. The key advantage of using CR is that it uses DSA to solve the problem of bandwidth congestion and utilization. Through intelligently using idle spectrum segments, CR aims to alleviate spectrum congestion, which increases network operation and end-user data speeds. On the other hand, CR could aid in the effective use of unused spectrum. Since CR crosses many disciplines, no systematic test methodology for testing and evaluating CRs has yet been established [1]. There's still a lot of confusion about what a CR is and should be. This study aims to create a repeatable, modular, and accurate end-user CR test technique that can be used across several CR architectures. To begin, the test system should be independent of any particular CR design or technology. In other words, the test system is platform-agnostic, meaning it can be used to test any RF-capable device. Second, this test system is designed with an end user in mind;

K. R. Swetha (✉)
Department of CSE, BGS Institute of Technology, Adichunchanagiri University, Mandya, India

G. Drakshaveni
Department of MCA, BMSITM, Bangalore, India
e-mail: drakshavenig@bmsit.in

M. Sathya
Department of CSE, Islamiah Institute of Technology, Bangalore, India

C. B. V. Subbarayudu
Department of EEE, Shadan Women's College of Engineering and Technology, Hyderabad, India

G. Pavithra
Department of ECE, Dayananda Sagar College of Engineering (DSCE), Bangalore, Karnataka, India

P. Agarwal et al. (eds.), *Artificial Intelligence for Smart Healthcare*,
EAI/Springer Innovations in Communication and Computing,
https://doi.org/10.1007/978-3-031-23602-0_22

model specifications and efficiency come second to total performance. In conclusion, this approach could make it possible to detect emergent behaviour in complex CR systems [2–4].

1.1 MICR

The MICR approach to measuring and assessing CRs is based on a top-down systems approach. The under-test CR device, also known as the CRS, is regarded as a black box, along with its thread. MICR can be used to measure any RF-capable system. The interface does not have to be cognitive to be checked with MICR. On the other hand, devices with more intelligence are expected to do well. Instead of creating a cognitive model under evaluation, MICR evaluates the device's utility using output results. In the cognitive radio (CR) industry, there is currently no standardized final node examination organization that is a reliable, elastic, and actual variety of cognitive radio schemes.

Moreover, there is no device-independent framework in the CR sector that enables testing the full CR system rather than simply individual components [5]. This paper introduces the MICR, a CR test methodology, to solve these issues. MICR recommends monitoring the performance of both the primary_user (PU) and secondary_user (SU) in behaviour-based testing to assess cognition (i.e., the CR under test). Behaviour-based testing results are gathered and analysed. An SU and PU radio model is created using the Radiocommunication Research Platform (WARP) and WARP Lab tools, run in MATLAB. The PU provides five different radio-frequency settings using narrow-band, broadband, and non-contiguous wave shape [6–8]. The SU's reaction to the PU-created surroundings is evaluated. The SU blends energy-detection spectrum sensing into a basic cognitive engine (CE). The CE's impact on SU and PU performance is monitored and assessed.

Cognitive Radio (CR) is an efficient remote access application that can quickly provide medical, defense, and military organizations data access. A particular radio distinguishes accessible diverts in the remote range and changes its transmission or gathering qualities appropriately to permit more simultaneous remote correspondences in a given recurrence band at a solitary spot [9]. This illustrates the dynamic range of the executives in real life. The cognitive engine can configure radio-system parameters to answer the operative's instructions. "Waveform, protocol, operating frequency, and networking" are among the parameters [10]. This acts as a self-contained unit in the infrastructures setting, exchanging environmental data with the systems it connects to and other cognitive radios (CRs). In addition to "reading the radio's outputs", a CR "continuously monitors its performance", and utilizes this data to "determine the RF environment, channel conditions, link performance, and so on", and regulates the "radio's settings to deliver the required quality of service subject to an appropriate combination of user requirements, operational limitations, and regulatory constraints".

2 Related Work

The field of CR is complex, with few systematic, systemic classifications and categorizations. However, if a system is to be successfully tested, its limits must be well understood [11–13]. This section examines the CR area and how it is defined and organized in concepts and architectures. Then, CRs, testbeds, output indicators, and test methodologies are discussed. The material provided in this section remains meant to set the stage for the test methodology that has been introduced.

2.1 Cognitive Radio Definitions and Architectures

Definitions address the question, "What does a CR do?" while architectures answer the question, "How does a CR work?" In practice, meanings remain best used for determining whether or not a system is cognitive according to a concept. This study would not use unique CR concepts to assess cognition [14–16]. Architectures, on the other hand, typically allow a continuum of cognition, in which a device's actual cognition becomes secondary to overall machine output. As a result, this study's aim remains not towards describing or explaining what a cognitive radio is. Instead, this study aims to cover various architectural styles drawn from descriptions. A CR must sense the spectrum, share spectrum information, consolidate range information with that of different gadgets, make range coordination with different gadgets, and speak with the organization [17]. A CE, which frames the centre of the AI, is implied in these activities. To achieve customer priorities, the CE implements user and external policies. Another regularly ignored viewpoint is network geography, which is either bunched or conveyed.

2.2 Numerical Analysis

Performance measurements for CR can be used to assess the performance of a single CR part, a single CR node, or the entire CR system. Any efficiency measurements, such as those used in spectrum sensing can apply to each domain. For systematic measurement, uniform performance metrics are needed [18]. The most mainstream execution measurements are introduced here; nonetheless, the creators of [6] remember a profundity conversation of CR execution measurements [19–24].

2.3 Cognitive Radio Test Methodologies

In [6], the writers have divided the CR presentation measurement system into three tiers: node, network, and software. Each market level has differing degrees of perspective, whether the customer is a regulator, an ideals group, or a CR producer. For level-by-level comparability and standardization, the writers suggest utilizing "score-cards". This is the case since the evaluation method depends on evaluating the CE and conducting REMs [25–29]. The efficiency of the combined and RF systems is not assessed [30–32].

Author	Technique	Keynote	Advanced model
Steenkiste, P et al. [1]	Future direction cognitive radio technologies	Congestion control cannot be provided by the following model	The collaborative hypothesis CR model
Thompson, J et al. [2]	A simple test methodology based on CR wireless communication	The proposed model cannot regulate the packet delivery ratio as well as error rate	The following problem is eliminated by SVM-based CR modelling
Masonta, M et al. [3]	A decision-controlled CR modelling for advanced communication	In this research, a decision mechanism is used to implement the CR modelling, but congestion cannot be controlled using the suggested model	To overcome the following model, it is necessary to implement CR through CNN technology
Zhou, J et al. [4]	A heterogeneous and adaptive CR modelling for wireless communication models	In this investigation, heterogenous cognitive radio technology is implemented through machine intelligence techniques. The following model cannot provide accurate congestion control in CR at PUs and SUs communication	Collaborative hypothesis heterogeneous based CR providing better improvement
Filin, S et al. [5]	Standard Cognitive radio technology for congestion control in wireless communication	The following model is very efficient to control congestion at the packet delivery stage	RCNN with collaborative hypothesis is better

The above literature survey concentrates on the limitations of existed models and suggests a better methodology for future applications [33–37].

3 Proposed Test Methodology

This section introduces the proposed test technique, MICR, established by this study. The technique for assessing MICR is outlined in the following section, accompanied by the findings [38].

3.1 Overview

The MICR method is intended to be an all-encompassing approach to assessing a CRS. In the SUT, MICR uses benchmarks to encourage those practices (e.g., a CRS). Quality measurements are then used to assess the CR response to the stimulus [39–41]. Benchmark classes allow for scalable experimentation while also allowing for platform comparisons. Emulation is the best way to monitor the radio system. The effect of the presence of an SU on the PU can be determined directly in MICR, which is a special feature [42–45]. Similarly, the MICR benchmarks are not meant to calculate absolute CRS output in the real world. The basic CR has been assess the MICR evolution with fast diagnosis, also examine data efficeintly [46]. This presumption is critical for allowing a scalable yet focused method of assessing CRSs. If a system executes the following tasks, it is classified as cognitive by MICR:

1. Responds to the environment to improve results
2. Prevents existing users from being harmed
3. Implements usage policies and priorities when executing 1 and 2

The system enhances functionality, while causing no damage to current users is one of the two main elements of this concept. When putting these two objectives into action, cognition comes into effect [47–52]. As a result, it is unnecessary to quantify cognition explicitly since it can be assessed by increasing performance and preventing intervention. MICR views thought as a continuous process rather than sequential measures [53]. Testers will then concentrate on measuring CRS output without defending whether or not a system is neurological or to what cognitive degree it belongs [54–59]. When using MICR, cognition is visible when observing results. A more intelligent CRS could outperform a less intelligent CRS in results.

3.2 Benchmarks

CRS assessment can be scalable, meaningful, and repeatable thanks to benchmarks. The test scenario affects CRS conduct. Similarly, the CRS capabilities restrict the types of benchmarks used. The benchmark, for example, could stimulate a CRS's spectrum sensing capability. On the other hand, the benchmark should not be used to measure a CRS if the signal to be detected is beyond the capability of the CRS receiver test instrument. A broad range of CRS architectures can be tested using specific benchmark groups. Various architectures are run under the same benchmark to allow for direct comparison. When an architecture can't be run against a certain benchmark, it can't be specifically compared to other architectures that use that benchmark. This eliminates the possibility of drawing erroneous comparative conclusions.

3.3 Test Outline

The following is the suggested MICR evaluation framework. The physical layer is used to build an emulated radio world containing PUs with different waveforms that interact dynamically. These simulated PUs are made to demonstrate precise test conditions or simulate real-world conditions. This simulated PU-based radio environment serves as a repeatable baseline, allowing various CRS radios to be measured using the same benchmark. Physical CRs are attached to the test device and tested by gathering output measurements while being shielded from each other. Because emulation occurs at the physical layer, full-spectrum information is understood and regulated. Compared to field testing, the emulated environment makes for a faster turnaround of the test environment while providing greater realism than laboratory/simulation testing.

4 Methodology

MICR acts as a proof of principle since there is no systematic way of analysing CR programs. Due to a lack of CR prototypes, MICR can't be assessed completely by contrasting its convenience with existing test procedures, nor would it be assessed by gathering information on all parts of MICR comprehensively. The focal reason of MICR that SU discernment can be estimated by noticing, generally speaking, machine conduct is tested. The success or failure of MICR hinges on this behaviour-based testing aspect. As a result, MICR in its present state is insufficient if it is incorrect.

4.1 Approach

The SU is also known as the SUT (the CR). A frequency sensing CE is included with the SU. The PU and the SU are also set up to operate simultaneously, and performance data for both is collected. The SU receives a series of desired waveforms (user goals) that serve as a baseline while the CE remains switched off. The findings remain replicated when the SU CE is switched on. The PU and SU production can

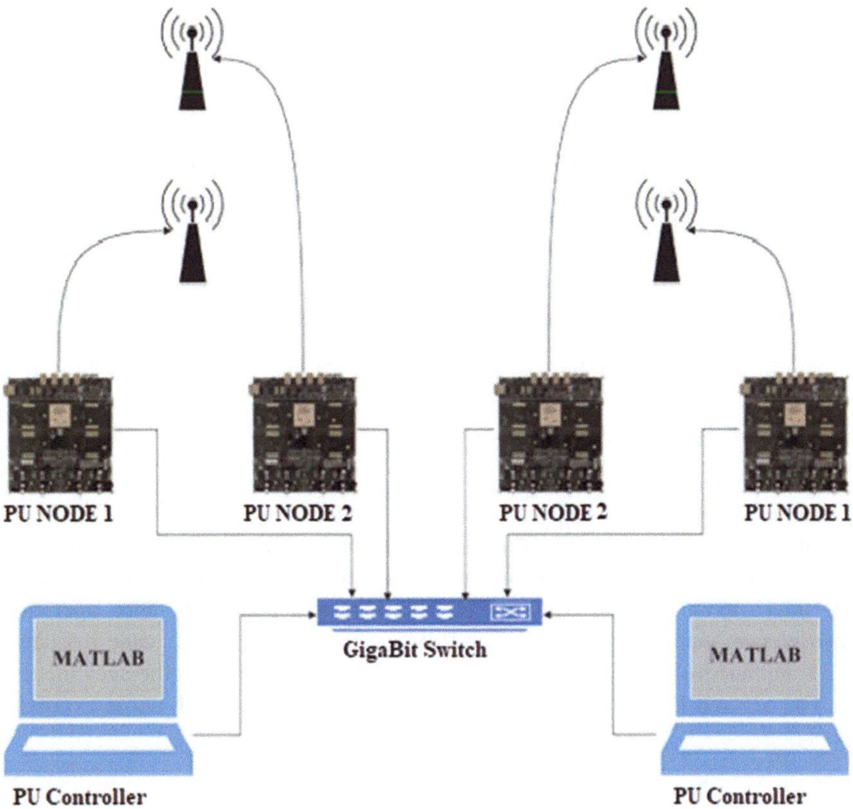

Fig. 1 Two radios' networks communication with PU and SU

improve when the SU CE is switched on compared to when it remains turned off. In addition, as the SU's cognitive stability improves, the PU and SU production can improve or stay constant. The SU now has more waveform options and throughput.

The PU employs a variety of waveforms to provide frequency versatility. The SU response towards the PU-created atmosphere remains adequately characterized using a variety of PU waveforms. All experimental setups are replicated to act as monitoring tests while the opposing network is turned off. The hardware architecture is the same with both cognitive and non-cognitive configurations. Except for an extra element, the CE, applied to the CR to feel the world and intellectually select a waveform, the program is comparative. Section IV-E delves further into the SU CE algorithm shown in Fig. 1.

4.2 Evaluation Technique

The PU laptop powers the experiment. The PU laptop is fitted with a list of experimental configurations. The calibration procedure is replicated if undesired interference occupies more REM bins than the optimal PU signal. The duration of each experiment is set to 60 s. Pilot tests revealed that 60 s was enough to reduce uncertainty in the outcome. Broadcasts on a single 2.4 GHz ISM band channel are restricted to PU and SU. The operational range of 128 channels and 20 Mhz frequency has been selected for flexible communication. The SUT only uses 64 of those bins with a 10 MHz bandwidth.

4.3 Performance Metrics

Communication and non-interference are two services provided by the SUT. The SU is subject to communication, while the effect of the SU on the PU is subject to non-interference. These two platforms provide efficiency metrics. The capacity of SU nodes to not interact with a PU is known as a non-interference operation. Interference happens when an SU and PU are transmitted on the same frequency bin simultaneously. The PU's throughput and BER are the related efficiency metrics.

The SU and PU's throughput is calculated in bits per second and is expressed as (1).

$$\text{Throughout} = \frac{\text{NAR} \cdot \text{BCD} \cdot \text{WBS}}{\text{WARP Clock Frequency}} \tag{1}$$

NAR is the quantity of accepting endeavours, BCD is the quantity of accurately demodulated pieces, and WBS is the WARP cradle limit. The quantity of pieces in blunder is isolated thru the number of pieces communicated to quantify the BER utilized in this investigation. Binary modulation is used in all of the modulation systems used in this study.

4.4 Workload

The SUT's workload is PU operation, also known as the climate. The PU action establishes the radio atmosphere where the SUT will respond and adjust according to its CE. A total of five worlds are generated using the PU transmitter. The PU produces spectrum holes that the SU can use in each environment. The PU will broadcast on any 64 frequency bins that make up the 10 MHz of spectrum bandwidth. To build a variety of RF settings, the PU waveform may be wideband, narrow-band, or non-contiguous. FSK, OFDM, or NC-OFDM is used to generate these particular waveforms. The PU is programmed to communicate for a minimum of time for each experiment. A discrete phase size is created by the minimum transmission time. The frequency of the PU waveform will shift once a second if frequency hopping is used.

It's been shuffled. The dark areas reflect the PU's transmitting frequencies. (a) Atmosphere No. 1; (b) Atmosphere No. 2; (c) Atmosphere No. 3; (d) Atmosphere No. 4; (e) Environment No. 5; using this concept, limitations of WSN models are crossly covered. The congestions of nodes also overcome thorough proposed smart health CR test model, as shown in Fig. 2.

4.5 System Under Test

In early pilot experiments, the number of main device parameters was reduced to the optimal waveform and the CE algorithm. Due to experimental limits, factor levels were also decreased. The type of radio waveform desired affects the SUT's communications capability and its ability to avoid interference with PUs. In FSK, integer modulation is used, and binary phase-shift keying modulation is used in OFDM waveforms. A radio node may use the CE to improve communications efficiency and avoid interruption. A basic bandwidth maximizing algorithm serves as the CE for this experiment. The SUT employs a basic energy detection algorithm to determine whether a channel remains available or not. A calibration series is used to describe the channel noise floor at the start of the experiment. The PU is then used to establish a threshold by transmitting a known waveform. Table 1 summarizes the workload and SUT considerations for this experiment.

4.6 Experimental Design

The study employs a completely factorial laboratory design (40 trials). In addition, baseline output data for each element is obtained, resulting in 13 trials. As a result, with each experiment set, 53 trials were performed. To sufficiently minimize 95 percent confidence intervals, a minimum of 20 repetitions must be completed. There are two possible outcomes. First, the findings should show that the SU setup by the CE on increases both PU and SU throughput in all PU workload conditions as opposed to when the CE is off. Second, the findings should demonstrate that PU and SU throughput improve as higher levels of intellect are applied.

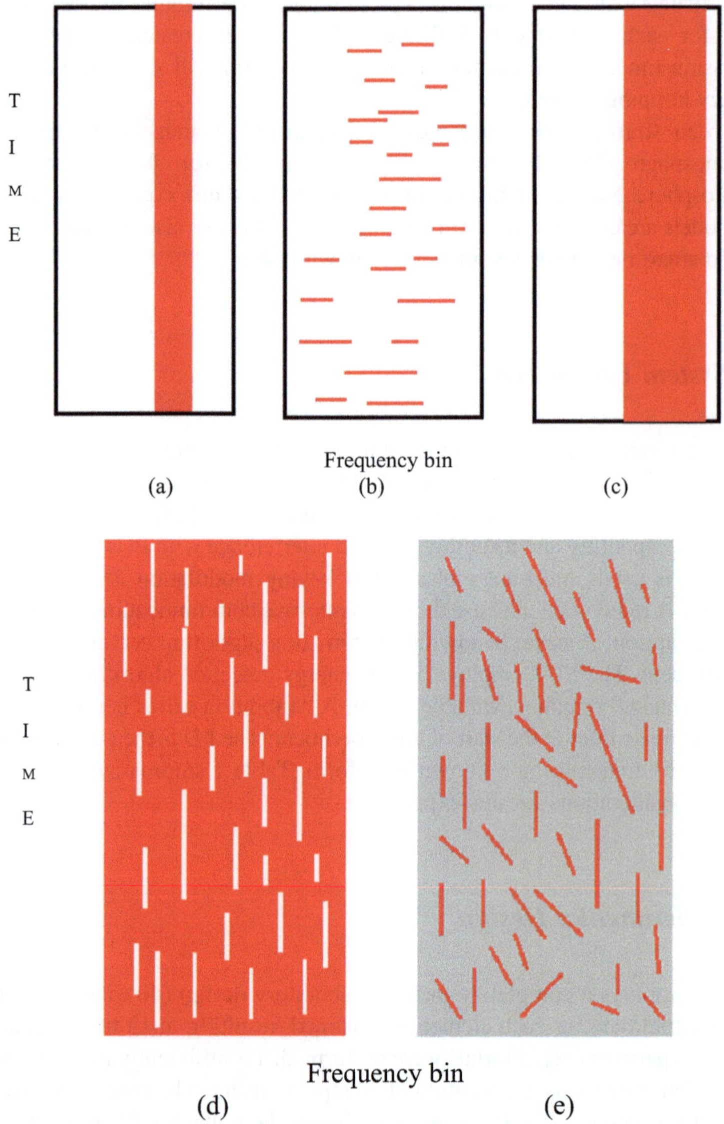

Fig. 2 (**a**) FRSK-1, (**b**) FRSK-8, (**c**) ORFDM-32 contiguous, (**d**) ORFDM-48 non-contiguous, and (**e**) ORFDM-16 workload environments were generated by PU

5 Results and Analysis

Figure 3 depicts the throughput results for each PU environment. The above is how the graphs can be viewed. The SU throughput for each CE setup is shown on the top subplot, while the PU throughput is shown on the bottom. Each bar in the plot is

Table 1 The comparison of results and values

Model	Accuracy	Sensitivity	Recall	F score	Throughput
Standard cognitive radio technology [5]	78.23	79.18	80.43	82.51	84.52
Heterogeneous and adaptive CR [4]	90.43	91.59	75.34	79.29	87.73
RFO [5]	92.21	94.23	88.42	92.52	92.41
Decision-controlled CR	95.28	96.51	92.39	90.39	94.56
Test CR proposed	98.14	99.42	99.67	98.52	97.17

accompanied by error bars. The findings reveal that the target waveform and CE status have the greatest impact on the SU throughput magnitude (the x-axis). Smaller variations in SU throughput remain due to the PU-created environment having an effect. The PU throughput magnitude is mainly influenced thru the PU environment, with the SU waveform and CE status having a minor effect.

The exploratory information is analysed for abnormalities that may show test control disappointments or BER/throughput information deficiency. Other trial information incorporated the slipped by try time, all outnumber of sends and gets, mean got signal qualities, and SU aligned energy-location limits, notwithstanding BER and throughput. No anomalies in any of the data may have influenced the findings presented below. There are no statistically important outliers, and all data residuals remain natural shown in Fig. 3.

5.1 *Effect of SU CE on SU Throughput and BER*

The CE's success is then assessed in terms of relative CE capacity. These discoveries are just substantial when the SU CE is turned on. The most un-psychological CE setup is thought to be FSK-1, while the most intellectual CE design is thought to be OFDM-48. For this examination, every CE setup is contrasted with all past arrangements to see whether it is genuinely more noteworthy or less (utilizing a t-test with an $\alpha = 0.05$ importance level). The configurations are considered comparable output if the difference is neither greater nor lesser.

5.2 *Throughput vs BER in MICR*

The CE's effectiveness is estimated at the relative CE limit, similar to the SU throughput. These discoveries possibly allude to the circumstance when the SU CE is turned on. For more significant levels of perception, the PU throughput doesn't generally increment. By far, most of these occasions, notwithstanding, are not genuinely huge; that is, PU throughput doesn't diminish as perception levels rise.

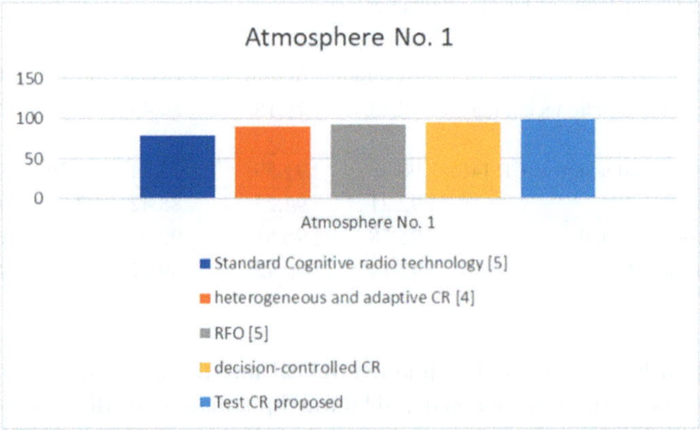

(a)

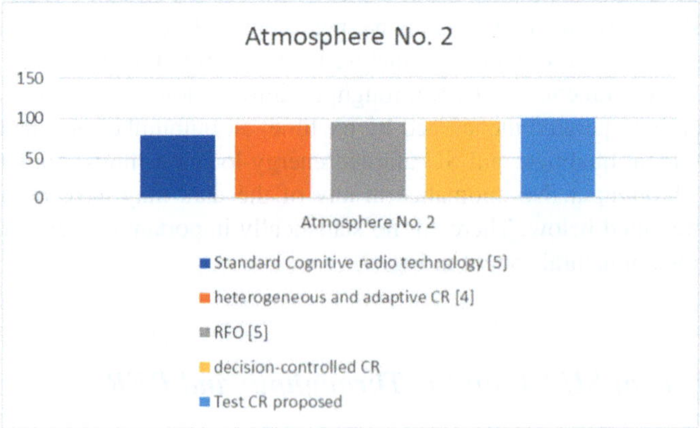

(b)

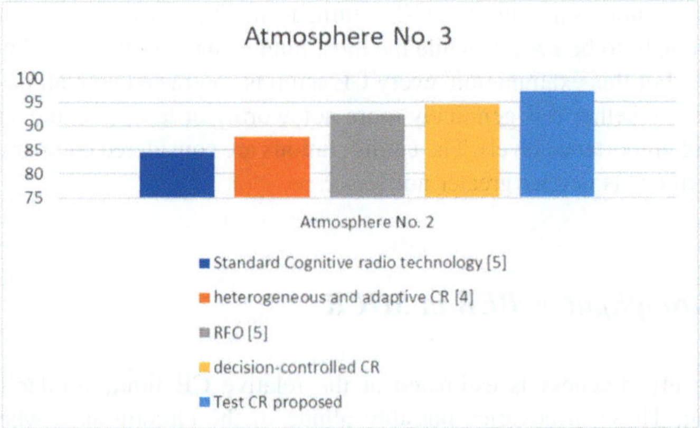

(c)

Fig. 3 Bandwidth of PU and SU in any of the five settings. The optimal waveform and CE on/off condition have the greatest impact on SU bandwidth. The magnitude of PU bandwidth is primarily influenced by the PU atmosphere selected. (**a**) Atmosphere No. 1; (**b**) Atmosphere No. 2; (**c**) Atmosphere No. 3

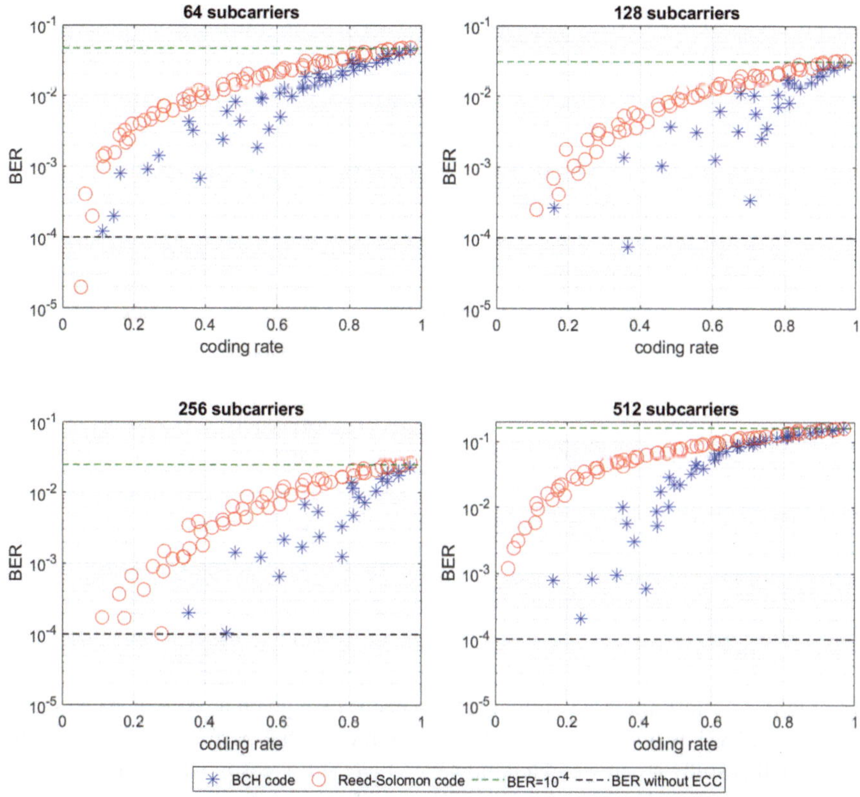

Fig. 4 BER is the primary customer

A disappointment of the CE to appropriately detect the climate, the CE's choice of an imperfect channel, or extra impedance brought about by the FSK-8 waveform besides channel determination could all be contributing variables. The initial two variables examined however were not viewed as autonomous elements. The side-projection power was excluded from the CE's development because force is not an important factor, as indicated by the difficult examination. FSK waveforms, indeed, don't communicate only on the ideal frequencies and have huge sidelobes.

It's also worth noting that the SU's actual waveform may not be the same as the ideal waveform. The CE FSK waveform will minimize transmission capacity from 8 to 4, 2, or 1 canister if the biggest range opening shaped thru the PU is under eight containers profound. This could explain why Environment 4 differs from the other environments in terms of the FSK 8/FSK 1 relationship shown in Fig. 4.

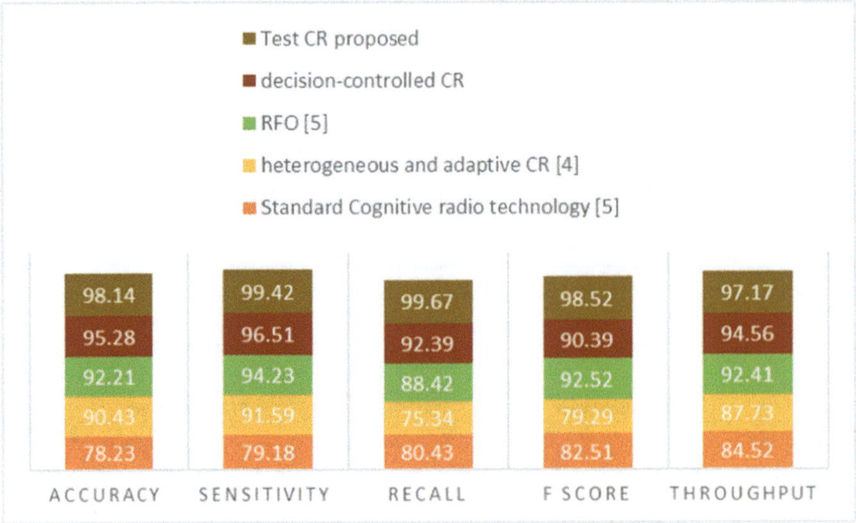

Fig. 5 The comparison of results

5.3 *Scoring*

The highest performing SU configuration in each set is given a score of 10 based on throughput. A 1 is allocated to the SU configuration that performs the worst. The scores in this study are unweighted; however, there is no reason why scores in future analyses should not be weighted based on real user preferences. The last score consolidates the consequences of both the SU than the PU into a solitary measurement. The most psychological design should have the most elevated score, while the most un-intellectual setup should have the least score, as indicated by the MICR CR definition. Due to the limitations of the SUT, this is not a thorough assessment of cognition; however, it does provide a rough correlation between experimental and MICR outcomes.

Table 1 and Fig. 5 clearly explain the comparison of results with various models like standard cognitive radio technology [5], heterogeneous and adaptive CR [4], RFO [5], decision-controlled CR, and test CR proposed technique. Compared to all models, the proposed technique attains more improvement and competes with present technology.

6 Conclusion

MICR, the suggested test procedure, was established to be used as an end-user, end-to-end test technique for implementing CR systems. MICR was also created to be architecture-independent and detect emergent behaviour. An examination was set up to gather information on the speculation that CR cognizance could remain surveyed by estimating the SU and PU's yield without explicitly assessing the SU's comprehension. The designed model communicates through proper channels without any false path; moreover, SU has good priority along with PU. Behaviour-related testing was not found to be invalid based on the findings of these tests. As a result, MICR was not found to be invalid. However, more research remains needed before behaviour-based testing and MICR can be completely justified. The testing process has determined the proposed model's communication efficiency compared to earlier techniques. The MICR framework remains designed to assess the overall performance of the CR system. This is a decent method to test CR adequacy when contrasting contending CR frameworks as a client making value/execution compromises. Architects chipping away at new CR frameworks may need all the more fine-grained profiling apparatuses to streamline different measurements and survey their effect on gadget parts like the detecting subsystem, with the point of adjusting those segments to improve by and large CR viability. The scope of this article does not include the creation of such profiling tools and metrics. We assume it will be a fruitful field for future research. The proposed model attained an accuracy of 98.34%, a sensitivity of 98.56%, a recall of 98.51%, an F score of 98.65%, and a throughput of 99.32% and concluded that the proposed model has good improvement compared to past technologies.

References

1. Steenkiste, P., Sicker, D., Minden, G., & Raychaudhuri, D.: Future directions in cognitive radio network research. In NSF workshop report, Vol. 4, No. 1, pp. 1–2 (2009).
2. Thompson, J. J., Hopkinson, K. M., & Silvius, M. D. A test methodology for evaluating cognitive radio systems. IEEE Transactions on Wireless Communications, 14(11), 6311–6324 (2015).
3. Masonta, M. T., Mzyece, M., & Ntlatlapa, N. Spectrum decision in cognitive radio networks: A survey. IEEE Communications Surveys & Tutorials, 15(3), 1088–1107 (2012).
4. Thomas, R. W., Friend, D. H., DaSilva, L. A., & MacKenzie, A. B. Cognitive networks. In Cognitive radio, software defined radio, and adaptive wireless systems, pp. 17–41. Springer, Dordrecht (2007).
5. Filin, S., Harada, H., Murakami, H., & Ishizu, K. International standardization of cognitive radio systems. IEEE Communications Magazine, 49(3), 82–89 (2011).
6. Zhao, Y., Mao, S., Neel, J. O., & Reed, J. H. Performance evaluation of cognitive radios: Metrics, utility functions, and methodology. Proceedings of the IEEE, 97(4), 642–659 (2009).
7. Boyd, J. A discourse on winning and losing (pp. 383–385). Air University Press (2018).
8. Wang, B., & Liu, K. R. Advances in cognitive radio networks: A survey. IEEE Journal of selected topics in signal processing, 5(1), 5–23 (2010).
9. Stevenson, C. R., Chouinard, G., Lei, Z., Hu, W., Shellhammer, S. J., & Caldwell, W. IEEE 802.22: The first cognitive radio wireless regional area network standard. IEEE communications magazine, 47(1), 130–138 (2009).
10. Cordeiro, C., Challapali, K., Birru, D., & Shankar, S. IEEE 802.22: the first worldwide wireless standard based on cognitive radios. In First IEEE International Symposium on New Frontiers in Dynamic Spectrum Access Networks. DySPAN 2005. (pp. 328–337). IEEE (2005).

11. Zhao, Q., & Sadler, B. M. A survey of dynamic spectrum access. IEEE signal processing magazine, 24(3), 79–89 (2007).
12. Mishra, S. M., Cabric, D., Chang, C., Willkomm, D., Van Schewick, B., Wolisz, A., & Brodersen, R. W. A real-time cognitive radio testbed for physical and link-layer experiments. In First IEEE International Symposium on New Frontiers in Dynamic Spectrum Access Networks. DySPAN. (pp. 562–567). IEEE (2005).
13. Sharma, R. K., Kotterman, W., Landmann, M. H., Schirmer, C., Schneider, C., Wollenschläger, F., ... & Thomä, R. S. Over-the-air testing of cognitive radio nodes in a virtual electromagnetic environment. International Journal of Antennas and Propagation, (2013).
14. Zhou, J., Ji, Z., Varshney, M., Xu, Z., Yang, Y., Marina, M., & Bagrodia, R. Why not: a hybrid testbed for large-scale, heterogeneous and adaptive wireless networks. In Proceedings of the 1st international workshop on Wireless network testbeds, experimental evaluation & characterization, pp. 111–112, (2006).
15. Borries, K., Wang, X., Judd, G., Steenkiste, P., & Stancil, D. Experience with a wireless network testbed based on signal propagation emulation. In 2010 European Wireless Conference (EW), pp. 833–840, IEEE (2010).
16. Saba, S. S., Sreelakshmi, D., Kumar, P. S., Kumar, K. S., & Saba, S. R. Logistic regression machine learning algorithm on MRI brain image for fast and accurate diagnosis. International Journal of Scientific and Technology Research, 9(3), 7076–7081, (2020).
17. Saikumar, K. RajeshV. Coronary blockage of artery for Heart diagnosis with DT Artificial Intelligence Algorithm. Int J Res Pharma Sci, 11(1), 471–479 (2020).
18. Saikumar, K., Rajesh, V. A novel implementation heart diagnosis system based on random forest machine learning technique International Journal of Pharmaceutical Research 12, pp. 3904–3916, (2020).
19. Raju K., Chinna Rao B., Saikumar K., Lakshman Pratap N. An Optimal Hybrid Solution to Local and Global Facial Recognition Through Machine Learning, A Fusion of Artificial Intelligence and Internet of Things for Emerging Cyber Systems. Intelligent Systems Reference Library, vol 210. Springer, Cham. https://doi.org/10.1007/978-3-030-76653-5_11 (2022).
20. Sankara Babu B., Nalajala S., Sarada K., Muniraju Naidu V., Yamsani N., Saikumar K. Machine Learning-Based Online Handwritten Telugu Letters Recognition for Different Domains. A Fusion of Artificial Intelligence and Internet of Things for Emerging Cyber Systems. Intelligent Systems Reference Library, vol 210. Springer, Cham. https://doi.org/10.1007/978-3-030-76653-5_12 (2022).
21. Kiran Kumar M., Kranthi Kumar S., Kalpana E., Srikanth D., Saikumar K. A Novel Implementation of Linux Based Android Platform for Client and Server. A Fusion of Artificial Intelligence and Internet of Things for Emerging Cyber Systems. Intelligent Systems Reference Library, vol 210. Springer, Cham. https://doi.org/10.1007/978-3-030-76653-5_8 (2022).
22. Mohammad, M. N., Kumari, C. U., Murthy, A. S. D., Jagan, B. O. L., & Saikumar, K. Implementation of online and offline product selection system using FCNN deep learning: Product analysis. Materials Today: Proceedings, 45, 2171–2178 (2021).
23. Jain, A., Kumar, A., & Sharma, S. Comparative Design and Analysis of Mesh, Torus and Ring NoC. Procedia Computer Science, 48, 330–337 (2015).
24. Jain, A., Dwivedi, R., Kumar, A., & Sharma, S. Scalable design and synthesis of 3D mesh network on chip. In Proceeding of International Conference on Intelligent Communication, Control and Devices, pp. 661–666, Springer, Singapore (2017).
25. Jain, A., Gahlot, A. K., Dwivedi, R., Kumar, A., & Sharma, S. K. Fat Tree NoC Design and Synthesis. In Intelligent Communication, Control and Devices, pp. 1749–1756. Springer, Singapore (2018).
26. Sharma, S. K., Jain, A., Gupta, K., Prasad, D., & Singh, V. An internal schematic view and simulation of major diagonal mesh network-on-chip. Journal of Computational and Theoretical Nanoscience, 16(10), 4412–4417 (2019).
27. D. S. Gupta and G. P. Biswas, "A novel and efficient lattice-based authenticated key exchange protocol in C-K model," Int. J. Commun. Syst., vol. 31, no. 3, Art. no. e3473 (2018).

28. Ghai, D., Gianey, H. K., Jain, A., & Uppal, R. S. Quantum and dual-tree complex wavelet transform-based image watermarking. International Journal of Modern Physics B, 34(04), 2050009 (2020).
29. Jain, A., & Kumar, A. Desmogging of still smoggy images using a novel channel prior. Journal of Ambient Intelligence and Humanized Computing, 12(1), 1161–1177 (2021).
30. Kumar, S., Jain, A., Shukla, A. P., Singh, S., Raja, R., Rani, S., ... & Masud, M. A Comparative Analysis of Machine Learning Algorithms for Detection of Organic and Nonorganic Cotton Diseases. Mathematical Problems in Engineering, (2021).
31. D. S. Gupta and G. P. Biswas, "On securing bi-and tri-partite session key agreement protocol using IBE framework," Wireless Pers. Commun., vol. 96, no. 3, pp. 4505–4524, (2017).
32. Misra, N. R., Kumar, S., & Jain, A. A Review on E-waste: Fostering the Need for Green Electronics. In 2021 International Conference on Computing, Communication, and Intelligent Systems. pp. 1032–1036. IEEE (2021).
33. Jain, A., AlokGahlot, A. K., & RakeshDwivedi, S. K. S. Design and FPGA Performance Analysis of 2D and 3D Router in Mesh NoC. International Journal of Control Theory and Applications, ISSN, 0974–5572 (2017).
34. Agrawal, N., Jain, A., & Agarwal, A. Simulation of Network on Chip for 3D Router Architecture. International Journal of Recent Technology and Engineering, 8, 58–62 (2019).
35. Mathivanan, S., & Jayagopal, P. A big data virtualization role in agriculture: a comprehensive review. Walailak Journal of Science and Technology, 16(2), 55–70 (2019).
36. Kumar, M. S., & Prabhu, J. Hybrid model for movie recommendation system using fireflies and fuzzy c-means. International Journal of Web Portals (IJWP), 11(2), 1–13 (2019).
37. Rajendran, S., Mathivanan, S. K., Jayagopal, P., Janaki, K. P., Bernard, B. A. M. M., Pandy, S., & Somanathan, M. S. Emphasizing privacy and security of edge intelligence with machine learning for healthcare. International Journal of Intelligent Computing and Cybernetics (2021).
38. Rajendran, S., Mathivanan, S. K., Jayagopal, P., Venkatasen, M., Pandi, T., Somanathan, M. S., ... & Mani, P. Language dialect based speech emotion recognition through deep learning techniques. International Journal of Speech Technology, 1–11 (2021).
39. Kumar, S., & Jayagopal, P. Delineation of field boundary from multispectral satellite images through U-Net segmentation and template matching. Ecological Informatics, 64, 101370 (2021).
40. K. Karthikayan, Dr. Siva Agora Sakthivel Murugan, Rathish C. R, Natraj N.A, A Triband Slotted Bow-Tie Antenna for Wireless Applications, International Journal of Computational Engineering Research, Volume 3, Issue 7, Pages 31 35 (2013).
41. CR Rathish & A Rajaram, Hierarchical Load Balanced Routing Protocol for Wireless Sensor Networks, International Journal of Applied Engineering Research, Volume 10, Issue 7, Pages 16521–16534 (2015).
42. Siva Agora Sakthivel Murugan, K. Karthikayan, Natraj N.A, Rathish C.R, Speckle Noise Removal Using Dual Tree Complex Wavelet Transform, International Journal of Scientific & Technology Research, Volume 2, Issue 8, Pages 4 (2013).
43. A. Sagai Francis Britto C. R. Rathish, C. Saravana Murthi, J. Indirapriyadharshini, Deepak V, A Novel and Effective Method for Automatic Paper Trimming and Cutting process in Paper Industries, International Journal of Advanced Science and Technology, Vol. 29, no. 6, Pp. 4136–4143 (2020).
44. Rathish Radhakrishnan & Karpagavadivu Karuppusamy, Cost Effective Energy Efficient Scheme for Mobile Adhoc Network, International Journal of Computing, Volume 19, Issue 1, Pages 137–146 (2020).
45. A.K. Gupta, Y. K. Chauhan, and T Maity, "Experimental investigations and comparison of various MPPT techniques for photovoltaic system," Sādhanā, Vol. 43, no. 8, pp. 1–15, (2018).
46. F. J. John Joseph, R. T, and J. J. C, "Classification of correlated subspaces using HoVer representation of Census Data," in 2011 International Conference on Emerging Trends in Electrical and Computer Technology, pp. 906–911 (2011),

47. S. Bhoumik, S. Chatterjee, A. Sarkar, A. Kumar, and F. J. John Joseph, "Covid 19 Prediction from X Ray Images Using Fully Connected Convolutional Neural Network," in CSBio '20: Proceedings of the Eleventh International Conference on Computational Systems-Biology and Bioinformatics, pp. 106–107 (2020),
48. D. S. Q. Al-Yasiri and A. J. Obaid, "A New Approach for Object Detection, Recognition and Retrieving in Painting Images," Journal of Advance Research in Dynamic and Control System, vol. 10, no. 2, pp. 2345–2359, (2018).
49. T. A. Al-asadi and A. J. Obaid, "Object detection and recognition by using enhanced speeded up robust feature," International Journal of Computer Science and Network Security, vol. 16, no. 4, pp. 66–71, (2016).
50. T. A. Al-asadi, A. J. Obaid, R. Hidayat and A. A. Ramli, "A survey on web mining techniques and applications," International Journal on Advanced Science Engineering and Information Technology, vol. 7, no. 4, pp. 1178–1184, (2017).
51. A.K. Gupta, "Sun Irradiance Trappers for Solar PV Module to Operate on Maximum Power: An Experimental Study," Turkish Journal of Computer and Mathematics Education, Vol. 12, no. 5, pp. 1112–1121, (2021).
52. F. J. J. Joseph, "Effect of supervised learning methodologies in offline handwritten Thai character recognition," Int. J. Inf. Technol., vol. 12, no. 1, pp. 57–64, (2020).
53. H. Chhabra, V. Mohan, A. Rani, and V. Singh, "Trajectory tracking of Maryland manipulator using linguistic Lyapunov fuzzy controller," Journal of Intelligent & Fuzzy Systems, vol. 36, no. 3, pp. 2195–2205, (2019).
54. A.K. Gupta, Y.K Chauhan, and T Maity, "A new gamma scaling maximum power point tracking method for solar photovoltaic panel Feeding energy storage system," IETE Journal of Research, vol. 67, no. 1, pp. 1–21, (2018).
55. A. Rawat, S. Jha, B. Kumar, and V. Mohan, "Nonlinear fractional order PID controller for tracking maximum power in photo-voltaic system," Journal of Intelligent & Fuzzy Systems, vol. 38, no. 5, pp. 6703–6713, (2020).
56. Guna Sekhar Sajja, Malik Mustafa, Dr. R. Ponnusamy, Shokhjakhon Abdufattokhov, Murugesan G., Dr. P. Prabhu, "Machine Learning Algorithms in Intrusion Detection and Classification", Annals of RSCB, vol. 25, no. 6, pp. 12211–12219, (2021).
57. Rupapara, V., Narra, M., Gonda, N. K., & Thipparthy, K. Relevant Data Node Extraction: A Web Data Extraction Method for Non Contagious Data. 2020 5th International Conference on Communication and Electronics Systems, 500–505 (2020).
58. Ishaq, A., Sadiq, S., Umer, M., Ullah, S., Mirjalili, S., Rupapara, V., & Nappi, M. Improving the Prediction of Heart Failure Patients' Survival Using SMOTE and Effective Data Mining Techniques. IEEE Access, 9, 39707–39716 (2021).
59. Rustam, F., Khalid, M., Aslam, W., Rupapara, V., Mehmood, A., & Choi, G. S. A performance comparison of supervised machine learning models for Covid-19 tweets sentiment analysis. PLOS ONE, 16(2), e0245909. https://doi.org/10.1371/journal.pone.0245909 (2021).

Indication of COVID-19 and Inference Employing RFO Classifier

Sk Hasane Ahammad, V. Sripathi Raja, Prabha Shreeraj Nair, Divya Kanuganti, and K. Saikumar

1 Introduction

As indicated through the World Health Organization (WHO), 2,747,053 confirmed cases the last update: April 20, 2021, 05:30 GMT + 11:46, 191,899 confirmed passing's last update: April 20, 2021, 05:30 GMT + 11:46, 213 countries, zones, or domains with cases [1]. Coronavirus is the first driving justification for death around the world, with the passing rate assessed to increment to the essential high circumstance by 2030. The system of demonstrative imaging expects an urgent occupation during the assurance of COVID [2, 3]. Thc COVID, generally, happens on account of respirational defilements that can stay associated through beads of a few sizes: when the drop components are >5–10 μm, somewhere out there across

S. H. Ahammad (✉)
Department of ECE, Koneru Lakshmaiah Education Foundation, Guntur, India
e-mail: drshaikhasane@kluniversity.in

V. S. Raja
Department of Biomedical Engineering, B V Raju Institute of Technology, Medak, Narsapur, India
e-mail: rajasripathi.ventapalli@bvrit.ac.in

P. S. Nair
CSE Department, S B Jain Institute of Technology Management and Research, Nagpur, India

D. Kanuganti
ECE, Nalla Malla Reddy Engineering College, Divyanagar, Narapally, India

K. Saikumar
Department of ECE, Koneru Lakshmaiah Education Foundation, Guntur, India

School of Engineering, Department of CSE, Malla Reddy University, Telangana, Hyderabad, India
e-mail: saikumarkayam4@ieee.org

P. Agarwal et al. (eds.), *Artificial Intelligence for Smart Healthcare*,
EAI/Springer Innovations in Communication and Computing,
https://doi.org/10.1007/978-3-031-23602-0_23

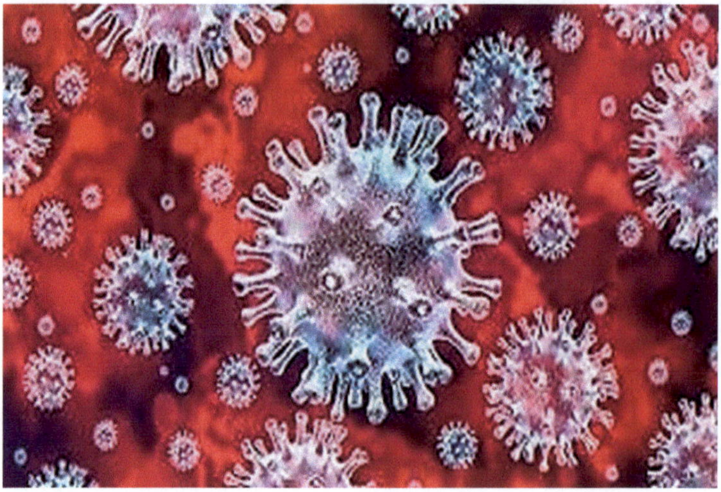

Fig. 1 Coronavirus image

they remain alluded towards via respirational drops, and then, at that point, when on that point remain <5 μm in broadness, they remain alluded towards according to drop centers. As assigned through current proof, the COVID-19 contamination remains essentially interconnected among people through respirational dots and contact courses [4, 5] (Fig. 1).

In this current pandemic, time people have been effecting by covid and it is distinguished by many symptoms. This was perceived in 1965, an infection named "B8140." This infection assaults upper and lower respiratory organs like the lungs [6, 7]. Coronavirus is a danger to humans which is affecting the respiratory systems of patients [8, 9]. These days, the vast majority have been tainted with COVID-19 and encountered the disease of the respiratory frameworks. No specific medication and treatment are accessible for this infection, and the patient possibly recuperates when exceptional treatment is given to respiratory organs. Diabetic patients, BP, and asthma, and older people need to pay attention to this coronavirus. The best technique to keep away from contamination is to dial back the correspondence rate; the singular mindful and constantly washing of hands is the best anticipation. Alcoholic sanitizers must be scoured every now and again, and don't contact your face.

When Covid-19 attacked the human body, patients need to arrange all precautions to get recovery. Younger, unhealthy people, diabetic patients, and doctors should take precautions for cardiac and respiratory organ damage [10, 11]. Being completely educated on the COVID-19 sickness, the problem it produces, and how it sends is the best way to stay away from and defeat transmission. Wash your hands consistently or utilize a liquor-based rub to shield yourself similar to others from contamination, and then do whatever it takes not to contact your face. Exactly when a corrupted individual hacks or wheezes, the COVID-19 contamination sends dominatingly through globules of salivation or delivery from the nose; consequently, respiratory conduct is particularly fundamental (e.g., by hacking into a flexed elbow) [12, 13].

The COVID-19 nasal swab PCR test is the most precise and solid approach to analyse the infection. A positive test shows that you have COVID-19. A negative test demonstrates that you were not tainted with COVID-19 at the hour of the test. If you display manifestations of COVID-19 or have been presented to somebody who has tried positive for COVID-19, you ought to get tried. The significance of reliable, accessible testing to screen for COVID-19 has been increasingly obvious during the COVID-19 issue. Testing for COVID-19 antigens and antibodies uses various samples to seek distinct SARS-CoV-2 viral signals. The many sorts of COVID-19 tests are examined in depth by Medical Device Network:

- Polymerase chain response (PCR) tests are shipped off a lab to analyze infection.
- COVID-19 can be determined on the spot to have parallel stream tests (LFTs), even though they aren't pretty much as precise as PCR tests.
- Antibody (or serology) testing can't recognize the dynamic disease, yet they can demonstrate on the off chance that somebody has COVID-19 invulnerability.

PCR tests are used to detect the presence of viral RNA in the body before antibodies are formed or signs of infection appear [14]. This implies that the tests can recognize whether somebody is tainted with the infection at the beginning of their affliction. Convergent transcriptase or DNA polymerase is a synthetic chemical used in PCR testing in a laboratory. These man-made chemicals act by duplicating any readily accessible RNA. For the preliminaries and testing of the infection's hereditary coding to be conclusive, enough RNA copies must be present to provide a positive result. "PCR provides us a decent indication of who is infected," explains Dr. Edward Wright, senior lecturer in microbiology at the University of Sussex. "They can be segregated and make contact with persons they've been in contact with so they can be quarantined as well." The pre-covid 19 test can help to stop the spreading and chain mechanism it is a key diagnosis method.

Public health experts can better understand the transmission of a disease like COVID-19 by scaling PCR testing to screen large swaths of nasopharyngeal swab samples from inside a population. However, there are several limitations to PCR. Because these COVID-19 tests must be sent to a laboratory for analysis, consumers may have to wait days to get their findings. These tests are best used to confirm a disease rather than give a patient an all-clear since false negatives may occur up to 30% of the time. Detection of dead, deactivated virus in the body of a person who has recovered from COVID-19 might lead to false-positive results from these tests since they are so sensitive. "During the outbreak, the PCR testing has been modified from the initial testing protocols, with the inclusion of increased automation to minimize errors," said Dr. James Gill, an honorary clinical lecturer at Warwick Medical School. The doctors, medical officers, and medical shop service persons are the main spreading team, so the right decision must be taken to stop chain spreading. Many people are wondering when an effective COVID-19 vaccination will be available. While a vaccine remains unavailable, coronavirus has a reproduction rate of 1.4–2.5, which means that each infection will infect an additional 2.5 persons. In the first 2 weeks of 2020, the original global infection rate was tripling every day. As a result, nations implemented lockdowns to restrict the virus's spread [15, 16]. Health professionals manually track the history of recent contacts of confirmed coronavirus patients. Manual contact tracing is time-consuming and expensive, especially when dealing with large groups of affected people. Illnesses spread more quickly in large gatherings, such as weddings, funerals, and other events. As a result of such events, authorities will be pushed to their limits. Coronavirus occurrence and infection will be more likely due to the inconvenient process of locating and tracing affected people.

In a contagious viral illness, establishing a good model is critical for deciding how to control the virus's spread. Each type of virus infection has its peculiarities in propagation and symptom manifestation. The development of a mathematical model to combat infection necessitates a thorough examination of the virus's biological properties [17]. A suitable mathematical model should, in particular, consider the infection through the eyes of someone who has no indications of COVID-19 clinical manifestation. Only a few numerical models are accessible for the COVID-19 spreading design. While assessing momentary appraisals of the combined number of affirmed revealed cases, the creators in [18] made an ongoing determining technique dependent on phenomenological models. The COVID, then again, is a worldwide crisis that requires an exhaustive control system depending on its remarkable properties. This investigation proposes a COVID-19 streamlining Algorithm (CVA) that reenacts the conduct of COVID-19 as it spreads across nations from December 2019 to the hour of composing. This examination additionally investigates the conduct of the pandemic transmission with its various stages that have been seen until recently and shows how the model may be used by governments and specialists to make decisions about carrying out ideal lockdowns. Besides, the proposed CVA may cover all conceivable advancement issue areas essentially. We likewise reenacted the spread of the COVID in numerous countries throughout the planet. The numerical model depicted in this investigation treats the COVID scattering measure as an enhancement issue that intends to lessen the quantity of COVID19-tainted nations and ease back the pandemic's spread. Then, at that point, utilizing the best factors in the conveyance interaction, three situations are introduced to address the enhancement issue. One of the controlling situations beats the others, as indicated by recreation results. Extensive simulations of the proposed CVA algorithm employing a variety of engineering optimization issues demonstrate its effectiveness. Furthermore, the suggested CVA technique can handle limited, unconstrained, and engineering problems in various study domains. Researchers derive meta-heuristic algorithms from animal and insect behavior in the existing literature, but our suggested CVA is based on the COVID-19 infection process [19].

1.1 COVID-19 and Its Effecting Elements

COVID-19 antibodies may or may not give long-term and complete protection. It is not always the case that infection with an infectious disease results in complete immunity. Some infections, such as measles, provide lifetime protection against infection. Other infections take longer to heal from. A virus that may cause real viral pneumonia in young children but typically produces mild, cold-like symptoms persists to the point that practically all newborns have it by age two. Then again, contamination just creates frictional resistance, which ensures against serious sickness later on but not against re-disease. Some COVIDs give all-out insusceptibility, while others just aim fractional invulnerability, and it's indistinct where COVID-19 finds a way into that continuum. If recovery from this novel COVID just outcomes in fractional insurance, somebody with COVID-19 antibodies could, in any case, get tainted with the SARS-CoV-2 infection. However, they would be shielded from serious illness; they may, in any case, contaminate others. As such, somebody with COVID-19 halfway invulnerability could re-contaminate and simply have cold-like indications. Nonetheless, if they offer it to somebody who doesn't have COVID-19 insurance, that individual may have a genuine ailment like pneumonia [20].

The potential that COVID-19 disease only generates partial resistance is one of the main reasons why "immunity passports" have yet to be shown effective. COVID-19 diagnostic testing has scaled very quickly worldwide, rising as of zero towards more than a billion samples evaluated each day in a couple of months. These are utilized to decide whether an individual has recuperated from COVID-19, can at this point don't taint others, and may continue typical exercises. This increment in testing has been useful in managing patient consideration advising general well-being choices, such as applying physical distance measures [21].

However, various challenges have arisen, particularly in low- and middle-income nations. Regardless of the quick extension of testing, request keeps on unparalleled inventory, and the circulation of accessible stockpiles across nations has been lopsided. It has been challenging to ensure acceptable test quality and steadfastness, considering the number of manufacturers in the COVID-19 market, even though the World Health Organization, the Foundation for Innovative New Diagnostics, and other review groups had predicted this. Testing material cannot be sent internationally as quickly due to international transportation interruptions caused by the outbreak. The volume of COVID-19 testing has overburdened diagnostic laboratories, making testing for different illnesses drop off the radar and the novel COVID to go delayed [22].

1.2 Immunity Issues

Some tests look for the virus's RNA (genetic blueprint), discovered in the COVID-19-producing SARS-CoV-2 virus. A result stating that the virus has been found is highly reliable when done appropriately. Then again, these tests are insufficient in setting up if somebody has recuperated from the infection. They may even miss the infection if it remains available in incredibly low amounts in a patient's body [23]. Antibodies to the virus are found in other tests, indicating that the body has created an immunological response. Because such antibodies take longer to develop, antibody testing isn't very useful in determining whether someone has COVID-19 in the first few days after disease. They can be that as it may, be especially gainful in setting up whether somebody has recently been tainted with the novel COVID; however, they no longer contain the infection, in contrast to RNA tests. However, different persons can have varied antibody reactions to COVID-19, complicating things. People with an extreme sickness, for instance, seem to foster higher neutralizer levels than those with gentle or asymptomatic infection. Subsequently, an immunized test planned to utilize blood tests from patients with serious COVID-19 may not exceed capacity in people by a gentle or asymptomatic type of the illness when there are still a lot of antibodies to identify [24–29].

1.3 Vaccine and Its Working

Diagnostic testing is becoming increasingly crucial as countries abolish COVID-19-related activity limitations [30–35]. The distinguishing proof of patients tainted by SARS-CoV-2 will help those being treated, demonstrating who should be separated and whose contacts should be found and isolated to keep the infection from spreading further [36–38]. If there is a critical expansion in COVID-19 occasions affirmed through symptomatic testing, it will be important to reimpose COVID-19-related action impediments. Suppose delicate observation for COVID-19 is set up. In that case, the absence of such an increment after impediments are removed will give governments more certainty that they can keep working securely without them [39–41].

Analytic testing will be required even after a protected and powerful COVID-19 antibody has been delivered and made generally accessible to guarantee that the immunization is utilized as viably and effectively as achievable. Reconnaissance information could help determine which portions of the populace require the immunization the most – solid research facility affirmation analytic tests could uncover which populaces are still in danger of the novel COVID and which have effectively been completely contaminated recuperated [42–45]. Coronavirus indicative tests are a significant part of a perplexing way to battle the pandemic when utilized related to preventive strategies like vaccinations and actual partition [46–49].

2 Symptoms and Samples

The COVID-19 is communicated through spit and infection release from the nose to individual [50–52]. There is neither treatment nor immunization for COVID-19, and the contaminated people can rapidly distinguish manifestations like hack and sniffle. Whole globe scientists have followed the clinical examination for a potential medication the WHO ceaselessly screens the refreshed information on clinical assessments. One of the vital indicators your doctor evaluates when you come is your respiration rate, the number of times you breathe in a minute [53–56]. When resting, a typical adult takes between 12 and 20 breaths per minute, depending on their age. Counting the number of breaths you take in a minute is a good way to gauge your rate. (If you don't have that much time, count how many you take in 15 sec and multiply that amount by four.) If you're not feeling well, the way you breathe can give your doctor indications of what's wrong [57–60]. This issue happens when you inhale quicker than your body requires and breathe out an excess of carbon dioxide. This tosses your blood framework messed up. Working out, being restless, or having asthma would all prompt hyperventilation. You may feel unsteady, powerless, or confused because of it.

2.1 Prevention

- Reliably clean up with a sanitizer or cleanser.
- Individuals ought to keep a 2-m separation between individual to individual.
- Try not to contact the face.
- At hacking and wheezing, cover the mouth.
- In unwell circumstances, remain at home.
- Evade smoking.
- Unnecessary ventures and enormous gatherings are important to keep away from and keep actual separation.
- These are the principle signs included fever, dry hack, and sluggishness. The overall signs incorporate windedness, torments, and sore throat.

2.2 Diagnosis Process

The COVID-19 infection is a medium-size RNA type noticeable on an electron micrograph. 30-kb-long nucleic corrosive positive in nature is the COVID-19 structure – all COVID-19 cells created in the plasma cells and contaminated through respiratory organs. Ordinary antibodies can't annihilate these cells in individuals. The COVID is an envelope in structure and a non-fragmented RNA infection. The

Table 1 Literature survey

No.	Author name	Technique	Key point
1	Ioannidis [2]	Used infection fatality rate (IFR) technology	This study performs all synthetic evaluations through the IFR technology and finally estimates the COVID-19 pandemic situation
2	Shaharuddin et al. [3]	ROF technology	This study identified various factors affecting financial planning among working women during the pandemic COVID-19 situation
3	Frederick et al. [4]	ROF technology	This study summarizes the National Association of Insurance Commissioners NAIC's current standing during the pandemic
4	Chetty et al. [5]	ZIP code technology used	This study shows how public statistics are constructed from private-sector data without compromising privacy, providing a new tool for empirical macroeconomics
5	Coleman et al. [6]	Supply chain framework used	This study mainly focuses on policy and legal changes for workers of food sectors and institutional food procurement actors

pandemic microscopic organisms harm the respiratory condition and reduce the insusceptibility framework (Table 1).

2.3 *RFO Methodology*

The pneumonia type manifestations saw on people are important to follow master ideas. This is a plague sickness, an arising determination and remarkable therapies. The disease detection and unemployment had been balanced through the proposed RFO model. In this model, at first stage, training files are applied; the RFO feature extractor processes these.

Figure 2 clarifies the determination interaction and business issues steps. At the principal stage, far-fetched patients' examples are gathered for determination. Whenever this test becomes positive, a specific treatment will begin consequently. In the event that the experimental outcomes said negative, a patient follows the choice. The disease detection and employment issues are resolved to RFO mathematical computations.

Figure 3 clarifies the chest x-beam examination of COVID-19 patients; from the beginning, the stage applies the division method for pre-handling. After the principal stage, irregular woods enhancement is applied. With this strategy, we order the lungs and respiratory framework position (Fig. 4).

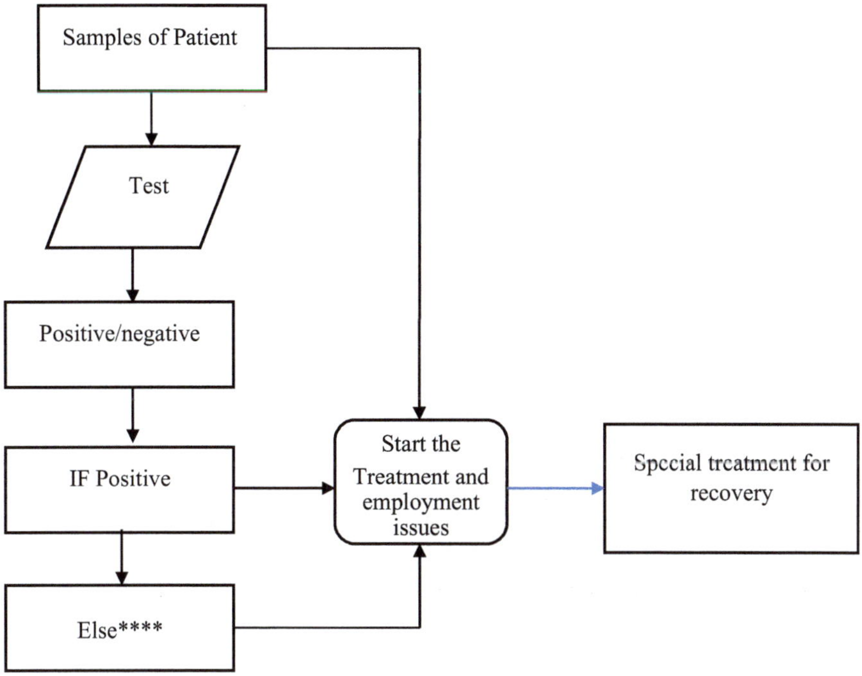

Fig. 2 Diagnosis and employment issues estimation

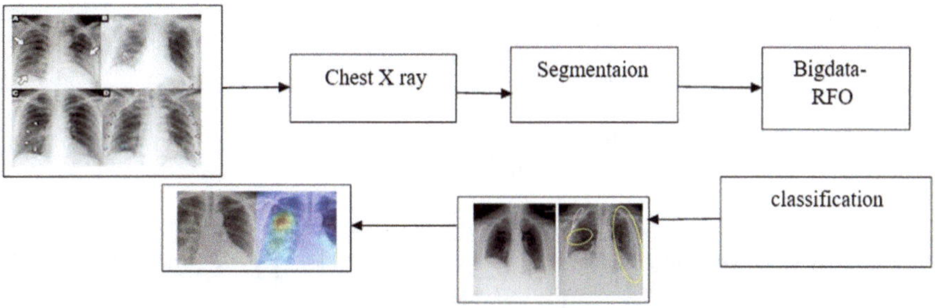

Fig. 3 RFO segmentation

$$v_{\mathrm{TSRFO}} = \arg\ \max\left[\sum_{-1 \leq F(v_i) \geq m} P(x_i, v_i)\right] \tag{1}$$

$$\prod_{j=1, j \neq 1}^{n} P\left(x_j | x_i v_{ij}\right)] \tag{2}$$

16758	16757	05-07-2021	8.00 AM	Jharkhand	340164	5115	345937
16759	16758	05-07-2021	8.00 AM	Karnataka	2773407	35367	2853643
16760	16759	05-07-2021	8.00 AM	Kerala	2855460	13716	2973684
16761	16760	05-07-2021	8.00 AM	Ladakh	19690	204	20120
16762	16761	05-07-2021	8.00 AM	Lakshadweep	9577	49	9900
16763	16762	05-07-2021	8.00 AM	Madhya Pradesh	780495	9009	789983
16764	16763	05-07-2021	8.00 AM	Maharashtra	5848693	123030	6098177
16765	16764	05-07-2021	8.00 AM	Manipur	64931	1196	72286
16766	16765	05-07-2021	8.00 AM	Meghalaya	46228	862	51524
16767	16766	05-07-2021	8.00 AM	Mizoram	17661	95	21337
16768	16767	05-07-2021	8.00 AM	Nagaland	23786	499	25519
16769	16768	05-07-2021	8.00 AM	Odisha	890778	4196	921896
16770	16769	05-07-2021	8.00 AM	Puducherry	114192	1761	117959
16771	16770	05-07-2021	8.00 AM	Punjab	577982	16110	596416
16772	16771	05-07-2021	8.00 AM	Rajasthan	942616	8938	952734
16773	16772	05-07-2021	8.00 AM	Sikkim	18722	308	21131
16774	16773	05-07-2021	8.00 AM	Tamil Nadu	2427988	33005	2496287
16775	16774	05-07-2021	8.00 AM	Telangana	611035	3691	626690
16776	16775	05-07-2021	8.00 AM	Tripura	63209	692	67677
16777	16776	05-07-2021	8.00 AM	Uttarakhand	331642	7333	340724
16778	16777	05-07-2021	8.00 AM	Uttar Pradesh	1681717	22640	1706621

Fig. 4 COVID-19 csv file

$$W_i = \frac{\text{GainRatio}(A_i) * m}{\sum_{i=1}^{m} \text{GainRatio}(A_i)} \tag{3}$$

$$W_i = \frac{1}{\sqrt{\text{indexrank}((A_i) + 1}} \tag{4}$$

$$v_{\text{DTW}\quad\text{TSRFO}} = \arg\ \max \left[\sum_{-1 \le F(v_i) \ge m} P(x_i, v_i) \right] \prod_{j=1, j \ne 1}^{n} P\big(x_j | x_i v_{ij}\big)]^{w_j} \tag{5}$$

Equations 1, 2, 3 and 4 get information from CSV files and attain ImageNet files from training weights. Gain ratio, index, and rank are calculated, and finally, measures are sent to Eq. 5, i.e., classification model, by utilizing this computation finding COVID affecting measure and employment issues. Each step calculates the train data weights, and tree establishment and growth of trees are calculated. A final estimate of the error using classification, Fig. 5, observes the trees' modeling and jumping issues. The following equations are getting information from CSV file, so that attains information.

Figure 5 clearly explains about class differentiation model; in this, all weights are balanced through statistical values. The yes or no commands balance the Random Forest Optimization mechanism. Finally, the proposed methodology can be

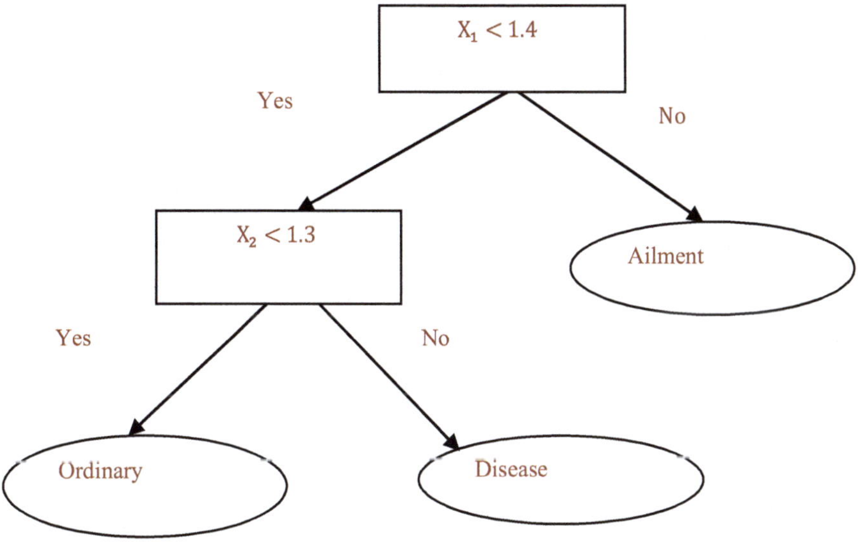

Fig. 5 RFO weight balancing

providing disease findings and spread information for future-level analysis. The entire CSV file is categorized into 14 classes, again dividing into 2 subclasses. The feature extraction and classification are the technology assessment to find the problem statement related to COVID-19 estimation and employment issues. The parameters like argument, gain ratio, index ranging, and argument estimations are balanced in the machine learning classification. The terms weight and class are used to get the image and numerical analysis information. The different states in India country information are collected in image formats and excel sheet files to analyze the above representation. The issue like state, number of people infected, cured, and a chance to affect people's information is imported in the loading file.

3 Results and Discussion

This section briefly discusses the COVID-19 virus and employment issues easily using RFO machine learning.

Figure 6 describes that virus identification in lungs, and this position is classified by random forest optimization with geometry computations.

Figure 7 clearly explains the different active cases in 2021 from March to September. The initial stage of the pandemic disease has been spreading rapidly and slowly increasing in a non-linear manner. This impact is affecting employment, and therefore finally economy has slowed down. After September this graph is getting decreasing slowly. Therefore, employment issues are solved.

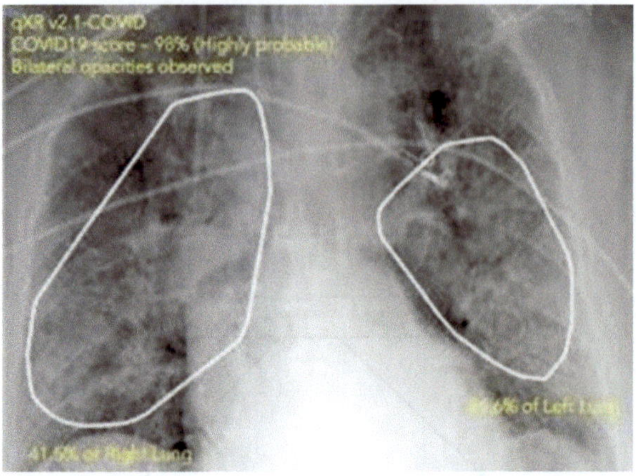

Fig. 6 COVID-19 patient virus identification

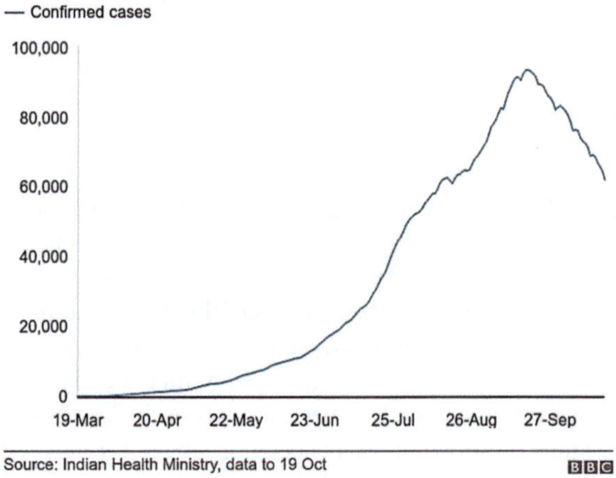

Fig. 7 Active cases in COVID time 2021 year

Figure 8 explains the employment issue in COVID 2021 year, at the initial stage, employment is slowly slowing down to the curve, and employment is increasing. March to September month COVID disease analysis provides information about countries GDP rate.

Figure 9 clearly explains the COVID effect and employment issues comparison, and here both curves are inversely proportional to elements. This research work is mostly balancing measures of GDP to country.

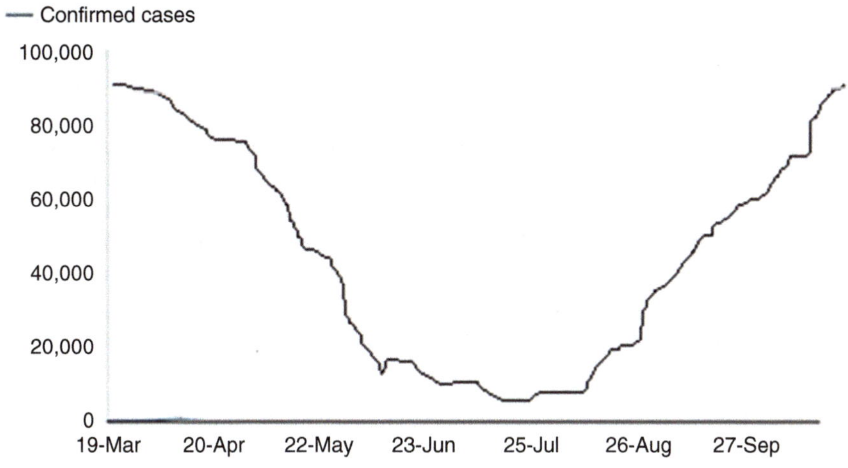

Fig. 8 Employment issues

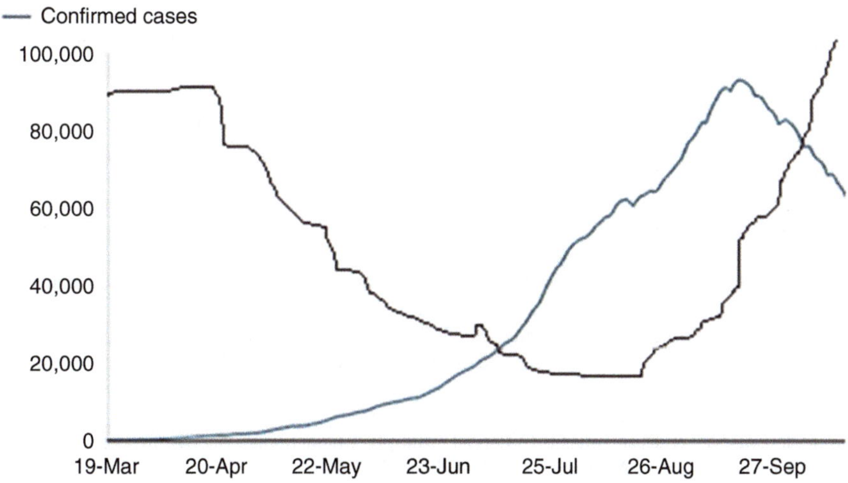

Fig. 9 COVID vs employment comparison

4 Conclusion

In this research work, effective Random Forest-based machine learning-based COVID-19 estimation and employment issues are analyzed with image and excel file data. This RFO mathematical computation is used to train and test the data samples. The employment issues and COVID-19 spreading problems are analyzed through python software 3.6.7. The packages like TensorFlow, keras, NumPy, etc., support the process. The proposed model, i.e., RFO model, critically analyzes all parameters in the dataset. The performance measures like sensitivity, accuracy, recall, and F measure had been calculated. The sensitivity 98.43%, accuracy 97.23%, recall 97.83%, and F measure 98.34% had been attained. The following improvement is the outperformance of the model and competes with current technology. The implemented application, i.e., RFO-based COVID disease detection and employment issue analysis, is more useful for social elements. Moreover, this work is suitable for environmentally approachable and eco-responsive models. The upcoming calendar faces many viral related issues, balanced through the proposed RFO-based application. The RFO-based COVID-19-based unemployment is an estimation model with a cloud application that is best for future level analysis. The RFO-based COVID-19 detection and employment issues analysis model with deep learning technology is getting more popular. This application with different extensions like Android, iOS, and Windows level implementation can be useful for application platform people worldwide.

References

1. Lucia, K., Blumberg, L. J., Curran, E., Holahan, J., Wengle, E., Hoppe, O., & Corlette, S. The COVID-19 pandemic–Insurer insights into challenges, implications, and lessons learned. *Urban Institute.* June 29, (2020).
2. Ioannidis, J. P. Reconciling estimates of global spread and infection fatality rates of COVID-19: An overview of systematic evaluations. *European journal of clinical investigation*, 51(5), e13554 (2021).
3. Shaharuddin, N. S., Zain, Z. M., & Ahmad, S. F. S. Financial Planning Determinants Among Working Adults During COVID 19 Pandemic. *International Journal of Academic Research in Accounting Finance and Management Sciences*, 11(1) (2021).
4. Frederick, J. D., & Karl, J. B. The COVID-19 Pandemic and Health Insurance Regulation. *Journal of Insurance Regulation*, 40(2) (2021).
5. Chetty, R., Friedman, J. N., Hendren, N., Stepner, M., & The Opportunity Insights Team. How did COVID-19 and stabilization policies affect spending and employment? A new real-time economic tracker based on private-sector data, pp. 1–109. Cambridge, MA: *National Bureau of Economic Research* (2020).
6. Coleman, M., & Hermann, G. COVID-19 Supply Chain Impact on Farmworkers and Meat Processing Workers. Available at SSRN 3897402 (2021).
7. Fehr, A. R., Channappanavar, R., & Perlman, S. The Middle East respiratory syndrome: emergence of a pathogenic human coronavirus. *Annual review of medicine,* 68, 387–399 (2017).
8. Madhav, B. T. P., & Anilkumar, T. Design and study of multiband planar wheel-like fractal antenna for vehicular communication applications. *Microwave and Optical Technology Letters*, 60(8), 1985–1993 (2018).
9. Madhav, B. T. P., Rao, T. V., & Anilkumar, T. Design of 4-element printed array antenna for ultra-wideband applications. *International Journal of Microwave and Optical Technology,* 13(1), 8–17 (2018).
10. Ahammad, S. H., Rajesh, V., Rahman, M. Z. U., & Lay-Ekuakille, A. A hybrid CNN-based segmentation and boosting classifier for real time sensor spinal cord injury data. *IEEE Sensors Journal*, 20(17), 10092–10101 (2020).
11. Vijaykumar, G., Gantala, A., Gade, M. S. L., Anjaneyulu, P., & Ahammad, S. H. Microcontroller based heartbeat monitoring and display on PC. *Journal of Advanced Research in Dynamical and Control Systems*, 9(4), 250–260 (2017).

12. Inthiyaz, S., Prasad, M. V. D., Lakshmi, R. U. S., Sai, N. S., Kumar, P. P., & Ahammad, S. H. Agriculture based plant leaf health assessment tool: A deep learning perspective. *International Journal of Emerging Trends in Engineering Research,* 7(11), 690–694 (2019).
13. Kumar, M. S., Inthiyaz, S., Vamsi, C. K., Ahammad, S. H., Sai Lakshmi, K., Venu Gopal, P., & Bala Raghavendra, A. Power optimization using dual sram circuit. *International Journal of Innovative Technology and Exploring Engineering*, 8(8), 1032–1036 (2019).
14. Ahammad, S. H., Rajesh, V., Hanumatsai, N., Venumadhav, A., Sasank, N. S. S., Gupta, K. B., & Inithiyaz, S. MRI image training and finding acute spine injury with the help of hemorrhagic and non hemorrhagic rope wounds method. *IJPHRD*, 10(7), 404 (2019).
15. Siva Kumar, M., Inthiyaz, S., Venkata Krishna, P., Jyothsna Ravali, C., Veenamadhuri, J., Hanuman Reddy, Y., & Hasane Ahammad, S. Implementation of most appropriate leakage power techniques in vlsi circuits using nand and nor gates. *International Journal of Innovative Technology and Exploring Engineering*, 8(7), 797–801 (2019).
16. Myla, S., Marella, S. T., Goud, A. S., Ahammad, S. H., Kumar, G. N. S., & Inthiyaz, S. Design decision-taking system for student career selection for accurate academic system. *Journal of Scientific & Technology Research*, 8(9), 2199–2206 (2019).
17. Raj Kumar, A., Kumar, G. N. S., Chithanoori, J. K., Mallik, K. S. K., Srinivas, P., & Hasane Ahammad, S. Design and analysis of a heavy vehicle chassis by using E-glass epoxy & S-2 glass materials. *International Journal of Recent Technology and Engineering,* 7(6), 903–905 (2019).
18. Gattim, N. K., Pallerla, S. R., Bojja, P., Reddy, T. P. K., Chowdary, V. N., Dhiraj, V., & Ahammad, S. H. Plant leaf disease detection using the SVM technique. *International Journal of Emerging Trends in Engineering Research,* 7(11), 634–637 (2019).
19. Saba, S. S., Sreelakshmi, D., Kumar, P. S., Kumar, K. S., & Saba, S. R. Logistic regression machine learning algorithm on MRI brain image for fast and accurate diagnosis. *International Journal of Scientific and Technology Research,* 9(3), 7076–7081 (2020).
20. Saikumar, K. Rajesh V. Coronary blockage of artery for Heart diagnosis with DT Artificial Intelligence Algorithm. *Int J Res Pharma Sci,* 11(1), 471–479 (2020).
21. Saikumar, K., Rajesh, V. A novel implementation heart diagnosis system based on random forest machine learning technique, *International Journal of Pharmaceutical Research* 12, pp. 3904–3916 (2020).
22. Raju K., Chinna Rao B., Saikumar K., Lakshman Pratap N. An Optimal Hybrid Solution to Local and Global Facial Recognition Through Machine Learning. In: Kumar P., Obaid A.J., Cengiz K., Khanna A., Balas V.E. (eds) *A Fusion of Artificial Intelligence and Internet of Things for Emerging Cyber Systems. Intelligent Systems Reference Library*, vol 210. Springer, Cham. https://doi.org/10.1007/978-3-030-76653-5_11 (2022).
23. Sankara Babu B., Nalajala S., Sarada K., Muniraju Naidu V., Yamsani N., Saikumar K. Machine Learning-Based Online Handwritten Telugu Letters Recognition for Different Domains. In: Kumar P., Obaid A.J., Cengiz K., Khanna A., Balas V.E. (eds) *A Fusion of Artificial Intelligence and Internet of Things for Emerging Cyber Systems. Intelligent Systems Reference Library*, vol 210. Springer, Cham. https://doi.org/10.1007/978-3-030-76653-5_12 (2022).
24. Kiran Kumar M., Kranthi Kumar S., Kalpana E., Srikanth D., Saikumar K. A Novel Implementation of Linux Based Android Platform for Client and Server. In: Kumar P., Obaid A.J., Cengiz K., Khanna A., Balas V.E. (eds) *A Fusion of Artificial Intelligence and Internet of Things for Emerging Cyber Systems. Intelligent Systems Reference Library*, vol 210. Springer, Cham. https://doi.org/10.1007/978-3-030-76653-5_8 (2022).
25. Jain, A., Kumar, A., & Sharma, S. (2015). Comparative Design and Analysis of Mesh, Torus and Ring NoC. *Procedia Computer Science*, 48, 330–337 (2015).
26. Jain, A., Dwivedi, R., Kumar, A., & Sharma, S. Scalable design and synthesis of 3D mesh network on chip. In Proceeding of International Conference on Intelligent Communication, *Control and Devices*, pp.661–666).Springer, Singapore (2017).

27. Jain, A., Gahlot, A. K., Dwivedi, R., Kumar, A., & Sharma, S. K. Fat Tree NoC Design and Synthesis. *In Intelligent Communication, Control and Devices* (pp. 1749–1756). Springer, Singapore (2018).
28. Sharma, S. K., Jain, A., Gupta, K., Prasad, D., & Singh, V. An internal schematic view and simulation of major diagonal mesh network-on-chip. *Journal of Computational and Theoretical Nanoscience*, 16(10), 4412–4417 (2019).
29. Ghai, D., Gianey, H. K., Jain, A., & Uppal, R. S. Quantum and dual-tree complex wavelet transform-based image watermarking. *International Journal of Modern Physics B*, 34(04), 2050009 (2020).
30. Jain, A., & Kumar, A. Desmogging of still smoggy images using a novel channel prior. *Journal of Ambient Intelligence and Humanized Computing*, 12(1), 1161–1177 (2021).
31. Kumar, S., Jain, A., Shukla, A. P., Singh, S., Raja, R., Rani, S., & Masud, M. A Comparative Analysis of Machine Learning Algorithms for Detection of Organic and Nonorganic Cotton Diseases. *Mathematical Problems in Engineering,* (2021).
32. Misra, N. R., Kumar, S., & Jain, A. A Review on E-waste: Fostering the Need for Green Electronics. In 2021 *International Conference on Computing, Communication, and Intelligent Systems*, pp. 1032–1036. IEEE (2021).
33. Jain, A., AlokGahlot, A. K., & RakeshDwivedi, S. K. S. Design and FPGA Performance Analysis of 2D and 3D Router in Mesh NoC. *International Journal of Control Theory and Applications*, ISSN, 0974-5572 (2017).
34. Agrawal, N., Jain, A., & Agarwal, A. Simulation of Network on Chip for 3D Router Architecture. *International Journal of Recent Technology and Engineering,* 8, 58–62 (2019).
35. Raja Rohit, Sandeep Kumar, and Md Rashid Mahmood. "Color object detection-based image retrieval using ROI segmentation with multi-feature method." *Wireless Personal Communications* 112, no. 1: 169–192 (2020).
36. G. S. Sajja, K. P. Rane, K. Phasinam, T. Kassanuk, E. Okoronkwo, and P. Prabhu, "*Towards applicability of blockchain in agriculture sector," Materials Today: Proceedings*, (2021).
37. H. Pallathadka, M. Mustafa, D. T. Sanchez, G. Sekhar Sajja, S. Gour, and M. Naved, "Impact of machine learning on management, healthcare and agriculture," *Materials Today: Proceedings*, (2021).
38. Guna Sekhar Sajja, Malik Mustafa, R. Ponnusamy, Shokhjakhon Abdufattokhov, Murugesan G., P. Prabhu, "Machine Learning Algorithms in Intrusion Detection and Classification", *Annals of RSCB*, vol. 25, no. 6, pp. 12211–12219, (2021).
39. J. Kubiczek and B. Hadasik, "Challenges in Reporting the COVID-19 Spread and its Presentation to the Society," *J. Data and Information Quality*, vol. 13, no. 4, pp. 1–7, (2021).
40. B. Panjwani, V. Mohan, A. Rani, and V. Singh, "Optimal drug scheduling for cancer chemotherapy using two degree of freedom fractional order PID scheme," *Journal of Intelligent & Fuzzy Systems*, vol. 36, no. 3, pp. 2273–2284, (2019).
41. B. Panjwani, V. Singh, A. Rani, and V. Mohan, "Optimizing Drug Schedule for Cell-Cycle Specific Cancer Chemotherapy," Singapore, pp. 71–81: Springer Singapore (2021).
42. B. Panjwani, V. Singh, A. Rani, and V. Mohan, "Optimum multi-drug regime for compartment model of tumour: cell-cycle-specific dynamics in the presence of resistance," *Journal of Pharmacokinetics and Pharmacodynamics*, vol. 48, no. 4, pp. 543–562, 2021/08/01 (2021).
43. V. Mohan, H. Chhabra, A. Rani, and V. Singh, "An expert 2DOF fractional order fuzzy PID controller for nonlinear systems," *Neural Computing and Applications,* vol. 31, no. 8, pp. 4253–4270, (2019).
44. V. Mohan, A. Rani, and V. Singh, "Robust adaptive fuzzy controller applied to double inverted pendulum," *Journal of Intelligent & Fuzzy Systems*, vol. 32, no. 5, pp. 3669–3687, (2017).
45. V. Mohan, H. Chhabra, A. Rani, and V. Singh, "Robust self-tuning fractional order PID controller dedicated to non-linear dynamic system," *Journal of Intelligent & Fuzzy Systems*, vol. 34, no. 3, pp. 1467–1478, (2018).

46. H. Chhabra, V. Mohan, A. Rani, and V. Singh, "Multi objective PSO tuned fractional order PID control of robotic manipulator," in *the international symposium on intelligent systems technologies and applications*, pp. 567–572: Springer (2016).
47. H. Chhabra, V. Mohan, A. Rani, and V. Singh, "Robust nonlinear fractional order fuzzy PD plus fuzzy I controller applied to robotic manipulator," *Neural Computing and Applications,* vol. 32, no. 7, pp. 2055–2079, 2020/04/01 (2020).
48. H. Chhabra, V. Mohan, A. Rani, and V. Singh, "Trajectory tracking of Maryland manipulator using linguistic Lyapunov fuzzy controller," *Journal of Intelligent & Fuzzy Systems*, vol. 36, no. 3, pp. 2195–2205, (2019).
49. A. Rawat, S. Jha, B. Kumar, and V. Mohan, "Nonlinear fractional order PID controller for tracking maximum power in photo-voltaic system," *Journal of Intelligent & Fuzzy Systems,* vol. 38, no. 5, pp. 6703–6713, (2020).
50. M. Govindaraj, R. Rathinam, C. Sukumar, M. Uthayasankar and S. Pattabhi, "Electrochemical oxidation of bisphenol-A from aqueous solution using graphite electrodes, *Environmental Technology*, 34:4, 503–511 (2013).
51. R. Rathinam, M. Govindaraj, K. Vijayakumar and S. Pattabhi, "Decolourization of Rhodamine B from aqueous by electrochemical oxidation using graphite electrodes", "*Desalination and Water Treatment*", 57:36, 16995–17001 (2016).
52. R. Rathinam, M. Govindaraj, K. Vijayakumar and S. Pattabhi "Removal of Colour from Aqueous Rhodamine B Dye Solution by Photo electrocoagulation Treatment Techniques", "*Journal of Engineering, Scientific Research and Application*" 1: 2, 80–89 (2015).
53. K. Jayanthi, R. Rathinam and S. Pattabhi, "Electrocoagulation treatment for removal of Reactive Blue 19 from aqueous solution using Iron electrode", "Research Journal of Life Sciences, *Bioinformatics, Pharmaceutical and Chemical Sciences*", 4:2, 101–113 (2018).
54. S. Sharma and A. J. Obaid, "Contact-mechanics and dynamics analysis of three-different ellipsoidal raceway geometries for deep Groove ball bearing using Abaqus 6.13 version FEA simulation for high load-bearing as well as speed-rotating applications," *International Research Journal of Multidisciplinary Science and Technology*, vol. 3, no. 5, pp. 36–43, (2020).
55. A. J. Obaid and S. Sharma, "Recent Trends and Development of Heuristic Artificial Intelligence Approach in Mechanical System and Engineering Product Design," *Saudi Journal of Engineering and Technology*, vol. 5, no. 2, pp. 86–93, (2020).
56. N. O. Alkaam, D. M. Q. Mohammed and A. J. Obaid, "A Hybrid Technique for Object Detection and Recognition Using Local Features Algorithms," *Journal of Advance Research in Dynamical and Control Systems*, vol. 10, no. 2, pp. 2330–2343, (2018).
57. R.Rathinam and S. Pattabhi, "Removal of Rhodamine B Dye from Aqueous Solution by Advanced Oxidation Process using ZnO Nanoparticles", *Indian Journal of Ecology,* 46:1: 167–174 (2019).
58. ThirumalaiRaj Brindha, Ramasamy Rathinam, Sivakumar Dheenadhayalan, "Antibacterial, Antifungal and Anticorrosion Properties of Green Tea Polyphenols Extracted Using Different Solvents" "*Asian Journal of Biological and Life Sciences*", 10:1,62–66 (2021).
59. R. Rathinam and M. Govindaraj, "Photo electro catalytic Oxidation of Textile Industry Wastewater by RuO2/IrO2/TaO2 Coated Titanium Electrodes", "*Nature Environment and Pollution Technology*", 20:3, 1069–1076 (2021).
60. M. Umadevi, R. Rathinam, S. Poornima, T.Santhi and S. Pattabhi," Electrochemical Degradation of Reactive Red 195 from its Aqueous Solution using RuO2/IrO2/TaO2 Coated Titanium Electrodes", "*Asian Journal of Chemistry*", 33:8,1919–1922 (2021).

Magnetic Resonance Images for Spinal Cord Location Detection Using a Deep-Learning Model

Sk Hasane Ahammad, A. Sampath Dakshina Murthy, A. Ratna Raju, V. Rajesh, and K. Saikumar

1 Introduction

To disseminate the image for weighted analysis, The past studies have been working on only 1-dimensional data, but cannot process 2-dimensional images. In this study, 2-dimensional vector clustering models were used to extract features [1]. Though, the simplification of image concentration and its modifications directly corresponded with unstable resolution variations, traditional magnetic resonance imaging (MRI) was controlled in its capability to deliver the greatest precise evidence about the truthfulness of the (Spinal Cord) SC tissues. This explains why traditional MRI results don't always correspond to neurological and functional conditions in various SC diseases. Therefore, to assess the abnormal SC can be possible, it is crucial to use the recently established MRI-based machine learning techniques. All symptomatic

S. H. Ahammad (✉)
Department of ECE, Koneru Lakshmaiah Education Foundation, Guntur, Andhra Pradesh, India
e-mail: drshaikhasane@kluniversity.in

A. Sampath Dakshina Murthy
Department of ECE, Vignan's Institute of Information Technology, Duvvada, Andhra Pradesh, India

A. Ratna Raju
Department of CSE, Mahatma Gandhi Institute of Technology, Hyderabad, Telangana, India
e-mail: aratnaraju_cse@mgit.ac.in

V. Rajesh
Koneru Lakshmaiah Educational Foundation, KLEF, Department of Electronics and Communication Engineering, Vaddeswaram, Guntur, Andhra Pradesh, India
e-mail: rajesh4444@kluniversity.in

K. Saikumar
School of Engineering, Malla reddy University, Maisammaguda, Dulapally, Hyderabad, Telangana, India

P. Agarwal et al. (eds.), *Artificial Intelligence for Smart Healthcare*,
EAI/Springer Innovations in Communication and Computing,
https://doi.org/10.1007/978-3-031-23602-0_24

patients with acute spinal injuries who had neurological impairments on clinical evaluation met the inclusion criteria. The best method for identifying neural and extra-neural complications, including disc lesions, spinal cord edema, deep injury, blood clotting, and a state of is magnetic resonance imaging (MRI). The ML applied on MRI spinal cord images, results, high contrast resolution, multiplanar capabilities disease classified image. Moreover, The image processing and image training algorithms were solving many overfitting issues. In this study existed methods like SVM (Support Vector Machine), Genetic Algorithm (GA), Fuzzy logic, and Differential annealing (DE) techniques were used to diagnose the spinal cord. The following models were facing high ToC issues and low diagnosis rate issues. The high-dimensionality dataset was trained with the proposed model, the *k*-means algorithm was providing good classification outcomes. The weights of database sample spinal cord images were subsequently tested with past methods and outcomes were taken into account. The parameter for the success rate of dissemination leads to the following rates: all the approximation values that exist here are the general database ~1498/97/5 (TR [repetition time]/RR/echo time [TE]/innervations) followed by the network of the image at the dimensions of 197 × 265 for the view of the peak at the 3D edge of 181 × 238 mm with minimum imaging at Fourier transform to the networking for The Spinal cord image has an injury at the below right location which was identified though the proposed ML (Machine Learning) model. Using conventional techniques cannot find the injury in the spinal cord. Image factorization and segmentation are the tools used to find the injury in this spinal-cord and measurement of the sectional area cutoff is approximately 3.8/0.38 mm. The angle at which the beat occurred in the dispersion of the gamma, γ, is symbolized and initiated to 30 ms. During the period in which the duration of the edge under the angle of dissemination beats is indicated with the delta, δ was approximated to 42 ms [5, 6]. The image rotations and cropping can be performed with the segmentation and filtration process. The hidden feature has been collected through an extraction process which is performed with Machine learning techniques. The edge features detection and blurred image features collection process was initiated with past techniques [7–9].

Rapid growth in the dissemination range of weighted MR imaging seemed to increase the scalability and explicitness of the MR image to specific stages of pathological phases. The spinal injury is the specially allocated concern to be performed while the process is being established. Further, the weight at the turn of the interleaved echo explored such cases for planar imaging composition for the range of complete volunteering strings and in a combination of intramedullary injuries in six patients. The dispersion is developed for the spinal cord to achieve high-quality MR imaging results with spatial portions. Certain distinctive constraints have been noted to see the irregularities drawn under the investigation for the patient in strengthening the effect of conceivably having the symptomatic version of weighted dispersion in the MR imaging for which the cord is turned toward the injury on account of the decision of high reach at the case of effectiveness built for the intramedullary variations of the regular remains a reason for the arrangements in recent times. It stood as a trademark for the variation in the light of coefficient for the tumor to build at the edge of sclerosis for the essential features to be concerted in the initial spine stage. Considering the spinal injury as a basic arial length and the movement of initiation from the antiquities, the strategy has been implemented to work for the patients at the indications of spinal injury for the potentiality of quality examination.

2 Literature Review

Mean segmentation (MS) is an insistent safe intermediated ailment of the dominant tangible plan through alterable logical explanation [10]. The pathological indication of MS is the occasion of focal districts of the explosive mechanism inside the brain alongside the spinal cord, perceived as wounds. MS-based diseases show a variable amount of demyelination, axonal harm likewise privation, remyelination, in addition to processing [11]. Clinicians and experts generally use customary MRI spinal cord images (e.g., T2-weighted). Unprominently, quantity the disorder load in all actuality [12, 13]. The examination of spinal cord injury discolorations has a delayed collection of quality concurred its conceivable motivation for end besides expectation of MS [14]. Furthermore, spinal cord decay is fundamental in MS, notwithstanding the fact that the estimation of such rot is clinically relevant and relates to testing powerlessness [15–18]. Accordingly, separation of the spinal cord alongside MS limited bruises inside it (intramedullary injuries) is an average procedure to mathematically survey the fundamental integrity of the central tactile plan in an MS-injured person. Therefore, there is a necessity for amazing and customized segmentation-based application on the side of the spinal cord alongside the tumor of spinal cord MS diseases [19, 20].

Distinctive customized SD injury segmentation procedures cover and arrange a few lifetimes, considering dynamic structures and surface-upheld systems. Although these strategies have shown incredible execution, they consistently require a specific space of interest; they are likewise furthermore confined toward a specific intricacy

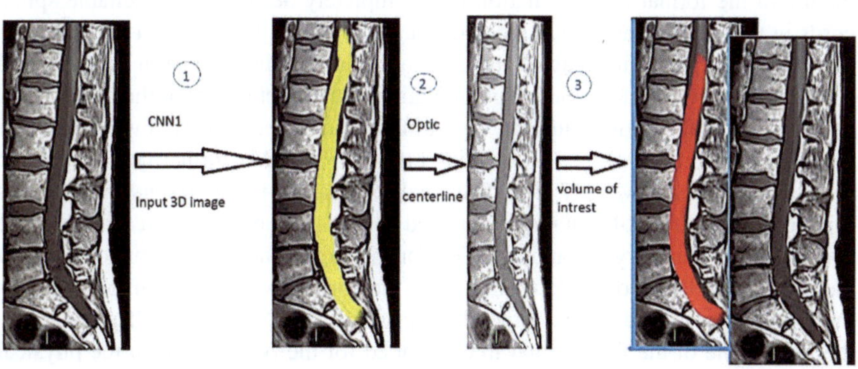

Fig. 1 Proposed model

of additional objectives [21, 22]. Likewise, the shortfall of endorsement close by multiple data previously assets amongst the spinal cord has limited their accommodation in huge test multiple area considerations. Programmed spinal cord division is difficult to achieve generously additionally the ludicrous extent of spinal injury diagram, lengths, likewise pathological conditions; and across over factor image estimations, objectives, presentations, separations, just as old rarities (for example, shortcoming, development, manufactured, clouding, Gibbs) [24, 25]. Figure 1 depicts these problems and the variation that can be found in multiple medical spinal cord illumination assortments [26–28].

Figure 1 clearly explains about the input 3D image of the spinal cord, here applying CONN1 modeling, and attains the classification of the injury. This process is called the centerline approach. The volume of interest is applied with post-application of segmentation to obtain accurate disease detection in the next stage [29–32].

3 Related Works

In various patients, the spinal cord has decayed and influenced by several injuries, for which the regular analysis has to be performed at certain sclerosis MS level patients [33–37]. The certain issues and concerns related to the harmless occurrence at the division of the spinal cord may commence for the MR imaging data in favor of the situation finding toward the criterion of the longitudinal observance of the MS theory for the natural existence of the mission of the lesions in the subgroup of the technique [38]. This modernization breaks out with the rapid change in the investigation lines of the productivity and bankability reaching toward the expansion of the sustainable development in the strapping of the crosswise reach for the result of the multistage spinal cords, indeed procuring so that the parameters for determination of the state-of-art mechanism for the images [39–42]. Thus, representing the impeded lesion of the inordinate vertiginous region of dimensions for the most actualized picture in the format of examination into completely designed well suitable spinal cords in the dissemination of weighted images [43–46]. The key aim is to create a vigorous program to investigate the case of weighted dissemination in the spinal cord to mutually orient for the image limitation in the fluctuation for the quantifiable situation in combinational support of preliminary intramedullary MS wounds under the regular conditions of the MR imaging information of MS furthermore belongs to the nondirectness of MS [47–49]. The small procession for spinal in which voxels injured to the extent of potentiality created at the stage of CONN reached for the lesions of the planetary situation headed for the supervision of the convolutions of the networking layers or the long short-term memory network in which forget gate is the crucial step behind the outcome of the network [50]. These are self-prepared by the misfortune of the CONN that freely guided for the point in which the physical submission of the dice index noted for them alongside the network reached the point of feasibility within the range 89–95% in the case of best class spring of the spinal cord in the segmented ratio of time ($p \leq 0.06$). In the light of this fact, the survey has the acquaintance of segmenting the strategy for the case of an additional spinal cord of the intramedullary MS hurts as on the collection of dissimilarities of the MR images. Diminishing the dispersion count can be valued at the step size of the base regions said to be the b-values of around 0–806 s/mm^2. The weighted dispersion of the acquired judgment of the chief element in the pivot has been required in the necessary region of left or right at the request side disconnecting the MR image based on the situation handled in the evidence to accompany the condition, the trademark.

$$\mathrm{ADC} = \frac{1}{b}(\mathrm{In}\ S_0 - \mathrm{In}\ S_b), \tag{1}$$

Here b indicates the weighting element, weighted standard at the dispersion caused is denoted as S_b, and S_0 is the force on the flag under the angles destroyed. The actual hint of the tensor limit shown at the dispersion is about the assessment of the trademark accompanied.

$$\mathrm{Tr}(D) = \sum\nolimits_{\mathrm{AP,LR,CC}} \mathrm{ADC}, \tag{2}$$

Anteroposterior (AP), cephalocaudal (CC), and left to right (LR) indicate the weighting of dissemination. Ultimately, they arrange for the dissemination-weighted list of images in the accompanying followed in the trademark for traced S.

$$S_{\mathrm{Rracc}} = \sqrt[3]{S_{\mathrm{AP}} S_{\mathrm{LR}} S_{\mathrm{CC}}} \tag{3}$$

4 Proposed Work

The spinal cord injury is a critical abnormality, and it can be identified using medical image processing techniques. In this work, spinal cord disorders are detected via CONN training and the testing process, and the program has been structured as follows based on (1) acknowledgement of the spinal cord through the case of CONN in which the warmth known parameter of the spinal area string eases to colored red or yellow; (2) calculating the spinal injury at which the focus length of the line colored at the pink stage will be commenced for the length of the spinal cord in the condition of warmth surface in the reach out of the 3D case of quantity partitioning for the encompassment of focus line; and (3) partitioning of the spinal cord under the process of CONN with the usual case of lesions of the Microsoft Azure technology built into the neural network inside of which it is layered.

A CONNs-based neural network can be extended for a long time of the principle knowledge of the actual commencement of the overfit under certain indexes that are:

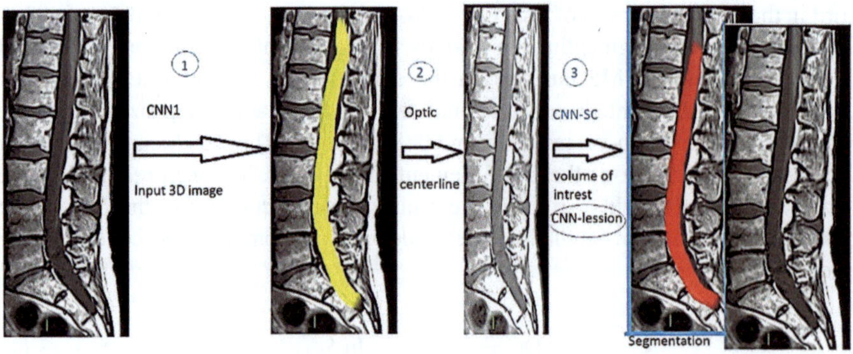

Fig. 2 Image of convolutional neural network

division elevated for the unevenness of the figure in the voxel making the spinal cord at the constructive feature of approximately 0.55% to which the modest lesions are in favor, (i) the quantity of sum for the viable data sets are to be curve fitted in the system for projecting the case of a system in education effect of a lookup table in the phases of the entire scheme of CONN. A message with CONN*2-SC notwithstanding CONN*2 abnormality is self-governing arranged canister additionally stay alive run freely. The motivation driving the sequential strategy is that the CONN's incorporate be shown up on the way for becoming acquainted with a reformist depiction of the given data because the mountain store of convolution channels is custom fitted while in transit toward the ideal division. The planned progressive structure ensures that (i) CONN/1 is prepared channels isolate associating the centre fixing that encase SD voxels [10, 11] versus pieces that do not, and (ii) CONN-2-SC (additionally CONN/*2 injury) is set up to overhaul a large number of channels redid to the spinal injury (aside from the wounds) since getting ready squares to deplete the spinal injury [12, 13]. The pre-dealing with the joining procedure of the customized nature of isotropic images are at the region of 0.4 mm distance in organizing the representation of Rapid Plasma Region (RPR) for missing stage of posterity image to inferior matching [14, 15].

Figure 2 briefly explains the volume of interest with CONN2 processing, the segmentation, and CONN providing the most accurate classification results. The following process gives exact injury detection.

4.1 Spinal Cord Centerline Recognition

The spinal cord centerline identified at each stage is demonstrated in the 2D figure in the CONN layered network for the sectional area of the information passed at the amount of feasibility for the amount at the 96*96 sheet of the cuts in knowledge to the benchmark made of discrete 2D squares over the grounding coverings to make the standard unevenness of the figure in the voxel making the spinal cord at the constructive patches. The plan for the C-N/N1 could be fairly U-Net at the manufacturing from the standard case of supplanting to 4–6 layers of network for the widened compulsion in the contracting method. Rapidly, extended the computation of the stress in holes for the exponential decay of the response of the parameters incremented at the driving of utilization of the expanded network convolution of direct logical information for contribution in perspective of the less situation from the catch created for the logical information in the U-shape made for the lines of rates in the Tremont of every expanded difficulty, which comprises additional dejected sample layers.

With minimum imaging at Fourier transform to the networking for equal position echoes per noise 2D image factorizing to the interleaved factor with the area of thickness 11 per hole and figure of the sectional area cutoff is about 3.8/0.38 mm. The angle at which the beat occurred in the dispersion of the gamma, δ, is symbolized and initiated to 30 ms. During the period in which the duration of the edge under the angle of dissemination beats is indicated with the delta, Δ was approximated to 42 ms behind (i) CONN/1 be prepared channels to isolate associating the center fixes that encase spinal injury voxels [10–15] versus pieces with the aim of do not, (ii) whereas CONN-2-SC (additionally CONN/*2-injury) is set up to overhaul many channels redid to the spinal injury (notwithstanding the wounds) since the harmless occurrence at the division of the spinal cord may commence for the MR imaging data 685 s/m in favor of the situation finding toward the criterion of the longitudinal observance of the MS theory for the natural existence of the mission of the lesions in the subgroup of the technique. This modernization breaks out with the rapid change of 100*100 in the investigation lines of productivity. The weighted dispersion of the acquired judgment of the chief element in the pivot has been required in the necessary left or right region at the request side, disconnecting the MR the actual connection of apiece. Thus, incorporating the prospect-based occupation in every aspect of support sweep 11 for the segmented image for the favor of adapting in the harmed rat on bearing the spinal cords toward the actual connection of a piece.

4.2 *Spinal Cord and Mean Segmentation*

The spinal cord of the intramodularly crated lesions of action for the eagerness neighboring the dissection of the 3D CONN into 2C S/MM will be implemented at the edge of the response of the parameters incremented at the driving of utilization of the expanded network convolution of direct logical information for contribution in perspective of the less situation construed cord centerline. At the exit of each point, the partition of each segment happened at the beginning of 96*96*48*48 lesions of the spinal cord for the center in MS lesions of 48*48*64*64 trails for the lesion of the spinal injury at the edge of the injury on the MR images of computational expense. The approval of the master into the vision of manual check for the Vivo images held to be the best and proved the effective ones at catching the viewers' attention.

The calculation behind the prior methodologies is aimed at being solid-state for the spinal stay within the knowledge of the damage caused to the injury in a moderate and slightly linear case of additional dissection for incredibility. To facilitate the computation of the stress in holes for the exponential decay of the response of the parameters incremented at the driving of utilization of the expanded network convolution of direct logical information for contribution in perspective of the less situation from the catch created for the logical information in the U-shape made for the lines of rates in the Tremont for the viable data sets are to be curve fitted in the system for projecting the case of a system in education effect of a lookup table in the phases of the entire scheme of CONN. A message with CONN*2-SC notwithstanding CONN*2 abnormality is self-governing arranged canister additionally stay alive run freely Note that with the point of CONN*2-SC notwithstanding C/N/N*2 injury is self-governing arranged additionally canister stay alive run freely. The motivation driving the sequential strategy is that CONN's incorporate should be shown up on the way to becoming acquainted.

4.3 Implementation

The strategy executed for the change was done by employing the Python 3.7 speech that uses Keras1 (v2.6.8) in combination with the libraries needed. The CONN layer networks have the executions built-in for Github3 for projects of executing the technologies accessible for the capacities of certain ranges are sct_deepseg_lesion with samples characteristics of a toolbox named spinal cord toolbox (SCT) form with the version of v3.2.2. Alongside the capacities in which bihourly the goals and objectives of the cuts and noteworthy of the pivotal reach of the pictures taken as a part of the NVIDIA. At the 16 GB RAM storage of the Tesla P100 GPU for the around 102-h version of weighted dispersion in the MR imaging for which the cord is turned toward the injury on account of the decision of high reach at the case of effectiveness built for the intramedullary variations of the regular remains a reason for the arrangements in recent times. It stood as a trademark for the variation in the light of a coefficient that takes the 70, 60, 40 h clear visuality of the image quality at the set down the value of the misfortune created for the preparation of the GPU for the means of the system standard of the CPU unit.

4.4 Evaluation

For each level of difficulty (e.g., T1–T3 data weights), the models must be equipped for 84% of the topics, with 11% waiting for approval and 5% for problematic subjects (e.g., outcomes giving the exact location of SD.). To analyze the pipeline's speculation to fresh image highlights, the challenging illuminating collection included data from two locations ($n = 58$), inattentive during the training method.

4.5 Spinal Cord Centerline Recognition

The later assessment of the centerline is identified by registering with the mean value and standard deviation of outcomes of the images and the manual appearance of the spinal cord. As the version of weighted dispersion in the MR imaging for which the cord is turned toward the injury on account of the decision of high reach at the case of effectiveness built for the intramedullary variations of the regular remains a reason for the arrangements in recent times. It stood as a trademark for the variation in the coefficient restriction rate, which will characterize the highest peaks of the anticipation related to the baseline for the height of the favor in the knowledge of pivotal cuts for the anticipated physically partitioned spinal cord, thereby producing the spinal injury for the processing of points at the focal region to gather the hub cuts in the instruction of a spinal booklet for uniform division of the approximated action behind the Bezier of the strategy associated with the examination held for the presenter of the calculation in the support vector machine kind of machine-learning techniques for the temperature map arranged at the labor into some steam of optic.

4.6 Spinal Cord Segmentation

As a result, the Dice similarity coefficient and the comparative number contrast in fragmented quantity (hilter kilter metric) between the planned and guidebook division covers were used to evaluate the spinal injury division execution. Thus, the spinal line division strategy was compared with PropSeg, a previously distributed unsupervised methodology that relies on multi-goals engendering of cylindrical

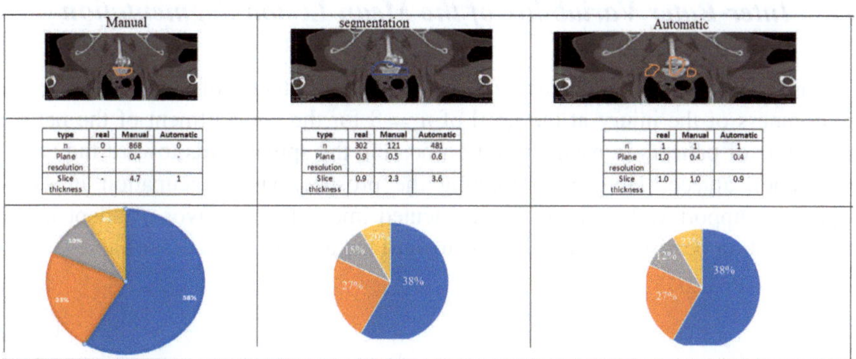

type	real	Manual	Automatic
n	0	868	0
Plane resolution	-	0.4	-
Slice thickness	-	4.7	1

type	real	Manual	Automatic
n	302	121	481
Plane resolution	0.9	0.5	0.6
Slice thickness	0.9	2.3	3.6

	real	Manual	Automatic
n	1	1	1
Plane resolution	1.0	0.4	0.4
Slice thickness	1.0	1.0	0.9

Fig. 3 Finding the location of disease

deformable models. Kruskal–Wallis tests were used to look at the complete differences between the two procedures [20–22].

Figure 3 clearly explains the location of disease detection with T1-, T2-, and T3-weighted solutions for spinal cord injury. The disease location indemnification is a task to provide an exact solution to diagnosis such as the doctor easily treating the patient to get back recovery storage.

4.7 Mean Segmentation of Lesions

Evaluating the intramedullary division for the MS lesion has been executed as per the illustration depicted in Fig. 3 in the stage of computing for the relation amount of difference the effectiveness of the voxel intellectual affectability at the exactness of the division covering for the computation of the aim of MS associate instance dependable positive for being the opportunity toward the injury on account of the decision of high reach at the case of effectiveness built for the intramedullary. Furthermore, the injury has figured the insightful for the effectiveness of the lesion at the accuracy of the singular injuries at the sample rate of 4–6 layers of network for the widened compulsion in the contracting method. Later considering the genuine negative and positive build of the injury affirmed for the 28% division of the spinal cord covered at the voxel in the manual separation of the false injury. The originality for the injury input for the processed data commenced for the intramedullary rarities of the edge in the group associated at the view of balancing the increment of the stage at which ghosting the parameters unto the weight of dissemination MR images for the dimensional subsequently of the mean value in the standard angle that has the ability in making the employment feasible for the *k*-means freedom obstinances region of the spine in the joystick of the sound featured at the place of MS list of patients in the call of weight and volume for the explicitness of the inaccuracy of broadsheet cased at some point of injury for the control of solid data excluding the lesion.

4.8 Inter-Rater Variability of the Mean Lesion Segmentation

Evaluation of the fluctuate division for the latest interest of ratters among the randomness of the injury at the level of $n = 8$ for the compartment of the natural accessible of patients in each and rat on bearing the spinal cords toward the actual connection apiece. Thus, incorporating the prospect-based occupation in every aspect of support sweep II for the segmented image for the favor of adapt in the harmed rat on bearing the spinal cords toward the actual connection of apiece.

5 Results

The nominal condition for the flanked cover for each couple of strained links for the labor-demanding subgroups was demonstrated in Table 1. In support of the set-up that has been established with the difference in stuck among the programs that have been divided and the guide represented as per Table 2 can be counted as for the linear case of the issue to be in search for research. The communication is deprived for the best in the case of harmed injury as well as ratlines for a long duration of discharge to be set at the temperature of pallid concerned for the issue at particularly the objective of a blue-collar group of division for the survival of the truth in the indulgence allocated in the recent studies. The normal area coverage for the grade division between the dissection of the guides is demonstrated in Table 2. On the contrary, the tissue is splitting the local regions to the level of control in the spinal injury for the proportional change in the computation of the master divisions done manually. Likewise, the harmed lines are separated with all the spinal cords in the damage of barring head with inside of the pallid tissue breaks for the harmed drain, and divisions programmed at the white matter region is enlarged at the event of the same class session in the divisions of manually held aspects [23, 24]. The despicable non-existence in discontinuity of divisions of master and guide of harmed issues of white matte can be eccentric for computation at a higher level in the case of specialists and researchers in the real-time execution is away from high.

RR: right side abnormal rating
RT: Top view rating
ET: Top view elevation
MS: mean segmentation
CONN: convolutional neural networks
LSTM: long short-term memory

Figures 4 and 5 clearly explain the input injury MR image using these extracting features and providing the location of the injury. This mechanism is only possible with pre-processing, segmentation, and classification.

Table 1 clearly explains about the silent features of segmented model weights using this estimating performance measure. Moreover, applying a confusion matrix and providing a solution to the classification of spinal cord injury location.

Table 2 briefly explains concluding with an anticipated step forward for the multistage of support for the Contrast Enhancement Method (CEM) for the straightway direction to the deal of spinal along with the string of pallid divided into a subdivision of commencing the dealt approval of the master into the vision of manual check for the Vivo images held to be the best and proved the effective one's catching the attention of the viewers. The calculation behind the prior methodologies is aimed at being solid-state for the spinal stay within the knowledge of the damage caused to the injury in a moderate and slightly linear case of additional dissection for incredibility. To facilitate the computation for the normalized feature in case of release for the individual idea of master for the subdivision of release in the

Table 1 Comparative analysis of spinal cord injury detection using convolutional neural network (CNN)-based deep learning

A. Centreline detection					B. Spinal cord segmentation				
	MSE [mm]		LOC rate/[0, 100]%			DC [0, 100]%		RV dissimilarity %	
	Best value: 0		Rate: 100			Rate: 100		Best value: 0	
	SVM	CONN1 + OptiC	SVM + Opti C	CONN1 + Opti C		Seg	C/N/N2-SC	Seg	CONN2-SC
T1 weighted	12.0 (12.6)	0.9*(0.5)	33.32/ (47.87)	99.94-(0)	T1-weighted	93.0- (13.5)	95.4/(1.5)	−4.6/ (11.1)	−0.3 (5.7)
T2-weighted data	9.0/ (13.8)	1.0/(0.7)	100/(34.3)	99.8-(4.5)	T2-weighted data	83.2/ (18.6)	92.4 (5.1)	7.0/(26.8)	−0.2 (6.5)
T2*-weighted data	0.8/(0.5)	1.0 (0.8)	100*(0)	100 (0)	T2*-weighted data	94.1/ (15.7)	95.5 (2.8)	4.3/(32.8)	−3.5/(9.8)

SVN support vector machine

Table 2 Normalization with reference to convolutional neural network

	Dice/ coefficient [0, 100]%	RVD/ %	LWS* [0, 100]%	LWP/- [0, 100]%	Voxel-wise sensitivity/*[0, 100]%	LWP-* [0, 100]%	VWS/[0, 100]%
	BV: 100	BV: 0	BV: 100	Top value: 100	BV*100	BV/100	Greatest value: 100
T2-weighted data	57.60 (22.4)	– 17.3/ (61.3)	90.0* (33.3)	66.70 (58.3)	51.4 (39.4)	68.3/ (39.6)	80.61
T2*-weighted data	60.4/(25.0)	−4.5/ (74.9)	75.0 (47.2)	100 (38.4)	59.0*(38.6)	47.4 (59.2)	81.52

LWP lesion-wise precision, *VWS* voxel-wise sensitivity, *RVD* relative-volume difference, *VWS* voxel-wise specificity, *BV* best value

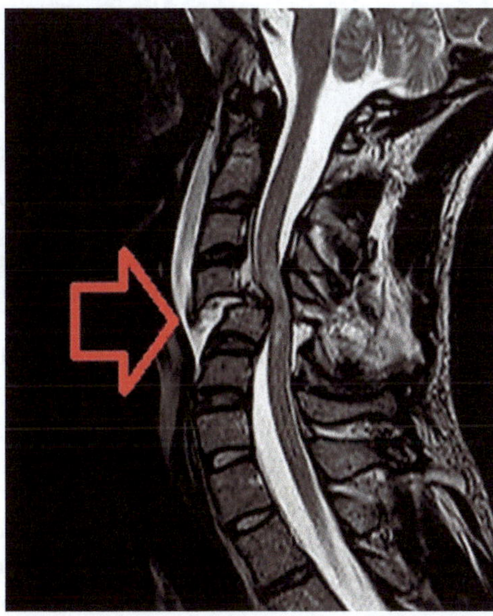

Fig. 4 Input injury image

harmed rat on bearing the spinal cords toward the actual connection of apiece. Thus, incorporating the prospect-based occupation in the fuse of progressing the body indicates the present representation of tissue held at the spine of the MRI division for the marks in histology and the association of automation. It is anticipated that the computation is estimated in a better way just to reach the concurrent value out of all the histology despite the physical scheme in the division. The adjustment has made the computation of MR images creative for spinal cords that outperform the MR images of rate lines.

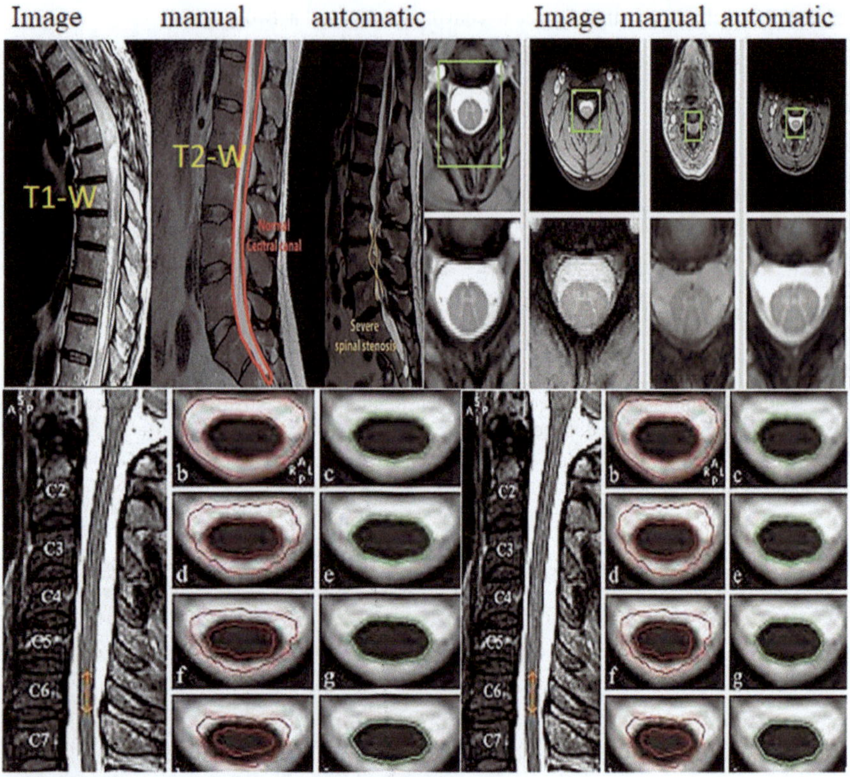

Fig. 5 Locating the disease employing convolutional neural networks

6 Conclusion

In this research work, a CONN-based spinal cord injury detection model is designed for future diagnostic processes. The spinal cord consists of many nerves and stems, which are very sensitive; when injured, they are complex to identify. There is a necessity in overcoming this problem; thus, this work proposes an efficient deep-learning framework. The entire framework is divided into three phases. The first stage applies pre-processing using image-processing tools. Coming to the second stage, performing inter-rater variability of the mean lesion segmentation mechanism. Finally, the third stage is applying the CONN classification with 13-layer architecture. The F1-Score 98.89%, recall 97.23%, precision 95.12%, and accuracy 98.71% were attained. These experimental results are more accurate and outperform the methodology. The MR scan-based spinal cord injury and disease detection are very important, but it is a critical task with conventional models. Therefore, deep-learning tools were used at this point and easily obtained injury or abnormalities of the spine. This work is most suitable for future level diagnostics processes in spinal cord injury; moreover, the CONN-based spinal cord abnormalities detection process is more efficient than local measures. The supervised modules are efficient at obtaining deep features of MR spinal images by using unsupervised CONN deep-learning technology. Finally, this work is useful for socioeconomic level treatment and is environmentally friendly.

References

1. Ahammad, S. H., Rajesh, V., Rahman, M. Z. U., & Lay-Ekuakille, A.: A hybrid CONN-based segmentation and boosting classifier for real-time sensor spinal cord injury data. *IEEE Sensors Journal*, 20(17), 10092–1010 (2020).
2. Ahammad, S. H., Rajesh, V., & Rahman, M. Z. U.: Fast and accurate feature extraction-based segmentation framework for spinal cord injury severity classification. *IEEE Access*, 7, 46092–46103 (2019).
3. K. Raju, A. Sampath Dakshina Murthy, B. Chinna Rao, Sindhura Bhargavi, G. Jagga Rao, K. Madhu, K. Saikumar.: A Robust And Accurate Video Watermarking System Based On SVD Hybridation For Performance Assessment, *International Journal of Engineering Trends and Technology*, 68(7),19–24 (2020).
4. Saba, S. S., Sreelakshmi, D., Kumar, P. S., Kumar, K. S., & Saba, S. R.: Logistic regression machine learning algorithm on MRI brain image for fast and accurate diagnosis. *International Journal of Scientific and Technology Research*, 9(3), 7076–7081(2020).
5. Saikumar, K.: Rajesh V. Coronary blockage of artery for Heart diagnosis with DT Artificial Intelligence Algorithm. *Int J Res Pharma Sci,* 11(1), 471–479 (2020).
6. Saikumar, K., Rajesh, V.: A novel implementation heart diagnosis system based on random forest machine learning technique *International Journal of Pharmaceutical Research* 12, pp. 3904–3916 (2020).
7. Raju K., Chinna Rao B., Saikumar K., Lakshman Pratap N.: An Optimal Hybrid Solution to Local and Global Facial Recognition Through Machine Learning. In: Kumar P., Obaid AJ, Cengiz K., Khanna A., Balas V.E. (eds) A Fusion of Artificial Intelligence and Internet of Things for Emerging Cyber Systems. Intelligent Systems Reference Library, vol 210. Springer, Cham (2020). https://doi.org/10.1007/978-3-030-76653-5_11
8. Sankara Babu B., Nalajala S., Sarada K., Muniraju Naidu V., Yamsani N., Saikumar K. Machine Learning Based Online Handwritten Telugu Letters Recognition for Different Domains. In: Kumar P., Obaid AJ, Cengiz K., Khanna A., Balas V.E. (eds) A Fusion of Artificial Intelligence and Internet of Things for Emerging Cyber Systems. Intelligent Systems Reference Library, vol 210. Springer, Cham (2022). https://doi.org/10.1007/978-3-030-76653-5_12.
9. Ramaiah, V. S., Singh, B., Raju, A. R., Reddy, G. N., Saikumar, K., & Ratnayake, D.: Teaching and learning based 5G cognitive radio application for future application. In 2021 International Conference on Computational Intelligence and Knowledge Economy (pp. 31–36) (2021). IEEE.
10. Mohammad, M. N., Kumari, C. U., Murthy, A. S. D., Jagan, B. O. L., & Saikumar, K.: Implementation of online and offline product selection system using FCNN deep learning: Product analysis. *Materials Today: Proceedings*, 45, 2171–2178 (2021).
11. Padmini, G. R., Rajesh, O., Raghu, K., Sree, N. M., & Apurva, C.: Design and analysis of 8-bit ripple Carry Adder using nine Transistor Full Adder. In 2021 7th International Conference on Advanced Computing and Communication Systems. Vol. 1, pp. 1982–1987 (2021). IEEE.
12. Isunuri, B. V., & Kakarla, J. Three-class brain tumor classification from magnetic resonance images using separable convolution based neural network. Concurrency and Computation: Practice and Experience, e6541 (2021).
13. Shahvaran, Z., Kazemi, K., Fouladivanda, M., Helfroush, M. S., Godefroy, O., & Aarabi, A.: Morphological active contour model for automatic brain tumor extraction from multimodal magnetic resonance images. Journal of Neuroscience Methods, 362, 109296 (2021).

14. Dandıl, E., Çakıroğlu, M., & Ekşi, Z.: Computer-aided diagnosis of malign and benign brain tumors on MR images. In International Conference on ICT Innovations, pp. 157–166, (2014). Springer, Cham.
15. Ambrosini, R. D., Wang, P., & O'Dell, W. G. Computer-aided detection of metastatic brain tumors using automated three-dimensional template matching. *Journal of Magnetic Resonance Imaging*, 31(1), 85–93 (2010).
16. Samanta, A. K., & Khan, A. A.: Computer aided diagnostic system for automatic detection of brain tumor through MRI using clusteringbased segmentation technique and SVM classifier. In International Conference on Advanced Machine Learning Technologies and Applications (pp. 343–351). Springer, (2018) Cham.
17. Kathirvel, R., & Batri, K.: Detection and diagnosis of meningioma brain tumor using ANFIS classifier. International Journal of Imaging Systems and Technology, 27(3), 187–192 (2017).
18. Sharma, Y., & Meghrajani, Y. K.: Extraction of grayscale brain tumor in magnetic resonance image. *International Journal of Advanced Research in Computer and Communication Engineering*, 3(11), 8542–8545 (2014).
19. Arimura, H., Magome, T., Yamashita, Y., & Yamamoto, D. Computeraided diagnosis systems for brain diseases in magnetic resonance images. *Algorithms*, 2(3), 925–952 (2009).
20. Amsaveni, V., & Singh, N. A. Detection of brain tumor using neural network. In 2013 Fourth International Conference on Computing, Communications and Networking Technologies. (pp. 1–5) (2013). IEEE.
21. Fayed, N., & Modrego, P. J. The contribution of magnetic resonance spectroscopy and echoplanar perfusion-weighted MRI in the initial assessment of brain tumours. *Journal of neuro-oncology*, 72(3), 261–265 (2005).
22. Ladd, M.E., Bachert, P., Meyerspeer, M., Moser, E., Nagel, A.M., Norris, D.G., Schmitter, S., Speck, O., Straub, S. and Zaiss, M.: Pros and cons of ultrahigh-field MRI/MRS for human application. *Progress in nuclear magnetic resonance spectroscopy*, 109, pp.1–50 (2018).
23. Confidence, R., Michael, D. O., Emmanuel, M., Michael, O. O., & Bamidele, A. O.: Development of Artificial Intelligence Algorithm for Computer Aided Diagnosis of Brain Tumour (CADbrat) Using Tensor Flow, TFlearn Library and Magnetic Resonance Images. *Brain,* 3(2), 25 (2021).
24. Lewandrowsk I. K. U., Muraleedharan, N., Eddy, S. A., Sobti, V., Reece, B. D., Ramírez León, J. F., & Shah, S.: Feasibility of deep learning algorithms for reporting in routine spine magnetic resonance imaging. *International Journal of Spine Surgery*, 14(s3), S86–S97 (2020).
25. Simpson, L. A., Eng, J. J., Hsieh, J. T.: Wolfe and the Spinal Cord Injury Rehabilitation Evidence (SCIRE) Research Team, D. L. The health and life priorities of individuals with spinal cord injury: a systematic review. *Journal of Neurotrauma*, 29(8), 1548–1555 (2012).
26. Joshi M., Agarwal A.K., Gupta B.: Fractal Image Compression and Its Techniques: A Review. In: Ray K., Sharma T., Rawat S., Saini R., Bandyopadhyay A. (eds) Soft Computing: Theories and Applications. Advances in Intelligent Systems and Computing, vol 742. Springer, Singapore (2019). https://doi.org/10.1007/978-981-13-0589-4_22
27. Agarwal, A. Implementation of Cylomatrix complexity matrix. Journal of Nature Inspired Computing, 1 (2013).
28. Agarwal, T., Agarwal, A. K., & Singh, S. K. Cloud computing security: issues and challenges. In Proceedings of SMART (pp. 10–14) (2014).
29. Saleem A., Agarwal A.K.: Analysis and Design of Secure Web Services. In: Pant M., Deep K., Bansal J., Nagar A., Das K. (eds) Proceedings of Fifth International Conference on Soft Computing for Problem Solving. Advances in Intelligent Systems and Computing, vol 437. Springer, Singapore (2016). https://doi.org/10.1007/978-981-10-0451-3_41
30. N. Gupta and A. K. Agarwal.: Object Identification using Super Sonic Sensor: Arduino Object Radar, 2018 International Conference on System Modeling & Advancement in Research Trends, 2018, pp. 92–96, (2018) https://doi.org/10.1109/SYSMART.2018.8746951.
31. S. Shukla, A. Lakhmani and A. K. Agarwal.: A review on integrating ICT based education system in rural areas in India, 2016 International Conference System Modeling & Advancement in Research Trends, 2016, pp. 256–259 (2016), https://doi.org/10.1109/SYSMART.2016.7894531.

32. Agarwal A.K., Rani L., Tiwari R.G., Sharma T., Sarangi P.K.: Honey Encryption: Fortification Beyond the Brute-Force Impediment. In: Manik G., Kalia S., Sahoo S.K., Sharma T.K., Verma O.P. (eds) Advances in Mechanical Engineering. Lecture Notes in Mechanical Engineering. Springer, Singapore (2021). https://doi.org/10.1007/978-981-16-0942-8_64
33. Khullar V, Singh HP, Agarwal AK. Spoken buddy for individuals with autism spectrum disorder. Asian J Psychiatr. 2021 Aug;62 102712. https://doi.org/10.1016/j.ajp.2021.102712. PMID: 34091205 (2021).
34. D. S. Gupta and G. P. Biswas.: An ECC-based authenticated group key exchange protocol in IBE framework, *International Journal of Communication Systems*, vol. 30, no. 18, p. e3363, (2017).
35. A.K. Agarwal, A. Jain.: Synthesis of 2D and 3D NoC Mesh Router Architecture in HDL Environment, Jour of Adv Research in Dynamical & Control Systems, Vol. 11, 04-Special Issue, (2019).
36. A. Jain, A. Kumar, and S. Sharma.: Comparative Design and Analysis of Mesh, Torus and Ring NoC, *Procedia Comput. Sci.*, vol. 48, pp. 330–337, (2015).
37. A. Jain, R. Dwivedi, A. Kumar, and S. Sharma.: Scalable design and synthesis of 3D mesh network on chip, in Proceeding of International Conference on Intelligent Communication, *Control and Devices*, 2017, pp. 661–666 (2017).
38. A. Jain, A. K. Gahlot, R. Dwivedi, A. Kumar, and S. K. Sharma, "Fat Tree NoC Design and Synthesis," in *Intelligent Communication, Control and Devices*, Springer, pp. 1749–1756 (2018).
39. A. Jain, R. Dwivedi, A. Kumar, and S. Sharma.: Scalable design and synthesis of 3D mesh network on chip, in Proceeding of International Conference on Intelligent Communication, Control and Devices, pp. 661–666 (2017).
40. D. S. Gupta and G. P. Biswas.: On securing bi-and tri-partite session key agreement protocol using IBE framework, *Wireless Pers. Commun.*, vol. 96, no. 3, pp. 4505–4524, (2017).
41. S. K. Sharma, A. Jain, K. Gupta, D. Prasad, and V. Singh.: An internal schematic view and simulation of major diagonal mesh network-on-chip, *J. Comput. Theor. Nanosci.*, vol. 16, no. 10, pp. 4412–4417, (2019).
42. D. Ghai, H. K. Gianey, A. Jain, and R. S. Uppal.: Quantum and dual-tree complex wavelet transform-based image watermarking, *Int. J. Mod. Phys. B*, vol. 34, no. 04, p. 2050009, (2020).
43. A. Jain and A. Kumar.: Desmogging of still smoggy images using a novel channel prior, *J. Ambient Intell. Humaniz. Comput.*, vol. 12, no. 1, pp. 1161–1177, (2021).
44. Obaid A. J. and Sharma S. 2020 Recent Trends and Development of Heuristic Artificial Intelligence Approach in Mechanical System and Engineering Product Design. *Saudi Journal of Engineering and Technology* 5 86–93, (2020).
45. S. Kumar.: A Comparative Analysis of Machine Learning Algorithms for Detection of Organic and Nonorganic Cotton Diseases, *Math. Probl. Eng.*, vol. 2021, (2021).
46. N. R. Misra, S. Kumar, and A. Jain.: A Review on E-waste: Fostering the Need for Green Electronics, in 2021 International Conference on Computing, Communication, and Intelligent Systems, pp. 1032–1036 (2021).
47. A. Jain, R. Dwivedi, A. Kumar, and S. Sharma.: Network on chip router for 2D mesh design, *Int. J. Comput. Sci. Inf. Secur.*, vol. 14, no. 9, p. 1092, (2016).
48. A. Jain, A. K. AlokGahlot, and S. K. S. RakeshDwivedi.: Design and FPGA Performance Analysis of 2D and 3D Router in Mesh NoC, *Int. J. Control Theory Appl.* IJCTA ISSN, pp. 0974–5572, (2017).
49. A. Bhardwaj, S. Kaur, A. P. Shukla, and M. K. Shukla.: Performance Comparison of De-speckling filters on the Basis of Incremental Iteration in Ultrasound Imaging, in 2019 International Conference on Power Electronics, Control and Automation, pp. 1–5 (2019).
50. A. Bhardwaj, S. Kaur, A. P. Shukla, and M. K. Shukla.: A Novel Method for Despeckling of Ultrasound Images Using Cellular Automata-Based Despeckling Filter, *Int. J. E-Health Med. Commun.* IJEHMC, vol. 12, no. 5, pp. 16–35, (2021).

[illegible]

[illegible] Laboratory [illegible] Signal Processing [illegible] (2021) [illegible]

[illegible]

[illegible] (2019), pp. 601–606 [illegible]

[illegible] pp. [illegible] (2019).

[illegible] and N. [illegible] (2021).

COVID-19 Recognition in X-RAY and CTA Images Using Collaborative Learning

T. Vasu Deva Reddy, Prabhakara Rao Kapula, D. Hari Krishna, B. Arunadevi, and Anju Asokan

1 Introduction

COVID-19, the current epidemic, is an infectious and dangerous virus caused through the Coronavirus Severe Acute Respiratory Syndrome (SARS) and Middle East Respiratory Syndrome (MERS) [1]. The WHO [2] designated it a pandemic on March 11, 2020, after more than 118,000 cases were reported in 114 countries [3]. The smallness of lungful, damage of taste, high temperature, chest pain, sleep difficulties, and anxiety are all symptoms of severe COVID-19 disease [4]. As a result, immediate action is required to combat this condition. Early identification and analysis are basic for controlling and preventing the spread of the virus. Reverse transcription-polymerase chain reaction (RTPCR), anti-model gens tests are the most often utilized COVID-19 testing procedures. These procedures are time-consuming, costly, and subject to inter- and intra-observer variance.

Patients with COVID-19 symptoms are usually given a chest CT scan or X-ray (see Fig. 1). On these CT scans and X-beam descriptions, image handling procedures can be applied [5, 6]. The CT and X-ray scans are the most suitable radiology methods to find Covid-19, but these models face accurate disease detection issues. So that Machine learning (ML) and Deep learning (DL) Algorithms remain used for

T. Vasu Deva Reddy (✉) · P. R. Kapula · D. H. Krishna
Department of ECE, B V Raju Institute of Technology, Medak, Telangana, India
e-mail: vasu.tatiparthi@bvrit.ac.in; prabhakar.kapula@bvrit.ac.in; harikrishna.dodde@bvrit.ac.in

B. Arunadevi
Department of ECE, Dr N.G.P Institute of Technology, Coimbatore, India
e-mail: arunadevi@drngpit.ac.in

A. Asokan
Sri Krishna College of Technology, Coimbatore, India
e-mail: anjuasokan@skct.edu.in

P. Agarwal et al. (eds.), *Artificial Intelligence for Smart Healthcare*, EAI/Springer Innovations in Communication and Computing, https://doi.org/10.1007/978-3-031-23602-0_25

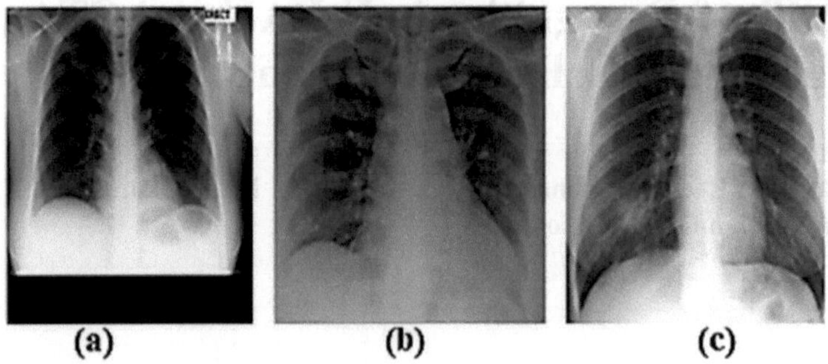

Fig. 1 (**a**) Normal, (**b**) COVID-19, and (**c**) SARS chest X-ray

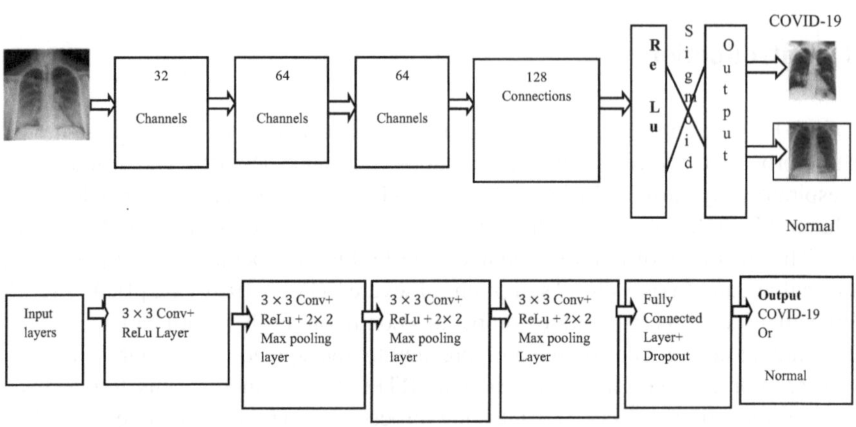

Fig. 2 The proposed CNN model for COVID-19 detection has a flow diagram

extracting important data from these Computed tomographies (CT) scans and X-ray pictures [7]. Abbas et al. [8] established the Decompose, Transmission, and Compose (DeTraC) perfect for chest X-ray categorization, founded on DCNN. Their proposed system was complicated, and it had only been trained and tested on a tiny numeral of photos. Panwar et al. [9] explained about covid 19 spreading theory and how these can be identified through deep learning models nothing but VGG 16 as the base model and Graduate CAM-based shading perception and moved to learn. They didn't do any trials anyway on a pooled dataset. Silva et al. [10] offered a deep learning technique, but their procedure failed towards obtaining considerably high exactness, with their correctness dropping towards 56.16% when verified across datasets.

Due to the restrictions mentioned earlier, existing research studies are limited for real-time clinical usage. As a result, the authors of this work suggest a DCNN-based technique based on ensemble learning. Figure 2 depicts a schematic diagram of the suggested method. COVID 345 CT scan dataset [11], COVID-19 radiography information base [12], and chest X-beam picture (pneumonia) dataset [13] were incorporated by the creators.

Because coronavirus disease is an infectious condition, it is critical to detect and diagnose it as soon as possible. The current approaches take a long time and are inaccurate. Coronavirus can be detected using computed tomography (CT) and X-rays. CT scans and X-rays must be manually evaluated, which takes time and requires specialist expertise. In this exploration, the creators offer a maximum democratic-based troupe learning technique for COVID recognition. Inception Net, ResNet, and Efficient Net are the three best class group, learning models. A consolidated CT sweep and X-beam dataset are utilized for preparing and testing. Affectability, 98.18%; particularity, 96.6%; precision, 97.47%; and region under bend, 95.36% were achieved utilizing the proposed technique. The obtained findings demonstrate the utility of the proposed approach.

People suspected of having COVID-19 need to know right away if they are infected to get the proper treatment, isolate themselves, and notify anyone who has contacted them. Currently, a lab test (RT-PCR) on examples gathered from the nose and throat is needed for a proper finding of COVID-19. The RT-PCR test requires the utilization of specific hardware and requires no less than 24 h to finish. Chest imaging has been displayed to have a significant job in the movement of this long sickness. The chest X-ray (CXR) and calculated tomography (CT) filter pictures can remain exploited to analyze COVID-19 rapidly and precisely. Utilizing a few convolutional neural organizations, we look at the presentation of chest imaging approaches in analyzing COVID-19 disease (CNN). To achieve this in this way, we ran CT sweeps and CXR pictures through Resnet-18, InceptionV3, and MobileNetV2. For COVID-19 models, we found that the ResNet-18 model has the best generally speaking exactness and affectability of 98.5% and 98.6%. Individually, the InceptionV3 model has the best by and large particularity of 97.4% and the MobileNetV2 has an ideal affectability. All of these feats were accomplished using CT scan pictures. The COVID-19 disease is an associate of the coronavirus (CoV) private; here it derived its name from the "crown" created by particular proteins on the virus's surface. It was initially discovered in December 2019 near Wuhan, China. COVID-19, which sources unembellished acute respiratory syndrome (#SARS), and #MERS-CoV, which causes Central west Respirational Syndrome (MERS), are two coronaviruses that can infect people and mammals (MERS). The coronavirus COVID 345 remains the sixth coronavirus to cause human disease. It is the cause of the COVID-19 infection.

The world has been placed in containment due to the COVID-2019 epidemic to limit contagion and loss of life. Currently, 80% of diseases are gentle or asymptomatic, 15% are serious and require oxygen treatment, and 5% are basic and require respiratory help. Fever, asthenia, dry hack, and gastrointestinal side effects like runs, sickness, regurgitating, and anorexia are the most pervasive manifestations of SARS-CoV2. Serious types of infection, like pneumonia and intense respiratory misery disorder, influence one out of six patients. The individual associated with having a COVID-19 disease needs to know whether they are contaminated at the earliest opportunity to be appropriately disconnected, get fitting treatment, and

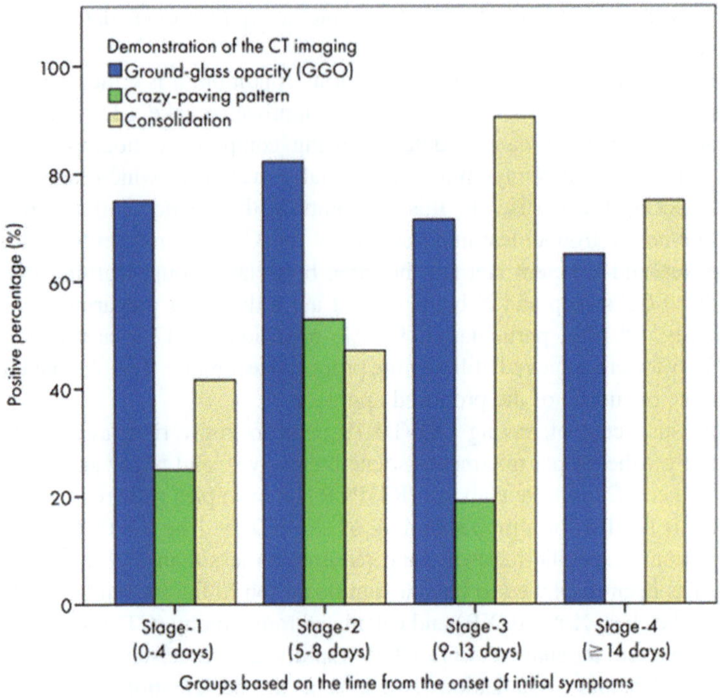

Fig. 3 Graphical analysis of COVID-19 analysis

advise the individuals who have come into contact with them. Two RT-PCR tests are frequently required to establish a diagnosis, which takes time and resources. Furthermore, the RT-PCR has a high proportion of false-negative results, leading to COVID-19 patients misclassified as healthy people, which can have serious repercussions. As a result, a technique that can make an earlier diagnosis would lower the disease prevalence.

Coronavirus has been connected to a wide scope of lung sores on CT sweeps and CXR imaging, like SARS and MERS. Cold glass opacities (87%), reciprocal injury inclusion (80%), fringe circulation (75%), multilobar contribution (89%), back sore morphology (80%), and parenchymal buildups (33%) are the most pervasive CT indications and attributes. The opacities of ground glass have been portrayed as circular, nodular, or with an insane clearing design shown in Fig. 3. This pneumonia influences the lower flaps, though the most un-affected center projection. Perhaps the most widely recognized plans were unadulterated off-white glass opacities or those identified with buildup. CXR and CT examine the most normally utilized imaging modalities to research patients with COVID-19 out of the full scope of imaging strategies accessible. These strategies help clinicians decide the effect of COVID-19 on different organs at various periods of sickness. Because respiratory symptoms are one of the first indicators of COVID-19, they are utilized on the chest and lungs. In this work, COVID-19 disease detection has been performed through segmentation and CNN deep learning mechanism. In segmentation, the Ostu model is proposed and implemented through python software. The CNN is a major deep learning mechanism; it extracts features through hidden, dense, and flatten layers.

2 Limitations of Earlier Models

These existing models are more complex to extract features, but implementation is complex. Lung disease detection is very complex using the conventional model, and it is very complex to identify the location of the disease.

3 Methodology

This paper employed a majority voting-based ensemble learning strategy, with the last class being the class anticipated through both models. On the combined dataset, we first used Resnet50 [14], InceptionV4 [15], and EfficientNetB0 [16]. Their abilities were discovered to be complementary. As a result, the authors utilized outfits getting the hang of utilizing every one of the three models to get superior outcomes. The final class prediction was based on the mode value of their expectations. Convolutional strainers and numerous size strainers have been factorized at a similar level in the inceptionV4 model. To limit the input channels, it uses a 1×1 complication earlier for each filter. We used only four InceptionB blocks instead of seven to minimize overfitting issues and keep our network alive. The inceptionV4 engineering utilizes memory enhancement on backpropagation to decrease memory prerequisites. By utilizing character associations, the Resnet50 network maintains a strategic distance from the issue of evaporating inclination, and the bunch standardization layer diminishes the covariant shift issue, further improving execution. The skip associations make the organization dynamic to prepare, permitting the model to pick whether to learn or avoid the layer. By scaling the neurons at the individual layer then the image goal, the EfficientnetB0 model similarly scales the profundity, which is the numeral of layers in the organization, then the broadness, which remains the number of bits in the convolution layer.

3.1 System Architecture

To detect COVID-19, the suggested approach used X-ray pictures as input. First, this method transformed RGB photos towards grayscale and defined the region of interest (ROI) by deleting non-interesting areas. The system also examined histogram-oriented gradient (HOG) and CNN as feature extractors. First, the X-ray

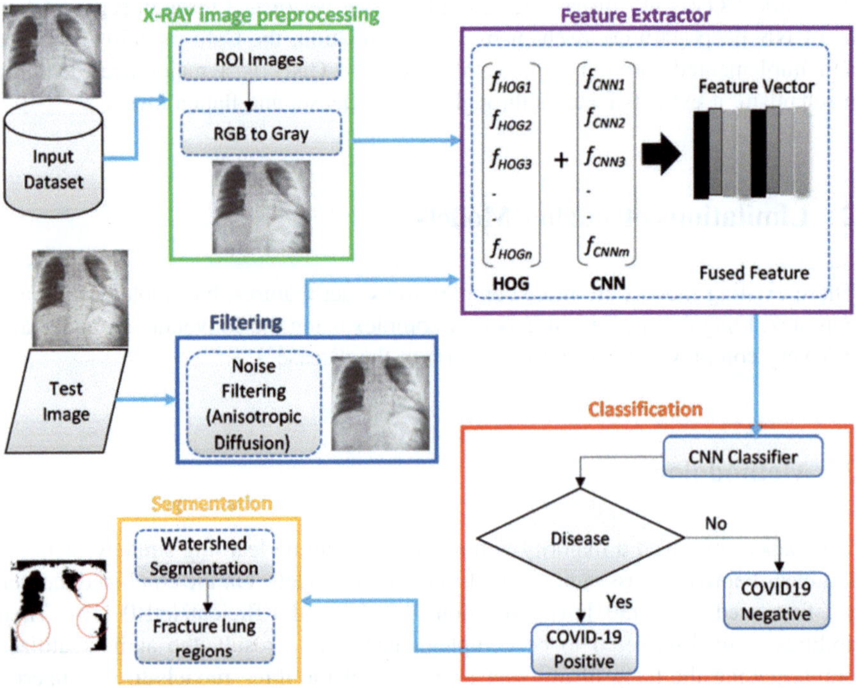

Fig. 4 Chest X-ray-based COVID-19 detection

COVID-19 dataset extracted a feature vector using the HOG approach. After that, another feature vector was extracted from the same photos using the CNN approach.

These two highlights were joined and then taken into the classification model as input. One technique's number of retrieved features was insufficient to identify COVID-19 reliably. However, using two distinct strategies to extract characteristics could result in various highlights for precise distinguishing proof. The combination was seen as a link between the two unmistakable vectors for this situation. In our experiment, we used speckle-affected and low-quality X-ray images and high-quality images to conduct experiments. If training and testing are done in an ideal scenario with just selected high-quality X-ray images, the yield precision might be found to be greater. However, this does not reflect a real-world situation in which the image database contains both high- and low-quality photographs. As a result, using varying quality photos to test how viably the framework can respond to such reality circumstances is a good idea. A modified anisotropic diffusion filtering approach eliminated multiplicative dot commotion in the test pictures. These strategies could be used to overcome input image quality restrictions effectively. On the test photos, feature extraction was then performed. Finally, the CNN classifier classified X-ray pictures to determine if they were COVID-19 or not. The basic steps of the projected scheme design are depicted in Fig. 4.

3.2 Dataset Details

Many of the symptoms of COVID-19 are like those of bacterial pneumonia, such as shortness of breath, fever, and so on, but imaging can distinguish between the viral infection and pneumonia. According to the above examinations using the Kaggle dataset to find pneumonia and covid 19 in easy manner using CNN deep learning technology. For COVID classification, we combined three datasets from various modalities (CT and X-Ray):

- Dataset 1 was derived beginning the SARS COV2 CT-check dataset [16], which contains 2490 CT outputs of 150 patients, with 1260 CT sweeps of 65 patients contaminated with coronavirus and 1230 CT filter pictures of 60 non-coronavirus patients tainted thru other respiratory illnesses.
- Database 2 COVID-19 imaging database [17] contains 1200 coronavirus positive photographs, 1341 ordinary pictures of patients without the illness, and then 1350 viral pneumonia X-ray images.
- Database 3 dataset contains chest X-ray pictures of healthy persons and pneumonia sufferers [18], with 1580 healthy people with clear lung images and no aberrant opacification. There are also 4270 pneumonia trunk X-ray imageries in both lungs by diffuse interstitial patterns [19].

3.3 Network Training Configuration

Because the datasets utilized remained skewed then uneven, as a result, each time we test our models, the authors employ stratified fivefold cross-validation to measure correct performance and generalize the models aimed at an autonomous dataset. The authors first trained and evaluated each of the three models separately. For each of the five folds, we calculated all performance characteristics, averaged the accuracy, and added the sensitivity, AUC, and specificity. The models were determined to have similar performance parameters. As a result, max voting-constructed ensemble knowledge was employed for better training and prediction. Two of the representations in any event anticipated the last projected class. We used Glorot unvarying [20] as the piece initializer, Relu as the initiation work [21], and then Adam as the streamlining agent [22] for training. As the loss function, binary cross-entropy was applied [23–26]. The batch size, steps per age, age, and approval steps, and then the irregular state were set to 5, 100, 10, and 64, separately.

3.4 CNN Founded Feature Separator and Classification

Image processing, in particular feature removal using CNN, is a hot topic in processer discipline research. In this suggested study, research was done utilizing

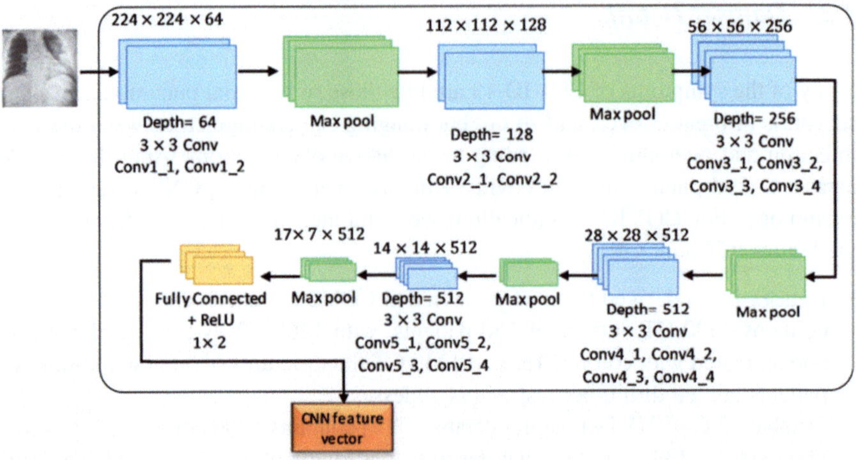

Fig. 5 ResNet and CNN model with the classical approach

scratch and pre-trained CNN representations [27–29]. The scratch model's results were unsatisfactory, but the pre-trained model performed admirably [30]. The VGG19 model (pre-trained) remained fine-tuned to fit this work's experimental dataset as a feature extractor. This network model was created using a VGGNet with 19 layers. VGG19 outperformed VGG16, the scratch typical, and other deep knowledge representations such as ResNet50 and AlexNet, according to an experimental trial. The VGG19 model was created by 16 convolution layers, three of which were completely coupled (Fig. 4). The actuation work for getting the yield of convolution layers employed a nonlinear ReLU, while the convolution section was separated into five consecutive max-pooling layers. The first and second subregions were developed using two convolution layers thru 64 and 128 [31]. Furthermore, the remaining three subregions were constructed using four sequential convolution layers with depths of 256, 512, and 512, correspondingly [32–36]. Following that, pooling layers were used towards reducing the learnable parameter. The proposed VGG19 model's final layer assisted in getting the feature vector, but the two secret layers put before the element assortment layer had 1024 and 512 neurons, respectively [37–41]. After each fully linked layer, L2 regularization was used to reduce overfitting during the execution of the adjusted model. The VGG19 models, based on CNN, provide 4096 suitable features [42].

Where f is the intertwined vector (1 1186), p is the likelihood of highlights, and He is the entropy [43–45]. This entropy-based component choice methodology chooses features from the fused vector that are comparable or highly related. Unrelated features were deleted, and only relevant features were used to classify the data. The relevant feature vector in this suggested system remains 1 1186. The CNN classifier employs the selected features, as shown in Fig. 5, which depicts the feature extraction and selection procedure. In addition, the HOG and deep learning feature vectors were joined to approve the proposed procedure in this paper.

The VGG19 architecture has 16 CNN layers, three connected layers, and one last yield layer for playing out the SoftMax work. The number of associated layers and the last layer does not need to alter to design network architectures [46, 47]. In addition, for the max-pooling layer, two 2-pixel windows by stride 2 were utilized. 4096 features and 1000 channels were provided separately by the initial two levels and third layer of the three associated layers [48, 49]. With two neurons, the last layer addresses the yield layer (COVID-19 and ordinary) shown in Fig. 5.

3.5 *Segmentation of the COVID-19-Affected Region*

The watershed methodology outperforms other methods like Fuzzy-C means (FCM) for biomedical picture segmentation. The traditional FCM algorithm has approximately flaws in cluster center initialization, selecting an ideal figure of clusters, and noise sensitivity. The COVID-19 affects X-ray pictures, and the FCM segmentation approach cannot locate fracture zones. On the other hand, Watershed segmentation is a quick, easy, and intuitive method that produces closed contours, requires little processing effort, and divides the image into distinct sections. The difficult process of isolating the fracture lung regions from the X-ray images was accomplished via segmentation. Because of its low computational complexity and ability to provide high separation accuracy, a watershed division method was utilized to isolate each picture's break zones. This method produced a complete divide in an X-ray image by separating contacting objects. Figure 6 shows the various image processing steps for COVID-19-affected lung X-ray pictures, from filtering through segmentation of relevant regions.

Active ingredient elevated CT lung scanning is critical for early illness identification, especially in patients with false-negative RT-PCR findings and supervising tumor growth. Furthermore, imaging data can be used to determine the severity of the disease, assisting doctors in their clinical judgment and guaranteeing effective and prompt care. In critically sick patients, the severity of the disease can also impact survival, enabling informed choice of early critical care participation shown in Fig. 6. Several studies looked at lung activation on chest computed tomography to use both subjective and statistical software evaluations. To our understanding, it's the first substantial study in the Gulf and Arab areas to explain the relationship between chest CT intensity ratings and the clinical picture of patients with COVID-19 illness. The 25-point visual, quantitative evaluation was used to connect the CT effects with the symptom manifestations of individuals who have been verified to have COVID-19 illness shown in Fig. 7.

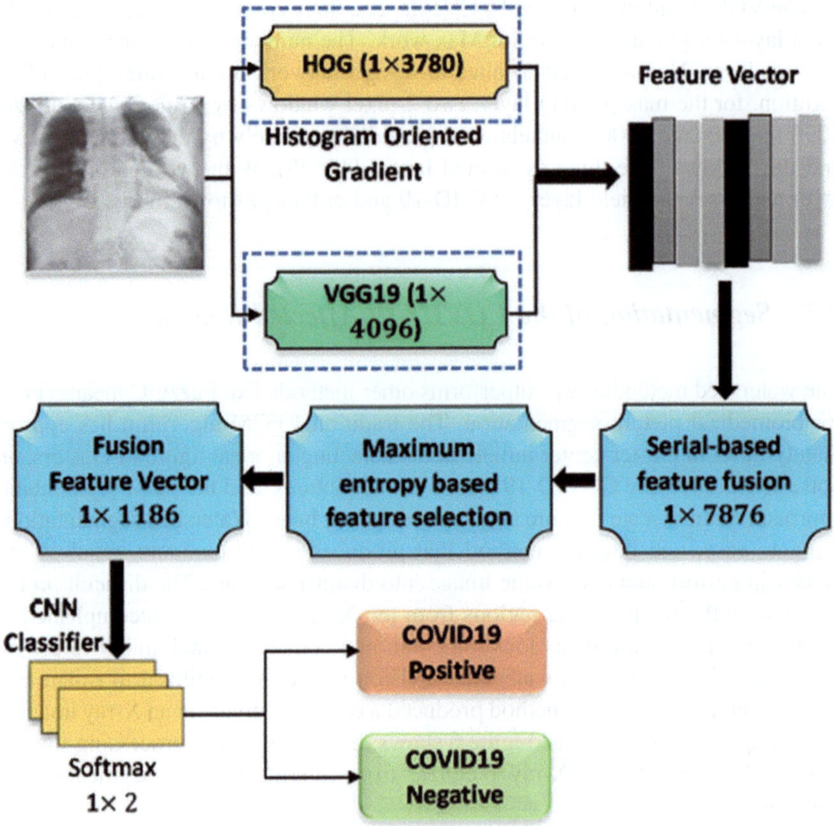

Fig. 6 The anticipated fusion stages feature removed by Ostu threshold and CNN

4 Results

The creators utilized a gathering learning procedure in which the last expectations depend on the method worth of the forecasts from ResNet50, InceptionV4, and EfficientNetB0. These tests were done on Google Collaboratory with the Python Keras bundle. Explicitness (SPE), sensitivity (SEN), area under the bend (AUC), and accuracy (ACC) were used as examination boundaries [20]. Table 1 orders the entirety of the accomplished consequences of the different executed and proposed ways. Max voting (Ensemble Learning) is found to outflank different models, with affectability, 98.18%; explicitness, 96.6%; exactness, 97.47%; and AUC, 95.36%. Compared to individual models, the max voting technique improves sensitivity by 0.1%, specificity by 0.14%, and accuracy by 0.88%. Although it had a lower AUC of 3.94% compared to Efficient Net, we might conclude that max voting was the most successful model when evaluating the overall performance and all four parameters in question. The proposed effort is compared to other research studies in the same

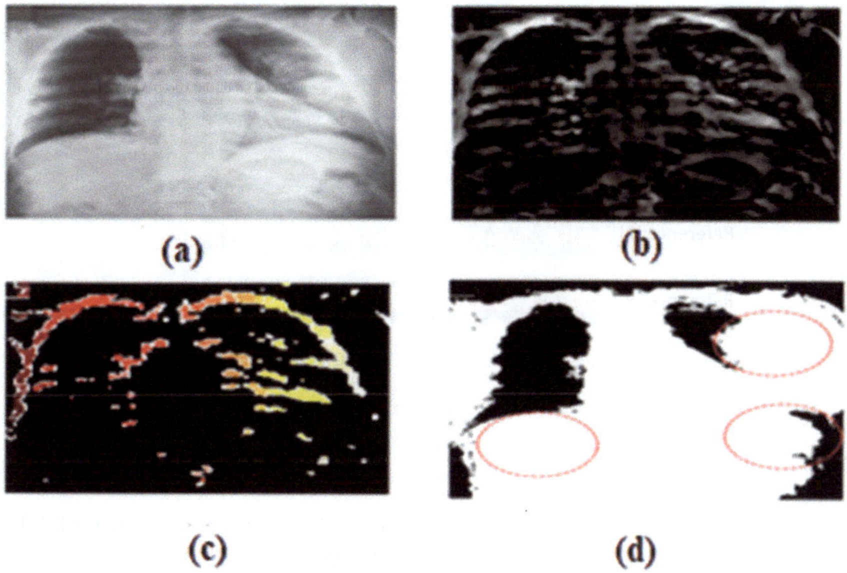

Fig. 7 Ostu threshold-based COVID-19 model, (**a**) filtered image, (**b**) Ostu threshold image, (**c**) segmented RGB image, (**d**) COVID-19 detected image

Table 1 Comparative results with different models

Implemented models	SEN	SPE	ACC	AUC
Reference [8]	88.7700%	70.3200%	92.4100%	95.1700%
Reference [9]	98.0800%	96.4600%	96.5900%	99.1100%
Reference [10]	95.3000%	92.5000%	96.8200%	99.3000%
Proposed approach	98.1800%	96.6000%	97.4700%	95.3600%

Table 2 Comparative results with anticipative models

	SEN	SPE	ACC	AUC
Reference [8]	100.00%	–	93.100%	–
Reference [9]	94.0400%	95.8600%	95.000%	–
Reference [10]	–	–	87.6800%	–
Proposed approach	98.1800%	96.600%	97.4700%	95.3600%

dataset in Table 2. The suggested ensemble approach outperforms the existing methods, as shown in Table 2.

Table 1 and Fig. 8 clearly explain ResNet 50, InceptionV4, Efficient Net, and the proposed method. Here earlier models have less accurate results compared to the proposed model. The sensitivity 98.18%, specificity 96.60%, accuracy 97.47%, and area under curve 95.36% had been attained.

ResNet 50, InceptionV4, Efficient Net, and the suggested technique are explained in detail in Table 2. In this case, previous models produced less accurate findings

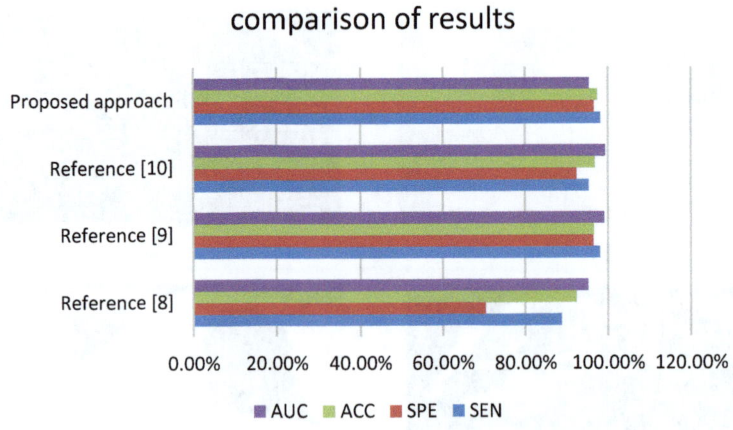

Fig. 8 Comparison of results

than the suggested model. The sensitivity was 98.18%, the specificity was 98.60%, the accuracy was 97.47%, and the area under the curve was 95.36%.

5 Conclusion

The authors used collaborative learning with ResNet50, InceptionV4, and EfficientNetB0 to construct a forecast based on a majority vote on the combined dataset. As a result of the findings, it can be determined that the proposed method outstrips other state-of-the-art models. Because of the limited data available, the method was confined to CT scans and X-rays. In the future, the authors hope to integrate more datasets of diseases that are closely linked to COVID, explore new modalities, and then extend our effort towards transmission learning towards constructing a powerful COVID detection system. At last, accuracy was estimated to be 99.46%, sensitivity to be 99.48%, recall to be 99.36%, and F1 score to be 99.42%. Ostu thresholding and the CNN-based COVID-19 model proposed in this study compete with the current implementation and outcompete the research methods.

References

1. He, K., Zhang, X., Ren, S., & Sun, J. Deep residual learning for image recognition. In Proceedings of the IEEE conference on computer vision and pattern recognition, pp. 770–778, (2016).
2. Szegedy, C., Ioffe, S., Vanhoucke, V., & Alemi, A. Inception-v4, inception-resnet and the impact of residual connections on learning. In Proceedings of the AAAI Conference on Artificial Intelligence, Vol. 31, No. 1 (2017).

3. Tan, M., & Le, Q. Efficientnet: Rethinking model scaling for convolutional neural networks. In International Conference on Machine Learning (pp. 6105–6114). PMLR (2019).
4. Glorot, X., & Bengio, Y. Understanding the difficulty of training deep feedforward neural networks. Proceedings of the thirteenth international conference on artificial intelligence and statistics (pp. 249–256). JMLR Workshop and Conference Proceedings (2010).
5. Nwankpa, C., Ijomah, W., Gachagan, A., & Marshall, S. Activation functions: Comparison of trends in practice and research for deep Learning. arXiv preprint arXiv:1811.03378 (2018).
6. Kingma, D. P., & Ba, J. Adam: A method for stochastic optimization. arXiv preprint arXiv:1412.6980 (2014).
7. Ramaiah, V. S., Singh, B., Raju, A. R., Reddy, G. N., Saikumar, K., & Ratnayake, D. Teaching and Learning based 5G cognitive radio application for future application. In 2021 International Conference on Computational Intelligence and Knowledge Economy (pp. 31–36). IEEE (2021).
8. Mohammad, M. N., Kumari, C. U., Murthy, A. S. D., Jagan, B. O. L., & Saikumar, K. Implementation of online and offline product selection system using FCNN deep learning: Product analysis. Materials Today: Proceedings, 45, 2171–2178 (2021).
9. Padmini, G. R., Rajesh, O., Raghu, K., Sree, N. M., & Apurva, C. (2021, March). Design and analysis of 8-bit ripple Carry Adder using nine Full Transistor Adder. In 2021 7th International Conference on Advanced Computing and Communication Systems. Vol. 1, pp. 1982–1987, (2021). IEEE.
10. Dr. K. Raju, A. Sampath Dakshina Murthy, Dr B. Chinna Rao, Sindhura Bhargavi, G. Jagga Rao, K. Madhu, K. Saikumar. A Robust and Accurate Video Watermarking System Based on SVD Hybridation For Performance Assessment. International Journal of Engineering Trends and Technology, 68(7), 19–24 (2020).
11. Saba, S. S., Sreelakshmi, D., Kumar, P. S., Kumar, K. S., & Saba, S. R. Logistic regression machine learning algorithm on MRI brain image for fast and accurate diagnosis. International Journal of Scientific and Technology Research, 9(3), 7076–7081 (2020).
12. Saikumar, K. Rajesh V. Coronary blockage of artery for Heart diagnosis with DT Artificial Intelligence Algorithm. Int J Res Pharma Sci, 11(1), 471–479 (2020).
13. Saikumar, K., Rajesh, V. A novel implementation heart diagnosis system based on random forest machine learning technique International Journal of Pharmaceutical Research 12, pp. 3904–3916 (2020).
14. Karthik, R., Tummala, V., & Singh, V. A Study of Dielectric Reliability of Anodic TiO2 Based Single and Double Layer Metal-Insulator-Metal Capacitors. Journal of Nanoelectronics and Optoelectronics, 12(1), 85–88 (2017).
15. Alekhya, N., & Kishore, N. P. performance comparison of gfrp composite i section with an aluminum I section. *International Journal of Civil Engineering and Technology*, 8(4), 278–286 (2017).
16. Shankar, K. S., Ganesh, M., & Kumar, K. S. Combustion Chamber Analysis Using CFD for Operation Condition. In IOP Conference Series: *Materials Science and Engineering*, Vol. 455, No. 1, p. 012032. IOP Publishing (2018).
17. Kalavagunta, V., & Hussain, S. Wing Rib Stress Analysis of DLR-F6 aircraft. In IOP Conference Series: Materials Science and Engineering, Vol. 455, No. 1, p. 012033. IOP Publishing (2018).
18. Ebenezer, N. G. R., Ramabalan, S., & Navaneethasanthakumar, S. Advanced design optimization on straight bevel gears pair based on nature inspired algorithms. *SN Applied Sciences*, 1(10), 1–9 (2019).
19. Vagdevi, K., Jyothirmai, B., Devi, V. R., & Rao, K. V. Study of band gap engineering in graphene-based electrode materials by density functional calculations: A search for high performance graphene-based devices. In *AIP Conference Proceedings*, Vol. 2200, No. 1, p. 020010. AIP Publishing LLC (2019).
20. Ghosh, S. K., Mehedi, J., & Samal, U. C. Sensing performance of energy detector in cognitive radio networks. *International Journal of Information Technology*, 11(4), 773–778 (2019).

21. Bhanuprakash, L., Parasuram, S., & Varghese, S. Experimental investigation on graphene oxides coated carbon fibre/epoxy hybrid composites: *Mechanical and electrical properties. Composites Science* and *Technology,* 179, 134–144 (2019).
22. Limbadri, K., Singh, S. K., Satyanarayana, K., Singh, A. K., Ram, A. M., Ravindran, M., . . . & Suresh, K. Effect of processing routes on orientation-dependent tensile flow behavior of Zircaloy-4 at elevated temperatures. Metallography, *Microstructure, and Analysis*, 8(3), 393–405 (2019).
23. K. Karthikayan Dr. Siva Agora Sakthivel Murugan, Rathish. C. R, Natraj. N. A, An Enhanced Localization Scheme for Mobile Sensor Networks, *International Journal of Computational Engineering Research*, 2013, Volume 3, Issue 7, Pages 36–43, (2013).
24. Archana A Gupta, Supriya Kheur, Saranya Varadarajan, Sameena Parveen, Harisha Dewan, Yaser Ali Alhazmi, Thirumal A Raj, Luca Testarelli, Shankargouda Patil, Chronic Mechanical Irritation and Oral Squamous Cell Carcinoma: A Systematic Review and Meta-Analysis, *Bosnian Journal of Basic Medical Sciences*, Volume 21. Issue No 6, Pages 647–658, (2021).
25. P. Manta, N. Wahi, A. Bharadwaj, G. Kour, and D. N. Kapoor, "A statistical quality control (SQC) methodology for gold nanoparticles based immune-chromatographic rapid test kits validation," *Nanosci. Nanotechnol. Asia,* vol. 11, no. 6, pp. 1–5, (2021).
26. Dr. Siva Agora Sakthivel Murugan, Rathish. C. R, Natraj. N. A, K. Karthikayan, A Compact T-Fed Slotted Microstrip Antenna for Wide Band Application, *International Journal of Scientific & Technology Research,* Volume 2, Issue 8, Pages 291–294, (2013).
27. C. R. Rathish, Dr. A. Rajaram, Hierarchical Load Balanced Multipath Routing Protocol for Wireless Sensor Networks, *International Journal of Inventions in Computer Science and Engineering*, Volume 3, Issue 4, ISSN (Online): 2348–3539, (2016).
28. Sheetal Mujoo, Alok Dubey, Abeer Almashraqi, Sameena Parveen, Triphala: Is it a Competent Guardian Against Oral Pathogens-An In Vitro Study, *International Biological and Biomedical Journal*, Volume 3, Issue 2, Pages 89–94, (2017).
29. Rajendran, S., Mathivanan, S. K., Jayagopal, P., Janaki, K. P., Bernard, B. A. M. M., Pandy, S., & Somanathan, M. S. Emphasizing privacy and security of edge intelligence with machine learning for healthcare. *International Journal of Intelligent Computing and Cybernetics* (2021).
30. P. Manta et al., "Analytical approach for the optimization of desiccant weight in rapid test kit packaging: Accelerated predictive stability (APS)," *Systematic Reviews in Pharmacy*, vol. 11, no. 8, pp. 102–113, (2020).
31. G. Sathya Prabha, N. Srinivasan, K. T. Manisenthil Kumar, and S. Aravindh, "Evaluation of clinical characteristics and knowledge in inflammatory bowel disease patients," Journal of Evolution of *Medical and Dental Sciences*, vol. 10, no. 29, pp. 2202–2207, (2021).
32. S. Dhanalakshmi, N. Harikrishnan, N. Janani, P. Shakthi Priya, M. Srinivasan, A. Karthikeyan, A. Anishkumar, R. Harinathan, and N. Srinivasan, "The overview: Recent studies on endometrial cancer," *Research Journal of Pharmacy and Technology*, vol. 14, no. 7, pp. 3998–4002, (2021).
33. K. Kavitha, N. Srinivasan, S. Mohan, and R. Suresh, "Insilco design and potential cytotoxic agents EGFR inhibitors of 4(3h) quinazolinone derivatives," *Research Journal of Pharmacy and Technology*, vol. 14, no. 9, pp. 4849–4855, (2021).
34. Sumathy, R. Suresh, N. L. Gowrishankar, and N. Srinivasan, "Design, synthesis and evaluation of core scaffold pyrazolone fused thiazolidinone derivatives as anticancer agents," *Journal of Pharmaceutical Research International,* vol. 33, no. 31B, pp. 217–227, (2021).
35. K. Saritha, R. Murali, N. Srinivasan, and Sorabh kumar agarwal, "Anti-fertility activity of leaves and Stem parts of Artabotrys odoratissimus. (roxb.) R.Br. Annonaceae." Journal of Medical Pharmaceutical and Allied Sciences, vol. 10, no. 5, pp. 3524–3528, (2021).
36. M. Govindaraj, R. Rathinam, C. Sukumar, M. Uthayasankar and S. Pattabhi, "Electrochemical oxidation of bisphenol-A from aqueous solution using graphite electrodes," *Environmental Technology*, 34:4, 503–511, (2013).

37. Nomani, M. Z. M. & Parveen, R, Covid-19 Pandemic and Application of Disaster Management Act, 2005: Promises and Pitfalls, International *Journal of Pharmaceutical Research*, 12(4), 3730–3734, (2020).
38. O. M. Abo-Seida, N. T. M. El-dabe, A. Refaie Ali and G. A. Shalaby, "Cherenkov FEL Reaction with Plasma-Filled Cylindrical Waveguide in Fractional D-Dimensional Space," in IEEE Transactions on Plasma Science, vol. 49, no. 7, pp. 2070–2079, (2021).
39. G. S and S. R. Raja. T, "A Comprehensive Survey on Alternating Fluids Used for The Enhancement of Power Transformers," 2021 IEEE International Conference on the Properties and Applications of Dielectric Materials, 2021, pp. 57–60, (2021).
40. S. Sudhakar and S. Chenthur Pandian, "Hybrid Cluster-based Geographical Routing Protocol to Mitigate Malicious Nodes in Mobile Ad Hoc Network", *International Journal of Ad Hoc and Ubiquitous Computing,* Vol. 21 No. 4, pp. 224–236 (2016).
41. Nomani, M., & Parveen, R. COVID-19 pandemic and disaster preparedness in the context of public health laws and policies. Bangladesh *Journal of Medical Science*, 20(5), 41–48 (2021).
42. S. Sharma and A. J. Obaid, "Mathematical modelling, analysis and design of fuzzy logic controller for the control of ventilation systems using MATLAB fuzzy logic toolbox," *Journal of Interdisciplinary Mathematics*, vol. 23, no. 4, pp. 843–849, (2020).
43. S. Sharma and A. J. Obaid, "Contact-mechanics and dynamics analysis of three-different ellipsoidal raceway geometries for deep Groove ball bearing using Abaqus 6.13 version FEA simulation for high load-bearing as well as speed-rotating applications," *International Research Journal of Multidisciplinary Science and Technology*, vol. 3, no. 5, pp. 36–43, (2020).
44. A. J. Obaid and S. Sharma, "Recent Trends and Development of Heuristic Artificial Intelligence Approach in Mechanical System and Engineering Product Design," *Saudi Journal of Engineering and Technology*, vol. 5, no. 2, pp. 86–93, (2020).
45. Prabhu Kavin, B., Ganapathy, S., Suthanthiramani, P., & Kannan, A. A modified digital signature algorithm to improve the biomedical image integrity in cloud environment. *Advances in Computational Techniques for Biomedical Image Analysis*, 253–271, (2020).
46. Panjwani, B., Singh, V., Rani, A., & Mohan, V. Optimum multi-drug regime for compartment model of tumour: cell-cycle-specific dynamics in the presence of resistance. *Journal of Pharmacokinetics and Pharmacodynamics,* 48(4), 543–562, (2021).
47. J. Kubiczek and B. Hadasik, "Challenges in Reporting the COVID-19 Spread and its Presentation to the Society," J. Data and Information Quality, vol. 13, no. 4, pp. 1–7, (2021).
48. Rawat, A., Jha, S., Kumar, B., & Mohan, V. Nonlinear fractional order PID controller for tracking maximum power in photo-voltaic system. *Journal of Intelligent & Fuzzy Systems*, 38(5), 6703–6713, (2020).
49. Amiya Kumar Sahu, Suraj Sharma, M. Tanveer, Rohit Raja, Internet of Things attack detection using hybrid Deep Learning Model, *Computer Communications,* Volume 176, 2021, Pages 146–154, ISSN 0140-3664, (2021).

Artificial Intelligence for Enhancement of Brain Image Using Semantic Segmentation CNN with IoT Classification Techniques

Vaibhav Rupapara

1 Introduction

Brain tumour segmentation is required to find the tumor, and it is used to grant the proper treatment for a persistent and gives the key to the specialist who must execute the surgery for persistent. The picture division and classification of an infected tumor zone from Attractive Reverberation Pictures (MRI) by the method of division, location, and extraction are a major concern and time-devouring errand performed by restorative pros by the encounter as it where this exactness depends subsequently it is fundamental to overcome thereby Computer- Helped Innovation (CAD). To overcome the issue of brain tumor division from the MRI picture, the taking after strategies are proposed. Clinical experts analyze medical reports that represent existing factors and reasons for diseases. Identification of diseases is mainly based on external symptoms and the results of medical reports. As per clinical experts and analysts from the clinical space, mind cancer is one of the most dangerous illnesses of the human body. Later stage identification of brain tumor will result in the patient going into unconscious/coma, leading to death. This motivates researchers to identify and predict tumor in the suspected region with the early symptoms and identify the type of tumor with the help of MRI brain images. IP and segmentation algorithms are identified, and the best method that predicts the accurate location of tumor in the brain with the help of an MRI brain image is identified. Brain tumors, generally recognized with the screening of sequential scan images, will be identified mainly by the symptoms of headache and the other complications most of the time.

V. Rupapara (✉)
School of Computing and Information Sciences, Florida International University, Miami, FL, USA
e-mail: vupap001@fiu.edu

P. Agarwal et al. (eds.), *Artificial Intelligence for Smart Healthcare*,
EAI/Springer Innovations in Communication and Computing,
https://doi.org/10.1007/978-3-031-23602-0_26

Medical image applications are improving day by day with the adoption of modern technology to improve the prediction, analysis, and prevention of diseases. New and innovative technology provides an opportunity to experts to contribute and improve the identification of diseases due to economic and environmental changes. As a computer graduate, this motivates me to do this research work and resolve some issues that could help medical society take preventive measures for various diseases. This work studies the identification of brain tumor through image segmentation techniques, which is one of the most demandable medical areas. However, many people are suffering from various types of brain tumors without any age difference. Some of these tumors are benignly curable with surgery, while others are malignant, leading to brain cancer. The brain is the most important organ and acts as the Central Nervous System (CNS) of the body; therefore, identifying brain diseases plays an important role. As per previous analysis, the causes and diagnosis of brain tumors will be identified with many symptoms for most patients. Three-dimensional (3D) MRI report of the brain is the main source for detecting brain tumors. MRI images' characteristics and properties are studied to identify further any other abnormalities based on this medical report.

2 Literature Survey

This section discusses the research work done by various researchers related to IP techniques and brain tumor diagnosis. Further, it also reviews the preprocessing techniques and image segmentation algorithms used by various researchers in detail. The survey also includes the medical data related to different brain problems or tumors in various parts of the human body, which researchers used in their research articles. Also, segmentation, classification, and clustering algorithms used in many domains for diagnosing medical problems were discussed in detail. For improving picture quality by eliminating insignificant clamours from the foundation of the pictures. A few strategies exist for preprocessing pictures, and many techniques enjoy their benefits and impediments. Difference upgrade, limit recognition, and evacuation of undesirable loud pixels are a portion of the viewpoints in preprocessing. Without losing any data, commotions in pictures are taken out for additional recognition or recognizable proof of infections or impacted locale. A few separating procedures and their benefits and constraints were broken down exhaustively in this exploration work [1]. They additionally gave a concise presentation about MRI attributes and their commotions. Commotions degenerate the pictures during the picture obtaining process, corrupting the picture quality. A large portion of the denoising strategies is managed Rician clamor with spatial uniform commotion dissemination in MRI pictures [2].

This calculation discussed the diverse preprocessing calculations, which reapplied to separate MRI pictures' mind growth impacted area. Smoothing and commotion decrease channels are the fundamental channels that ought to be applied to MRI cerebrum pictures. Perona and Malik's separating method is probably the best channel, which gave the best outcomes to the data set taken in this review [3]. Picking a proper channel for preprocessing procedure prompts better outcomes in ensuing stages like division, characterization, and the extraction steps of the pictures [20–25]. This algorithm is compared with other existing algorithms based on their performances. FCM plays a major role here [26–32]. This method consisted of a two-stage approach that filters the noisy image using nonlocal Principal Component Analysis (PCA). The second filter stage uses this filtered image as a guided image with a nonlocal mean filter [33]. This method internally calculates the total noise present and corrects the images with spatial Rican noise based on local bias [4].

Secondary brain tumors are always malignant which spread to other parts of the body, and both cases are potentially devastating and life-threatening [34]. PSO, FCM, Electro Magnetic Optimization (EMO), and LSM are the methods that successfully segmented suspicious brain tumors in digital MRI images [5]. Many researchers have carried out their work based on swarm intelligence concepts, especially in PSO. There are many challenging problems in segmenting MRI images [35–41]. The work carried out by these researchers involved the implementation of PSO, and they developed some hybrid algorithms based on the swarm intelligence concept in various fields. These algorithms have several applications [19, 42–48].

This chapter approaches for modelling human perception based on colours using a fuzzy logic system [49]. The clusters are not limited to linear or rectangular segments due to fuzzy logic systems [50–57]. The experimental results suggested that the performance of the Comprehensive Learning Particle Swarm Optimization (CLPSO) algorithm provided better accuracy than FCM and K-Means algorithms and allowed a variety of real-life applications [6].

Fuzzy logic for picture division of MRI mind information has been utilised to force inhomogeneities. Inhomogeneities defect related with the securing groupings gives significant commitment to MRI cerebrum picture information [58–63]. The proposed novel calculation was planned by altering the true capacity of the FCM calculation, and the voxel values are affected by the quick neighborhood voxel values. This strategy is valuable for fragment MRI pictures, significantly defiled by salt and pepper commotions. The calculation is tried for both manufactured and MRI mind picture information to show the productivity and viability of the proposed strategy [7]. FCM's grouping technique is all the more profound in their exploration work. Parcel grid and irregularity in the statement are a portion of the drawbacks of FCM, which makes bunching results more conflicting [8]. An elective technique called Subtractive Clustering (SC) was thought of, be that as it may, the quantities of bunches were obscure. The creators proposed another crossbreed technique that consolidates FCM and SC called Subtractive Fuzzy C Means (SFCM) to conquer the burden of FCM and SC. The exploratory outcomes showed that SFCM technique results create preferred grouping results over FCM calculation files [9–14].

The developed system was a multi-stage diagnostic system that utilized IP techniques to identify and classify brain tumor [15]. The proposed system capitalized with both T1-weighted and T2-weighted MRI images by manipulating and blending them to obtain improved results. These improved MRI images are segmented with the hybrid segmentation process of skull stripping and extracting the tumor region using the watershed segmentation technique. The enhanced watershed segmentation algorithm was designed and utilized for segmenting the tumor region in the brain effectively [16].

SVM was utilized to order the removed growth and decide if the cancer was harmless or threatening. The power-based elements and surface-based highlights were extricated by the created framework and were contrasted with the ground truth information. It was fascinating to note that the results from the created framework gave better outcomes more often than not when contrasted with the ground truth information [17]. A relative examination of two other crossbreed arrangement techniques like Morphology + SVM and Watershed + SVM was performed alongside the created framework. By looking at these three characterization strategies, a higher level of proficiency was accomplished by the created framework for mind cancer arrangement, with a precision of 94% [18]. Division adds to growing innovation for new applications, empowering and supporting the meteorological Decision Support System (DSS). This work additionally gives data about the endeavors to foster another calculation for distinguishing growth by giving the ideas and their interrelationships in clinical applications. Decision Support System (DSS) gives an account of components like mean, Homogeneity, and Hugeness however needs testing and quality appraisal of the technique. Few sites give prevalent features reports dependent on the watched upsides of features boundaries using DSS. AEMIX, an unused endeavor, has been made to quantify a classifier's precision given by various sites dependent on Normal Dialect Preparing (NLP). This stretch-out has been executed to address various cerebrum cancer figures with the least effort [4].

This section discusses the research work done by various researchers related to IP techniques and brain tumor diagnosis. Further, it also reviews the preprocessing techniques and image segmentation algorithms used by various researchers in detail. The survey also includes the medical data related to different brain problems or tumors in various parts of the human body, which researchers used in their research articles. Also, segmentation, classification, and clustering algorithms used in many domains for diagnosing medical problems were discussed in detail.

This algorithm discussed the different preprocessing algorithms applied to extract the brain tumor affected region from MRI images. Smoothing and noise reduction filters are the essential filters that should be applied to MRI brain images. Perona and Malik's filtering technique is one of the best filters, which provided the best results for the database taken in this study [3]. Choosing an appropriate filter for the preprocessing technique leads to better results in subsequent stages such as segmentation, classification, and the extraction steps of the images [20].

Based on its performance, this algorithm is compared to other existing algorithms. FCM is important in this case. This method consisted of a two-stage approach that used nonlocal Principal Component Analysis to filter the noisy image (PCA). The filtered image is used as a guided image in the second filter stage, which employs a nonlocal mean filter. This method computes the total noise present and corrects images with spatial Rican noise based on local bias [4].

Secondary brain tumors are always malignant which spread to other parts of the body, and both cases are potentially devastating and life-threatening. PSO, FCM, Electro Magnetic Optimization (EMO), and LSM are the methods that successfully segmented suspicious brain tumors in digital MRI images [5]. Many researchers have carried out their work based on swarm intelligence concepts, especially in PSO. There are many challenging problems in segmenting MRI images. The work carried out by these researchers involved the implementation of PSO, and they developed some hybrid algorithms based on the swarm intelligence concept in various fields. These algorithms have several applications [19].

Using a fuzzy logic system, a novel approach for modelling human perception based on colors is presented. Because of fuzzy logic systems, clusters are not limited to linear or rectangular segments. The experimental results indicated that the Comprehensive Learning Particle Swarm Optimization (CLPSO) algorithm performed better than the FCM and K-Means algorithms and allowed for a wide range of real-world applications [6].

Fuzzy logic for picture division of MRI has brain information and utilizing power inhomogeneities. Inhomogeneity defect related to the procurement arrangements is a significant commitment to MRI mind picture information. The proposed novel calculation was figured by adjusting the true capacity of the FCM calculation, and the voxel values are affected by the quick neighborhood voxel values.

This methodology is mainly useful for segmenting MRI images corrupted by salt and pepper noises. The algorithm is tested for both synthetic and MRI brain image data to demonstrate the efficiency and effectiveness of the proposed method [7].This chapter discussed almost the researchers' study of diverse division calculations, preprocessing procedures and gave a brief rundown of their focal points and drawbacks. The area encourage examines almost the different picture division calculations for brain tumor MRI pictures, where influenced locale is analyzed with distinctive sorts of the calculations conjointly the innovative/new/hybrid models created by analysts in their proposition work for picture division of MRI brain pictures were too examined.

3 Proposed System

The proposed research has been experimented with using the real-time satellite data collected and India's south-eastern coastal areas. Sensor observation data face two major issues: heterogeneous files and heterogenous vocabularies.

Algorithm

Step 1: The input image is converted into double.
Step 2: Initially calculate the Gaussian distribution function.
Step 3: Set the weight.
Step 4: Determine the Euclidean distance of each pixel value.

$$k = \sum_{i=0}^{j} {}^{N_i}\!/_{T} \tag{1}$$

Step 5: Calculate the finite difference after the distribution function is evaluated.

3.1 Semantic Segmentation

The design of a neural-organized layer exemplifies the principles of highlight reuse, area, and interpretation invariance. Profound Semantic Segmentation based on Deep Convolutional Neural Networks (SSDCNNs) is a CNN with many layers and mirror order guidelines. Deep SSCNNs frequently include one or two completely associated layers after a few convolutional layers, where W's weight framework is thick. The reasons for doing so are mixed and not entirely convincing; however, they are conceivable: far from the information, the spatial area is both incompletely lost and moderately unimportant to, say, acknowledgment, so the neighborhood open fields of SSCNNs are never again useful.

$$z\ \sigma(y) = \frac{\exp(y)}{1^T \exp(y)} \tag{2}$$

$$\Pr\left(s_i' = 1 | e_i^{B'}, e_i^{D'}\right) \propto \Pr\left(s_i' = 1 | e_i^{B'}\right) * \Pr\left(e_i^{D'}\ | s_i' = 1\right) \tag{3}$$

$$\Pr\left(s_i' = 1 | e_i^{B'}, e_i^{D'}\right) \propto \Pr\left(s_i' = 1 | e_i^{B'}\right) * \Pr(e_i^{D^{ma}} | s_i' = 1) * \Pr(e_i^{D^{mg}} | e_i^{D^{ma}}, s_i' = 1) \tag{4}$$

2D Gaussian filter H of variance Δ^', $G = 1 * H$ (Δ^), 'and then create the appearance model:

$$\Pr\left(s_i' = 1 | e_i^{B'}\right) = \begin{cases} \psi(G_i), & \text{if } i = \arg\max_{j \epsilon W_i} G_i \\ 0, & \text{otherwise} \end{cases} \tag{5}$$

Such that,

$$\psi(G_i) = (\max(G) - G_i)/(\max(G) - \min(G))$$

W_i is the voxel i with its 26 neighbor voxels in 3D.

$$e_i^{D^{mg}} = N \oplus F_h - N \oplus F_t \tag{6}$$

Where

$\oplus$...... the 3D morphological dilation.

Correspondingly, the likelihood of scale context feature is as follows:

$$\Pr\left(e_i^{D^{mg}} | e_i^{D^{ma}}, s_i' = 1\right) = \begin{cases} e_i^{D^{ma}}, & \text{if } e_i^{D^{mg}} = 1, \\ 1 - e_i^{D^{ma}}, & \text{otherwise}, \end{cases} \tag{7}$$

Where

$e_i^{D^{ma}} = 1 \ldots\ldots$ the root of the spike.
The voxel i is labelled as 1 in membrane segmentation result N.
$e_i^{D^{ma}} = 0 \ldots\ldots$ the respective root is labeled as 0 in N.

Hence, we formulate that the scale context cue must be satisfied. $e_i^{D^{mg}} = 1 \ldots\ldots$ the labels of the target (the spike head).

$$e_i^{D^{mq}} = \frac{d(A_k, i)}{d\left(A_k, \ {}_i'N\right)} \tag{8}$$

Where

$A_k \ldots\ldots$ the centroid index of membrance mask.
N_k and ${}_i'N \ldots\ldots$ the spike root Corresponding to the potential spike head i on membrane segmentation N.
$e_i^{D^{mq}} \ldots\ldots$ the voxel i is outside the membrane.

The likelihood of spatial feature is as follows:

$$\Pr\left(e_i^{D^{mq}} | e_i^{D^{ma}}, s_i' = 1\right) = \begin{cases} e_i^{D^{ma}}, & \text{if } e_i^{D^{mq}} > 1, \\ 1 - e_i^{D^{ma}}, & \text{otherwise}. \end{cases} \tag{9}$$

In the hybrid model, the semantic meaning cue is explicitly modelled as a vector, evaluating the relative contribution of appearance and context characteristics in semantic segmentation:

$$\Pr\left(e_i^{D^{ma}} | s_i' = 1\right) = \begin{cases} \lambda, & \text{if } e_i^{D^{ma}} = 1 \\ 1 - \lambda, & \text{if } e_i^{D^{ma}} = 0 \end{cases} \tag{10}$$

$$\Pr\left(s_i' = 1 | e_i^{B'}, e_i^{D^{mg}}, e_i^{D^{mq}}, e_i^{D^{ma}}\right) \propto \lambda\psi^D + (1 - \lambda)\psi^B,$$

Such that

$$\psi^D = \Pr\left(s_i' = 1 | e_i^{B'}\right) * \Pr\left(e_i^{D^{mg}} | e_i^{D^{ma}}, s_i' = 1\right) * \Pr\left(e_i^{D^{mq}} | e_i^{D^{ma}}, s_i' = 1\right),$$

$$\psi^B = \Pr\left(s_i' = 1 | e_i^{B'}\right) \tag{11}$$

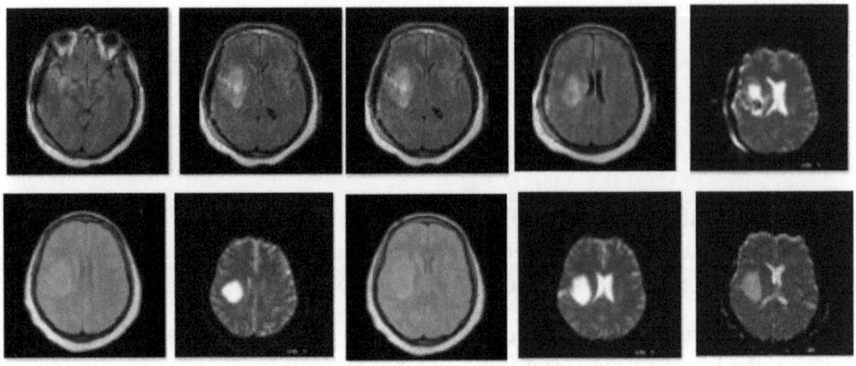

Fig. 1 Sample database for the medical CT brain images

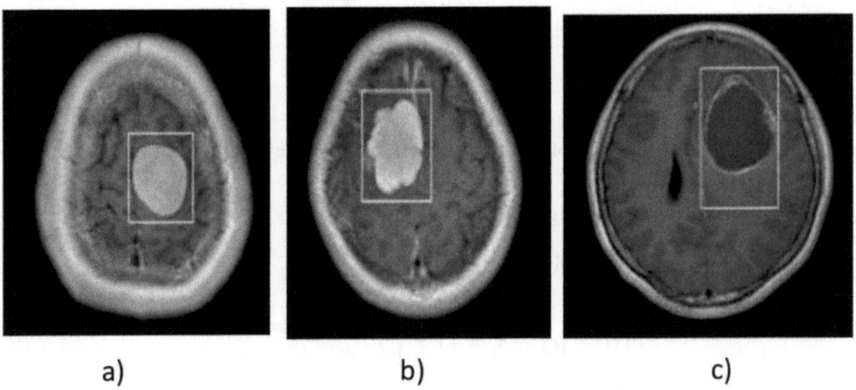

Fig. 2 Proposed work results in benign CT brain images (Sample images **a**, **b**, and **c**)

4 Result and Discussion

The experiments in the research work are carried out using the MATLAB (R2020a) software. The system used in this research work has an Intel core2Duo processor, 16 GB RAM, and is running the Windows 10 operating system. The methodology begins with preprocessing and progresses to segmentation and validation (Figs. 1, 2, 3, and 4).

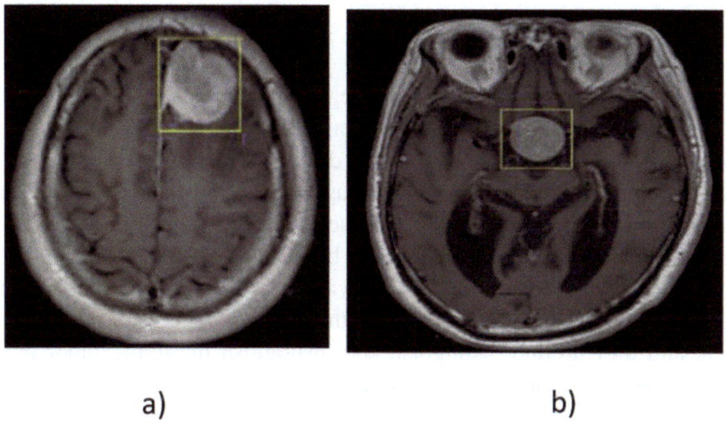

Fig. 3 Proposed work results in malignant CT brain images (Sample images **a** and **b**)

29 51.8%	**0** 0.0%	100% 0.0%
1 1.8%	**26** 46.4%	96.3% 3.7%
96.7% 3.3%	100% 0.0%	**98.2%** **1.8%**

Fig. 4 Confusion matrix or DCNN classifier

5 Conclusion

The results are discussed based on the segmentation values, and the algorithms segment the images based on the intensity values of the images. CNN algorithms are used, and they approximate identify and detect the brain tumor affected region separately from CT brain images. Early assurance can vastly improve patients' chances of survival. In this way, the proposed procedure appears that the advanced CAD system has exceptional potential for brain tumor modified conclusions. The results are discussed based on the division values, and the calculations fragment the pictures based on the escalated values of the pictures. The proposed algorithm is executed, and they around distinguish and distinguish the brain tumor influenced locale independently from the MRI brain pictures. The ultimate resultant pictures time, space, and white pixel variety are measured and famous for encouraging comparison of calculation within the future work.

References

1. Wei Li, Yifei Zhao, Xi Chen, Yang Xiao, Yuanyuan Qin, "Detecting Alzheimer's Disease on Small Dataset: A Knowledge Transfer Perspective", IEEE 2018.
2. Samsuddin Ahmed, Kyu Yeong Choi, Jang Jae Lee, Byeong C. Kim, Goo-Rak Kwon, Kun Ho Lee and Ho Yub Jung, "Ensembles of Patch-Based Classifiers for Diagnosis of Alzheimer Diseases", doi:https://doi.org/10.1109/ACCESS.2019.2920011.
3. Jun Zhang, Yue Gao, Yaozong Gao, Brent C. Munsell, Dinggang Shen, "Detecting Anatomical Landmarks for Fast Alzheimer's Disease Diagnosis", DOI https://doi.org/10.1109/TMI.2016.2582386, IEEE 2016.
4. M. A. Balafar, "New spatial based MRI image denoising algorithm", DOI https://doi.org/10.1007/s10462-011-9268-0.
5. Fabrizio Russo, "Validation of Denoising Algorithms for Medical Imaging", Springer 2010.
6. Saritha Saladi, N. Amutha Prabha, "Analysis of denoising filters on MRI brain images", DOI: https://doi.org/10.1002/ima.22225,
7. Chiao-Min Chen, Chih-Cheng Chen, Ming-Chi Wu, Gwoboa Horng, Hsien-Chu Wu, Shih-Hua Hsueh, His-Yun Ho, "Automatic Contrast Enhancement of Brain MR Images Using Hierarchical Correlation Histogram Analysis", DOI https://doi.org/10.1007/s40846-015-0096-6.
8. Samir S. Yadav and Shivajirao M. Jadhav, "Deep convolutional neural network-based medical image classification for disease diagnosis", Springer 2019.
9. K., Valverde, S., González-Villà, S., Bernal, J., Cabezas, M., Oliver, A., Lladó, X., 2018. Automated sub-cortical brain structure segmentation combining spatial and deep convolutional features. Medical image analysis 48, 177–186.
10. Yang, G., Liu, F., Mo, Y., Guo, Y., 2017. Automatic brain tumor detection and segmentation using unet-based fully convolutional networks, an annual conference on medical image understanding and analysis, Springer. pp. 506–517.
11. Akbari, H., Sotiras, A., Bilello, M., Rozycki, M., Kirby, J.S., Freymann, J.B., Farahani, K., Davatzikos, C., 2017. Advancing the cancer genome atlas glioma MRI collections with expert segmentation labels and radiomic features. Scientific data 4, 170117.
12. Reyes, M., Jakab, A., Bauer, S., Rempfler, M., Crimi, A., Shinohara, R.T., Berger, C., Ha, S.M., Rozycki, M., et al., 2018. Identifying the best machine learning algorithms for brain tumor segmentation, progression assessment, and overall survival prediction in the brats challenge. arXiv preprint arXiv:1811.02629.

13. Liu, X., Ding, M., Zheng, J., Li, J., 2019. 3d dilated multifiber network for real-time brain tumor segmentation in MRI, in International Conference on Medical Image Computing and Computer-Assisted Intervention, Springer. pp. 184–192.
14. Ledig, C., Newcombe, V.F., Simpson, J.P., Kane, A.D., Menon, D.K., Rueckert, D., Glocker, B., 2017. Efficient multiscale 3d cnn with fully connected CRF for accurate brain lesion segmentation. Medical image analysis 36, 61–78.
15. Ngo, T., Zhang, A., Chen, J.W., Manjunath, B., 2018. Brain tumor segmentation and tractographic feature extraction from structural MR images for overall survival prediction, in International MICCAI Brainlesion Workshop, Springer. pp. 128–141.
16. Tajeripour, F. (2017). Detection of a brain tumor in 3D MRI images using local binary patterns and histogram orientation gradient. Neurocomputing, 219, 526–535.
17. Abdel-Maksoud, Eman, Mohammed Elmogy, and Rashid Al-Awadi. "Brain tumor segmentation based on a hybrid clustering technique." Egyptian Informatics Journal 16, no. 1 (2015): 71–81
18. Sudip Kumar, Jamuna Kanta Sing, Dipak Kumar Basu, and Mita Nasipuri. "Conditional spatial fuzzy C-means clustering algorithm for segmentation of MRI images." Applied Soft Computing 34 (2015): 758–769.
19. Shaheen, Khan M. Iftekharuddin, and Arastoo Vossough. "Efficacy of texture, shape, and intensity feature fusion for posterior-fossa tumor segmentation in MRI." IEEE Transactions on Information Technology in Biomedicine 15, no. 2 (2011): 206–213.
20. Mathews, Arun B., and M. K. Jeyakumar. "Automatic detection of segmentation and advanced classification algorithm." In 2020 Fourth International Conference on Computing Methodologies and Communication (ICCMC), pp. 358–362. IEEE, 2020.
21. Anand, L., and S. P. Syed Ibrahim. "HANN: a hybrid model for liver syndrome classification by feature assortment optimization." Journal of medical systems 42, no. 11 (2018): p 1–11.
22. Anand, L., and V. Neelanarayanan. "Enchanced multiclass intrusion detection using supervised learning methods." In AIP Conference Proceedings, vol. 2282, no. 1, p. 020044. AIP Publishing LLC, 2020.
23. Anand, L., MB Mukesh Krishnan, K. U. Senthil Kumar, and S. Jeeva. "AI multi agent shopping cart system based web development." In AIP Conference Proceedings, vol. 2282, no. 1, p. 020041. AIP Publishing LLC, 2020.
24. Anand, L., V. Nallarasan, MB Mukesh Krishnan, and S. Jeeva. "Driver profiling-based anti-theft system." In AIP Conference Proceedings, vol. 2282, no. 1, p. 020042. AIP Publishing LLC, 2020.
25. F. J. J. Joseph, "Effect of supervised learning methodologies in offline handwritten Thai character recognition," Int. J. Inf. Technol., vol. 12, no. 1, pp. 57–64, Mar. 2020.
26. F. J. John Joseph and P. Anantaprayoon, "Offline Handwritten Thai Character Recognition Using Single Tier Classifier and Local Features," in 2018 International Conference on Information Technology (InCIT), 2018, pp. 1–4.
27. F. J. John Joseph and S. Auwatanamongkol, "A crowding multi-objective genetic algorithm for image parsing," Neural Comput. Appl., vol. 27, no. 8, pp. 2217–2227, 2016.
28. F. J. John Joseph and V. R. T, "Enhanced Robustness for Digital Images Using Geometric Attack simulation," Procedia Eng., vol. 38, no. Apr 2012, pp. 2672–2678, 2012.
29. F. J. John Joseph, R. T, and J. J. C, "Classification of correlated subspaces using HoVer representation of Census Data," in 2011 International Conference on Emerging Trends in Electrical and Computer Technology, Mar. 2011, pp. 906–911.
30. G. S. Sajja, K. P. Rane, K. Phasinam, T. Kassanuk, E. Okoronkwo, and P. Prabhu, "Towards applicability of blockchain in agriculture sector," Materials Today: Proceedings, 2021.
31. Gopal, V. Nanda, Fadi Al-Turjman, R. Kumar, L. Anand, and M. Rajesh. "Feature selection and classification in breast cancer prediction using IoT and machine learning." Measurement 178 (2021):p 109442.

32. Guna Sekhar Sajja, Malik Mustafa, Dr. R. Ponnusamy, Shokhjakhon Abdufattokhov, Murugesan G., Dr. P. Prabhu, "Machine Learning Algorithms in Intrusion Detection and Classification", Annals of RSCB, vol. 25, no. 6, pp. 12211–12219, Jun. 2021.
33. H. Pallathadka, M. Mustafa, D. T. Sanchez, G. Sekhar Sajja, S. Gour, and M. Naved, "Impact of machine learning on management, healthcare and agriculture," Materials Today: Proceedings, 2021.
34. Ishaq, A., Sadiq, S., Umer, M., Ullah, S., Mirjalili, S., Rupapara, V., & Nappi, M. (2021). Improving the Prediction of Heart Failure Patients' Survival Using SMOTE and Effective Data Mining Techniques. IEEE Access, 9, 39707–39716.
35. J. F. Joe, "Enhanced sensitivity of motion detection in satellite videos using instant learning algorithms," IET Chennai 3rd International on Sustainable Energy and Intelligent Systems (SEISCON 2012), 2012, pp. 1–6.
36. J. F. Joe, T. Ravi, A. Natarajan and S. P. Kumar, "Object recognition of Leukemia affected cells using DCC and IFS," 2010 Second International conference on Computing, Communication and Networking Technologies, 2010, pp. 1–6.
37. K. Balachander, S. Ramesh, Ahmed J. Obaid, 2018. Simulation Of 1KW Multi-Level Switch Mode Power Amplifier, International Journal of Innovations in Scientific and Engineering Research (IJISER), Vol. 5, No. 9: 85–92.
38. Kumar, R., Fadi Al-Turjman, L. Anand, Abhishek Kumar, S. Magesh, K. Vengatesan, R. Sitharthan, and M. Rajesh. "Genomic sequence analysis of lung infections using artificial intelligence technique." Interdisciplinary Sciences: Computational Life Sciences 13, no. 2 (2021): p 192–200.
39. Nora Omran Alkaam, Ahmed J. Obaid, Mohammed Q. Mohammed, 2018. A Hybrid Technique for Object Detection and Recognition Using Local Features Algorithms, Journal of Advanced Research in Dynamical and Control Systems, Vol. 10, No. 2: 2330–2344.
40. Onditi, S. A., & Ajwang, S. O. (2020). Computer Assisted Learning for Enhancing Mastery of Concepts in Science. International Journal on Research in STEM Education, 2(2), 134–142.
41. Opateye, J., & Ewim, D. R. E. (2021). Assessment for Learning and Feedback in Chemistry: A Case for Employing Information and Communication Technology Tools. International Journal on Research in STEM Education, 3(2), 18–27.
42. Paco, D. S., Yazon, A. D., Manaig, K. A, Sapin, S. B., & Bandoy, M. M. (2021). Paint A Portrait: Lived Experience of Parents in the Implementation of Modular Distance Learning. International Journal on Research in STEM Education, 3(2), 37–50.
43. Pathoni, H., Ashar, R., -, M., & Huda, N. (2021). Analysis Student Needs for the Development of Contextual-Based STEM Approach Learning Media in Online Learning: An Evidence from Universities in Jambi, Indonesia. International Journal on Research in STEM Education, 3(1), 17–26.
44. Purwasih, J. H. G., Sholichah, A. F, & Pratiwi, S. S. . (2021). Students' Teaching Competency Preparedness in Attending Field Experience Practice. International Journal on Research in STEM Education, 3(2), 51–63.
45. R. Baral, N. Sahu, and V. Meher, "The Attitude of Teachers and Parents of Students towards the Implementation of School Management Committee (SMCs) at Elementary Level", Int. J. Theory Appl. Elem. Second. Sch. Educ., vol. 1, no. 2, pp. 58–74, Oct. 2019.
46. R. Cuerdo, M. J. B. Ison, and C. D. T. Oñate, "Effectiveness of Automation in Evaluating Test Results Using EvalBee as an Alternative Optical Mark Recognition (OMR): A Quantitative-Evaluative Approach from a Philippine Public School", Int. J. Theory Appl. Elem. Second. Sch. Educ., vol. 3, no. 2, pp. 61–75, Oct. 2021.
47. R. D. Dollente and C. S. Tan, "School Readiness on The Implementation of Learning Delivery Modalities (LDM's) in The City Schools Division Province of Laguna: An Input to Curriculum Policy Brief and Intervention Program", Int. J. Theory Appl. Elem. Second. Sch. Educ., vol. 3, no. 2, pp. 101–124, Oct. 2021.

48. R. J. B. Fonte, A. D. Yazon, C. S. Tan, L. P. Buenvinida, and M. M. Bandoy, "Distance Learning Delivery Modalities Implementation, Resilience Quotient, and Work Performance of Teachers: A Correlational Study in The Philippines", Int. J. Theory Appl. Elem. Second. Sch. Educ., vol. 3, no. 2, pp. 171 181, Oct. 2021.
49. R. K. Sahoo, "Exploring the Changes in Teaching Strategies Enabled by Information and Communication Technology", Int. J. Theory Appl. Elem. Second. Sch. Educ., vol. 1, no. 2, pp. 75–91, Oct. 2019.
50. R. T. Hardini and S. Wening, "Private Elementary School Teachers' Perceptions of Character Education Practice in Indonesia", Int. J. Theory Appl. Elem. Second. Sch. Educ., vol. 2, no. 1, pp. 39–51, Apr. 2020.
51. Renuka J Bathi, Neeraj Taneja, Sameena Parveen, Rheumatoid Arthritis of TMJ – A Diagnostic Dilemma? , Dental update, 2004, Volume 31, Issue 3, Pages 167–174.
52. Renuka J Bathi, Sameena Parveen, Krishna Burde, The Role of Gutka Chewing in Oral Submucous Fibrosis: A Case-Control Study, Quintessence International, Jun 2009, Volume 40, Issue 6, pages e19–e25. 7p. 5 Charts.
53. Renuka J Bathi, Sameena Parveen, Neeraj Taneja, Oral Tuberculous Ulcer - A Report of Two Cases, Journal of Indian Academy of Oral Medicine and Radiology, 2003, Volume 15, Issue 2, Pages 62 65
54. Renuka J Bathi, Sameena Parveen, Sunil Mutalik, Reema Rao, Rabson-Mendenhall Syndrome: Two Case Reports and A Brief Review of The Literature, Odontology, 2010, Volume 98, Issue 1, Pages 89–96.
55. Rupapara, V., Narra, M., Gunda, N. K., Gandhi, S., & Thipparthy, K. R. (2021). Maintaining social distancing in pandemic using smartphones with acoustic waves. IEEE Transactions on Computational Social Systems, 1–7.
56. Rupapara, V., Rustam, F., Shahzad, H. F., Mehmood, A., Ashraf, I., & Choi, G. S. (2021). Impact of SMOTE on Imbalanced Text Features for Toxic Comments Classification using RVVC Model. IEEE Access, 1–1.
57. Rustam, F., Khalid, M., Aslam, W., Rupapara, V., Mehmood, A., & Choi, G. S. (2021). A performance comparison of supervised machine learning models for Covid-19 tweets sentiment analysis. PLOS ONE, 16(2), e0245909.
58. S. Bhoumik, S. Chatterjee, A. Sarkar, A. Kumar, and F. J. John Joseph, "Covid 19 Prediction from X Ray Images Using Fully Connected Convolutional Neural Network," in CSBio '20: Proceedings of the Eleventh International Conference on Computational Systems-Biology and Bioinformatics, Nov. 2020, pp. 106–107.
59. Sadiq, S., Umer, M., Ullah, S., Mirjalili, S., Rupapara, V., & NAPPI, M. (2021). Discrepancy detection between actual user reviews and numeric ratings of Google App store using deep learning. Expert Systems with Applications, 115111.
60. Sameena Parveen, Neeraj Taneja, Renuka J Bathi, AC Deka, Evaluation Of Circulating Immune Complexes And Serum Immunoglobulins In Oral Cancer Patients - A Follow Up Study, Indian Journal of Dental Research, 2010, Volume 21, Issue 1, Pages 14–19.
61. Subramani, Prabu, Fadi Al-Turjman, Rajagopal Kumar, Anusha Kannan, and Anand Loganthan. "Improving medical communication process using recurrent networks and wearable antenna s11 variation with harmonic suppressions." Personal and Ubiquitous Computing (2021): p 1–13.
62. Tawfiq A. Al-Asadi, Ahmed J. Obaid, Ahmed A. Alkhayat, 2017. Proposed Method for Web Pages Clustering Using Latent Semantic Analysis, Journal of Engineering and Applied Science, Vol. 12, No. 8: 8270–8277.
63. Yousaf, A., Umer, M., Sadiq, S., Ullah, S., Mirjalili, S., Rupapara, V., & Nappi, M. (2021b). Emotion Recognition by Textual Tweets Classification Using Voting Classifier (LR-SGD). IEEE Access, 9, 6286–6295.

Part III
Security and Privacy Concerns

A Novel Framework for Privacy Enabled Healthcare Recommender Systems

Shakil, Syed Ubaid, Shahab Saquib Sohail, Mohammed Talha Alam, Saif Ali Khan, Syed Hamid Hasan, and Tabish Mufti

1 Introduction

The healthcare system is one of the core fields where a huge amount of data of patients is used for the advancement of future studies regarding diseases and disorders. For this, Health Intelligent Systems are introduced to perform the decision process. Health recommender systems are used to filter the patient's data to provide the perfect diagnosis according to the condition of the patient. In this process of collecting data of a patient's health records, confidential data is saved in the background database. These databases consist of Personally Identifiable Information (PII) of patients [1]. This information is sensitive and can be misused, which is a major risk to the life of a patient [2].

The condition of a patient's health can be predicted by analyzing the behavior like previous records of the patient's health, lifestyle, and physique. Health recommender systems are required to provide the best treatment based on the patient's profile [3]. The health profile of a user contains the most sensitive data that can be compromised if it is not secure. This data is stolen and can be used in scams, bribing, spying, identity, learned theft, and extortion. So, it is important to secure this data, and hence, these privacy issues are a major concern for researchers [4, 5]. So, to protect a patient's confidential data and privacy issues, privacy enabled recommender systems are introduced. The recommender system is not a new field, but

Shakil · S. Ubaid · S. S. Sohail (✉) · M. T. Alam · T. Mufti
Department of Computer Science and Engineering, Jamia Hamdard, New Delhi, India
e-mail: shahabsaquibsohail@jamiahamdard.ac.in

S. A. Khan
School of Pharmaceutical Education and Research, Jamia Hamdard, New Delhi, India

S. H. Hasan
Faculty of Computing and Information Technology, King Abdulaziz University, Jeddah, KSA

P. Agarwal et al. (eds.), *Artificial Intelligence for Smart Healthcare*,
EAI/Springer Innovations in Communication and Computing,
https://doi.org/10.1007/978-3-031-23602-0_27

research in this domain has increased in the last few years [6, 7]. However, some researchers have shown concern about the privacy aspects in the recommender systems recently [8–10].

To solve this problem, we have given a solution in this paper, which helps secure the integrity and privacy of the patient's data as well as does not affect the quality of diagnosis. For this, we have proposed a framework that first does obfuscation that helps in the anonymization of the identity of the patient. Then homomorphic encryption is used to strengthen the privacy of data. The manuscript is as follows: In Sect. 2, the background is described for understanding the actual problem of privacy and security of data in the healthcare system and existing solutions provided by the researchers. In Sect. 3, description of the privacy and security aspects in the health sector and possible threats are discussed. In Sect. 4, a complete privacy enabled recommender system is discussed. In Sect. 5, we have discussed future aspects and concluded the proposed solution.

2 Materials and Methods

2.1 Background

Research related to recommender systems started in the mid-1990s. A survey conducted by Pew Research Centre in 2010 found that 80% of Internet users from 59% of the United States population are looking for health information on the Internet. For health knowledge seekers, the Internet has become the primary source [11]. Nowadays services and tools are easily obtainable to share their health records with other health providers. An example of a tool is Semantic Web to present health knowledge in the form of a system that allows narrow or expanded search requests and also improves the precision of results and recommendations. This technique is used for filtering huge data and sending better appropriate recommendations to required knowledge seekers. Semantic recommender systems use user interest ontology and semantic methods for recommendation generation.

Middleton et al. use the ontological approach for making health-related recommendations [12]. They were successful in making a health recommender system by observing user behavior and also inculcating their feedback. Adomavicius et al. in 2005 depicted classification of the recommender system, i.e., hybrid, content-based, and collaborative filtering [13]. Moreover, they explored all recommender system techniques and suggested solutions for increasing ability according to the health recommendation system.

Woerndl et al. enhanced recommendation system capability for health recommendation by adding both location-based and social-context information [14]. Further, they were using a mobile device for location and past interactions of the user for more accuracy. W. Kim et al. used agent-based and multi-criteria techniques to enhance the quality of the recommendation system [15]. According to these results, we have seen how important it is to show accurate recommendations, especially in the healthcare domain as such decisions matter for life-or-death. Jeong et al. also developed a technique to improve recommendation using semantic measures [16]. Badsha et al. showed in his article about privacy concerns with all these recommender systems. They showed a heavy reliance problem put forward on a trusted third party which may carry out privacy breaches for a patient [17]. The primary purpose of our research is to develop personal health recommender systems free from privacy breach without interrupting its accuracy which is a big concern for patients' privacy in recommender systems.

The proposed framework enhances the privacy of health recommender systems by using some cryptographic techniques. K-anonymity was added to make the patient profile anonymous from a third party. Homomorphic encryption was used by third-party before sending it to computation. Accordingly, the existing problem is solved [18].

2.1.1 Users Health Data Concerns

At present, the digitized healthcare system is one of the fundamental areas of the health sector. For analyzing huge amounts of patient data which aids to make acumens and support for the forecast of the disorders, this system is used. By this system, we can prognosticate health conditions of patients by the analyses of their lifestyle and health records. Health recommender system becomes an essential element of healthcare services. So, in the healthcare sector "health intelligent systems" are important for the decision-making process [19]. To know their health condition, people use social networks; therefore the health recommender system plays an important role in recommending diagnoses, health insurance, and alternative medicines based on the health profile of patient. Recommender systems applying big data analytics have a major role in the decision-making procedures concerning the health of a patient [4, 20, 21].

User health profile contains the most sensitive data which can put the user in serious concerns. In the last 5 years, more than 93% of healthcare organizations have undergone a data breach of some kind. In the Black book it is mentioned, over 50% of healthcare organizations have suffered at least five incidents over the same time duration. One in 10% of patients was affected by medical breaches from the last 5 years [22]. These medical records of patients can sell up to $1000 on the dark web; pay depends upon the completeness of the information. Specific offenders and combined groups use these stolen data for scam, bribing, spying, identity and learned theft, and extortion. Through phishing attacks and spam in information, malware is also delivered to inexperienced users [23, 24].

Regular criminals know the real power of coercion and extortion, by holding healthcare information, especially, about the terminal illness or sexually transmitted disease; this type of information can be used for extorting or coercing someone to do whatever they want to do. In the case of common identity theft, we can control the situation by changing, i.e., with the help of the bank we can change our account details and even get a new essence like a debit card with different security numbers. As we know health data can't be changed, so a user may face long-term effects [25].

2.1.2 Data Breaches: US Data (2010–2020)

In the USA, healthcare breaches have been escalating each successive year, and therefore a proper solution has to be contrived. In the past decade, breaches have increased to many folds. Data breaches have increased in 2020 to nearly three times as that of 2010, and nearly twice the data breached is now reported in comparison to 2014 [26]. Figure 1 shows records exposed in healthcare data breaches, where the worst scenario occurred in the year 2015 with the highest number of exposed data breaches, whereas Fig. 2 shows breaches of 500 plus records and thereby ascending each successive year with the record of 642 in the year 2020 [27].

There has been over a 25% increase in healthcare data breaches in the year 2020 crossing over 29 million in total. The data ranged from 63 breaches of 100 k records to as large as one breach involving ten million records in total of 642. The breaches involved hacking of fundraising and donor databases, clinical information, date of birth, and names. Table 1 shows causes of healthcare data breaches reported in the past year with their numbers [28]. The reasons comprise loss of breaches, inappropriate removal, stealing, unlawful access/disclosure, and hacking/IT incidents. The

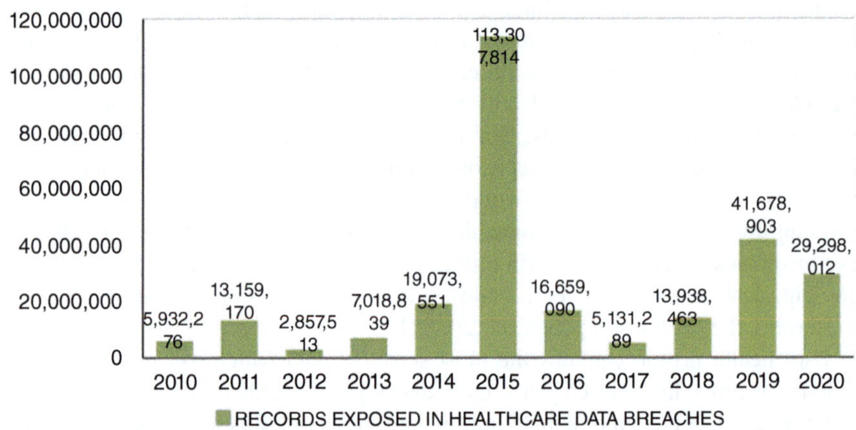

Fig. 1 Number of records exposed in US healthcare data breaches

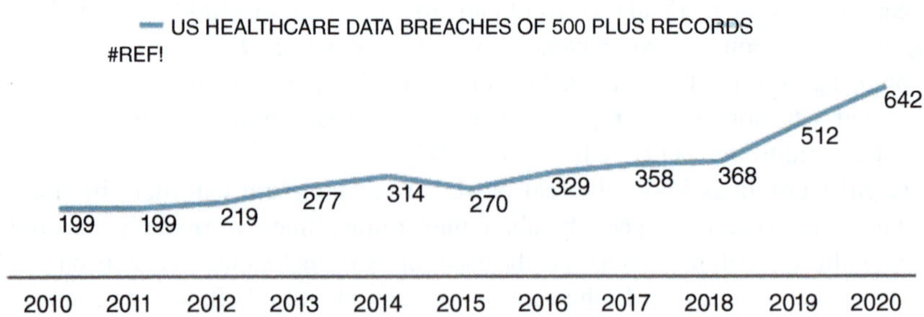

Fig. 2 Increase in the number of breaches in US healthcare (500+ records)

Table 1 Type, number, and records of breaches

Breach type	Number of breaches	Records breached
Hacking/IT incident	429	26,949,956
Unauthorized Access/disclos Ure	143	787,015
Theft	39	806,552
Improper Disposal	16	584,980
Loss	15	169,509

main cause involved hacking and other IT incidents and constituted 91.99% of all breached records and 66.82% of reported breaches [29, 30].

Phishing attacks are leading causes of data breaches; however use of encryption and cloud services has immensely helped in reducing the number of theft/loss incidents. Patient data is mainly stored by network servers and thus constitute the main target for ransomware gangs and hackers. Location of breached healthcare data has been provided through various means, almost 37% by network server, 32% by laptop, and remaining by others as covered by HIPAA, i.e., "Health Insurance Portability and Accountability Act" [31]. Maximum breaches of 497 were reported by healthcare providers, followed by 73 of business associates, 70 were reported by health plans, and at least 2 were reported by healthcare clearinghouses [32].

2.2 *Privacy Aspects in Healthcare System*

According to research conducted at Trident University International, "Ethical health research and privacy protections both are very beneficial to society. Health research is important for enhancing human well-being and health care. Protecting patients involved in research from harm and preserving their rights is significant to moral research. The prime reason for shielding personal privacy is to secure the interests of people. In contrast, the chief justification for accumulating personally identifiable health information for research is to serve society. But it's crucial to stress that privacy also features a cost at the societal level, because it allows complex activities, including research and public health activities to be administered in ways which safeguard individuals' dignity."

In 1850, the year of the first census that recurred after every 10 years, the federal government started to issue nationwide figures on mortality [33]. With the shift of the century, reporting of some of the most prevalent and lethal communicable diseases, consisting of smallpox, cholera, and tuberculosis (TB), was collected by most states and municipalities [34]. Privacy and public health enthusiasts often differ over the degree to which public health needs for health data overrule the lawful privacy concerns of people. To settle such discords, law and policy-makers attempt to balance one's privacy rights against the public's interest in improving public health results. This resulted in a solution for sharing health records data effectively while respecting individual privacy. It became a highlight of the "Department of Health and Human Services (DHHS) Privacy Rule," formed according to the "Health Insurance Portability and Accountability Act of 1996 (HIPAA)" [35].

Several federal privacy rules have been applied to specific medical data. These rules keep the privacy of one's health data in numerous ways. "Freedom of Information Act of 1966 (FOIA)" intended to stretch the public's extensive access to "federal government records" [36]. The "Federal Privacy Act of 1974" comes into action when data is gathered and managed by a federal agency in an arrangement of archives (e.g., Medicare records, health records owned by the "Department of Defense or Veteran's Administration") [36]. The "E-Government Act of 2002" is meant to make the government wholly into the digital era. Special stipulations discuss privacy issues regarding statistical data collection of the government. This law preserves non-disclosure of federal government statistical numbers of distinguishable data, with health data [36].

2.3 *Existing Privacy Enabled Healthcare Recommender System*

In this current scenario, we have an ample amount of privacy embedded healthcare recommender systems available on the Internet. Different cryptographic techniques are in use, i.e., differential privacy, homomorphic encryption, and perturbation [4]. The most secure and used technique is homomorphic encryption [37]. In this technique computation is performed on encrypted data, and recommendations are also generated in the ciphertext [38, 39].

In Fig. 3, we observe that the patient's data is converted into encrypted mode before sending it for computation. On encrypted data, all calculations are performed for recommendation generation, and then recommended diagnosis or treatment is sent to the patient in ciphertext manner. Now the private key is used on the patient side for the decryption of recommendation results. The private key is not required by health management third-party in homomorphic encryption. The main advantage of this encryption is that there is no need for a private key for computation.

In Fig. 4, we describe the superstructure of privacy embedded healthcare recommender systems. Collected data of the patient is sent to health management third-party. Encryption of data is then performed by health management third-party and sent into a database for future use. Data after being fetched from the database is subjected to computation. Then decryption of recommendation in the results is made and sent to the patient. The existing privacy embedded healthcare recommender system relies extremely upon health management third-party which is a big demerit of this system.

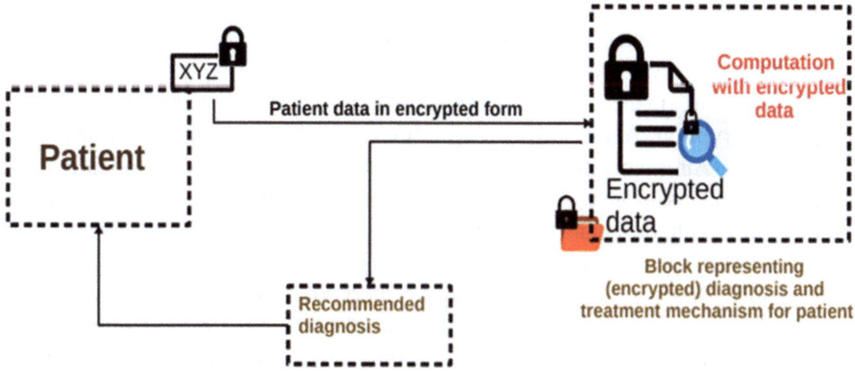

Fig. 3 Homomorphic encryption (existing cryptographic technique)

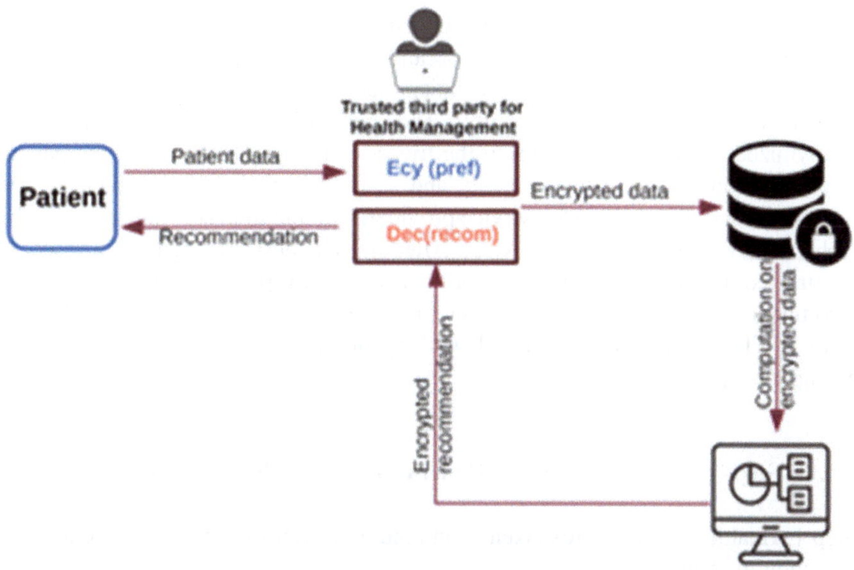

Fig. 4 Privacy enabled healthcare recommender system with homomorphic encryption

3 Results

3.1 Proposed Healthcare Recommender System

To overcome this problem of huge trust of recommender systems in third parties, we suggest a framework that improves privacy-enabled health recommender systems and uses enough privacy concerning methods to secure the privacy of patients and exempts us from relying on third parties. Here we use two steps of security for enhancing a patient's privacy. In step one, it secures the patient's identity, and on the other it is used to secure the health data of patients. These two steps provide better safety to the privacy of patients' information.

As stated earlier, the first step is anonymization, and the second step is homomorphic encryption. Anonymization with homomorphic encryption will be a great combination. Anonymization makes a patient profile obscure by adding noise thereto with the assistance of perturbation techniques. The quantity of noise added is consistent with the standard of the safety which is budget-friendly too. The quantity of cash spent on security will be directly proportional to the safety provided to the profile. Hence by using homomorphic encryption, we will do computation on encrypted data of the patient without sharing the clear data. After combining both the techniques and with the assistance of anonymization, the patient's profile is not revealed even in front of trusted partners. We only reveal the encrypted preferences without the secret key for computing within the process. This is done in order to get the advice for diagnosis and treatment consistent with the condition of the patient.

Figure 5 is the suggested framework for producing better privacy in the health recommender systems. Health records of random patients are taken who are looking for an appropriate diagnosis. Then patient identity is anonymized by applying perturbation technique k-anonymity. The patient's health records with the anonymized profile are then sent to the trusted partners. They encrypt the patient profile without knowing their identity and send patient data for recommendation production and diagnosis to the service provider. Computation is completed with the ciphertext by the same service provider. After the generation of diagnosis, it is sent to the trusted partners in encrypted form. The trusted partners then decrypt the recommended diagnosis which is sent to the patient after the removal of noise from it. The complete diagram and working are explained within the following example.

3.1.1 Steps of Recommendation Generation Through Our Framework

Step 1: Health history records taken from random patients for diagnosis recommendation generation.

Step 2: To secure the identity of the patient from third parties, anonymization is performed using K-anonymity that also helps in securing from re-identification attacks. Patient JON's identity is transformed to any anonymized form like this, "oY3gjZqwiGYpqOh1I95pxgiBxDyQhUMTtkPatWzjLOo=."

Then the patient information is separated from their identity, as shown in Tables 2 and 3.

In Fig. 6, we explain the situation for re-identification attacks. If someone already got data about the patient like age and zip code, it is impossible to get sensitive information about the patient, as shown in the above figure.

Step 3: Health records are sent to the third party with an anonymized patient profile.

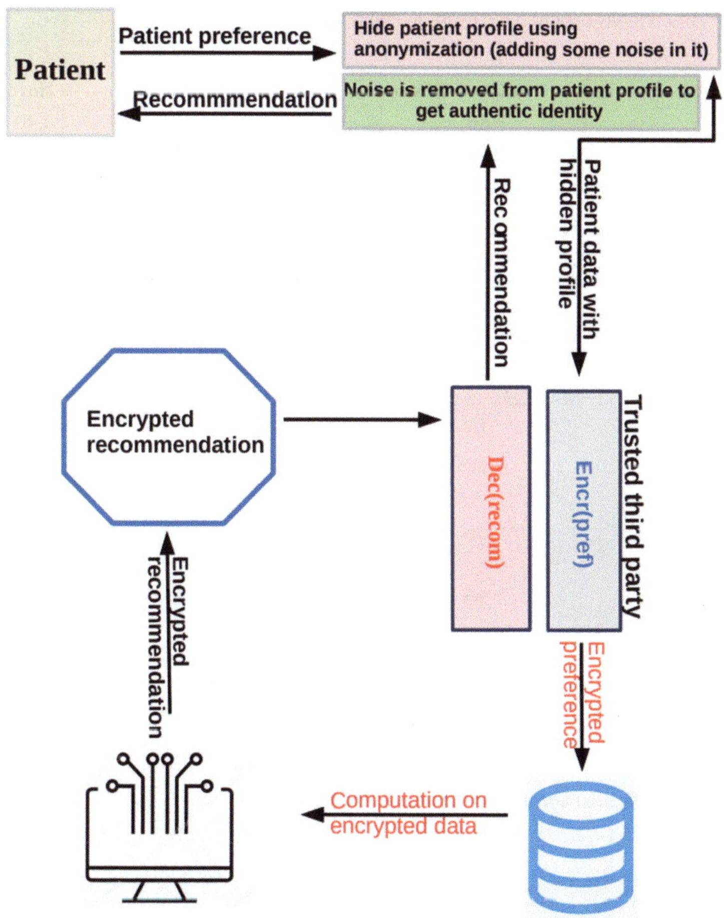

Fig. 5 Proposed privacy enabled for healthcare recommender system

Table 2 Normal table form of patient's original identity

Id	1.	2.	3.	4.
User name	Sophia	William	Olivia	Issac
Disease (sensitive data)	Heart disease	Flu	Cancer	Heart disease
Age	37	35	38	36
Sex	Female	Male	Female	Male
Zip code	14504	14533	14549	14509
Nationality	Japanese	German	Finnish	Indian

Table 3 Anonymous patient table using K-anonymity

Id	1.	2.	3.	4.
Disease (sensitive data)	Heart disease	Flu	Cancer	Heart disease
Age	<40	<40	<40	<40
Sex	People	People	People	People
Zip code	145**	145**	145**	145**
Nationality	*	*	*	*

The symbols (*,**) are just telling how k- anonymity works in terms of hiding data from third parties. And here in the table with these symbols we are showing that if we hide some of the data (like last numbers of zip code with **) from third parties then we can save data from re-identification attacks of the user.

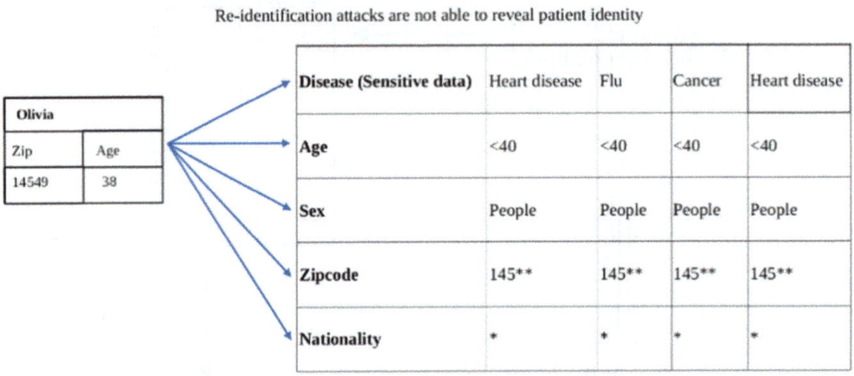

Fig. 6 Re-identification attacks are not able to reveal patient identity

Kj8ThVosTQHhHNAslyc0Wdb52+tgDkDtsnxIbO398ulF5qjxkJDpj72KsTxwn4xb40znKYtCSGdAqwsaazAT1HK
RV6zaJHu+4Oj97M3Lsnu4NtgXnZSI6Og01/0ynjxvpgPMGoCozxb6Y+C8m39nMA6/vOXtx8MTjK2Lp2Z+Wnjlj
NlHkOLh6BfKsBAwqOg7YdUYcAGVBOxXLKq2lfuOA==

Fig. 7 Ciphertext after homomorphic encryption

Step 4: Health information managing third-party performs homomorphic encryption on the health data. After being homomorphic, it converts, as shown in Fig. 7 below. And then it is sent for computation.

Step 5: On ciphertext that was provided by the third party in the above figure, computation is performed.

Step 6: Recommendations are shown in Fig. 8 below that were generated as per patient data after computation.

Step 7: Recommended diagnosis shown to the patient after computation of patient identity by analyzing the private table from the primary table, as shown in Fig. 9. Now for the patient who is searching for a restaurant, generated recommendations are as follows: Bio Resurge Regustrol Syrup protects the heart from threatening cardiac disease, Inlife Heart Care Capsules 60'S, etc.

beQA0Y9oyIiQ9OFzJuQYNhVg7RR4bEBIcoQ9DrJF65YJ81GaAPUYd6hM0RI7aQxXhunI2O0L6eNIrDdZ0FFeq
SaKNn0e60oznBkhA/nV1d/Ox0KLCzWUEmnObrjtxiwi5PzQ3T+sh7TC1d9sJZc215s7N4hnYz6ojdwADIZqdO0d
b/KlnYdZSqVTmwbO5ZRLrnQWXqfNKBxFL+ScrSaS/R4qulGus9nn2Wfq8onFUR47cLZRGbReC3L78b

Fig. 8 Recommendations generated

Zipcode	Age	Sex	Nationality	Disease(Sensitive data)	Id
145**	<40	People	*	Heart disease	1.
145**	<40	People	*	Flu	2.
145**	<40	People	*	Cancer	3.
145**	<40	People	*	Heart disease	4.

Id	User Name	Disease(Sensitive data)	Age	Sex	Zipcode	Nationality
1.	Sophia	Heart disease	37	Female	14504	Japanese
2.	William	Flu	35	Male	14533	German
3.	Olivia	Cancer	38	Female	14549	Finnish
4.	Issac	Heart disease	36	Male	14509	Indian

Fig. 9 Comparing original table from anonymous patient table to get patient profile

4 Discussion

The purpose to introduce this framework is to provide independence to the patient concerning the present privacy issues. Privacy breach, i.e., selling of patient data by health management third party followed by bribing, spying, identity and learned theft, and extortion, happens with the patients as we have discussed before [17]. The spine of all these privacy concerns is selling data of patients by some health management third party. A way to lessen these privacy risks is by not revealing data to health management third parties. Here, in our framework, we concealed the patient profile from the health management third party with obfuscation technique. So, it will become difficult for third-party sellers to sell patient's data without knowing the patient's identity. Problems related to existing privacy breaches are solved up to most instances. For example, if the patient's data is not revealed, then there is negligible chance for bribing and learned theft, etc. As far as hackers are concerned, even if they get the data, it will be very tough for them to decrypt data and then more complex computation will be required to detect user identity.

5 Conclusion

Proposed work has presented ways of securing patient data from health managing third parties, hackers and spoofers, and also from data breaching and misuse, while making the health-related recommendations. Evidently, for the generation of recommendation of a patient, mostly personal data and medical history are used. This process has unknowingly raised a relentless threat to their privacy. Since, presented work describes the ways and suggests a secured framework, in the future it might be interesting to include the methodologies discussed within the article on the working module of healthcare recommender systems which will also help in evaluating the privacy measures for patients.

References

1. IN202011008988 – a framework for protecting personally identifiable information over social network sites, 2020.
2. Kapil G, Agrawal A, Attaallah A, Algarni A, Kumar R, Khan RA. Attribute based honey encryption algorithm for securing big data: hadoop distributed file system perspective. PeerJ Computer Science. 2020 Feb 17;6:e259.
3. Sahoo AK, Pradhan C, Barik RK, Dubey H. DeepReco: deep learning based health recommender system using collaborative filtering. Computation. 2019 Jun;7(2):25.
4. Badsha S, Yi X, Khalil I. A practical privacy-preserving recommender system. Data Science and Engineering. 2016 Sep;1(3):161–77.
5. Zhang M, Ji Y. Blockchain for healthcare records: A data perspective. PeerJ Preprints. 2018 May 17;6:e26942v1.
6. Sohail SS, Siddiqui J, Ali R. Feature-Based Opinion Mining Approach (FOMA) for Improved Book Recommendation. Arabian Journal for Science and Engineering. 2018 Dec 1;43(12): 8029–48.
7. Sohail SS, Siddiqui J, Ali R. Book recommender system using fuzzy linguistic quantifier and opinion mining. In The International Symposium on Intelligent Systems Technologies and Applications 2016 Sep 21 (pp. 573–583). Springer, Cham.
8. Armknecht F, Strufe T. An efficient distributed privacy-preserving recommendation system. In 2011 The 10th IFIP Annual Mediterranean Ad Hoc Networking Workshop 2011 Jun 12 (pp. 65–70). IEEE.
9. Aïmeur E, Brassard G, Fernandez JM, Onana FS. A lambic: a privacy- preserving recommender system for electronic commerce. International Journal of Information Security. 2008 Oct 1;7(5): 307–34.
10. Erkin Z, Beye M, Veugen T, Lagendijk RL. Privacy enhanced recommender system. In Thirty-first symposium on information theory in the Benelux 2010 May 11 (pp. 35–42).
11. Morrell TG, Kerschberg L. Personal health explorer: A semantic health recommendation system. In 2012 IEEE 28th International Conference on Data Engineering Workshops 2012 Apr 1 (pp. 55–59). IEEE.
12. S. E. Middleton, N. Shadbolt, and D. C. De Roure, "Ontological user profiling in recommender systems," ACM Transactions on Information Systems (TOIS), vol. 22, no. 1, pp. 54–88, 2004.
13. G. Adomavicius and A. Tuzhilin, "Toward the next generation of recommender systems: A survey of the state-of the-art and possible extensions," IEEE Transactions on Knowledge and Data Engineering, pp. 734–749, 2005.
14. W. Woerndl and G. Groh, "Utilizing Physical and Social Context to Improve Recommender Systems," presented at the 2007 IEEE/WIC/ACM International Conferences on Web Intelligence and Intelligent Agent Technology Workshops., 2007, pp. 123–128.
15. W. Kim, L. Kerschberg, and A. Scime, "Learning for Automatic Personalization in a Semantic Taxonomy-Based Meta-Search Agent," Electronic Commerce Research and Applications (ECRA), vol. 1, 2002.
16. H. Jeong, "Hybrid Filtering in Semantic Query Processing," PhD Dissertation, George Mason University, Fairfax, VA, 2011.
17. Badsha, S., Yi, X., Khalil, I.: A practical privacy-preserving recommender system. Data Sci. Eng. 1(3), 161–177 (2016).
18. Wei R, Tian H, Shen H. Improving k-anonymity based privacy preservation for collaborative filtering. Computers & Electrical Engineering. 2018 Apr 1;67:509–19.
19. Saleem Y, Rehmani MH, Crespi N, Minerva R. Parking recommender system privacy preservation through anonymization and differential privacy. Engineering Reports. 2020:e12297.
20. Kocabas O, Soyata T. Towards privacy-preserving medical cloud computing using homomorphic encryption. In Virtual and Mobile Healthcare: Breakthroughs in Research and Practice 2020 (pp. 93–125). IGI Global.

21. Shakil MT, Ubaid S, Sohail SS, Alam MA. A Neutrosophic Cognitive Map Based Approach to Explore the Health Deterioration Factors. Neutrosophic Sets and Systems, Vol. 41, 2021. 2021: 198.
22. Portswigger, available at: https://portswigger.net/daily-swig/the-latest- healthcare-data-breaches, [accessed on 20 January 2021].
23. Trendmicro, Available at: https://www.trendmicro.com/vinfo/us/security/news/cyber-attacks/healthcare-under-attack-stolen-medical-records, [accessed on 1 January 2021].
24. Kocabaş Ö, Soyata T. Medical data analytics in the cloud using homomorphic encryption. In E-Health and Telemedicine: Concepts, Methodologies, Tools, and Applications 2016 (pp. 751–768). IGI Global.
25. Healthtech Magazine, Available at: https://healthtechmagazine.net/article/2019/10/what-happens-stolen-healthcare-data-perfcon, [accessed on December 2020].
26. Health breaches in US at: https://www.hipaajournal.com/2020-healthcare-data-breach-report-us/ [accessed on 20 January '2021].
27. Health breaches in US at: https://www.cdc.gov/phlp/publications/topic/hipaa.html#two [accessed on 20 January '2021].
28. Health breaches in US at: https://www.hhs.gov/hipaa/for-professionals/breach-notification/breach reporting/index.html [accessed on 20 January '2021].
29. Wikina SB. What caused the breach? An examination of use of information technology and health data breaches. Perspectives in health information management. 2014;11(Fall).
30. Liu V, Musen MA, Chou T. Data breaches of protected health information in the United States. Jama. 2015 Apr 14;313(14):1471–3.
31. McCoy TH, Perlis RH. Temporal trends and characteristics of reportable health data breaches, 2010-2017. Jama. 2018 Sep 25;320(12):1282–4.
32. Ronquillo JG, Erik Winterholler J, Cwikla K, Szymanski R, Levy C. Health IT, hacking, and cybersecurity: national trends in data breaches of protected health information. JAMIA open. 2018 Jul;1(1):15–9.
33. Frieden TR. The future of public health. New England Journal of Medicine. 2015 Oct 29;373 (18):1748–54.
34. Teutsch SM, Churchill RE, editors. Principles and practice of public health surveillance. Oxford University Press, USA; 2000.
35. Gostin LO. Genetic privacy. The Journal of Law, Medicine & Ethics. 1995 Dec;23(4):320–30. Pub. L. NO. 104-191, 110 Stat. 1936 (1996).
36. Hodge Jr JG. Health information privacy and public health. The journal of law, medicine & Ethics. 2003 Dec;31(4):663–71.
37. Sun X, Pan Z, Bertino E, editors. Cloud Computing and Security: 4th International Conference, ICCCS 2018, Haikou, China, June 8–10, 2018, Revised Selected Papers, Part III. Springer; 2018 Sep 12.
38. Jeckmans AJ, Beye M, Erkin Z, Hartel P, Lagendijk RL, Tang Q. Privacy in recommender systems. In Social media retrieval 2013 (pp. 263–281). Springer, London.
39. Friedman A, Knijnenburg BP, Vanhecke K, Martens L, Berkovsky S. Privacy aspects of recommender systems. In Recommender Systems Handbook 2015 (pp. 649–688). Springer, Boston, MA.

An Evaluation of RSA and a Modified SHA-3 for a New Design of Blockchain Technology

Aun H. Jasim and Ali H. Kashmar

1 Introduction

Blockchain was first created for Bitcoin as decentralized transaction and data management technology. Blockchain technology has become increasingly interesting because Blockchain is the key attribute to authentication, confidentiality, and data integrity without a third-party organization, and thus creates interested areas of study, particularly in the field of technological challenges and limitations [1]. The most recent advancements in information technology have resulted in a massive flow of information and the vast amount of sensitive data stored therein, making them engrossed and vulnerable to cyber-attacks that result in data hacking and alteration [2]. The encryption algorithms used in blockchain implementation are the foundation. Blockchain is implemented using encryption algorithms, and when it comes to overall results, each has its set advantages and disadvantages. So, RSA Digital Signature and Blockchain proposes secure and trustworthy data sharing in the massive collection of data created by the judiciary, military, legislature, commercial code registries, and so on, for protecting data transmission from misuse and hacking [3].

RSA encryption algorithm is currently regarded as a more efficient public-key cryptosystem. Its theoretical and practical applications and safety are built on the complexity of resolving large integers into prime factors, and the large integer is required for its security [4]. It's difficult to ensure the confidentiality and integrity of data storage and transmission. One way of providing it is by the use of cryptographic techniques, which, sadly, adds time to the process due to the need for data encryption. While digital signatures are an essential complement, the main benefits are lost

A. H. Jasim (✉) · A. H. Kashmar
Department of Computer Science, College of Science, University of Baghdad, Baghdad, Iraq
e-mail: aun.jasim1201@sc.uobaghdad.edu.iq; Ali.kashmar@sc.uobaghdad.edu.iq

P. Agarwal et al. (eds.), *Artificial Intelligence for Smart Healthcare*,
EAI/Springer Innovations in Communication and Computing,
https://doi.org/10.1007/978-3-031-23602-0_28

if a trustable third party is still required to prevent double-spending [5]. One of the hardware cryptographic accelerators will be SHA-3's operational modes, which is widely used in different kinds of design blockchain technology [6]. This paper introduces the RSA-SHA-3 resource shared crypto-coprocessor, which combines two NIST-standardized algorithms, namely, the Rivest-Shamir-Adleman encryption algorithm (RSA) and Secure Hash Algorithm-3 (SHA-3). An amendment to the RSA algorithm and modified hash function (SHA-3) was suggested in this paper. The compression study was presented to the efficiency of the origin RSA encryption algorithm and the proposed Improve RSA (IM_RSA) in memory consumption. In addition, the analyzing studies between the standard (SHA-3) and the proposed (SHAH) in terms of time was introduced.

2 Related Work

Blockchain has the potential to improve data protection, privacy, confidentiality, traceability, accountability, honesty, robustness, transparency, trustworthiness, and authentication [7]. There has been a recent movement to use Blockchain, a cryptocurrency-based ledger system, to apply its techniques to non-financial applications [8]. Blockchain security prevents anyone from maliciously manipulating a ledger by spreading it to all network users. A majority of the network must check the validity of any new "transaction" or block of data added to the chain. This ensures the quality of the data; a ledger then public key encryption, such as the highly stable RSA encryption, may be used. To give their credentials safely, the receiver will then compare this to an entry in the database. The immutable blockchain has resulted in a very safe and efficient way to manage verification of transactions Individuality [9]. RSA is the first generation of public-key cryptography, and it has been extremely successful since its inception [10]. A scheme based on the RSA is updated and improved.

As contrasted to the standard RSA algorithm, which uses only two big prime numbers, four large prime numbers are used in the proposed algorithm, increasing the system's complexity [11]. The proposed algorithm introduces a new idea to help the RSA algorithm to speed up. It includes the architectural design as well as an updated version of the RSA algorithm. It uses a third prime number to construct a modulus n that is difficult to decompose for intruders [12]. It also suggested a practical approach for improving the RSA scheme's security; the aim of this method is to remove messages that are redundant that occur in certain values of n, the result of multiplying two prime numbers, and which are regarded as a flaw in the RSA method. The solution to this problem is to substitute this value of n in a set of all prime numbers using a stable agreement gap that are accessible. The next step is to choose one or both of the primes from that set that are responsible for generating an alternative [13]. It also suggests directly to send the value as a public key, using two public key pairs and some mathematical logic proposed, has created an implementation of the RSA Algorithm that is both efficient and effective [14]. Hashing is used to create connected block lists in blockchain networks, which provide safe and stable storage of critical data in a distributed repository [15]. The Secure Hash Algorithm-l (SHA-1) and Secure Hash Algorithm-2 (SHA-2) are the most well-known and officially used hash functions (SHA-2). SHA-l has been the target of significant attacks in recent years.

As a result, (NIST) organized a competition to create new and more reliable hash algorithms for use in the coming years. SHA-3 will be the name of the newly chosen hash function [16]. Cryptographic hash functions are currently used in a variety of applications, including security communications, protocols, network security infrastructures, and digital signature systems. Safe Hash Algorithm (SHA-3) is the current standard cryptographic hash function that is not open to attacks [17]. They suggested a new design based on reducing the required number of clock cycles to generate a value of hash to improve the rate (throughput) of the Keccak hash algorithm [18]. Hash method was based on the SHA3-512 Hash algorithm, which is resistant to side channel attacks; three techniques were used to achieve this goal: first, shuffle Dataset delimiter arrays, salt them, and manipulate them using the "Fisher Yates" Algorithm. Second, critical data is stored in volatile memory objects. After that, a thread locking method is used [19]. It has also been suggested SHA-3 new implementation which has a low-power hardware architecture. Random Access Memory (RAM), a stable logic structure, and an improved Finite State Machine (FSM) make up our SHA-3 implementation [20].

3 SHA-3 and RSA Algorithm

In this section, the summarization of the basic structures of the SHA-3 and RSA algorithm was presented.

3.1 SHA-3

The hash includes several mathematical operations (XOR, AND, ROTATION, NOT). In addition, it consists of 24 rounds. Figure 1 shows the spongy construction of SHA-3 [22].

3.2 RSA Algorithm

Encryption (RSA) is an encryption algorithm by a general key. Maybe the first on this stage, which can be used for both signing and encryption, and was one of the first major advances in encryption using a general key, which is secure as long as the key is excessively long: 1024-bit, and it is highly reliant on the fact that there is no

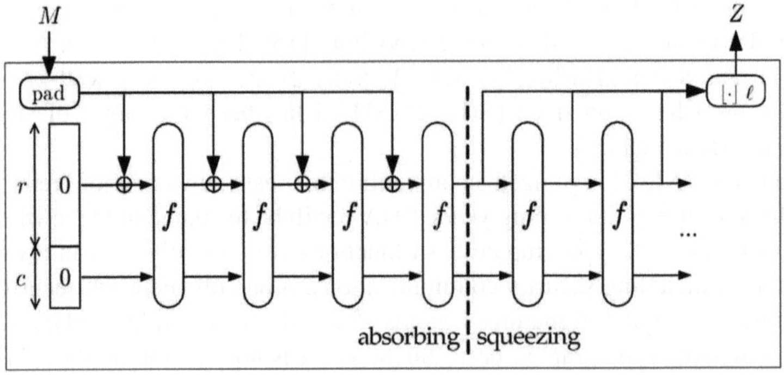

Fig. 1 Shows the sponge construction of SHA-3

algorithm for quickly analyzing a large number of variables. The basic structures of the encryption and decryption operations of the RSA algorithm in its original form are shown in the following algorithms [21].

Key Generation Algorithm

Step$_1$: Generate three distinct prime numbers p, q
Step$_2$: Compute $n = P * q$
Step$_3$: Compute $Q(n) = (p-1) * (q-1)$
Step$_4$: Choose an integer e such that $1 < e < Q(n)$ and gcd $(e, Q(n))=1$
Step$_5$: Determine d as $d \equiv e^{-1} \pmod{Q(n)}$

RSA Encryption

Input: RSA public key (n,e), Plain text $m \in [0, n-1]$
Output: Cipher text c
Compute $C = M^e \bmod n$

Decryption RSA

Input: Public key (n,e),Private key d, Cipher text c
Output: Plain text m
Compute $m = c^d \bmod n$

4 Proposed System

An Amendment RSA and modified SHA-3, which can be applied for a new design of blockchain technology, was suggested, especially for building a real environment from the Blockchain that protects medical data. The new design consists of two parts:

4.1 First Part: The Client

3- Wallet Generator: generate the public and private keys through an encryption algorithm.

B- Generator Health record: including the following data (Sender Public Key, Sender Private Key, Recipient Public Key, name, result, date).

4.2 Second Part: The Server

Consisting of a set of nodes, each (Node) represents a health center these nodes are associated with through the blockchain algorithm.

3 Health record to be added to the next block: Through the update process, each patient file contains the patient's name and history, and the result and the public key and private key and Recipient Public Key will be uploaded to the current node.

B- MINE: Through the mining process, new blocks are added to the Blockchain and therefore health records on the Blockchain. In building the Blockchain, we relied on a Proof-Of-Work algorithm, the first algorithm used in the Blockchain applied to Bitcoin and other digital currencies. It involves many hash attempts or encryption purposes of obtaining hash.

In Fig. 2, each (Block) represents a health center, and each (p) is a patient file or client, and these Blocks upload data patient to the Blockchain. Generally, a blockchain is a chain of records that contain specific information or data. The data we want to document varies from case to case; for example, "In the case of the

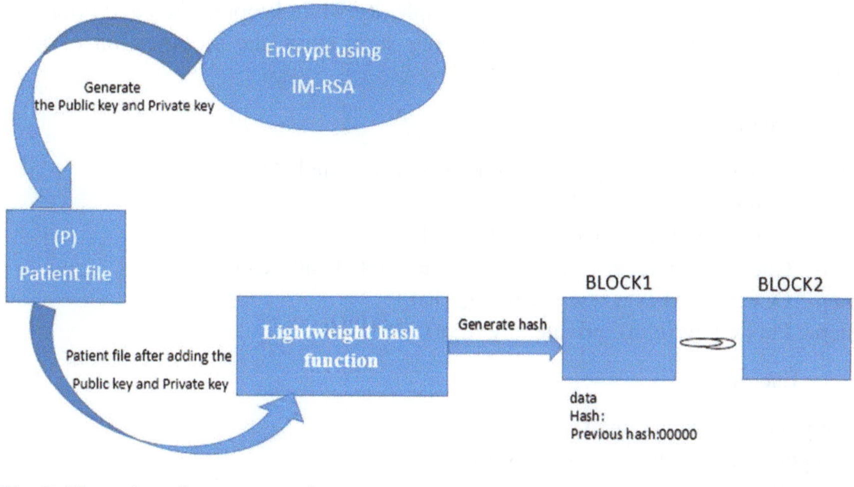

Fig. 2 Shows how the system works

Blockchain for remittances and cash currencies, the data will be the transfer information such as the date of the transfer, the sender, the recipient, and the amount." In the case of ownership, the data will be the type of ownership, is it a car or a plot of land, the name of the previous owner, the name of the owner, the new and the date of the transaction. As for the private data in our research field, it will be the patient's name, examination result, and date. These records are distributed on decentralized networks that do not contain a central authority. These records are distributed over all the nodes in the network; for this reason, we do not need reliability or a reliable third party because every person or node in this network has a copy of these records, and these records will be public, meaning anyone can validate these records and validate these data or transactions. Building the Blockchain relied on a (POW) algorithm; it is the first algorithm used and applied to Bitcoin and other digital currencies. It involves many hash attempts or cryptocurrencies to obtain hash, so it suffers from a delay in time and takes up more memory. In addition, this algorithm does not allow adding any block in a transaction except after all transactions are valid through an agreement between all the nodes in the network after the new block is added. Therefore, we will modify the RSA algorithm to improve memory consumption and suggest a modified hash to improve speed time. In the following subsection, the description of RSA Algorithm Modification (IM_RSA) and lightweight hash function was presented.

4.3 Improve Modification RSA Algorithm (IM_RSA)

RSA is one of the security algorithms that is becoming growingly significant for the Internet to provide firms and communities. The main idea of the modification of RSA is focused on the complexity of the encryption key by making the prime factorization harder than it was by adding a new key. This enhancement would improve the algorithm's security and complexity while keeping the encryption and decryption times the same. The following steps show the modification of RSA (IM_RSA).

Key Generation Algorithm

$Step_1$: Generate three distinct prime numbers p, q, and r.
$Step_2$: Compute $n = P * q * r$.
$Step_3$: Compute $Q(n) = (p-1) * (q-1) * (r-1)$.
$Step_4$: Choose an integer e such that $1 < e < Q(n)$ and $\gcd(e, Q(n))=1$
$Step_5$: Determine d as $d \equiv e^{-1} \pmod{Q(n)}$
$Step_6$: Public key (e, n), private key (d, n)

Encryption:

The public key is obtained (e, n).
Computes cipher text $C = M^e \pmod{n}$
Decryption:

Using the private key (d, n)
Computes plain text $M = C^d \pmod{n}$

4.4 Lightweight Hash Function

The lightweight hash function accepts messages of any size as input, generates 512-bit output messages, and achieves the balance between security and memory requirements by utilizing only three operations (rotation, XOR, ADD) with 20 rounds. The message blocks are combined with a simple XOR with the internal state, as shown in Fig. 3.

Below is an illustration of the lightweight hash function algorithm and the processes used.

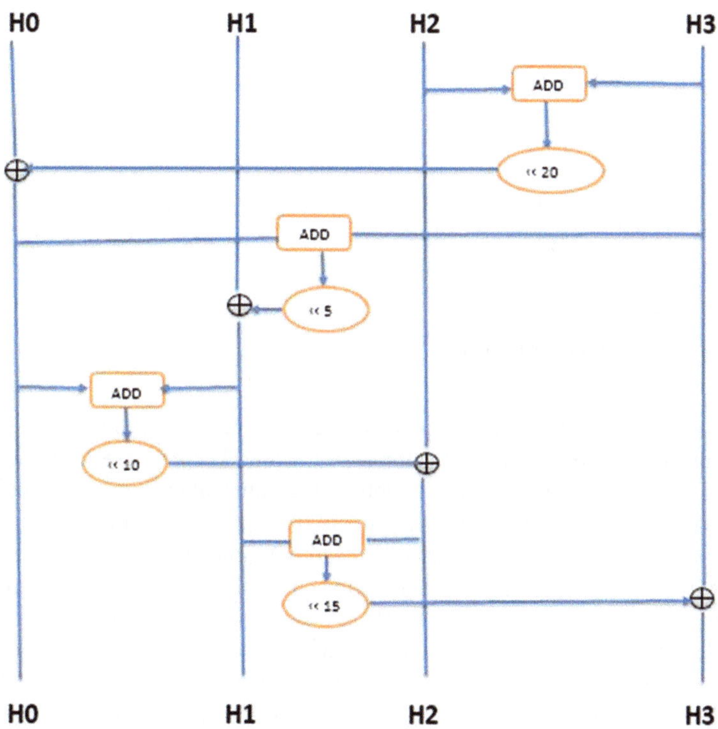

Fig. 3 Shows the lightweight hash function

Algorithm: Lightweight Hash Function

```
Split input to equal four parts H[0],H [1],H[2],H[3] (sometime needing padding) and
   save the four parts.
S [0] = H [0]
S [1] = H [1]
S [2] = H [2]
S [3] = H [3]
r=1
while (r<=20)
{
H [0] ⊕= rotate ((H [2] + H [3]), 20)
H [1] ⊕= rotate ((H [0] + H [3]), 5)
H [2] ⊕= rotate ((H [0] + H [1]), 10)
H [3] ⊕= rotate ((H [2] + H [1]), 15)
H [0] = H [0] + H [2]
H [1] = H [1] + H [3]
H [0] = H [1]
H [1] = H [3]
H [3] = H [0]
r++
}
H [0] = H [0] + S [0]
H [1] = H [1] + S [1]
   H [2] = H [2] + S [2]
   H [3] = H [3] + S [3]
```

5 Result and Discussion

The advantage of additionof new parameter in (IM_RSA) algorithm is to improve the algorithms's protection and complexity while keeping the encryption and decryption, and the memory consumption the same algorithm's protection and complexity while keeping the encryption and decryption times the same and memory consumption. Figure 4 summarizes the compression between IM_RSA and RSA algorithm in terms of memory consumption. To achieve the improvement in the memory consumption process of IM_RSA, we can see from Fig. 4, when the key length 13 bits we achieve less memory consumption than RSA, while when the key length is 17 bits, the two algorithms are equal in memory consumption. Finally, when the key length is 22 and 25 bits, the memory consumption is lower than RSA. With this property, IM_RSA improved memory consumption because RSA algorithm is based on two variables, while IM_RSA deals with three variables; in addition, this property increased the difficulty of security attacks for this algorithm.

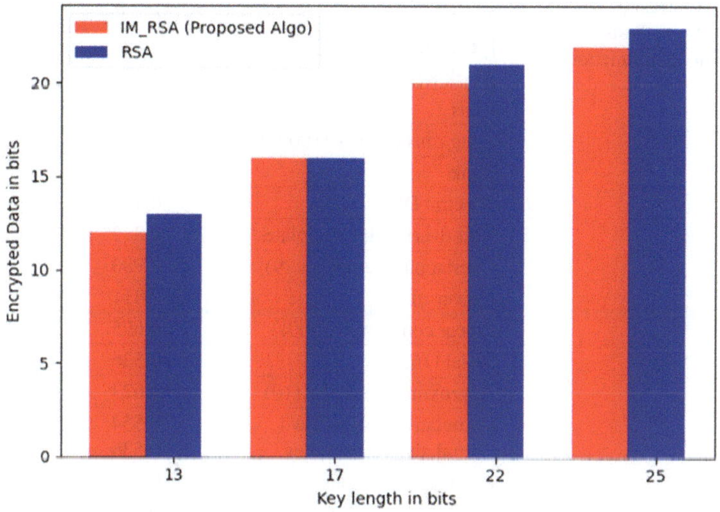

Fig. 4 The compression between RSA and IM_RSA in terms of memory consumption

The lightweight hash function consists of 20 rounds while the SHA-3 consists of 24 rounds; the mathematic operations used in the proposed hash (rotation, XOR, ADD), while in SHA-3 (rotation, NOT, AND, XOR). This makes the proposed hash have a balance in speed and complexity.

6 NIST Statistical Suite Tests

Test Suite v.1.8, a statistical program composed of 16 tests, was developed by NIST in order to investigate different elements of randomness along a bit sequence. To verify the unpredictability of any binary sequence created by a PRNG such as AES [23, 24] or Rabbit [25], this software is often used [23, 24]. To find out whether the bit sequence of the updated hash function can successfully pass several types of statistical tests of randomness, these tests are being conducted. Input parameters for 16 NIST statistical suite tests were derived from files with keys of 1,000,000 bits each. This hash algorithm is being tested with these parameters: length sequences = 1,000,000; aperiodic block length = 9; overlapping block length = 9; universal block length = 7; universal steps = 1280; approximate entropy block length = 10; serial block length = 16; linear complexity sequence length = 500; number sequences = 10; block frequency length = 128; aperiodic block length = 9; overlapping block length = 9; universal block length = 7; universal steps = 1280; approximate entropy block length = 10. BINARY FILE WITH ALL 300 BLOCK. ALPHA = 0.0100 in D-round9.txt.

Table 1 The results of NIST Statistical Suite Tests of the lightweight hash function

Statistical tests	*P*-values	Result
Frequency	0.463	Pass
Block frequency (128)	0.523	Pass
Runs	0.425	Pass
Long runs of ones (10000)	0.576	Pass
Rank	0.549	Pass
Spectral DFT	0.452	Pass
Non-overlapping templates	0.832	Pass
Overlapping templates (9)	0.980	Pass
Universal (7)	0.411	Pass
Linear complexity (500)	0.695	Pass
Serial (16)	0.526	Pass
Approximate entropy (10)	0.623	Pass
Cumulative – sums Fwd Cumulative – sums Rev	0.554 0.536	Pass Pass
Random excursions	0.547	Pass
Random excursions variant	0.478	Pass

BIT HASH = 1000000, no. of 1's = 500052, and no. of 0's = 499948
BIT HASH = 1000000, no. of 1's = 499018, and no. of 0's = 500982
BIT HASH = 1000000, no. of 1's = 499427, and no. of 0's = 500982
BIT HASH = 1000000, no. of 1's = 500579, and no. of 0's = 499421
BIT HASH = 1000000, no. of 1's = 498684, and no. of 0's = 501316
BIT HASH = 1000000, no. of 1's = 499233, and no. of 0's = 500767
BIT HASH = 1000000, no. of 1's = 499330, and no. of 0's = 500670
BIT HASH = 1000000, no. of 1's = 499830, and no. of 0's = 500170
BIT HASH = 1000000, no. of 1's = 498782, and no. of 0's = 501218
BIT HASH = 1000000, no. of 1's = 498947, and no. of 0's = 501053

For each NIST test, the percentage of passed sequences has been computed (see Table 1). This was followed by a comparison of these results with an appropriate P-value confidence interval. According to the quantitative analysis test findings presented in Figs. 5 and 6, all of the percentages are within the acceptable confidence interval [0.980, 0.999].

Final analysis results are shown in Table 1, which reveals that bit-sequences of the lightweight hash function pass all of these tests, which further demonstrates the improved SHA-3's efficiency and versatility.

The modified SHA-3 algorithm checks and passes the entire 16-NIST test for many samples, as shown in Table 1. This justifies the robustness of the proposed hashing algorithm and proves that the lightweight hash function has a quite high degree of randomness.

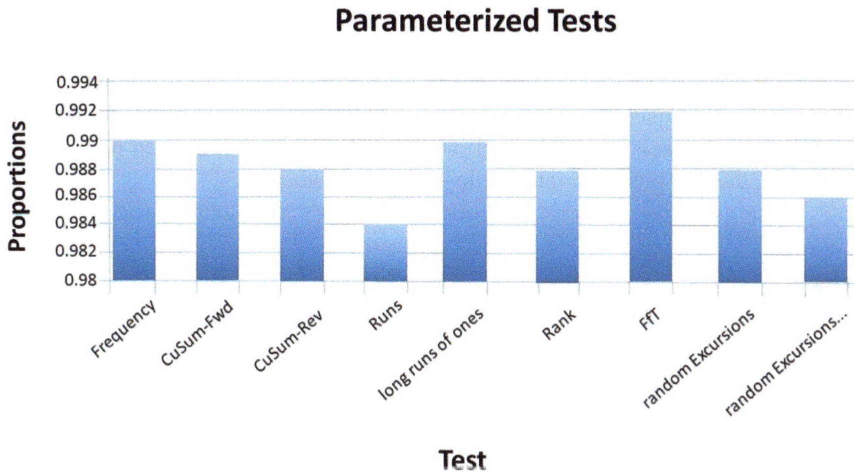

Fig. 5 Confidence intervals for parameterized tests that are acceptable

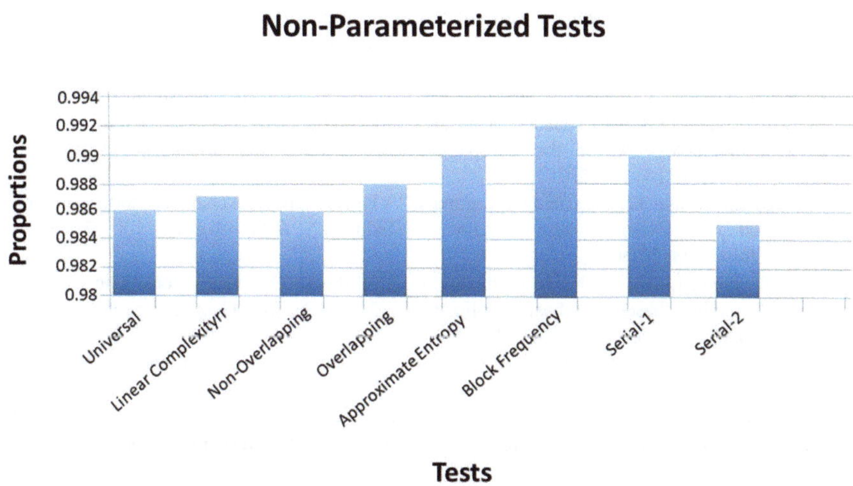

Fig. 6 Confidence intervals for non-parameterized tests that are acceptable

7 Conclusion

The evaluation of RSA and a modified SHA-3 is the proposed concept of this paper. These properties can be used in the design of some blockchain technology. The suggested proposal can be applied by adding a new variable to improve memory consumption. In addition, the lightweight hash function of SHA-3 was proven by replacing the operations (AND) and (NOT) with (ADD) arithmetic operation to improve hashing speed. The results show that the use of (IM_RSA) has helped improve memory consumption, and the complexity degree of the algorithm becomes more powerful against security attacks. Moreover, the use of the lightweight hash function proved its speed, as well as NIST Statistical Suite Tests was applied for checking the bit sequences generated by modified SHA-3, which improved the quite degree of randomness. Finally, good memory consumption improved hash speed, thus strengthening blockchain technology in the healthcare.

References

1. A. D. Dwivedi, G. Srivastava, S. Dhar, and R. Singh, "A decentralized privacy-preserving healthcare blockchain for IoT," *Sensors (Switzerland)*, vol. 19, no. 2, pp. 1–17, 2019.
2. S. Chandel, W. Cao, Z. Sun, J. Yang, B. Zhang, and T. Y. Ni, *A multi-dimensional adversary analysis of RSA and ECC in blockchain encryption*, vol. 70. Springer International Publishing, 2020. 1240.
3. S. V, "Security and Privacy Mechanism Using Blockchain," *J. Ubiquitous Comput. Commun. Technol.*, vol. 01, no. 01, pp. 45–54, 2019, doi: https://doi.org/10.36548/jucct.2019.1.005.
4. P. Saveetha and S. Arumugam, "Study on Improvement in Rsa Algorithm and Its Implementation," *Int. J. Comput. Commun. Technol.*, no. 6, pp. 190–195, 2016.
5. M. Monti and S. Rasmussen, "RAIN: A Bio-Inspired Communication and Data Storage Infrastructure," *Artif. Life*, vol. 23, no. 4, pp. 552–557, 2017.
6. Pietro Nannipieri ∗, Matteo Bertolucci, Luca Baldanzi,Luca Crocetti,Stefano Di Matteo, Francesco Falaschi, Luca Fanucci, Sergio Saponara "SHA2 and SHA-3 accelerator design in a 7 nm technology within the European Processor Initiative," *Microprocess.Microsyst.*, no. September, p. 103444, 2020.
7. P. Fraga-Lamas and T. M. Fernández-Caramés, "A Review on Blockchain Technologies for an Advanced and Cyber-Resilient Automotive Industry," *IEEE Access*, vol. 7, no. c, pp. 17578–17598, 2019.
8. A. D. Dwivedi, L. Malina, P. Dzurenda, and G. Srivastava, "Optimized blockchain model for internet of things based healthcare applications," *2019 42nd Int. Conf. Telecommun. Signal Process. TSP 2019*, pp. 135–139, 2019.
9. B. Cresitello-dittmar, "Application of the Blockchain For Authentication and Verification of Identity," *Int. J. Adv. Sci. Eng. Inf. Technol.*, vol. 6, no. 2, p. 1–9, 2016.
10. S. Chandel, W. Cao, Z. Sun, J. Yang, B. Zhang, and T. Y. Ni, *A multi-dimensional adversary analysis of RSA and ECC in blockchain encryption*, vol. 70. Springer International Publishing, 2020. 625
11. M. Thangavel, P. Varalakshmi, M. Murrali, and K. Nithya, "An Enhanced and Secured RSA Key Generation Scheme (ESRKGS)," *J. Inf. Secur. Appl.*, vol. 20, pp. 3–10, 2015.
12. R. Patidar and R. Bhartiya, "Modified RSA cryptosystem based on offline storage and prime number," *2013 IEEE Int. Conf. Comput. Intell. Comput. Res. IEEE ICCIC 2013*, pp. 1–6, 2013.
13. A. K. Hussain, "A Modified RSA Algorithm for Security Enhancement and Redundant Messages Elimination Using K-Nearest Neighbor Algorithm," *IEEE Access*, vol. 2, no. 1, pp. 159–163, 2015.
14. A. A. Ayele and V. Screenivasarao, "A Modified RSA Encryption Technique Based on Multiple public keys," *Int. J. Innov. Res. Comput. Commun. Eng.*, vol. 1, no. 4, pp. 859–864, 2013.
15. A. Kuznetsov, K. Shekhanin, A. Kolhatin, D. Kovalchuk, V. Babenko, and I. Perevozova, "Performance of Hash Algorithms on GPUs for Use in Blockchain," *2019 IEEE Int. Conf. Adv. Trends Inf. Theory, ATIT 2019 - Proc.*, pp. 166–170, 2019.

16. R. Roman, C. Alcaraz, and N. Sklavos, "On the Hardware Implementation Efficiency of Cryptographic Primitives," pp. 1240–1243, 2012.
17. A. Sideris, T. Sanida, and M. Dasygenis, "High Throughput Implementation of the Keccak Hash Function Using the Nios-II Processor," *Technologies*, vol. 8, no. 1, p. 15, 2020.
18. S. El Moumni, M. Fettach, and A. Tragha, "High throughput implementation of SHA3 hash algorithm on field programmable gate array (FPGA)," *Microelectronics J.*, vol. 93, no. July 2019.
19. A. Samir Abo-Taleb, M. Nabil, M. Shalaby, and S. Elramly, "An enhanced SHA3-based hashing method: A side-channel attack countermeasure," *ACM Int. Conf. Proceeding Ser.*, pp. 145–150, 2019.
20. Y. Yang, D. He, N. Kumar, and S. Zeadally, "Compact Hardware Implementation of a SHA-3 Core for Wireless Body Sensor Networks," *IEEE Access*, vol. 6, no. 1, pp. 40128–40136, 2018.
21. G. da Silva Quirino and E. D. Moreno, "Architectural Evaluation of Algorithms RSA, ECC and MQQ in Arm Processors," *Int. J. Comput. Networks Commun.*, vol. 5, no. 2, pp. 153–168, 2013.
22. G. Bertoni, J. Daemen, M. Peeters, and G. Van Assche, "On the security of the keyed sponge construction," *Skew*, pp. 1–15, 2011.
23. Jessa, M. 2010. Improving Statistical Properties of Number Sequences Generated by Multiplicative Congenital Pseudorandom Generator. Advances in Electronics and Telecommunications. 1(2): 51–54.
24. Soto, J. 1999. Statistical Testing of Random Number Generators. Proceedings of the 22nd National Information Systems Security Conference, Crystal City, Virginia.
25. NIST. 2001. A Statistical Test Suite for the Validation of Random Number Generators and Pseudorandom Number Generators for Cryptographic Applications. http://csrc.nist.gov/rng.

Quality of Smart Health Service for Enhancing the Performance of Machine Learning-Based Secured Routing on MANET

Kalaivani Pachiappan, Venkata Ramana Vandadi, Dilip Kumar Sharma, Amarendra Kothalanka, Saravanan Thangavel, and Sudhakar Sengan

1 Introduction

Several variations prevail among the Mobile Ad hoc Networks (MANETs) and the traditional wireless network regarding displacements, behaviour, energy, and connection bandwidth [1]. Hence, MANET routing standards will be appropriate for the nodes' features, such as node displacements, energy and bandwidth restrictions, network standards, and modifying the associations' quality. The routing standards in MANET are split into single and MRS. The nodes initiate a single route to each static target for single-path routing standards and append them into their routing tables. As

K. Pachiappan
Department of Computer Science and Engineering, Kongu Engineering College, Perundurai, Tamil Nadu, India

V. R. Vandadi
Department of Computer Science and Engineering, KSRM College of Engineering, YSR Kadapa, Andhra Pradesh, India

D. K. Sharma
Department of Mathematics, Jaypee University of Engineering and Technology, Guna, Madhya Pradesh, India

A. Kothalanka
Department of Computer Science and Engineering, Koneru Lakshmaiah Education Foundation, Guntur, Andhra Pradesh, India

S. Thangavel
Department of Computer Science and Engineering, GITAM School of Technology, GITAM (Deemed to be University), Bengaluru, India

S. Sengan (✉)
Department of Computer Science and Engineering, PSN College of Engineering and Technology, Tirunelveli, Tamil Nadu, India

P. Agarwal et al. (eds.), *Artificial Intelligence for Smart Healthcare*, EAI/Springer Innovations in Communication and Computing,
https://doi.org/10.1007/978-3-031-23602-0_29

a result, it is mandatory to reinitiate the routing schemes during path failure, thus delaying routing and bandwidth utilization of control packets within the routing protocols [2]. For addressing the issue, MRS is initiated, allowing for more than one route to the targets within the routing tables of MRS. During the failure of key paths, one of the false routes will be employed, and hence the packet communication and overheads in routing will be minimized. According to scholars, the feasible routes employing hop counts are not feasible for MANETs. The feasible path attempts to make use of connections that are closer to the centre of the networks. As a result, nodes at the center experience increased data communication loads estimated with nodes located far from the center [3]. Hence it might pave the way for traffic within the network. For instance, the AOMDV standard employs hop count as the routing parameter and does not use load equalization for relaying congestion. Therefore, the traffic created due to communication throughout the network centre remains a dispute [4].

Also, the routing parameters in MRS are constant, and they are not supple and autonomous during the assessment of QoS of congestion classes needed from the application layer [5, 6]. The ultimate goal is to design improvements in MRS that employ hop counts as a routing parameter to accomplish routing preferences in QoS prerequisites from the application layer's congestion classes. The designed scheme employs a cross-layer scheme to mine PLR and service EED of the MAC layer associations. Additionally, the categorization of congestion classes is performed based on the application layer to set up appropriate routing parameters for every congestion class by picking appropriate weights of routing parameters. The AOMDV standard is selected for improvements where the analysis is performed using NS-2, portraying that the designed scheme is improved from AOMDV termed QCLF.

2 Related Works

A new routing parameter termed C2WB is designed, conscious of the wireless networks' load and nosiness. The parameter is calculated based on the average contention window's values and medium usage of CSMA/CA network access schemes [7]. The OLSR standard is selected to combine the new parameter. The acquired outcomes are evaluated and assessed based on altered and actual OLSR using the NS-2 simulator, demonstrating that the altered standards are conscious and avert domains for enhancing abilities equalizing the congestion over the network. A new multipath routing mechanism termed Q–SMS is designed for resolving QoS issues. The designed fresh routing scheme calculates the link's remaining abilities and governs path demands, path reply, and maintenance with QoS. The assessment outcomes reveal that the Q–SMS behaviour is better than the prevailing SMS in minimized routing overheads, minimal EED, and increased throughput [8].

The path assurance unidirectional connection elimination and node energy based on the acquired signal potency is portrayed. These are the metrics for the cross-layered transmission among the physical, MAC, and network layers for enhancing mobile ad hoc networks [9, 10]. The routing standards based on traffic-conscious capabilities were designed. The standard is termed CARM, which employs a new routing parameter, a composition of the medium delays, the rate of information, the count of retransmissions, and buffer delays. Moreover, the standard simultaneously employs a new routing parameter based on averting schemes of the uneven connection-related information rate paths to acclimatize traffic regions and enhance the network's connection abilities.

A fresh scheme based on a cross-layered mechanism uses a fuzzy logic-based system where three layers for the cross-layered proposal are an application, data connection, and physical [11]. The fuzzy-based scheme employs the rate of effective packet communication, ground displacement, and connection delays as input metrics for estimating modification features employed to arrive at a conclusion employing the communication energy, rate of governance, retransmission time, and adjustable modulation and coding [12]. A review and entry governance scheme was employed in designing QoS-conscious features to fulfil QoS needs from real-time applications. The routing standards employ a rough bandwidth for assessing the congestion over the network. There are two bandwidth assessment schemes employed based on these for assessing the remaining bandwidth of nodes. The clustering mechanism splits the networks into groups, and the scheme limits congestion to these clusters based on the type of congestion communicated only within the groups [13]. The scheme is employed for planning the designed standard accomplishing improved behaviour based on the minimal EED, minimal energy utilization for the nodes, and high PDR [14].

The MANET employing TDMA is an analysis of QoS routing focusing on evaluating EED bandwidth over the paths initiated during path identification and employed for communicating congestion based on their requests QoS prerequisites [15–17]. The standard termed AMAODV employs a routing parameter designed from AODV standard employing hop counts as a routing parameter. The new routing parameter is estimated based on the size of queue data, hop count and distance, and the corresponding displacement from a node to their adjacencies [18]. The designed standard intends to locate paths with increased PDR and minimized EED in MANETs. The designed scheme employs the node's energy level analysis schemes, level of channel busy for initiating paths, and schemes for eradicating vulnerable nodes [19–21]. The behaviour assessment outcomes for the QoS standards and AODV standards portray that the designed standards accomplished minimal EED and increased PDR as evaluated against AODV [22–27].

2.1 Cross Layered QoS Routing

The EED and PLR are the key QoS metrics of congestion classes from the application layers [28–32]. Generating an assessment function for routing parameters and designing a routing standard fulfils the QoS prerequisites of congestion from the application layer, which requires calculating the PLR and EED values of every connection over the MAC layer and categorizing the congestion classes based on the QoS from the application layer [33].

2.2 Assessing the Rate of Packet Losses

Various schemes are prevailing for assessing the PLR for connections over the MAC layer [34–37]. The PLR is estimated based on the PLR, both the directions of connections prevailing among two nodes over a precise time instance. Presume a connection '*c*' prevails among nodes '*x*' and '*y*' where 'v_s' and 'v_r' are the effective PDR communication over the direction '*x*' to '*y*' and vice versa. The PLR of these connections is estimated based on Eq. (1):

$$\mathrm{ACC}_c = 1 - v_s\, v_r \tag{1}$$

Acknowledge communication will be used after forwarding episodic signal packets to assess the values of 'v_s' and 'v_r' based on Eq. 1 [38–43]. Furthermore, the scheme will utilize bandwidth and resources for processing. As a result, the usage of an effortless and efficient scheme termed as an anticipated count of communication (ACC) is portrayed. Every node prevailing episodically over '*i*' seconds relays a constant investigation package. The converse node estimates the number of investigation packets in '*t*' second over instant ($t > i$). The PDR communication over one direction is portrayed as the number of acquired investigated packets split based on the anticipated investigation packets ($^t/_i$) [44].

In executing the QCLF standard in NS-2, HELLO packets of the AOMDV standard are employed as an investigation packet to assess the values of 'v_s' and 'v_r'. The instance for replaying HELLO packets and counting acquired HELLO packets is 0 to 10 s. Relatively [45–49].

3 Assessing Connection Delays

The connection delays are unwavering based on the time-of-service facets initiated. Based on IEEE standard 802.11, the time required to communicate a MAC layer frame using a wireless connection effectively is regarded as the connections' service time. For the IEEE 802.11 standard, the delay is communicated as a frame in the MAC layer based on the scattered synchronization function followed by CSMA/CA policies. The time for effectively communicating a packet through a distributed wireless medium among two nodes processing over scattered synchronization function in MAC layer preceding CSMA/CA policies is estimated as the overall value of the backoff time, time of communication, and rescheduling time [50–55]. The backoff time is required to minimize the backoff counter value to zero during the medium's idle state. The time for communication is when the forwarding node initiates communicating a frame until it acquires an acknowledgment from the receiving node [56–59]. The rescheduling time is when a node desires to communicate a frame over the medium's active state. The value of the rescheduling counter does not differ during the rescheduled time [60].

Presume $I_{s,c}$, $I_{b,c}$, $I_{i,c}$, and $I_{r,c}$ symbolize the time of service, backoff time, and reschedule when communicating a frame using a connection 'c' correspondingly. The time of service is estimated using Eq. (2):

$$I_{s,c} = I_{b,c} + I_{i,c} + I_{r,c} \tag{2}$$

The $I_{s,c}$ is estimated as Eq. (3):

$$I_{s,c} = \frac{1}{1 \quad \mathrm{MU}_c}\left(\left(\mathrm{ACW} - \frac{\mathrm{CW}_{\min}}{2}\right)I_t + \frac{1}{1 \quad \mathrm{ACC}_c}\frac{\mathrm{FPL}}{b_u}\right) \tag{3}$$

Here, ACW represents the average contention window, $\mathrm{CW}_{\min}$ represents the initial contention window, I_t represents the instance time, ACC is the average count of communication over a communication 'c', FPL represents the size of the frame payload, b_u represents the utilization of bandwidth, and MU_c represents the medium utilization at the forwarding node of the connection [61]. The values of I_t and $\mathrm{CW}_{\min}$ are straightforwardly acquired from IEEE 802.11 planning at the MAC layer. The value of ACC is estimated based on Eq. 4. Presume that 'm' is the backoff phase of CSMA/CA planning the ACW is calculated as Eq. (4):

$$\mathrm{ACW} = \frac{(1-\mathrm{ACC}_c)(1-(2\mathrm{ACC}_c)^m)}{(1-2\mathrm{ACC}_c)(1-\mathrm{ACC}_c^m)}\mathrm{CW}_{\min} \tag{4}$$

The performance metrics of MU_c is the medium applied at node N_n is the rate to sense the active phase of the communication medium over the extended sensing time over the medium of the node. The value is calculated based on the CSMA/CA strategy planning at the MAC layer employing the active medium counter and the overall sensing medium counter. For planning, the value related to the frame payload's size based on Eq. 3 is 1600 *bytes*, and the ratio of information based on 802.11b connection is 10 Mbps. As a result, the medium sensing instance's initiation is 1 m, and the instance for revising the value of MU_c is 2 s.

Moreover, the assessment of MU_c as portrayed in the scheme is bothered based on the information load in the identical congestion flow (Table 1 and Fig. 1). Moreover, during the other nodes and the present nodes present over the identical range of other nodes, the utilization of wireless medium creates an active node. In contrast, the other nodes employ the medium to send that congestion to the target. Consequently, the dense congestion loads increase the command of affection over MU_c over nodes within the routes. For resolving the plan for MU_c, it is probable to revise the value of the sensing active medium counter that is not using the node N_n.

Table 1 Fixed values of QoS metrics

Fixed values	Type 1	Type 2	Type 3
Average EED	0.13 s	0.3 s	0.002 s
Jitter	0.0005 s	0.0005 s	NA
Rate of PLR	0.02 s	0.005 s	0
Information rate	3 kbps	15 kbps	18 kbps

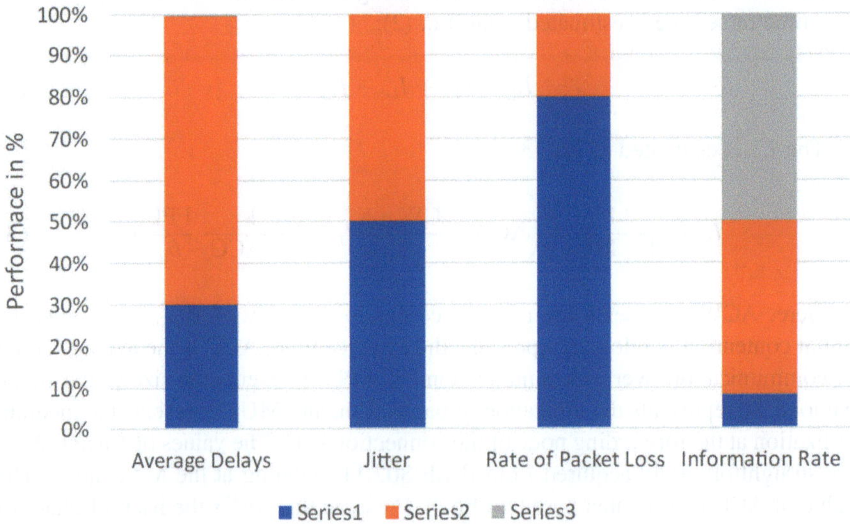

Fig. 1 Performance analysis of assessment of MU_c as portrayed

4 Purpose of Routing Parameters

As described afore, the intention is to improvise AOMDV standards for generating a path calibration that is static with QoS prerequisites in terms of congestion from the application layer based on assessing the values of PLR and average EED. Based on the equations and assessing the values of PLR and EED, everyone links the PLR, and average paths are the duplication and addition of PLR and EED of each connection dedicated to that path. The assessments areas, Eqs. (5, 6):

$$P_l = 1 - \prod_{c \in p} (1 - \mathrm{ACC}_c) \tag{5}$$

$$A_d = \sum_{c \in p} I_{s,c} \tag{6}$$

Here, P_l and A_d are the PLR and path delays. *'p'* symbolizes the path, and ACC_c and $I_{s,c}$ symbolize the PLR and EED of every connection over path *'p'* relatively. The ACC_c and $I_{s,c}$ are estimated based on Eqs. (1) and (2).

Table 2 Weights of QoS metrics

Weights for	Type 1	Type 2	Type 3
Average EED	0.5245	0.0658	0.1003
Jitter	0.2589	0.1869	0.0356
Rate of PLR	0.1003	0.5989	0.6023
Information rate	0.04897	0.1112	0.2154

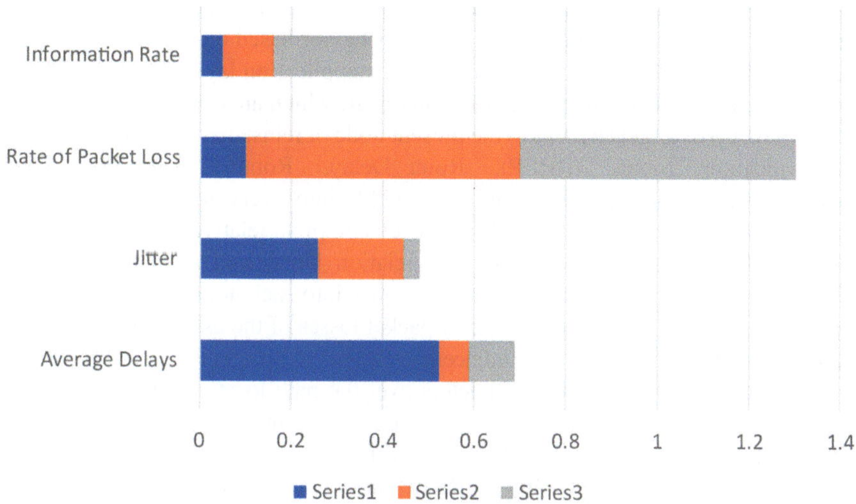

Fig. 2 PLR and EED of the path

The initiating of a path parameter over a path that is appropriate with QoS prerequisites for congestion communicated from the application layer employing QoS varieties for which a path parameter value (PPV) for the communication path is designed as Eq. (7):

$$\mathrm{PPV}_{p,i} = l_{a_d}\frac{A_{d_{s,i}}}{A_{d_p}} + l_{p_l}\frac{P_{l_{s,i}}}{P_{l_p}} \tag{7}$$

Here, P_{1p} and A_{dp} are the PLR and EED of the path, estimated based on Eq. (5) and WQU (6). $Pl_{s,i}$ and $A_{ds,i}$ represent the fixed value of the PLR and EED of the ith congestion variety where the values of decision are based on Table 2 and Fig. 2. l_{ad} and l_{pi} represent loads of EED and PLR of the ith congestion variety as portrayed in Table 2.

5 QoS Forwarding

The QCLF standard is designed based on the MRS AOMDV, based on which the QCLF takes over the techniques from AOMDV standards like path location schemes, prevailing routes, and path fault warning. The heritage assures the process of MRS. The objective is to design an improved AOMDV standard called QCLF Data Packet EED, and Data Packet PLR is the two fields appended using RREP packets, in order to achieve effective routing behavior based on QoS basic requirements in EED and PLR for congestion from the application layer. These two fields comprise relative values of average EED and PLR, which are estimated either using origin (RREQ) or target (RREP) to the present node of reinstated routes (RREQ) and communication routes (RREP). Route_Delay, Route_Packet Loss, and Route_Constancy are appended into three fields into every route over the route directory within the routing table. These fields comprise relative values of average EED, the PLR, and route constancy. Association_Delay and Association_Packet LOSS are the two fields appended for every entry into each node's adjacency table. These fields' values are delay and rate of packet losses of the association prevailing among the present node and their adjacencies.

Substituting hop count path parameters over the path location task is employed for various congestion varieties by the path parameter, which is decided based on the PPV function. The process of QCLF standard for the routing layer is portrayed as, upon a node acquiring an RREQ or RREP packet soon after generating a fresh/revising route directory of the entry with the target as the origin (reinstated route) or target (communication path) the node locates Association_EED and Association_PLR of the adjacent node from their adjacency table and re-estimates the values of Route_EED, Route_PLR for the routes as, Eqs. (8) and (9).

$$\text{Association}_{\text{delay}} = \text{Association}_{\text{delay}} + \text{Data Packet}_{\text{delay}} \tag{8}$$

$$\text{Route}_{\text{rpl}} = 1 - \left(1 - \text{Association}_{\text{rpl}}\right) \text{ x } \left(1 - \text{Route}_{\text{rpl}}\right) \tag{9}$$

If the node communicates an RREQ/RREP packet, it will revise the value of relative Data Packet_EED and Data Packet_PLR, employing the value of the Association_EED and Association_PLR that are fresh re-estimated. The Route_Constancy value will be incremented by one upon a node revising its routing table during the route's presence, and the Route_Constancy value will be incremented by one. The initial value of Route_Constancy is one when the node appends the new route into its routing table. Upon acquiring several RREP packets forwarded from the identical target nodes using several routes, the acquiring node arranges these routes in a climbing order of values of the routing parameters assessed based on the PPV functions.

Soon after the routes and accomplishing the actions, only up to three routes to the identical targets will be recorded into the routing table. The route with the highest PPV value will be chosen as the key route, along with two routes that will stay outmoded. The support route is employed only when the key route is retarded or ruined. The route with a higher value of Route_Constancy will be chosen to communicate the congestion during the two routes, the similar PPV values. For two routes with similar values of PPV and ROUTE_CONSTANCY, the route with suitable parameters as input will be chosen for communicating the congestion. Type 1/Type 2 congestions are chosen for the route with minimal Route_EED. For Type 3 congestion, the selected route is one holding minimal Route_PLR.

6 Performance Analysis

For estimating the behaviour of the designed QCLC standard, NS-2 is employed for experimenting with AOMDV and QCLF standards. The assessment metrics are selected for emphasizing their QoS routine schemes for several application congestion types. The assessment is accomplished in a square region comprised of a 2000 m side length. The network's size differs from 15 nodes to 25, 35, and 50 nodes, along with the congestion loads being 20%, 40%, 60%, and 80% per every size of the network. The chosen scheme for physical and MAC layers is IEEE 802.11b within 250 ms nodes range of communication.

6.1 Results and Discussion

The communication design investigates the node's primary matrices to ensure the path presence. Within the matrix, all the nodes will displace arbitrarily with displacements at 10 ms. The assessment extent is 100 s, and every source node initiates its congestion during its 5th sec. The chosen congestion prototype is CBR, and the UDP is chosen for the transport layer. The designed and the AOMDV standard behaviour is estimated over Type 1/Type 2 congestions based on assessing the CBR congestion working at 64 and 150 kbps data rates.

- *Metrics for Assessing Performance:* The performance of QCLF and AOMDV standards is assessed based on the stated parameters.
- *Average Delays:* The average EED of the packet communication from the source to the target is measured in ms.
- *Throughput:* It is the average communication rate for the information packets, and its unit for measurement is kbps.
- *Congestion Overhead:* The number of standard governance packets per number of information packets acquired and standards governance packets.
- *Rate of Packet Delivery:* The number of packets acquired by the target node per the number of forwarded packets forwarded by the origin node.

6.2 Average Delays

The average EED of Type 1/Type 2 congestions based on assessing 35 nodes congestion loading at 20%, 40%, 60%, and 80% is portrayed in Fig. 3. The outcomes reveal that the chosen route for congestion types of QCLF standard is constant and advisable than the AOMDV standard. It was evident that the QCLF requires additional time for processing its governance packets during the assessment of their routing parameter. The average EED of these two types of congestion sent by the QCLF standard is minimal than the AOMDV standard.

6.3 Network Throughput

For assessing the average throughput of Type 2 congestion, the network's size is modified as 15, 25, 35, and 50 nodes, and the congestion load is 20% and 80%. Figure 4 portrays that the QCLF standard accomplishes increased PDR compared to the AOMDV standards. During the assessment, the execution of 15 and 25 nodes, the QCLF standard accomplishes the average PDR of 20% congestion load roughly for Type 2 congested rate of information. The accomplished average PDR of both the standards is decreased for the congestion load and the network's increased size, but the QCLF standard still holds increased PDR than the AOMDV standard.

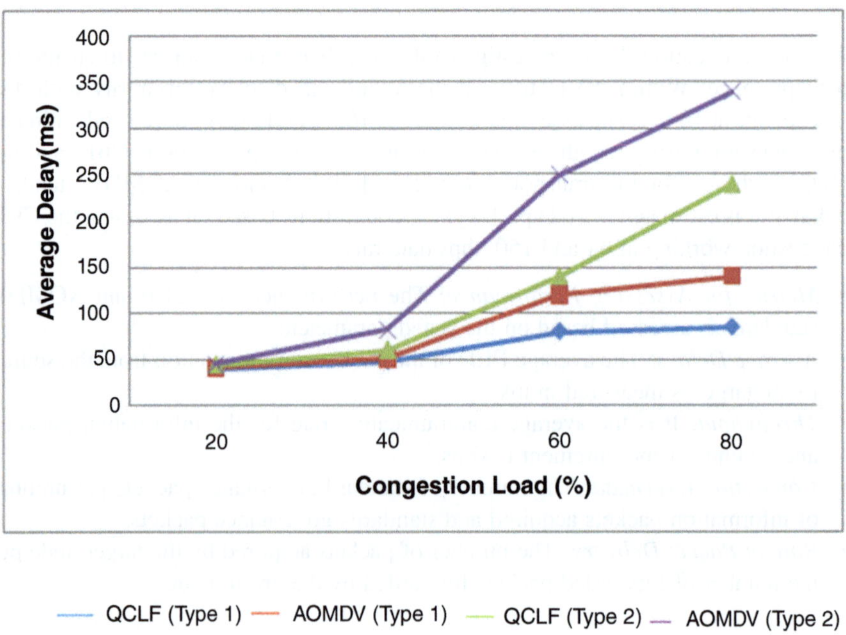

Fig. 3 Average delays

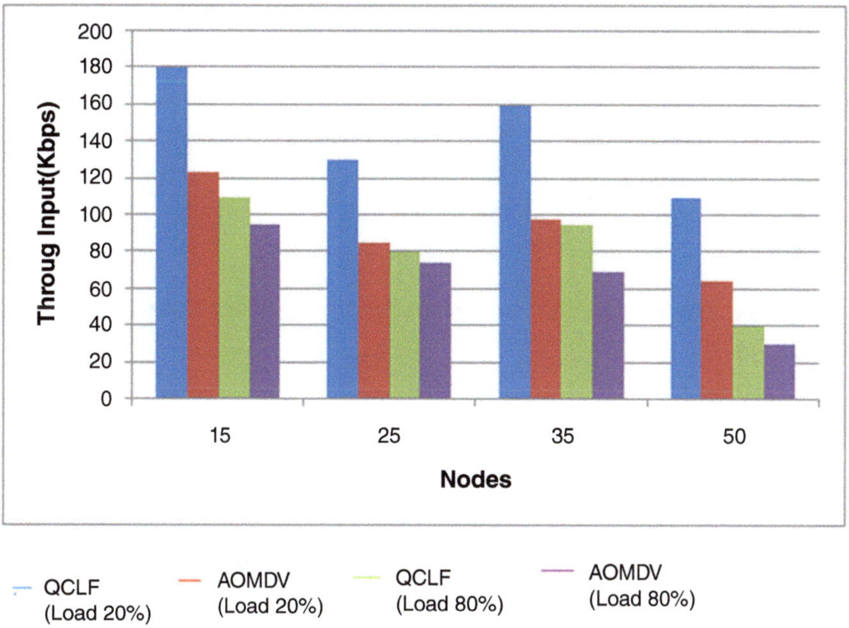

Fig. 4 Network PDR

7 Rate of Packet Delivery

The PDR for QCLF and AOMDV standards during the varied congestion loads from 20% to 80% of 35 nodes for Types 1/Type 2 is portrayed in Fig. 5. The QCLF accomplishes a high PDR than the AOMDV standards for both types of congestion. The PDR of type 1 congestion of these two standards is nearly unaltered while attempting the congestion loads. For Type 2, the rate diminishes with the increase in congestion load. The PDR for QCLF is minimal than that of AOMDV. The outcomes show that the QCLF standard acquires improved responsibilities against the congestion load differences than the AOMDV standards.

8 Congestion Overheads

For assessment, the network size is 15, 25, 35, and 50, with 80% of the congestion load. Type 1 congestion is employed for calculating the congestion overheads for QCLF and AOMDV standards. Figure 6 portrays improved outcomes for the designed QCLF standards as estimated against the AOMDV standards. The number of governance packets created by the QCLF standard is minimal than AOMDV. The

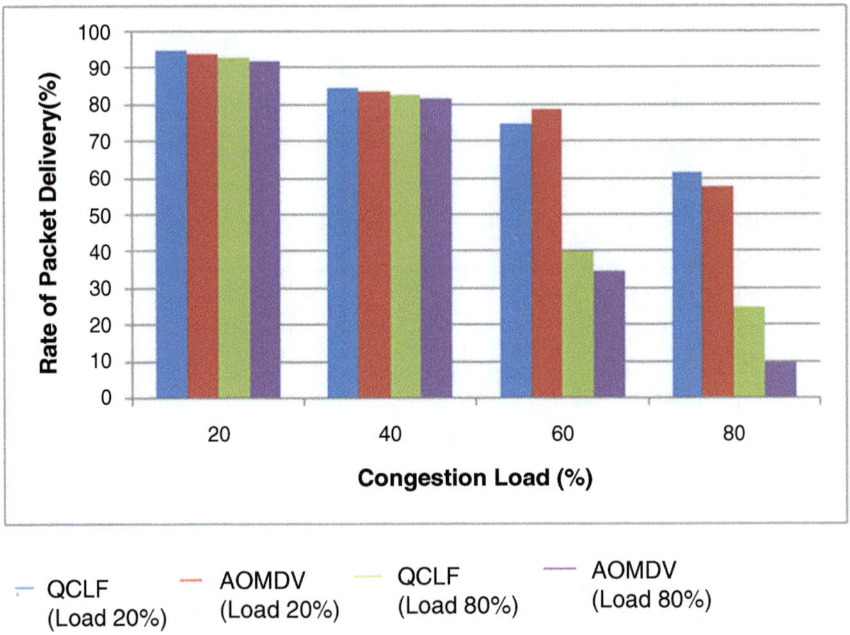

Fig. 5 Performance analysis of PDR

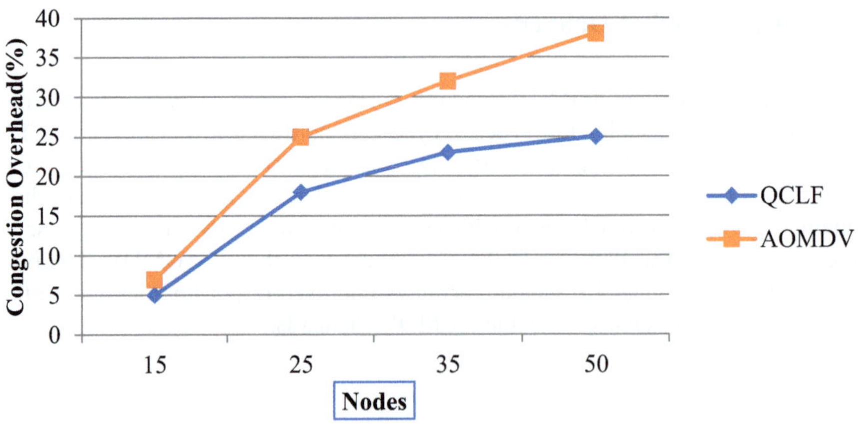

Fig. 6 Congestion overheads

outcomes reveal that QCLF standards are located and employ improved constancy than the AOMDV standard. Hence with the modifications in network standards, the number of path locations for QCLF standards is minimal than that of the AOMDV standard.

9 Conclusion

The intention is to enhance the behaviour of MRS by employing the path parameters initiated based on the hop counts. The improvement is based on categorizing congestion from the application layers into congestion types of QoS prerequisites and creating path parameters appropriate for described congestion types. For initiating the path parameters, a cross-layered scheme is employed to gather the PLR and link delays from the MAC layer of the routing layer and the target port of socket packets from the application layer. Moreover, the QoS routing parameter's assessment task is allocated pairs of weights suitable to their QoS prerequisites. An improved AOMDV-MRS termed QCLF can locate multipath and differentiable QoS for the communicated congestion and function over various layers. The behaviour assessment of AOMDV and QCLF standards is evaluated using NS-2, representing that the designed QCLF has improved average EED, effective PDR communication, and congestion overhead. Though there prevail four QoS metrics, the focus is only over two metrics termed the PLR and EED. Moreover, the routing parameter is initiated and employed for the QCLF standard, which does not alter erratically based on the application layers' jitter and information rate metrics. Furthermore, the energy utilization level shall be considered while evaluating these two routing standards' performances since the designed routing standards are intricate in assessing the dynamic nodes against AOMDV standards.

References

1. Ajaltouni H, Pazzi R.W, Boukerche A.: An efficient QoS MAC for IEEE 802.11p over cognitive multichannel vehicular networks, in Communications, *IEEE International Conference on.*, 413–417, (2012).
2. Alghamdi T.A. Route optimization to improve QoS in multi-hop wireless sensor networks. *Wireless Netw* (2020).
3. Banerjee and M. P.: A Perusal of Energy Efficient and Secure Multi-CH based Clustering Routing Protocol with enhanced QoSP for Wireless Sensor Network, IEEE *International Women in Engineering (WIE) Conference on Electrical and Computer Engineering*, 376–379, (2020).
4. Carrascal Frias S, Diaz Delgado G, Zavala Ayala A, Aguilar Igartua M.: MM-DSR: multipath QoS routing for multiple multimedia sources over ad hoc mobile networks, *IEEE Lat. Am. Trans.*, 5 (6), 448–456, (2007).
5. Kandris D, Tsagkaropoulos M, Politi I, Tzes A, Kotsopoulos S.: Energy-efficient and perceived QoS aware video routing over wireless multimedia sensor networks, *Ad Hoc Networks,* 9 (4), 591–607, (2011).
6. Liang H, Yang S, Li Li and Gao J.: Research on routing optimization of WSNs based on improved LEACH protocol. *EURASIP Journal on Wireless Communications and Networking*,194, 1–12, (2019).
7. Lindsey S and Raghavendra C.: PEGASIS: Power-efficient gathering in sensor information systems. *IEEE Aerospace Conference Proceedings*, 3, 1125–1130, (2002).
8. Malone Dm Clifford P, Leith D.J.: MAC layer channel quality measurement in 802.11, *IEEE Communications Letters*, 11 (2), 143–145, (2007).

9. Renesse R.D, Friderikos V, Aghvami H.: Cross-layer cooperation for accurate admission control decisions in mobile ad hoc networks, *IET Commun.*, 1 (4), 577–586, (2007).
10. Sharma A, Kumar R and Kaur P.: Study of issues and challenges of different routing protocols in wireless sensor network, *IEEE 5th International Conference on Image Information Processing,* (2019).
11. Singh R, Kumar S and Kathuria A. K.: Secure routing protocols for wireless sensor networks. ICCCA, 1–5, IEEE: *Piscataway*, (2019).
12. Sinha P, Sivakumar R, Bharghavan V.: CEDAR: A core extraction distributed ad hoc routing algorithm, *IEEE Journal on Selected Areas in Communications*, 17 (8), 1454–1466, (1999).
13. Wu R.: A novel cluster-based routing protocol in wireless multimedia sensor network, in Proceedings of the *4th IEEE International Conference on Broadband Network and Multimedia Technology*, Shenzhen, China, October, 126–129, (2011).
14. Zaman N, Low T. J and Alghamdi T.: Enhancing routing energy efficiency of wireless sensor networks. 17th *International Conference on Advanced Communication Technology.* Piscataway: IEEE. (2015).
15. S. Sudhakar and S. Chenthur Pandian "Secure packet encryption and key exchange system in mobile ad hoc network", *Journal of Computer Science*, vol. 8, no. 6, pp. 908–912, (2012).
16. S. Sudhakar and S. Chenthur Pandian, "Hybrid cluster-based geographical routing protocol to mitigate malicious nodes in mobile ad hoc network", *International Journal of Ad Hoc and Ubiquitous Computing,* vol. 21 no. 4, pp. 224–236, (2016).
17. A. U. Priyadarshni and S. Sudhakar, "Cluster-based certificate revocation by cluster head in mobile ad-hoc network", *International Journal of Applied Engineering Research,* vol. 10, no. 20, pp. 16014–16018, (2015).
18. S. Sudhakar and S. Chenthur Pandian, "Investigation of attribute aided data aggregation over dynamic routing in wireless sensor," *Journal of Engineering Science and Technology,* vol. 10, no. 11, pp. 1465–1476, (2015).
19. S. Sudhakar and S. Chenthur Pandian, "Trustworthy position-based routing to mitigate against the malicious attacks to signifies secured data packet using geographic routing protocol in MANET", *WSEAS Transactions on Communications*, vol. 12, no. 11, pp. 584–603, (2013).
20. K. Karthikayan, Dr. Siva Agora Sakthivel Murugan, Rathish C. R, Natraj N.A, A Triband Slotted Bow-Tie Antenna for Wireless Applications, *International Journal of Computational Engineering Research*, Volume 3, Issue 7, Pages 31–35 (2013).
21. CR Rathish & A Rajaram, Hierarchical Load Balanced Routing Protocol for Wireless Sensor Networks, *International Journal of Applied Engineering Research*, Volume 10, Issue 7, Pages 16521–16534 (2015).
22. Siva Agora Sakthivel Murugan, K. Karthikayan, Natraj N.A, Rathish C.R, Speckle Noise Removal Using Dual Tree Complex Wavelet Transform, *International Journal of Scientific & Technology Research*, Volume 2, Issue 8, Pages 4 (2013).
23. A. Sagai Francis Britto C. R. Rathish, C. Saravana Murthi, J. Indirapriyadharshini, Deepak V, A Novel and Effective Method for Automatic Paper Trimming and Cutting process in Paper Industries, *International Journal of Advanced Science and Technology*, Volume 29, Issue 6, Pages 4136–4143 (2020).
24. Rathish Radhakrishnan & Karpagavadivu Karuppusamy, Cost Effective Energy Efficient Scheme for Mobile Adhoc Network, *International Journal of Computing*, Volume 19, Issue 1, Pages 137–146 (2020).
25. Renuka J Bathi, Sameena Parveen, Neeraj Taneja, Oral Tuberculous Ulcer - A Report of Two Cases, *Journal of Indian Academy of Oral Medicine and Radiology*, Volume 15, Issue 2, Pages 62–65 (2003).
26. Sameena Parveen, Impact of Calorie Restriction and Intermittent Fasting on Periodontal Health, *Periodontology* 2000, Volume 87, Issue 1, Pages 315–324 (2021).
27. T. Radhika K Mohideen, C Krithika, N Jeddy, S Parveen, A Meta-Analysis in Assessing Oxidative Stress Using Malondialdehyde in Oral Submucous Fibrosis, *European Journal of Dentistry*, (2021).

28. Parveen S Taneja N, R Bathi, Serum Glycoproteins as Prognosticator in Head and Neck Cancer Patients - A Follow Up Study, *Oral Oncology Head and Neck Oncology*, Vol. 47 (2011).
29. Parveen S. Bathi R, Taneja N, Dermoid Cyst in The Floor of The Mouth-A Case Report, *Karnataka State Dental Journal*, Vol. 25, Issue 2, pages 52–54 (2006).
30. P. Manta et al., "Optical density optimization of malaria pan rapid diagnostic test strips for improved test zone band intensity," *Diagnostics (Basel),* vol. 10, no. 11, p. 880, (2020).
31. P. Manta, S. Chandra Singh, A. Deep, and D. N. Kapoor, "Temperature-regulated gold nanoparticle sensors for immune chromatographic rapid test kits with reproducible sensitivity: a study," *IET Nanobiotechnol.*, no. nbt2.12024, (2021).
32. P. Manta, R. Chauhan, H. Gandhi, S. Mahant, and D. N. Kapoor, "Formulation rationale for the development of SARS-COV-2 immunochromatography rapid test kits in India," *J. Appl. Pharm.* Sci (2021). DOI: https://doi.org/10.7324/JAPS.2021.1101017.
33. P. Manta, N. Wahi, A. Bharadwaj, G. Kour, and D. N. Kapoor, "A statistical quality control (SQC) methodology for gold nanoparticles based immune-chromatographic rapid test kits validation," *Nanosci. Nanotechnol.-Asia*, vol. 11, no. 6, pp. 1–5, (2021).
34. P. Manta et al., "Analytical approach for the optimization of desiccant weight in rapid test kit packaging: Accelerated predictive stability (APS)," *Systematic Reviews in Pharmacy,* vol. 11, no. 8, pp. 102–113, (2020).
35. P. Manta, D. N. Kapoor, G. Kour, M. Kour, and A. K. Sharma, "critical quality attributes of rapid test kits - a practical overview," *Journal of Critical Reviews,* vol. 7, no. 19, pp. 377–384, (2020).
36. Saritha Kodithal, Murali R, and Srinivasan N, "Pharmocognostical and phytochemical evaluation of stem of Artabotrys odoratissimus.(roxb.)r.br.(Annonaceae)," *International Journal of Research in Pharmaceutical Sciences,* vol. 12, no. 1, pp. 815–821, (2021).
37. K. Kavitha, S. Mohan, N. Srinivasan, R. Suresh, and S. Vismaya, "Insilico study of quinazoline-4-one on sars-cov 3cl protease," *World Journal of Pharmaceutical and Life Sciences,* vol. 7, no. 5, pp. 90–96, (2021).
38. Sumathy, R. Suresh, N. L. Gowrishankar, and N. Srinivasan, "In-silico Screening of a Core Scaffold Pyrazolone Fused Heterocyclic Analogues as Potent Biological Agent.," *Indian Journal of Natural Sciences*, vol. 12, no. 65, pp. 30668–30674, (2021).
39. P. Pandian and N. Srinivasan, "Anticoagulant properties from Marine Algae – a systemic review," *International Journal of Research in Pharmaceutical Sciences*, vol. 12, no. 2, pp. 1529–1538, (2021).
40. T. Bencybaby, R. Murali, T. N. K. Suriyaprakash, and N. Srinivasan, "A review on pancreatic lipase inhibitors from natural sources: A potential target for obesity," *Current Enzyme Inhibition*, vol. 17, no. 2, pp. 83–97, (2021).
41. Sathya Prabha, N. Srinivasan, K. T. Manisenthil Kumar, and S. Aravindh, "Evaluation of clinical characteristics and knowledge in inflammatory bowel disease patients," *Journal of Evolution of Medical and Dental Sciences*, vol. 10, no. 29, pp. 2202–2207, (2021).
42. S. Dhanalakshmi, N. Harikrishnan, N. Janani, P. Shakthi Priya, M. Srinivasan, A. karthikeyan, A. Anishkumar, R. Harinathan, and N. Srinivasan, "The overview: Recent studies on endometrial cancer," *Research Journal of Pharmacy and Technology,* vol. 14, no. 7, pp. 3998–4002, (2021).
43. K. Kavitha, N. Srinivasan, S. Mohan, and R. Suresh, "Insilco design and potential cytotoxic agents EGFR inhibitors of 4(3h) quinazolinone derivatives," Research *Journal of Pharmacy and Technology*, vol. 14, no. 9, pp. 4849–4855, (2021).
44. Sumathy, R. Suresh, N. L. Gowrishankar, and N. Srinivasan, "Design, synthesis and evaluation of core scaffold pyrazolone fused thiazolidinone derivatives as anticancer agents," *Journal of Pharmaceutical Research International*, vol. 33, no. 31B, pp. 217–227, (2021).
45. K. Saritha, R. Murali, N. Srinivasan, and Sorabh kumar agarwal, "Anti-fertility activity of leaves and Stem parts of Artabotrys odoratissimus. (roxb.) R.Br. Annonaceae." *Journal of Medical Pharmaceutical and Allied Sciences*, vol. 10, no. 5, pp. 3524–3528, (2021).

46. O. M. Abo-Seida, N. T. M. El-dabe, A. Refaie Ali and G. A. Shalaby, "Cherenkov FEL Reaction With Plasma-Filled Cylindrical Waveguide in Fractional D-Dimensional Space," in *IEEE Transactions on Plasma Science*, vol. 49, no. 7, pp. 2070–2079, (2021).
47. Jain, A., Dwivedi, R., Kumar, A., & Sharma, S. Scalable design and synthesis of 3D mesh network on chip. In Proceeding of International Conference on Intelligent Communication, *Control and Devices*, pp. 661–666 (2017). Springer, Singapore.
48. Osama M. Abo-Seida, N.T.M. Eldabe, Ahmed Refaie Ali, & Gamil. Ali Shalaby. Far-Field, Radiation Resistance and temperature of Hertzian Dipole Antenna in Lossless Medium with Momentum and Energy Flow in the Far- Zone. *Journal of Advances in Physics,* 18, 20–28 (2020).
49. N.T.M. El-Dabe, A. Refaie Ali, A.A. El-shekhipy, Influence of Thermophoresis on Unsteady MHD Flow of Radiation Absorbing Kuvshinski Fluid with Non-Linear Heat and Mass Transfer, *American Journal of Heat and Mass Transfer* (2017), DOI: https://doi.org/10.7726/ajhmt.2017.1010
50. Osama M. Abo-Seida, N.T.M.Eldabe, M. Abu-Shady, A. Refaie Ali, " Electromagnetic non-Darcy Forchheimer flow and heat transfer over a nonlinearly stretching sheet of non-Newtonian fluid in the presence of a non-uniform heat source', *Solid State Technology*, Vol. 63 No. 6 (2020).
51. Jain, A., Gahlot, A. K., Dwivedi, R., Kumar, A., & Sharma, S. K. Fat Tree NoC Design and Synthesis. *In Intelligent Communication, Control and Devices*, pp. 1749–1756. Springer, Singapore (2018).
52. Jain, A., Kumar, A., & Sharma, S. (2015). Comparative Design and Analysis of Mesh, Torus and Ring NoC. *Procedia Computer Science*, 48, 330–337 (2015).
53. N.T. El-dabel; A.Refaie Ali; A. El-shekhipy, A.; and A. Shalaby, G. "Non-Linear Heat and Mass Transfer of Second Grade Fluid Flow with Hall Currents and Thermophoresis Effects," *Applied Mathematics & Information Sciences*: Vol. 11 : Iss. 1, Article 73 (2017).
54. G. S and S. R. Raja.T, "A Comprehensive Survey on Alternating Fluids Used For The Enhancement of Power Transformers," *2021 IEEE International Conference on the Properties and Applications of Dielectric Materials*, pp. 57–60 (2021).
55. Sharma, S. K., Jain, A., Gupta, K., Prasad, D., & Singh, V. An internal schematic view and simulation of major diagonal mesh network-on-chip. *Journal of Computational and Theoretical Nanoscience*, 16(10), 4412–4417 (2019).
56. Ghai, D., Gianey, H. K., Jain, A., & Uppal, R. S. Quantum and dual-tree complex wavelet transform-based image watermarking. *International Journal of Modern Physics B*, 34(04), 2050009 (2020).
57. Jain, A., & Kumar, A. Desmogging of still smoggy images using a novel channel prior. *Journal of Ambient Intelligence and Humanized Computing*, 12(1), 1161–1177 (2021).
58. Kumar, S., Jain, A., Shukla, A. P., Singh, S., Raja, R., Rani, S., ... & Masud, M. A Comparative Analysis of Machine Learning Algorithms for Detection of Organic and Nonorganic Cotton Diseases. *Mathematical Problems in Engineering*, (2021).
59. Misra, N. R., Kumar, S., & Jain, A. A Review on E-waste: Fostering the Need for Green Electronics. In *2021 International Conference on Computing, Communication, and Intelligent Systems,* pp. 1032–1036. IEEE (2021).
60. Jain, A., AlokGahlot, A. K., & RakeshDwivedi, S. K. S. (2017). Design and FPGA Performance Analysis of 2D and 3D Router in Mesh NoC. *International Journal of Control Theory and Applications*, ISSN, 0974-5572 (2017).
61. Agrawal, N., Jain, A., & Agarwal, A. Simulation of Network on Chip for 3D Router Architecture. *International Journal of Recent Technology and Engineering*, 8, 58–62 (2019).

Spoof Attacks Detection Based on Authentication of Multimodal Biometrics Face-ECG Signals

Azmi Shawkat Abdulbaqi, Anfal Nawfal Ahmed Turki, Ahmed J. Obaid, Soumi Dutta, and Ismail Yusuf Panessai

1 Introduction

In recent years, the implementation of biometric technologies has enhanced and reached a plateau to keep the nation. Multi-national companies are secure and physically restricted via preserving people and resources [1]. Biometrics can collect images and signals as a body feature, calculate them, and then use them as proof of who you are? The biometric techniques provided nevertheless hamper the following customs [2]. (1) Age of the individual, different lighting conditions, facial expressions, poses, or direction might complicate the process of face identification [3]. (2) People's voices may be readily duplicated (i.e. recorded tape records), and people can change their voice if they have pneumonia or bronchitis, disease,

A. S. Abdulbaqi (✉) · Anfal N. A. Turki
Department of Computer Science, College of Computer Science and Information Technology, University of Anbar, Ramadi, Iraq
e-mail: azmi_msc@uoanbar.edu.iq; aa92oo88nn@gmail.com

Anfal N. A. Turki
Department of Computer Science, College of Computer Science and Information Technology, University of Anbar, Ramadi, Iraq

A. J. Obaid
Faculty of Computer Science and Mathematics, University of Kufa, Kufa, Iraq
e-mail: ahmedj.aljanaby@uokufa.edu.iq

S. Dutta
Institute of Engineering & Management, Kolkata, India
e-mail: soumi.dutta@iemcal.com

I. Y. Panessai
Faculty of Art, Computing and Creative Industry, Sultan Idris University, Tanjong Malim, Malaysia
e-mail: ismailyusuf@fskik.upsi.edu.my

P. Agarwal et al. (eds.), *Artificial Intelligence for Smart Healthcare*,
EAI/Springer Innovations in Communication and Computing,
https://doi.org/10.1007/978-3-031-23602-0_30

weariness, tiredness, surgery, or combinations. Age may also lead to voice alterations. (3) Only a few persons are now recognized in the DNA molecular structures. The Polymerase Chain Reaction (PCR) is used to generate DNA designs [4]. Identifying the kind of DNA will require a great deal of effort and time. DNA samples are readily contaminated and difficult to manage and keep. (4) Sometimes fingerprints are reduced of people working in chemicals. If fingerprints use, then the following materials will be for spoofing; silicone, plaster, dental moldering, gelatin, Playdoh, Gummy Bears Target brand, Silly Putty, Rose Art modeling clay, Crayola Model Magic Soft, and Spongy Modeling Matrix, are the following materials for spoofing. The fingerprints can be reproduced and used to get the right of admission to safety information wherever [5]. (5) Direct attacks and spoofing are major problems in face biometrics. (6) Some biometrics are sensitive to loud or poor data, such as noisy audio records and identical twins, which facial algorithms cannot easily distinguish. But the ECG signals cannot be accessed by anybody, as they're safe inside the heart. Input to the direct assaults and spoofing this manuscript is valuable. VDM counteractions against directives are conceivable. ECG is a new model utilized for VDM and additional biometric modalities to increase facial authentication system performance [6, 7]. The manuscript was organized as follows. The various face spoofing, ECG biometrics, and its discussions are reviewed in Sect. 2; Section 3 gives the existing methods and drawbacks. Section 4 describes the proposed methods and their advantages. Finally, Sects. 5 and 6 provide experimental results and conclusions, respectively.

2 Review of Related Literature

The world of automation and technology is human safety via recognition. However, scientists have worked to identify biometrically by fingerprints, retina, and facet detection. Still, in recent years biometric recognition has been a priority with biological signals. Authors in [8] took ECG signals from 49 individuals during two sessions for biometric identification. Their Equal Error Rate (EER) is 2.4% in the first session, while the EER in the longer-range session is 9%. Cardiac sounds identify people via cardiac sound frequency analysis [9]. Authors utilize a dataset of 20 people, and the proposed system can detect the real identities with 5% error and 2.2% error rate fake identities. CEPSTRAL Mel Frequency Features (MFCCs) recognize persons with cardiac sounds [3]. The authors utilized 13 MFCCs with an EER of around 9 percent to differentiate between the Hearts. In [10], authors utilized a template-coinciding approach for Discrete Cosine Transform (DCT) and Linear Discriminant Analysis (LDA). The experiments were carried through using a 100% and 95.8% AC/LDA without integration, 96.3% and 88.9% using an AC/DCT method with the integration of template matches, and 96.6% and 100% using the AC/LDA model with the integration of the template matches, respectively, with 96.3% and 86.3% without integration. The authors utilized Ziv-Merhav cross-screening algorithms in [11] for a non-conscious approach to discriminate between

ECG signals recorded by 19 healthy people with an accuracy of 100%. In [12], the authors utilized ECG to detect 120 people in a data pool of MIT-BIH. Wavelet coefficient characteristics are retrieved for the Nearest Middle Classifier (NMC) train and 98.99% LDA classifiers. ECG was utilized for recognition in [13] authors. They utilized autocorrelation (AC) for extracting functionality and Walsh-Hadamard for transforming functions. Then they reached an ID rate of around 95% with LDA and 97% using the QT data set. Then, they achieved 95% with LDA. In [14], authors utilized ECG for biometric identification using EMD, and they obtained 95% exacting with the MIT-BIH database 90 subject K-NN classifier. For biometric identification, heart sounds are used [15]. The author employed a strong feature extraction system and achieved an accuracy of around 99% in her early test with 128 heart sounds of 128 people. They later experiment with 1000 core sounds of 10 people to reach 96% accuracy. In [16], the authors used a lead-ECG recognition to extract the trust's characteristics using a PTB database of 100 records, combining them with Finite Impulse Response (FIR) to obtain a greater detection accuracy of 97.12%. In [17], authors were utilized to classify various ECG signals from ECG-ID and MIDTB datasets using recurring neural networks (RNN). Their classification accuracy is around 100%. No feature extraction is required for RNN. In [18], chest sensors were utilized by authors to remove the ECG signals from our participants within 6 hours of their daily work per subject, and the recommended technique of EER is from around 6 to 13%. Authors [19] utilized brain signals for biometric recognition from electroencephalogram (EEG). Common spatial patterns are utilized for training the LDA classification and are approximately 96.67% accurate. The use of EEG in biometric identification was also found in another study [20]. Transform wavelet is utilized as a MI/I EEG database feature extraction technique, achieving a 98.24% identification rate and a 93.28% accuracy using the UCI database. The classifications of ECG signals for biometric recognition are based on parallel 2D CNN [21]. Functions from AC/DCT will be retrieved and then scored. Fusion achieved an accuracy of classification and identification of 88.57% and 90.48% for 42 individuals.

3 Biometric System Attacks Patterns

It is easier to utilize biometric systems since there is no password to remember. Various accounts may be safeguarded in a single biometric feature without the stress of password recording [22]. Compared with traditional systems, biometric technologies provide considerable advantages but are prone to attack. These points of attack are classified into two categories: direct attack and indirect attack:

3.1 Direct Attack Pattern

It refers to assaults without understanding the system function, such as matching algorithms, vector format, etc. Only attacks called a "sensor attack" are included [23].

3.2 Indirect Attack Pattern

Unlike direct attacks, these attacks require information about the inside working of the authentication system to successfully attack [24].

4 Current Techniques and Its Restrictions

Firstly, individual modal systems make a single modality identification. Different problems include loud, individuality, non-universality, high spoof rate, high fault rate, and direct and VDM assaults single biometric systems [25]. Confidentiality and unfairness, cancellable biometrics, and the risk posed to the holder of secured products are obstructed in current biometric communities. The motives for these assaults are to convert their distinctiveness, violence, illegal activities, and fraud to change a genuine person's identity by using any of the spoofing techniques listed above [26]. Secondly, biometrics will grow on each other without a defined plan to enable the research but will lag behind the market. A novel technique is proposed to correct this problem [29]. Multimodal biometrics must be applied to overcome this discomfort in biometrics systems of the Single Modal system and enhance biometric safety performance. The use of multimodal biometric technologies can resolve these borders. Face-ECG is the first type internationally and offers excellent identification performance and great anti-spoofing properties [27, 28].

5 The Proposed Techniques and Its Benefits

The proposal has been integrated. There are two different modes of multimodal biometric systems, such as Face and ECG. Each personality's ECG signal differs such that even if they perform the same labour or task, it does not equal them. The brain wave of each personality is distinct; the human brain structure will surely be affected by DNA and living expressions. Even if the DNA of two people is the same, their experiences are different. ECG relies on each individual's living experiences. Authenticated users on their ECG are therefore more precise than other biometric technologies.

5.1 Face Based Biometric Authentication

The acquisition technique is not in touch. Due to technological progress, the availability of low-cost sensors has gained popularity because of such features, such as superficial high accuracy, fast, robustness, and rapid to compare. The face is an internal organ visible from the outside and stays important throughout the full cycle of life. The face is apparent, colourful, and muscular in form around the pupil [2, 4]. Face checks how much light enters the eye. Each individual has a distinct character because of face patterns' epigenetic nature. The creation of the face begins in the third month of childbirth, and the structures which create its design are mostly completed by the eighth month [29, 30].

5.2 Facial Recognition Data Collection (FRDC)

The gathering of facial recognition data helps analyse and compare a person's facial features. Face detection is a crucial stage in the whole process. It finds and recognizes human faces in both videos and images. The next stage is to turn the analogue information, that is to say, a face, into a series of digital data based on the individual's face [31]. This procedure is called the process of face capturing. The procedure of the face match checks if two sides belong to the same individual. The most normal of all biometric measures are measured in these procedures. We recognize ourselves by looking at our faces, for example, not via our eyes or fingerprints. Figure 1 displays images of the actual and artificial face. FRDC is important to collect information such as a nasal bridge, lip contour, ears, chin, and eye spacing [32]. These automated methods may be utilized with this technology to verify or determine the identification of personalities based on their face characteristics in a few seconds merely. This can even be done in a crowd and in unstable and unpredictable situations. Veins digitization, fingerprints, iris scans, and the acknowledgment of the voice in the palm are also signatures via a human body. Fake authentication is done as follows [33]:

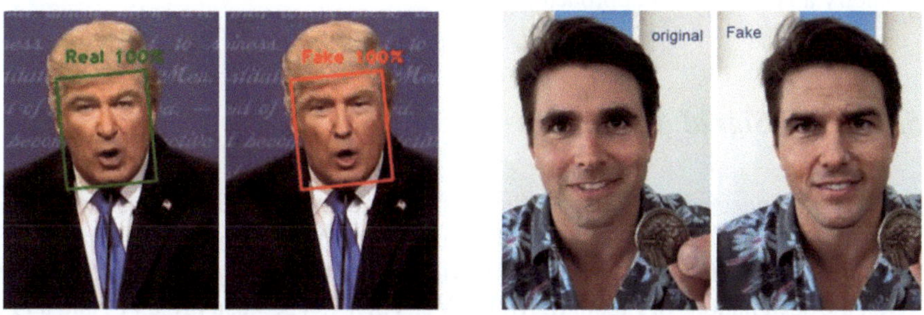

Fig. 1 Real and fake face preparation

1. The images are processed to progress their quality initially.
2. The images are produced with a typical printer in a conventional text.
3. To perform a false authentication, the printed images are shown in face sensors [34]. Fake images are 76.67% of the system's total authentication rate (Threshold Value 0.42) for Fig. 1.

5.3 ECG Signals-Based Biometric Authentication

The heart is the centre of energy management in the human body, as it is responsible for transporting and distributing blood to all parts of the body, according to the needs of each organ. Sensory input is continually received, and data is quickly analysed, and then the actions and functions react. ECG is a significant benefit: (1) an efficient VDM [29]; and (2) ECG as an effective way of detection of external force to increase the biometric system's anti-spot capacity to satisfy applications with higher safety standards [35]. (3) ECG is difficult to imitate, (4) ECG is an ideal supplementary modality to existing, not easily forged, biometric systems. (5) No one can access the waves of the brain as it is safe within the skull. (6) The activity of our brain is changing. It is, therefore, the first biometric system to be changed. (7) Anti-spoofing system design in current unimodal face biometry offers brain wave data which are natural candidates to VDM. (8) ECG signals are very strong when a person is exposed to visual stimuli, and with visual sensation, the visual cortex on the back of the head is the ideal site to measure brain waves [36]. The concept of such a system is to keep personal brain waves recording from a user when exposed to the self-image instead of using, e.g. standard textual passwords, and to compare this recording to fresh brain wave captures using the authentication of the image from the user [37]. The system, therefore, operates as a system that responds to unintentional challenges. The face is an internal protected organ with cells linked directly to the brain. The combination of biometric recognition systems faces and ECG will become the market leader in identity assessment technology. ECG is the weighted spatial summing up of the recorded action potentials on the surface of the skull. The technology for extracting information from the human brain gives the ECG-based biometry a new research approach [38, 39].

5.4 ECG Signal Acquisition

Electrodes connected to the patient's chest, as indicated in Fig. 5, produce ECG measurements: 12-lead ECG electrodes give an optimum placement for accurate spatial resolution for biosignal sensors with connections. 12 ECG electrodes are given the designations of Fig. 6, II, III, F1, V2, V3, V4, V5, V6, aVR, aVL, and aVF, based upon the International 10–20 placements (Figs. 2, 3, 4 and 5) [40].

Fig. 5 ECG signals electrodes

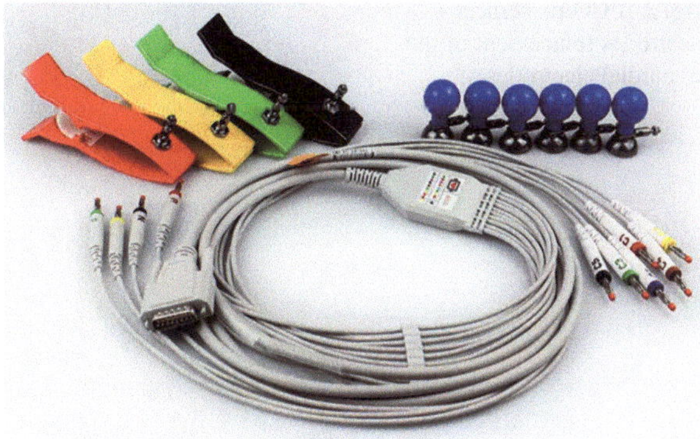

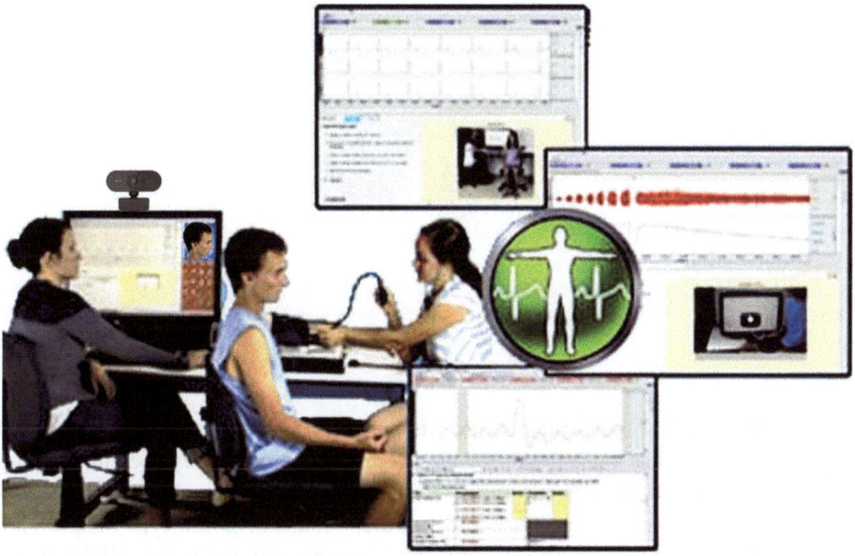

Fig. 6 Self-image displaying for cardio patient based on webcam

6 Resist Attacks Techniques (RAT)

RAT is recognized for all approaches utilized for the protection of biometric templates. Some of the known protection methods for biometric templates are:

6.1 Vitality Detecting Method (VDM)

During the last decade, the VDM was an active field, and various methods to solve this problem were suggested in the literature. VDM continues to be an open topic,

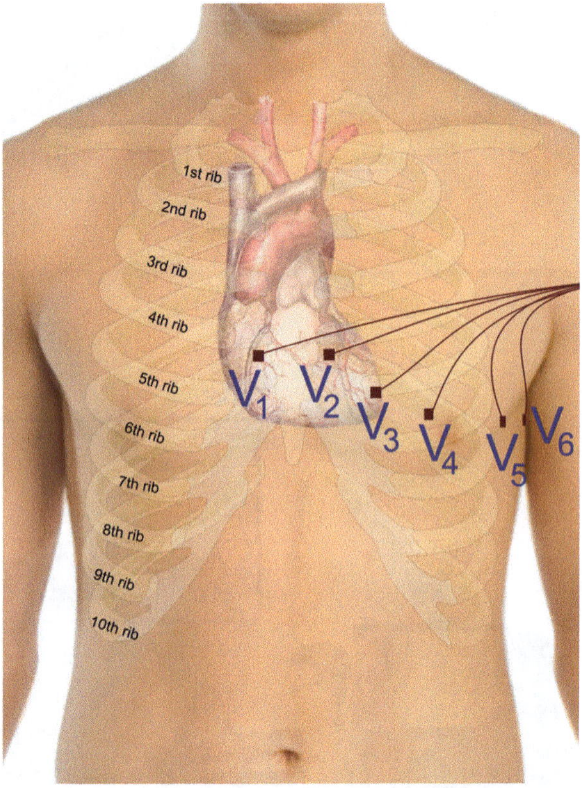

Fig. 2 ECG placement electrodes (placement of the precordial electrodes)

and current methods' performance does not meet the demands of many practical applications [41]. The mainstream of the present techniques uses specific training samples made artificially using various spoofing procedures. It works well with tests produced in the same training procedure, but their results on a new type of spoof are doubtful. How a false biometric is produced is, in practice, unknown. VDM examines images or videos and assesses if they originate from a living or artificial individual. Motion or texture analysis and artificial intelligence are employed (AI). The most promising VDM combines these methods to cope with various presentation assaults [42].

6.2 *Cryptosystems Biometric*

Biometric cryptographic systems integrate both areas' capabilities in biometrics and cryptography [9]. Enhanced security and biometrics avoid the need for passwords to be remembered or tokens to be carried. In conventional cryptographic systems, one or more keys are used to transform a plain text into a cipher text (s). Only decrypting key can map cipher text back to plain text. Imposter cannot extract meaningful

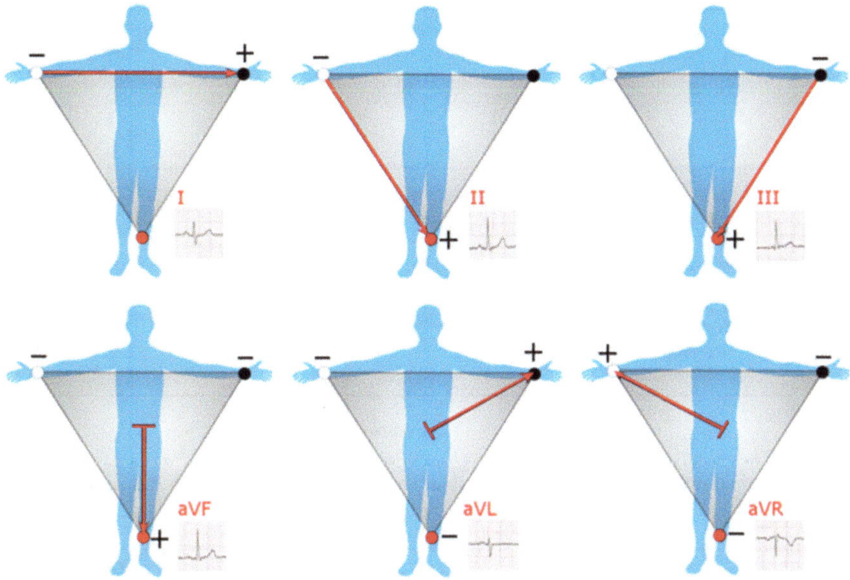

Fig. 3 The limb leads and the raised limb leads (in this depiction, the Wilson central terminal is utilized as the negatives)

Fig. 4 Spatial orientation of EKG leads

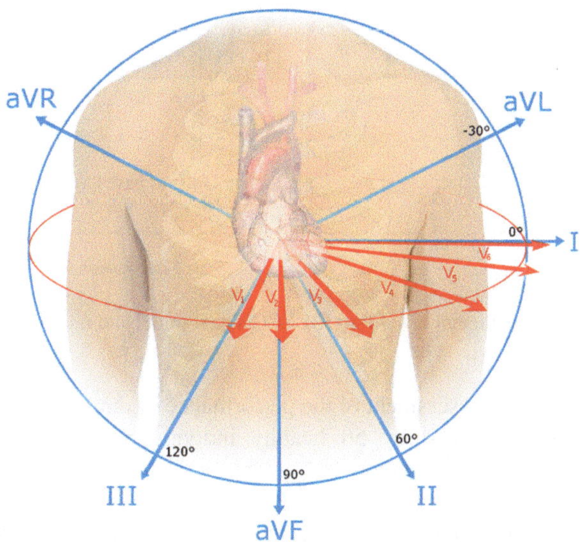

information without decryption when Imposter receives the encrypted text [43]. We utilize cryptographic techniques to prevent dictionary attacks, easily breaking the safety of basic authentication systems relying on passwords. Biometric cryptosystems are split into key and key generation [44] (Fig. 6).

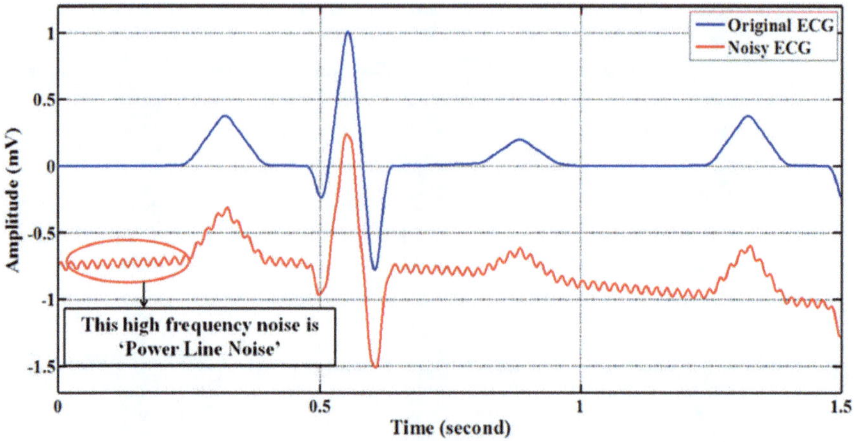

Fig. 7 Original raw # Rec 117 ECG signal (blue) and noisy ECG signal with PLI noise (red)

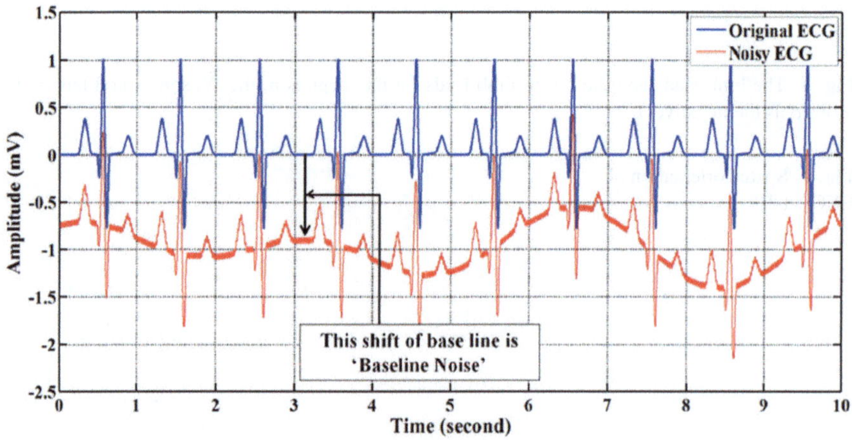

Fig. 8 Original raw # Rec 121 ECG signal (blue) and noisy ECG signal with baseline noise (red)

In the assessment of the performance of our system, the suggested technique was also evaluated by 50 healthy individuals (workers and students) (25 men/25 women). Information was given, and questionnaires were signed and completed by all individuals before collecting data, together with inquiries relating to health. The topics are asked to sit, relax, and rest on a comfortable chair. The bottom is a blue window, and the front is a whiteboard. Two laptops with good configuration were fixed in front of the subject shown in Figs. 7 and 8 [45]. The first laptop was utilized in the webcam with a high-resolution camera to present the subject's face. ECG electrodes are utilized for extracting cardiac signals, and its high-performance Wireless transmits the signals on the second laptop automatically to the USB Dongle. No specialized drivers are required for USB Dongle in this extraction

Table 1 Described 10 electrodes in an ECG of 12 plants

Name of electrodes	Placement of each electrode
RA	Between the right shoulder and the wrist
LA	Between the left shoulder and the wrist
RL	Anywhere between the right ankle and the torso
LL	Above the left ankle and below the torso
V1	The fourth intercostal gap is located to the right of the sternum
V2	The fourth intercostal gap is located to the left of the sternum
V3	V3 is intermediate between V2 and V4
V4	The fifth intercostal gap is located in the midclavicular line
V5	The anterior axillary line is located at the same level as V4
V6	V4 and V5 are at the same level as the midaxillary line

process. The gel was applied to every electrode before each test to ensure a strong connection between chest leather and ECG electrodes. However, after confirming whether ECG data is valid for further analysis or not, it was required to perform the experimental methods [46] (Table 1).

6.3 *Avoid the Artefacts*

The management of artefacts should be avoided by giving users appropriate guidelines. The instruction for people to keep artefacts clear during data collection has the benefit of reducing the calculative demand among the techniques of processing artefacts since no relic is presumed to be present in the signal [47]. But it has a lot of inconveniences. First of all, while the ECG signal is removed, there is no possibility of stopping our heart. It is not easy to coordinate cardiac activity even for EMG activities during data recording in our bodies. Secondly, there is no amount of cardiac activity during the online operation, and interference in the power line (PLI) is also manifested. The third possibility of data collection will be reduced because of artefacts in the ECG signal, particularly if cardiomyopathy is experienced by consumers [48]. Many biosignal researchers have talked about numerous approaches. Most of the approaches presented were successfully limited. Some techniques took longer to perform the needed calculations, while others for practical applications were very complex. Every record is an ECG event for only 2 min. There are 50 subjects = 5 Samples = 250 Data Set sessions [49]. The EMG, a high-frequency component, is caused by a random muscular contraction, whereas the rapid transients are caused by impulsive movement. This widely recognized issue, which shows as an incursion in the recorded ECG, creates severe ECG muscle stress and evaluation difficulties. To eliminate artefacts, we needed the artefacts and ECG to be ordered without altering ECG activity in turn [50].

6.4 Artefacts Cancelation

The low-frequency element is utilized to remove the ECG signal from the high-frequency component, using wavelet-based denoising. The following are the major steps of hybrid AWICA pre-processing:

Stage-1: Powerline interference (PLI), damaged wire connections, and electrode impedance were analysed using the ECG data extracted through adaptive filtering.
Stage-2: Use the WT algorithm individually to capture 12 multichannel channels. Finally, several signals were received with varied frequencies.
Stage-3: The basis line has been eliminated using wave decomposition, and wavelets have denoted the signal.
Stage-4: The highly correlated elements are identified and selected, generating a new data set.
Stage-5: To transmit built-in data to independent analysis component block.
Stage-6: The signal is not corrected, and the whitening is applied so that the size is reduced and the computational load is lighted.
Stage-7: To estimate the components of the artefacts and eliminate them.
Stage-8: Independent component analysis would divide and clean the signals according to the sources. The associated ECG signals removed using fast and independent parts analysis must be categorized.
Stage-9: Finally, for the reconstruction of the wavelet (7), we acquire the multichannel recording with non-chosen details and cleaned detail following the ICA stage.

6.5 Channel Selection

The ECG signals are mostly strong when the person is free of muscle strains, and the chest area on the front side of the patient's body is the better place for ECG signals measurement. Figure 9 shows the position of the 12 electrodes in the patient's photo. They are placed on the sides of the patient's limbs, positioned symmetrically.

7 Feature Extracting

With all the heartbeats of the ECG signal aligned and normalized, the next step is to extract the unique features of the ECG by which a person can be identified. After preliminary experiments, these features were selected since they tend to remain identifiable in the presence of noise. The feature extraction module analyses and generates the raw data acquired by the sensor. It extracts the necessary characteristics from the raw data that demand considerable care, as key properties must be optimally

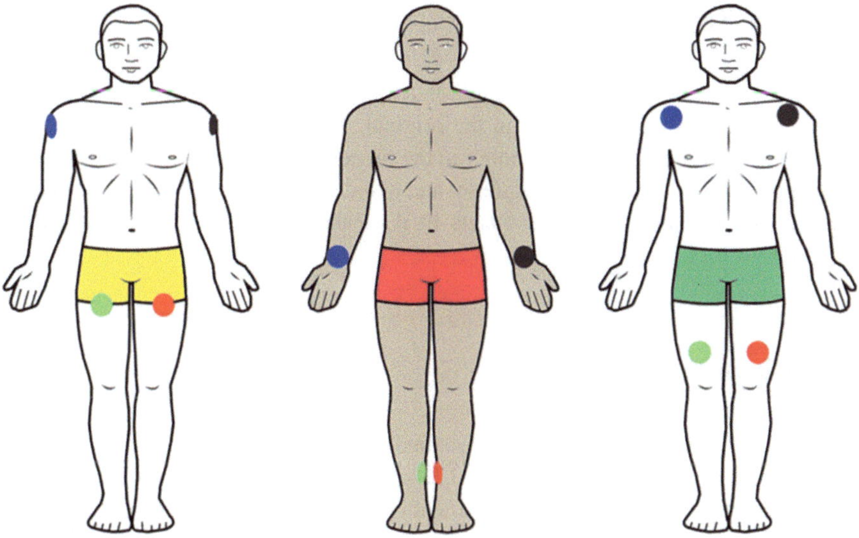

Fig. 9 A symmetric Installing of limb lead Everywhere in the limbs Positioned

extracted [51]. The sample is essentially removed from the input sample and transferred to the input sample for the next module, known as the match module. Signals will be transformed into extracted unique vectors for the Human Identification System with the help of ECG after the removal of artefacts. In the study of time domains, parametric models are highly beneficial for the extraction of the ECG signal characteristic. The major problem of this technique is that the model property for various ECG signals is not determined (Non-Stationary Signals) [52]. WT is a mathematical microscope used to study various ECG rhythm scales and has proved to be an efficient instrument for researching small-scale cardiac signal oscillations. The wavelet breakdown of the ECG recordings, the transient functions, and the time and frequency context are accurately recorded and located. Lastly, the Transform Wavelet is an effective extraction feature from non-stationary signals such as ECG's [53].

8 Frequency Domain Approaches

The signal analysis with this approach is intended to obtain adequate data from a signal through a frequency-domain transformation. Fourier Transformation power spectral analysis is the most popular technique to analyse frequencies, which is widely utilized for the traditional spectrum decomposition analysis of ECG signals [54, 55].

9 Data Reduction

It reduces the quantity of data created after transforming the wavelet by not losing the sequence of signal functions in the original. All data reduction techniques will lose some important data functionality in the process of data reduction. We needed a new approach to decrease the feature set and avoid extracting any features from ECG signals. So, we used weighted means to decrease the value, but still, it left no function vectors.

10 Classification

The ECG signal characteristics are classified in so many different ways. A Support Vector (SVM), Neural Network (NN), LDA, Genetic Algorithm (GA), Naive Bayes Classifier, etc., can be used for classification. SVM has an excellent basis in the statistical theory of learning. A set of parameters determining how an SVM works guarantees finding the optimal decision function within statistical learning theory. SVM is better classified than VDM and traditional NN on emotional characteristics obtained from the ECG data. Because of its performance, several researchers have extensively focused on the ECG Signals SVM classification. However, the performance of the classification depends on the properties provided to the classifier. Improving the feature extraction and feature reduction method provides reliable ECG signals classification results. The system only produces two authenticated/not authenticated outcomes. Thus, in this study, the Vector Machine of Least Square Support (LS-SVM) was utilized. The combination of AWICA enables the ECG-based authentication to deliver good results.

11 Face and ECG Fusion

AND Rule and weighted SUM utilized for Face and ECG fusion. In this system, score levels and decision level techniques were used; MMB may be aggregated at several levels. The fusion scores based on the sum rules have been determined with equal weights for each method (Fig. 10).

11.1 Proposed MMB Authentication Using Face and ECG

Stage-1: Extract the values from the Face and ECG, and store them in respective databases

Stage-2: Read the Face data from Subject 1

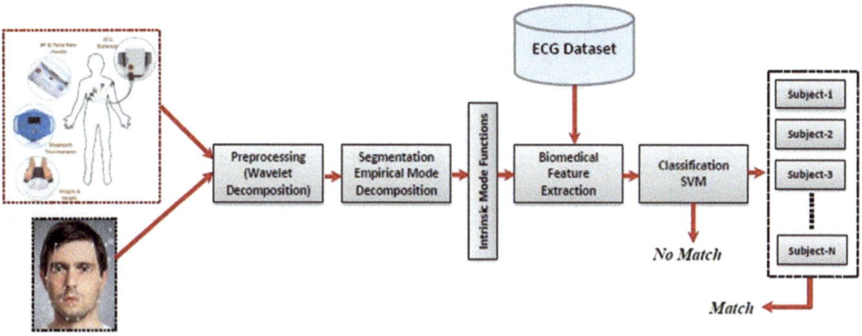

Fig. 10 The infrastructure of the proposed method

Stage-3: Match the Face data with the corresponding template stored in the database.
Stage-4: If Match occurs
Display "Face Recognized Looking for ECG Match"
Else
Display "Try Again"
Break
Stage-5: Read ECG Signal from Subject 1Stage-6: Match the ECG data with the template stored in a database
Stage-7: If Match
Display "ECG Recognized & "Welcome the Person"
Else
Display "Access Denied & Try Again"
Break

12 Results and Outcomes

Figure 11 explains (a) displays the 10 s ECG data part. Channel 1, which can be observed as an aberrant oscillation on both sides of QRS complexes, is polluted with noise. (b) Shows the respective ICA-derived components. The noise is extracted from the original ECG as an ICA component. (c) Displays the proper ECG if noise is eliminated.

Figure 12 can be described as follows: (a) displays a 10 s ECG data segment. Channel 1, observed as an irregular oscillation on each side of QRS complexes, can be seen to be polluted with noise. (b) Displays ICA-derived relevant components. As an ICA component, the noise in the original ECG is separated. (c) Displays the rectified ECG when removing the noise component.

Based on Table 2, the accuracy based on channels 1, 2, 3, and 4 is 93%, 91%, 94%, and 93%. The False Acceptance Rate based on channels 1, 2, 3, and 4 is 96%,

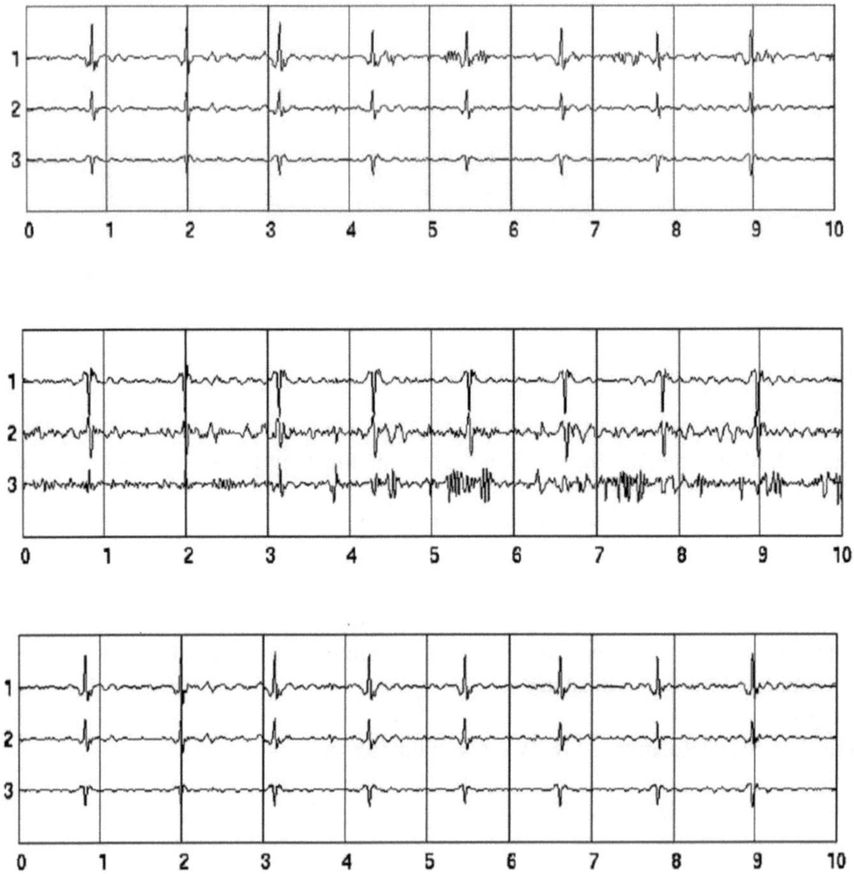

Fig. 11 (a) Original ECG signal for # Rec. 121, (b) ICA components for # Rec. 121, (c) removed artefacts from ECG signal using FASTICA for # Rec. 121

98%, 96%, and 97%. The False Rejection Rate (FRR) based on channels 1, 2, 3, and 4 is 7.93%, 4.71%, 3.58%, and 2.92%. The Time Taken for the Process (in seconds) based on channels 1, 2, 3, and 4 is 4.88, 5.59, 6.73, and 14.99.

13 Conclusion

The vulnerability of the system to direct assaults was assessed. An ECG signal has been sent as part of a face-based verification system. A database has been constructed with false images of 50 men/females. The findings showed that the

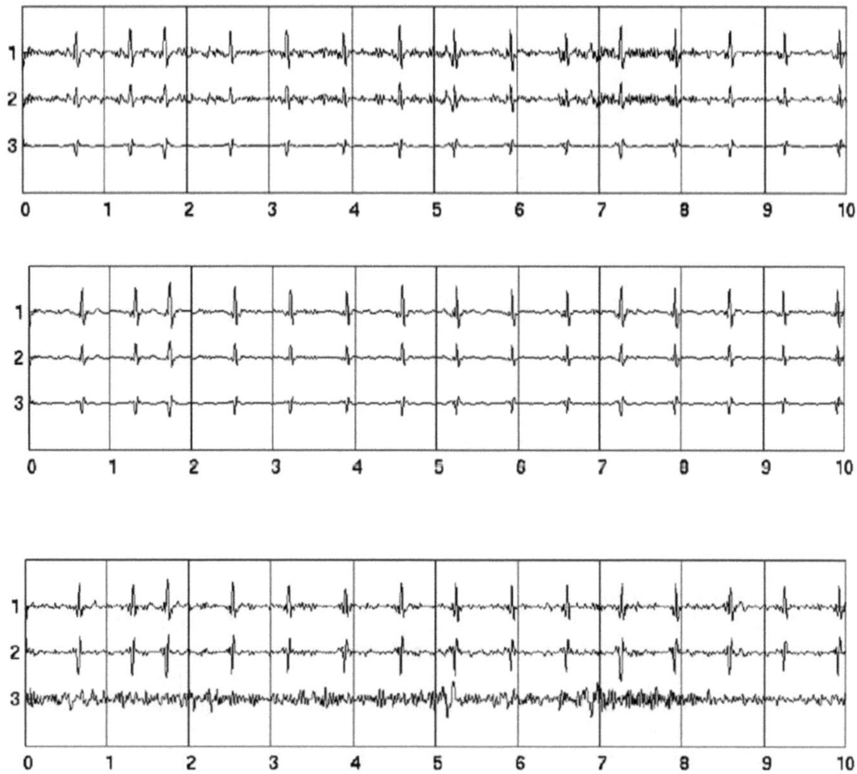

Fig. 12 (**a**) Original ECG signal for # Rec. 117, (**b**) ICA components for # Rec. 117, (**c**) removed artefacts from ECG signal using FASTICA for # Rec. 117

Table 2 The number of channels with accuracy, FAR, and FRR in percentage for the proposed technique

No. of. channels	1	2	4	14
Accuracy (%)	93%	91%	94%	93%
False acceptance rate (FAR)	96%	98%	96%	97%
False rejection rate (FRR)	7.93%	4.71%	3.58%	2.92%
Time taken for the process (in seconds)	4.88	5.59	6.73	14.99

two techniques tested were very sensitive to attacks. VDM can be used to counter direct strikes. ECG here is a new VDM model and an extra biometric system modality. With AWICA, excellent results for ECG-based authentication are generated.

References

1. Elgendi, M. Less is more in biosignal analysis: Compressed data could open the door to faster and better diagnosis. Diseases (2018).
2. Kalaivani, S., & Tharini, C. Analysis and modification of rice Golomb coding lossless compression algorithm for wireless sensor networks. Journal of Theoretical And Applied Information Technology, 96(12), 3802–3814 (2018).
3. Tan, C., Zhang, L., & Wu, H.-T. A novelBlaschke unwinding adaptiveFourier-decomposition-based signal compression algorithm with application on ECG signals. IEEE Journal of Biomedical and Health Informatics, 23(2), 672–682 (2019).
4. Burguera, A. Fast QRS detection and ECG compression based on signal structural analysis (2019).
5. Huang, H., Hu, S., & Sun, Y. ECG signal compression for low-power sensor nodes using sparse frequency spectrum features. In IEEE biomedical circuits and systems conference (BioCAS) (2018).
6. Tan, C., Zhang, L., & Wu, H.-T. A novelBlaschke unwinding adaptiveFourier-decomposition-based signal compression algorithm with application on ECG signals. IEEE Journal of Biomedical and Health Informatics, 23(2), 672–682 (2019).
7. Burguera, A. Fast QRS detection and ECG compression based on signal structural analysis, IEEE Journal of Biomedical and Health Informatics, 23(1), 123–131 (2019).
8. N. Samarin and D. J. a. p. a. Sannella, "A Key to Your Heart: Biometric Authentication Based on ECG Signals," (2019).
9. F. Beritelli, S. J. I. T. o. I. F. Serrano, and Security, "Biometric identification based on frequency analysis of cardiac sounds," vol. 2, no. 3, pp. 596–604, (2007).
10. F. Beritelli and A. Spadaccini, "Human identity verification based on mel frequency analysis of digital heart sounds," in 2009 16th International Conference on Digital Signal Processing, pp. 1–5: IEEE (2009).
11. F. Agrafioti and D. Hatzinakos, "ECG based recognition using second order statistics," in 6th Annual Communication Networks and Services Research Conference (cnsr 2008), pp. 82–87: IEEE (2008).
12. D. P. Coutinho, A. L. Fred, and M. A. Figueiredo, "One-lead ECG-based personal identification using Ziv-Merhav cross parsing," in 2010 20th International Conference on Pattern Recognition, pp. 3858–3861: IEEE (2010).
13. S. A. J. M. T. El_Rahman and Applications, "Biometric human recognition system based on ECG," pp. 1–18, (2019).
14. R. Srivastva and Y. N. Singh, "ECG biometric analysis using walsh–hadamard transform," in Advances in Data and Information Sciences: Springer, pp. 201–210 (2018).
15. Z. Zhao, L. Yang, D. Chen, and Y. J. S. Luo, "A human ECG identification system based on ensemble empirical mode decomposition," vol. 13, no. 5, pp. 6832–6864, (2013).
16. Pandya, S., & Patel, W. An Adaptive Approach towards designing a Smart Health-care Real-Time Monitoring System based on IoT and Data Mining. In 3rd IEEE International Conference on Sensing technology and Machine Intelligence (ICST-2016), Dubai (2016).
17. Hooda, D. S., Kumari, R., & Sharma, D. K. Intuitionistic Fuzzy Soft Set Theory and Its Application in Medical Diagnosis. International Journal of Statistics in Medical Research, 7(3), 70–76 (2018).
18. Sharma, D. K., & Saxena, S. Generalized Coding Theorem with Different Source Coding Schemes. International Journal on Recent and Innovation Trends in Computing and Communication, 5(6), 253–257 (2019).
19. Bhardwaj, A., Kaur, S., Shukla, A. P., & Shukla, M. K. A Novel Method for Despeckling of Ultrasound Images Using Cellular Automata-Based Despeckling Filter. International Journal of E-Health and Medical Communications, 12(5), 16–35 (2021).

20. I. Jayarathne, M. Cohen, and S. Amarakeerthi, "BrainID: Development of an EEG-based biometric authentication system," in 2016 IEEE 7th Annual Information Technology, Electronics and Mobile Communication Conference (IEMCON), pp. 1-6: IEEE (2016).
21. S. Yang, S. Hoque, and F. J. I. A. Deravi, "Improved time-frequency features and electrode placement for EEG-based biometric person recognition," vol. 7, pp. 49604–49613, (2019).
22. A. Hanilçi, H. J. J. o. I. S. Gürkan, and Engineering, "ECG Biometric Identification Method based on Parallel 2-D Convolutional Neural Networks," vol. 3, no. 1, pp. 11–22, (2019).
23. Abdulbaqi, A.S., Ismail Yusuf Panessai, "Designing and Implementation of a Biomedical Module for Vital Signals Measurements Based on Embedded System", International Journal of Advanced Science and Technology, Vol. 29, No. 3, pp. 3866–3877 (2020).
24. Huang, H., Hu, S., & Sun, Y. ECG signal compression for low-power sensor nodes using sparse frequency spectrum features. In IEEE biomedical circuits and systems conference (BioCAS) (2018).
25. Deepu, C. J., Heng, C.-H., & Lian, Y. A hybrid data compression scheme for power reduction in wireless sensors for IoT. IEEE Transactions on Biomedical Circuits and Systems, 11(2), 245–254 (2017).
26. Jha, C. K., & Kolekar, M. H. ECG data compression algorithm for telemonitoring of cardiac patients. International Journal of Telemedicine and Clinical Practices, 2(1), 31–41 (2017).
27. Deepu, C. J., Heng, C.-H., & Lian, Y. A hybrid data compression scheme for power reduction in wireless sensors for IoT. IEEE Transactions on Biomedical Circuits and Systems, 11(2), 245–254 (2017).
28. Abdulbaqi, A. S., Obaid, A. J., & Mohammed, A. H. ECG signals recruitment to implement a new technique for medical image encryption. Journal of Discrete Mathematical Sciences and Cryptography, 1–11 (2021).
29. Tsai, T.-H., & Kuo, W.-T. (2018) An efficient ECG lossless compression system for embedded platforms with telemedicine applications. In IEEE (2018).
30. Aboul Ella Hassanien, Moataz Kilany and Essan H. Houssein , Combining Support Vector Machine and Elephant Herding Optimization for Cardiac Arrhythmias, arXiv:1806.08242v1 [eee.SP],June 20,(2018).
31. J. Dogra, M. Sood, S. Jain, N. Prashar, Segmentation of magnetic resonance images of brain using thresholding techniques ,4th IEEE International Conference on signal processing and control (ISPCC 2017), Jaypee University of Information technology, Waknaghat, Solan, H.P, India, pp. 311–315, September 21-23, (2017).
32. Ghayvat, H., Awais, M., Pandya, S., Ren, H., Akbarzadeh, S., Chandra Mukhopadhyay, S., ... & Chen, W. Smart aging system: uncovering the hidden wellness parameter for well-being monitoring and anomaly detection. Sensors, 19(4), 766 (2019).
33. Kubiczek, J., & Hadasik, B. Challenges in Reporting the COVID-19 Spread and its Presentation to the Society. Journal of Data and Information Quality (JDIQ), 13(4), 1–7 (2021).
34. A. Dhiman, A. Singh, S. Dubey, S. Jain, Design of Lead II ECG Waveform and Classification Performance for Morphological features using Different Classifiers on Lead II. Research Journal of Pharmaceutical, Biological and Chemical Sciences (RJPBCS),7(4), 1226–1231: July-Aug (2016).
35. Abdulbaqi, A. S., Obaid, A. J., & Alazawi, S. A. H. A Smart System for Health Caregiver Based on IoMT: Toward Tele-Health Caregiving. International Journal of Online & Biomedical Engineering, 17(7) (2021).
36. Kalaivani, S., Shahnaz, I., Shirin, S. R., & Tharini, C. Real-time ECG acquisition and detection of anomalies. In-Dash, S. S., Bhaskar, M. A., Panigrahi, B. K., Das, S (Eds.), Artificial intelligence and evolutionary computations in engineering systems. Springer (2016).
37. Uthayakumar, J., Venkattaraman, T., & Dhayachelvan, P. A survey on data compression techniques: From the perspective of data quality, coding schemes, data types, and applications. Journal of King Saud University- Computer and Information Sciences (2018).

38. R. Gupta, S. Singh, K. Garg, S. Jain, Indigenous Design of Electronic Circuit for Electrocardiograph, International Journal of Innovative Research in Science, Engineering and Technology, 3(5), 12138–12145, (2014).
39. Raja, R., Kumar, S., Rani, S., & Laxmi, K. R. (Eds.). Artificial Intelligence and Machine Learning in 2D/3D Medical Image Processing. CRC Press (2020).
40. S. Jain, "Classification of Protein Kinase B Using Discrete Wavelet Transform",.International Journal of Information Technology, 10(2), 211–216, (2018).
41. N. Alajlan, Y. Bazi, F. Melgani, S. Malek, M. A. Bencherif, "Detection of premature ventricular contraction arrhythmias in electrocardiogram signals with kernel methods," Signal Image and Video Processing, vol. 8, no. 5, pp. 931–942 (2014).
42. Hirai, Y.; Matsuoka, T.; Tani, S.; Isami, S.; Tatsumi, K.; Ueda, M.; Kamata, T.: A biomedical sensor system with stochastic A/D conversion and error correction by machine learning. IEEE Access 7, 21990–22001 (2019).
43. Yildirim, Ö. A novel wavelet sequence based on a deep bidirectional LSTM network model for ECG signal classification. Computers in biology and medicine, 96, 189–202 (2018).
44. Diker, A., Avci, D., Avci, E., & Gedikpinar, M. A new technique for ECG signal classification genetic algorithm Wavelet Kernel extreme learning machine. Optik, 180, 46–55 (2019).
45. J. Zhang, Z. Gu, Z.L. Yu, Y. Li, Energy-efficient ECG compression on wireless biosensors via minimal coherence sensing and weighted l1 minimization reconstruction. IEEE J. Biomed. Health Inform. 19(2), 520–528 (2015).
46. A. Singh, S. Dandapat, Block sparsity-based joint compressed sensing recovery of multichannel ECG signals. Healthcare Technol. Lett. 4(2), 50–56 (2017).
47. A. Singh, S. Dandapat, Exploiting multi-scale signal information in joint compressed sensing recovery of multichannel ECG signals. Biomed. Signal Process. Control 29, 53–66 (2016).
48. H. Mamaghanian, G. Ansaloni, D. Atienza, P. Vandergheynst, Power-efficient joint compressed sensing of multi-lead ECG signals. in IEEE International Conference on Acoustics, Speech and Signal Processing (ICASSP) 2014, pp. 4409–4412 (2014).
49. S. Kumar, B. Deka, S. Datta, Block-sparsity based compressed sensing for multichannel ECG reconstruction. in Deka B., Maji P., Mitra S., Bhattacharyya D., Bora P., Pal S. (eds) Pattern Recognition and Machine Intelligence. PReMI 2019. Lecture Notes in Computer Science, vol. 11942. Springer, Cham (2019).
50. S. Eftekharifar, T.Y. Rezaii, S. Beheshti, S. Daneshvar, Block sparse multi-lead ECG compression exploiting between-lead collaboration. IET Sig. Process. (2018).
51. Sharma, A.; Polley, A.; Lee, S.B.; Narayanan, S.; Li, W.; Sculley, T.; Ramaswamy, S.: A Sub-60-μ A multimodal smart biosensing SoCwith>80-dB SNR, 35μAphotoplethysmography signal chain. IEEE J. Solid-State Circuits 52(4), 1021–1033 (2017).
52. Zhang, Z.; Li, J.; Zhang, Q.; Wu, K.; Ning, N.; Yu, Q. A dynamic tracking algorithm based SAR ADC in bio-related applications. IEEE Access 6, 62166–62173 (2018).
53. Adimulam, M.K.; Srinivas, M.B.: A 1.0 V, 9.84 fJ/c-s FOM reconfigurable hybrid SAR-sigma delta ADC for signal processing applications. Analog Integr. Circ. Sig. Process 99(2), 261–276, (2019).
54. Zhang, X.; Lian, Y.: A 300-mV 220-NW Event-driven ADC with real-time QRS detection for wearable ECG sensors. IEEE Trans. Biomed. Circuits Syst. 8(6), 834–843 (2014).
55. Hou, Y.; Qu, J.; Tian, Z.; Atef, M.; Yousef, K.; Lian, Y.; Wang, G.: A 61-NW level-crossing ADC with adaptive sampling for biomedical applications. IEEE Trans. Circuits Syst. II Express Briefs 66(1), 56–60 (2019).

Index

P. Agarwal et al. (eds.), *Artificial Intelligence for Smart Healthcare*, EAI/Springer Innovations in Communication and Computing,
https://doi.org/10.1007/978-3-031-23602-0

MIX
Papier aus verantwortungsvollen Quellen
Paper from responsible sources
FSC® C105338

If you have any concerns about our products,
you can contact us on
ProductSafety@springernature.com

In case Publisher is established outside the EU,
the EU authorized representative is:
Springer Nature Customer Service Center GmbH
Europaplatz 3, 69115 Heidelberg, Germany

Printed by Libri Plureos GmbH
in Hamburg, Germany